POLYPEPTIDE HORMONES

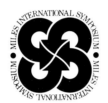

MILES INTERNATIONAL SYMPOSIUM SERIES

Polypeptide Hormones

Miles International Symposium Series
Number 12

Editors

**Roland F. Beers, Jr.,
M.D., Ph.D.**
Miles Laboratories, Inc.
Elkhart, Indiana

Edward G. Bassett, Ph.D.
Miles Laboratories, Inc.
Elkhart, Indiana

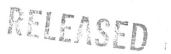
Raven Press ■ New York

Raven Press, 1140 Avenue of the Americas, New York, New York 10036

Made in the United States of America

Library of Congress Cataloging in Publication Data

Main entry under title:

Polypeptide hormones.

(Miles international symposium series; no. 12)
Based on a 3-day conference held at the Johns Hopkins
Medical Institutions and sponsored by Miles Laboratories.
Includes bibliographical references and index.
1. Peptide hormones—Congresses. I. Beers, Ronald F.
II. Bassett, Edward Graham, 1927–   III. Miles
Laboratories, Inc., Elkhart, Ind. IV. Series. [DNLM:
1. Hormones—Congresses. 2. Peptides—Congresses.
W3 MI543 no. 12 1979 / WK185 M643 1979p]
QP572.P4P64   599.01'927   79–66512
ISBN 0–89004–462–7

Preface

The importance of hormones as a class of chemical compounds that provide a regulatory function in many physiological processes cannot be overstated. Intensive studies of the biosynthesis, structure, transport, and role of polypeptide and protein hormones have been limited to the past four decades, many of them derived from the pioneering work of Choh H. Li beginning in 1938.

Although there is a wealth of information about the structural determinants of hormonal activity (the number, sequence, and identity of the amino acids of which hormones are comprised), their mode of action is still not well understood. There are many current research and clinical studies under way in an attempt to reveal, at the molecular level, the basis of endocrine diseases resulting from the excessive, deficient, or untimely release and/or availability of hormones.

Wishing to initiate, support, and improve contact among clinicians and researchers interested in polypeptide hormones, Miles Laboratories sponsored the development of this volume and the symposium on which it is based, inviting internationally recognized leaders to participate in the Twelfth Miles International Symposium.

Of interest to a wide array of workers in the medical and allied disciplines, this volume represents highlights of laboratory and clinical studies including some of the most recent advances in the biological synthesis, transport, receptors, and cellular response of polypeptide hormones, and discussions among the participants.

We are hopeful that this volume and the symposium on which it is based will launch productive communication (and perhaps collaboration) among researchers. This volume will be of interest to endocrinologists, cell biologists, pharmacologists, synthetic organic chemists, and other biomedical scientists.

Roland F. Beers, Jr.
Edward G. Bassett

Acknowledgments

Under the General Chairmanship of Dr. Roland F. Beers, Jr., the Program Committee consisting of Drs. Christian B. Anfinsen, Stephen R. Bloom, Karl A. Folkers, Choh H. Li, Andrew V. Schally, and Nathan Trainin organized the 3-day conference on which this volume is based for the discussion of the most recent multidisciplinary studies of polypeptide hormones. Coordinator of the Symposium was Dr. Edward G. Bassett. The conference was held at the Johns Hopkins Medical Institutions and was attended by a large number of biomedical investigators and other professionals from a wide array of disciplines.

We are especially grateful to Walter Ames Compton, M.D., Chairman of the Board of Directors of Miles Laboratories, Inc., for his continued support of and interest in these Symposia.

The editors extend grateful thanks to the contributors for assisting in the prompt publication of their manuscripts. The discussions included in this volume have been edited by the Session Chairmen. Within the time allotted for editing, it was not possible for each discussant to proofread his remarks; if error or misunderstanding of remarks has resulted, the Editors take full responsibility.

Contents

Section D: Pituitary Hormones

Section E: Gastrointestinal Hormones

Contributors

Christian B. Anfinsen
Laboratory of Chemical Biology
National Institute of Arthritis, Metabolism
    and Digestive Diseases
National Institutes of Health
Bethesda, Maryland 20205

Rene Arentzen
Division of Biology
City of Hope National Medical Center
Duarte, California 91010

A. Arimura
Veterans Administration Medical Center
New Orleans, Louisiana 70146

A. Astaldi
Central Laboratory of the Netherlands
    Red Cross Blood Transfusion Service
1006 AD Amsterdam, The Netherlands

G. C. B. Astaldi
Central Laboratory of the Netherlands
    Red Cross Blood Transfusion Service
1006 AD Amsterdam, The Netherlands

J. F. Bach
INSERM Unit 25
Necker Hospital
75730 Paris Cedex 15, France

M. A. Bach
INSERM Unit 25
Necker Hospital
75730 Paris Cedex 15, France

N. Barden
MRC Group in Molecular Endocrinology
Hospital Center
Laval University
Quebec G1V 4G2, Canada

M. Beaulieu
MRC Group in Molecular Endocrinology
Hospital Center
Laval University
Quebec G1V 4G2, Canada

Roland F. Beers, Jr.
Miles Laboratories, Inc.
Elkhart, Indiana 46515

Hemendra N. Bhargava
Department of Pharmacognosy and
    Pharmacology
University of Illinois Medical Center
Chicago, Illinois 60680

D. Blanot
Peptide Laboratory
C.N.R.S. Institute of Biochemistry
Paris-Sud University
91405 Orsay, France

Stephen R. Bloom
Royal Postgraduate Medical School
Hammersmith Hospital
London W12 0HS, England

P. Boregeat
MRC Group in Molecular Endocrinology
Hospital Center
Laval University
Quebec G1V 4G2, Canada

Cyril Y. Bowers
Tulane University School of Medicine
New Orleans, Louisiana 70112

E. Bricas
Peptide Laboratory
C.N.R.S. Institute of Biochemistry
Paris-Sud University
91405 Orsay, France

Stephanie Broome
The Biological Laboratories
Harvard University
Cambridge, Massachusetts 02138

Michael J. Brownstein
Unit on Neuroendocrinology
Laboratory of Clinical Science
National Institute of Mental Health
Bethesda, Maryland 20205

Don H. Catlin
Departments of Pharmacology and
*   Medicine*
Center for the Health Sciences
University of California, Los Angeles
Los Angeles, California 90025

R. C. C. Chang
Veterans Administration Medical Center
New Orleans, Louisiana 70146

William L. Chick
Elliot P. Joslin Research Laboratory
Harvard Medical School
Boston, Massachusetts 02115

J. Choay
Choay Institute
92120 Montrouge, France

Walter Ames Compton
Miles Laboratories, Inc.
Elkhart, Indiana 46515

David H. Coy
Department of Medicine
Tulane University School of Medicine
New Orleans, Louisiana 70112

Jan Dahmen
Institute for Biomedical Research
University of Texas at Austin
Austin, Texas 78712

M. Dardenne
INSERM Unit 25
Necker Hospital
75730 Paris Cedex 15, France

G. J. Dockray
Physiological Laboratory
University of Liverpool
Liverpool L69 3BX, England

Argiris Efstratiadis
Department of Biological Chemistry
Harvard Medical School
Boston, Massachusetts 02115

V. P. Eijsvoogel
Central Laboratory of the Netherlands
*   Red Cross Blood Transfusion Service*
1006 AD Amsterdam, The Netherlands

Bruce W. Erickson
Rockefeller University
New York, New York 10021

Marian Evinger
Roche Institute of Molecular Biology
Nutley, New Jersey 07110

A. Facchini
Institut of Normal Human Anatomy
University of Bologna
Bologna, Italy

L. Ferland
MRC Group in Molecular Endocrinology
Hospital Center
Laval University
Quebec G1V 4G2, Canada

Louis B. Flexner
Department of Anatomy
University of Pennsylvania School of
*   Medicine*
Philadelphia, Pennsylvania 19174

Karl A. Folkers
Institute for Biomedical Research
University of Texas at Austin
Austin, Texas 78712

Jerry D. Gardner
Digestive Diseases Branch
National Institute of Arthritis, Metabolism
 and Digestive Diseases
National Institutes of Health
Bethesda, Maryland 20205

Robert H. Gerner
Department of Psychiatry
Center for the Health Sciences
University of California, Los Angeles
Los Angeles, California 90024

Walter Gilbert
The Biological Laboratories
Harvard University
Cambridge, Massachusetts 02138

M. Godbout
MRC Group in Molecular Endocrinology
Hospital Center
Laval University
Quebec G1V 4G2, Canada

Allan L. Goldstein
Department of Biochemistry
School of Medicine and Health Sciences
George Washington University
Washington, D.C. 20037

Gideon Goldstein
Ortho Pharmaceutical Corporation
Raritan, New Jersey 08869

David V. Goeddel
Division of Molecular Biology
Genentech, Inc.
South San Francisco, California 94080

David A. Gorelick
Department of Psychiatry
Center for the Health Sciences
University of California, Los Angeles
Los Angeles, California 90024

Herbert L. Heyneker
Division of Molecular Biology
Genentech, Inc.
South San Francisco, California 94080

Paula L. Hoffman
Department of Physiology and Biophysics
University of Illinois Medical Center
Chicago, Illinois 60680

Toyahara Hozumi
Division of Biology
City of Hope National Medical Center
Duarte, California 91010

W. Y. Huang
Veterans Administration Medical Center
New Orleans, Louisiana 70146

Ka Kit Hui
Departments of Pharmacology and
 Medicine
Center for the Health Sciences
University of California, Los Angeles
Los Angeles, California 90024

Keiichi Itakura
Division of Biology
City of Hope National Medical Center
Duarte, California 91010

David M. Jacobowitz
Laboratory of Clinical Science
National Institute of Mental Health
Bethesda, Maryland 20205

Robert T. Jensen
Digestive Diseases Branch
National Institute of Arthritis, Metabolism
 and Digestive Diseases
National Institutes of Health
Bethesda, Maryland 20205

Abba J. Kastin
Endocrinology Section
Veterans Administration Medical Center
New Orleans, Louisiana 70146

Maria Kenez-Keri
Hormone Research Laboratory
University of California, San Francisco
San Francisco, California 94143

György Keri
Hormone Research Laboratory
University of California, San Francisco
San Francisco, California 94143

Baruch Klein
Department of Cell Biology
Weizmann Institute of Science
Rehovot, Israel

Israel Kleir
Department of Cell Biology
Weizmann Institute of Science
Rehovot, Israel

F. Labrie
MRC Group in Molecular Endocrinology
Hospital Center
Laval University
Quebec G1V 4G2, Canada

Catherine Lau
Ortho Pharmaceutical Corporation
Don Mills, Ontario M3C 1L9, Canada

M. Lavoie
MRC Group in Molecular Endocrinology
Hospital Center
Laval University
Quebec G1V 4G2, Canada

Johann Leban
Institute for Biomedical Research
University of Texas at Austin
Austin, Texas 78712

Maria Lebek
Institute for Biomedical Research
University of Texas at Austin
Austin, Texas 78712

C. Y. Lee
Department of Biochemistry
Chinese University of Hong Kong
Shatin, N.T., Hong Kong

P. Lefrancier
Choay Institute
92120 Montrouge, France

C. J. M. Leupers
Central Laboratory of the Netherlands
Red Cross Blood Transfusion Service
1006 AD Amsterdam, The Netherlands

Choh Hao Li
Hormone Research Laboratory
University of California, San Francisco
San Francisco, California 94143

Peter Lomedico
The Biological Laboratories
Harvard University
Cambridge, Massachusetts 02138

Teresa L. K. Low
Department of Biochemistry
School of Medicine and Health Sciences
George Washington University
Washington, D.C. 20037

Thomas J. Lukas
Rockefeller University
New York, New York 10021

Elsa Lundanes
Institute for Biomedical Research
University of Texas at Austin
Austin, Texas 78712

Russell McCandliss
Roche Institute of Molecular Biology
Nutley, New Jersey 07110

Chester A. Meyers
Department of Medicine
Tulane University School of Medicine
New Orleans, Louisiana 70112

Imre Mezo
Department of Medicine
Tulane University School of Medicine
New Orleans, Louisiana 70112

Giuseppe Miozzari
Division of Molecular Biology
Genentech, Inc.
South San Francisco, California 94080

William Murphy
Department of Medicine
Tulane University School of Medicine
New Orleans, Louisiana 70112

Stephen P. Naber
Elliot P. Joslin Research Laboratory
Harvard Medical School
Boston, Massachusetts 02115

Mary V. Nekola
Department of Medicine
Tulane University School of Medicine
New Orleans, Louisiana 70112

Thomas L. O'Donohue
Department of Pharmacology
Howard University
Washington, D.C. 20059

Masahiro Ohta
Institute for Biomedical Research
University of Texas at Austin
Austin, Texas 78712

Escipion Pedroza
Department of Medicine
Tulane University School of Medicine
New Orleans, Louisiana 70112

Sidney Pestka
Roche Institute of Molecular Biology
Nutley, New Jersey 07110

J. M. Pleau
INSERM Unit 25
Necker Hospital
75730 Paris Cedex 15, France

Julia M. Polak
Royal Postgraduate Medical School
Hammersmith Hospital
London W12 0HS, England

Michael B. Prystowsky
Rockefeller University
New York, New York 10021

Salvatore Raiti
National Pituitary Agency
University of Maryland School of
  Medicine
Baltimore, Maryland 21201

J. Ramachandran
Hormone Research Laboratory
University of California, San Francisco
San Francisco, California 94143

Georg Rampold
Institute for Biomedical Research
University of Texas at Austin
Austin, Texas 78712

T. W. Redding
Veterans Administration Medical Center
New Orleans, Louisiana 70146

Ronald E. Ritzmann
Department of Physiology and Biophysics
University of Illinois Medical Center
Chicago, Illinois 60680

Michael J. Ross
Division of Molecular Biology
Genentech, Inc.
South San Francisco, California 94080

Menachem Rubinstein
Roche Institute of Molecular Biology
Nutley, New Jersey 07110

Maoki Sakura
Institute for Biomedical Research
University of Texas at Austin
Austin, Texas 78712

Curt A. Sandman
Endocrinology Section
Veterans Administration Medical Center
New Orleans, Louisiana 70146

Andrew V. Schally
Department of Medicine
Tulane University School of Medicine
New Orleans, Louisiana 70112

P. Th. A. Schellekens
Central Laboratory of the Netherlands
Red Cross Blood Transfusion Service
1006 AD Amsterdam, The Netherlands

Peter H. Seeburg
Department of Molecular Biology
Genentech, Inc.
South San Francisco, California 94080

Alan Sloma
Roche Institute of Molecular Biology
Nutley, New Jersey 07110

Gerard P. Smith
Department of Psychiatry
New York Hospital–Cornell Medical
Center
White Plains, New York 10605

Stanley Stein
Roche Institute of Molecular Biology
Nutley, New Jersey 07110

Michael O. Thorner
Department of Internal Medicine
University of Virginia School of Medicine
Charlottesville, Virginia 22908

Gary B. Thurman
Department of Biochemistry
School of Medicine and Health Sciences
George Washington University
Washington, D.C. 20037

Richard Tizard
The Biological Laboratories
Harvard University
Cambridge, Massachusetts 02138

Nathan Trainin
Department of Cell Biology
Weizmann Institute of Science
Rehovot, Israel

C. Turkelson
Veterans Administration Medical Center
New Orleans, Louisiana 70146

Tehila Umiel
Department of Cell Biology
Weizmann Institute of Science
Rehovot, Israel

T. van Bemmel
Central Laboratory of the Netherlands
Red Cross Blood Transfusion Service
1006 AD Amsterdam, The Netherlands

Lydia Villa-Komaroff
Department of Microbiology
University of Massachusetts Medical
School
Worcester, Massachusetts 01605

Wolfgang Voelter
Institute for Organic Chemistry
Tübingen University
D-7400 Tübingen, West Germany

Roderich Walter
Department of Physiology and Biophysics
University of Illinois Medical Center
Chicago, Illinois 60680

P. Wijermans
Central Laboratory of the Netherlands
Red Cross Blood Transfusion Service
1006 AD Amsterdam, The Netherlands

Brigitte Wittmann-Liebold
Max-Planck-Institute for Molecular
Genetics
D-1000 Berlin 33 (Dahlem), West
Germany

Daniel G. Yansura
Division of Molecular Biology
Genentech, Inc.
South San Francisco, California 94080

James E. Zadina
Endocrinology Section
Veterans Administration Medical Center
New Orleans, Louisiana 70146

Polypeptide Hormones, edited by
R. F. Beers, Jr. and E. G. Bassett.
Raven Press, New York © 1980.

1. Welcoming Remarks

Walter Ames Compton

Miles Laboratories, Inc., Elkhart, Indiana 46515

It is indeed a pleasure to welcome you all to this, the 12th Miles International Symposium, a series begun 12 years ago, back in 1967. At that first meeting, a day and a half program held at the New York Hilton, we considered transfer of genetic information in protein synthesis and the synthesis, structure, and function of messenger RNA. Generally, the focus of all of our Symposia has been various aspects of molecular biology running through the most exciting period of its development as a new bioscience. The Symposia generally have placed special emphasis on the chemistry and rationale of genetics and, recently, of immuno-biochemistry. Last year we dealt with mechanisms of pain and analgesia; in 1976 at the Massachusetts Institute of Technology, our Symposium was entitled "Impact of Recombinant Molecules on Science and Society" and we addressed the area of hot debate and active concern in the interface of this new life science with matters of social concern.

This year, at our 12th conference, we are dealing with the current, very high level of interest regarding polypeptide hormones and their involvement in cellular biology, immunology, endocrinology, and pharmacology. It is of interest to note that 10 years ago, at our third Symposium, the subject was "Polypeptides—Their Enzymatic and Chemical Synthesis and Their Role in Immunological Processes"; if time permitted, it would be of great interest to review in some detail the papers presented at that time. I shall, however, note just a few of them.

On the first day we heard Ephraim Katchalski (later known as Ephraim Katzir), then of the Weizmann Institute of Science, the President of Israel in recent past, present a paper on the chemical synthesis of polypeptides. He was followed by a report about synthetic studies on staphylococcal nuclease that was co-authored by Christian B. Anfinsen, Chairman of today's opening session. Finally, I should be remiss not to remark that at that meeting we enjoyed the assistance as Co-chairman of the Symposium, Michael Sela, then of the Weizmann Institute of Science and currently its President.

Unfortunately, it was not until the following year that we began the practice of publishing the full proceedings of the Symposia, and the many interesting papers of the 1967–1969 Symposia, together with their critical discussions, are not available.

We do thank you for coming and hope that you enjoy the conference and find it rewarding.

Polypeptide Hormones, edited by
R. F. Beers, Jr. and E. G. Bassett.
Raven Press, New York © 1980.

2. Introduction

Roland F. Beers, Jr.

Miles Laboratories, Inc., Elkhart, Indiana 46515

I usually make a few opening remarks at these Symposia, to set, hopefully, the stage of thinking, not necessarily directing the line of thinking, but at least providing a framework in which to consider some of the dominant questions and issues that might arise during the course of the proceedings. The area of polypeptide hormones represents, to a certain extent, a deviation from the traditional directions in which the field of molecular biology has proceeded.

The research enterprise in the field of molecular biology has been dominated since the Second World War by what may be broadly defined as molecular genetics with primary emphasis on the information systems of the cell involved in polypeptide synthesis. The success in elaborating the complicated mechanisms of polypeptide synthesis, beginning with the description of the Watson-Crick double helix of DNA and culminating in recombinant DNA research, has tended to obscure the simple fact that polypeptides and proteins constitute the essential and necessary components of the structure and machinery of the cell. An understanding of the normal and pathological processes of the cell and of higher organisms must include an understanding of the characteristics and role of polypeptides.

We have witnessed, during the past 10 years, a resurgence in research on the polypeptide field that is reminiscent of the late 1940s. It is worth noting that many of the techniques used to study nucleic acids were first developed for the study of protein structure and amino acid sequencing. This volume is devoted to a distinct class of polypeptides demonstrating hormonal-like activity. This is in some respects reminiscent of the messenger role of RNA.

Schwyzer (1) has suggested the term *sychological* to distinguish them from larger polypeptides (proteins) whose secondary and tertiary structures are essential for biological activity.

There is another possible distinction that is reflected in the kinds of research pursued in the late 1940s and today. Proteins were thought of as carriers of functional groups essential for biological activity. This found very popular support in the study of enzymes. The main characteristic distinguishing enzymes from other catalysts was the topological role of the protein carrier in providing a structural basis for optimal positioning of the functional group. Allosterism proved to be a very useful concept to explain the functions of such topological changes in proteins.

3

In the simpler polypeptides the topological configurations of functional groups do not appear to be as important. Rather, the amino acid sequences are critical for biological activity. Whatever conformational features are required for biological activity are established at the receptor site rather than by any unique conformation of the polypeptide established by the amino acid sequence, hydrogen bonds, disulfide bridges, and so forth.

The first section of this volume is devoted to *in vivo* and *in vitro* polypeptide synthesis. It addresses itself to biological systems with major emphasis on recombinant DNA technology. The examples selected for presentation include proteins such as insulin and interferons, which are outside the area of polypeptides as defined earlier, but do provide an excellent opportunity to assess the practical problems of polypeptide synthesis with recombinant DNA techniques.

Dr. Folkers' section addresses itself to chemical synthetic routes, primarily by solid phase procedures. It will be very interesting to see which of these two technologies, biological or chemical, will prevail in the production of polypeptides for therapeutic use.

The four areas of hormonal research covered in the succeeding sections have been selected somewhat arbitrarily. Dr. Schally's treatment of the hypothalamic hormones overlaps that of Dr. Li's on the pituitary hormones, two highly productive areas of polypeptide hormone research that have already been recognized by the Nobel committee.

Dr. Bloom's discussion of gastrointestinal hormones reflects a very rapid pace of development that is unique because of the site of their origins. Indeed, the notion of gastrointestinal hormones is a relatively new concept.

Finally, Dr. Trainin's section on thymic hormones represents another rapidly developing field. They are unique for their demonstrated role in immunocompetence and for potential major therapeutic advances in the future.

REFERENCE

1. Schwyzer, R. (1977): ACTH: A short introductory review. *Ann. N.Y. Acad. Sci.*, 297:3–26.

Polypeptide Hormones, edited by
R. F. Beers, Jr. and E. G. Bassett.
Raven Press, New York © 1980.

3. Introduction to Section A: Biological Synthesis of Peptide Hormones

Christian B. Anfinsen

Laboratory of Chemical Biology, NIAMDD, National Institutes of Health, Bethesda, Maryland 20205

The preparation of polypeptide hormones for clinical use and basic studies on mechanism of action has classically involved either the isolation of such materials from very large quantities of animal tissues or, in favorable cases, organic synthesis. For only a limited number of compounds such as ACTH and glucagon has it been possible, to date, to prepare sizable amounts of dependably homogeneous material by the classic techniques of the peptide chemist. Even in the case of insulin, the isolation of the hormone from pancreatic tissue has economic advantages over the synthetic preparation of this substance by proven methods. The increasing elegance of classic synthetic methods and of the solid-phase procedure of Merrifield and his colleagues may soon make the chemical production of large hormones and a variety of lymphokines commercially competitive. However, the most exciting possibilities at the moment stem from recent developments in the field of messenger RNA translation and the cloning of bacterial cells for specific gene recombinant properties. I would not like to predict at the present time whether the chemist or the bacterial cell will win the race. Speaking as a chemist, I still feel that the mass production of kilo quantities by the patient coupling of amino acids is the most straightforward and dependable alternative. Nevertheless, as the title of this opening section, which is devoted to various aspects of the new genetic technology, indicates, we must begin to take very seriously the biological synthesis of long polypeptide chains.

One approach has not been specifically included among the subjects for discussion—the production of large polypeptides and small proteins in large scale cultures of eukaryotic cells. I would like to describe very briefly the current efforts in quite a number of laboratories around the world that are involved with the stimulation of eukaryotic cells in culture by viruses or synthetic double-stranded RNA preparations to produce the clinically promising interferon molecule. As a representative example I will summarize, for my colleagues Drs. Pamela Bridgen, Mark Smith, and Kathryn Zoon, the status of such efforts in our own laboratory.

The total protein content of 200 to 800 liters of the induced Namalwa B-lymphocyte cultures, after removal of cells in a cream separator, can be precipitated with relatively little loss by addition of trichloroacetic acid (TCA). A 200-liter batch normally contains on the order of 0.5 to 1.0 mg of interferon, based on biological assay. Interferon is purified in our own particular set of purification steps as summarized in Table 1. In recent experiments, a step involving chromatography on sulfopropyl-Sephadex has been added before the step involving L-tryptophyl-L-tryptophan-Affi-gel 10 with no significant loss in recovery. The final material obtained on the preparative slab gel has an activity profile as shown in Fig. 1. The major interferon band exhibits a molecular weight of approximately 18,000 with the suggestion of one or two much less abundant components with molecular weights on the order of 20,000 to 22,000 daltons. On elution of the major band, and rerunning on a second SDS gel, a single band is obtained with a molecular weight of approximately 18,000 daltons as shown in Fig. 2. The standard proteins on the left of this figure are bovine serum albumin, soybean trypsin inhibitor, and apomyoglobin. This apparently homogeneous material yields an amino acid composition that is summarized in Table 2. The value for glycine is indeterminate due to large amounts of this amino acid in the slab gel buffer. The value for ½ cystine has very recently been found to be 2 per 155 amino acid residues, tryptophan probably 1, and proline on the order of 4 to 5. A particularly interesting aspect of the amino acid analyses is that the composition shown in Table 2 is extremely similar to what has been reported for mouse interferon and for both human leukocyte and fibroblast interferons. It is particularly encouraging that human interferon can now be produced in homogeneous form, a condition that is strongly supported by preliminary automatic sequence analysis on both the fibroblast material

TABLE 1. *Purification of human lymphoblastoid interferon[a]*

Fraction	Specific activity (units/mg)	Cumulative recovery (%)
Trichloroacetic acid (5% w/v)	$1–2 \times 10^3$	75
Sephadex G-25	$1–2 \times 10^3$	68
Immunoabsorbant-affinity chromatography	$1–5 \times 10^5$	48
Millipore Pellicon ultrafiltration	$1–5 \times 10^5$	48
Sephadex G-150	$1–5 \times 10^6$	29
Millipore Pellicon ultrafiltration	$1–5 \times 10^6$	29
Glycosidase treatment, pH 6.0	$1–5 \times 10^6$	29
L-Tryptophyl-L-tryptophan-Affi-gel 10	$0.8–2.0 \times 10^7$	18
SDS-PAGE	$2–4 \times 10^8$	10

[a] The large scale growth and viral induction of the human lymphoblastoid cells, "Namalva," has been possible through the cooperation of the group at the Frederick Cancer Research Center under the expert direction of Dr. Frederick Klein.

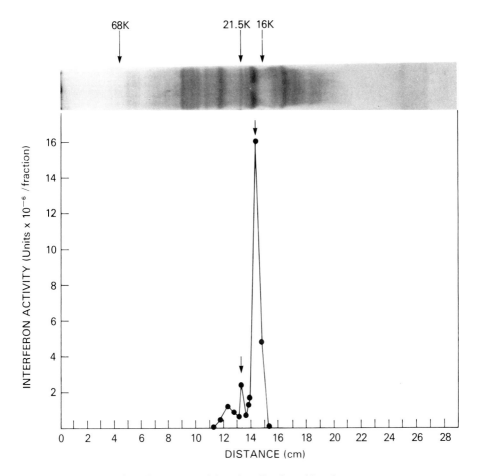

FIG. 1. Preparative slab gel purification of interferon.

isolated by Dr. Ernest Knight at the DuPont Co. and on our own lymphoblastoid preparation. Serious attempts using organic synthesis are still in the distant future, but such efforts have at least now become a credible possibility.

Section A is heavy with considerations of the techniques being developed for the production of peptide hormones through genetic engineering employing bacterial cells. A complete coverage is limited because of our time restrictions. In addition to the work summarized by Drs. David Goeddel, Peter Seeburg, and Lydia Villa-Komaroff, that there has been considerable success with other materials, including hormones from the parathyroid and thyroid in the laboratory of Dr. John Potts.

Dr. Sidney Pestka, from the Roche Institute of Molecular Biology, discusses another type of approach with potentials not only for eventual use of bacterial

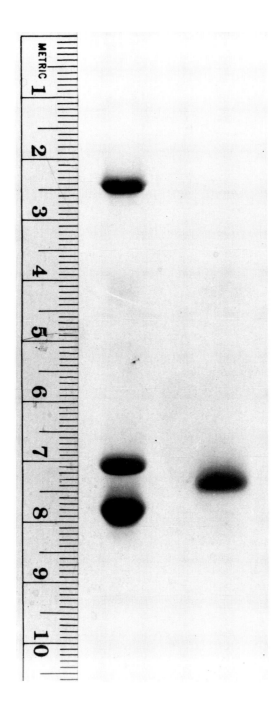

FIG. 2. SDS gel purification of the major interferon band; marker proteins at the left.

TABLE 2. *Amino acid composition of human lymphoblastoid interferon*[a]

Amino acid	Residues/155 amino acids residues[b] $(X \pm SD)$[c]
Asx	16.3 ± 0.7
Thr	7.8 ± 0.6
Ser	11.0 ± 1.4
Glx	24.6 ± 1.9
Pro	N.D.[d]
Gly	N.I.[e]
Ala	10.4 ± 1.5
Cys	N.D.
Val	9.1 ± 1.4
Met	1.6 ± 0.8
Ile	7.4 ± 0.4
Leu	16.0 ± 1.2
Tyr	4.2 ± 1.3
Phe	8.1 ± 1.2
His	N.D.
Lys	13.2 ± 1.2
Arg	10.5 ± 1.2
Trp	N.D.

[a] Amino acid analyses were done at the National Geophysical Laboratories, Washington, D.C. by Dr. P. E. Hare using high-performance liquid chromatography of *o*-phthalaldehyde derivatives of amino acid residues and a fluorescence detection system. (From ref. 1.)

[b] Based on the molecular weight of 18,500, the number of amino acid residues in interferon is 155.

[c] The mean of seven determinations of the amino acid composition of interferon eluted from SDS gels.

[d] Not determined.

[e] Not integrated.

cloning techniques but also for direct translation of isolated interferon messenger RNA. I am certain the chapters that follow will most certainly be highly interesting and likely to stimulate active discussion.

REFERENCES

1. Hare, P. E. (1977): Subnanomole-range amino acid analysis. In: *Methods of Enzymology, Vol. 47: Enzyme Structure, Part E,* edited by C. H. W. Hirs and S. N. Timasheff, pp. 2–18. Academic Press, New York.

Polypeptide Hormones, edited by
R. F. Beers, Jr. and E. G. Bassett.
Raven Press, New York © 1980.

4. Use of Chemically Synthesized DNA for the Bacterial Production of Human Growth Hormone

David V. Goeddel, Herbert L. Heyneker, Giuseppe Miozzari,
Michael J. Ross, Peter H. Seeburg, Daniel G. Yansura, *Rene
Arentzen, *Toyhara Hozumi, and *Keiichi Itakura

*Division of Molecular Biology, Genentech, Inc., South San Francisco, California 94080; and
Division of Biology, City of Hope National Medical Center, Duarte, California 91010

Recombinant DNA technology has made possible the microbial production of mammalian polypeptide hormones. One method is to prepare enzymatically DNA complementary to mRNA from a specific gland and to insert this complementary DNA (cDNA) into a bacterial plasmid encoded gene. Using this approach, rat proinsulin (14) and rat pre-growth hormone (13) have been expressed in *E. coli* as chimeric proteins fused to the bacterial β-lactamase. A shortcoming of this approach is that it has not yet been possible to process proteolytically such fusion proteins to yield the mature natural hormones.

The alternative approach has been to synthesize chemically DNA fragments that can be assembled to form a gene coding for the desired peptide hormone and attach this gene to a bacterial gene on a plasmid. By incorporating a methionine residue in the synthetic plan, the peptide of choice is produced as a tail attached to a larger protein, and can be efficiently released by treatment with cyanogen bromide. The larger protein (β-galactosidase being the current preference) protects the smaller peptide from proteolytic degradation. This approach was successfully used for the synthesis in *E. coli* of somatostatin (7) and human insulin A and B chains (2,5), none of which contain methionine. Peptides with methionine residues could be produced by this approach, using a protease-susceptible amino acid for attachment to the precursor protein (assuming that the peptide is resistant to that protease). Larger polypeptide hormones might be stable in bacteria and, if so, could be synthesized directly in a nonprecursor form. Since it is theoretically possible to synthesize chemically a gene of any size, the major disadvantage of this approach is the length of time involved.

By combining the above approaches of cDNA molecular cloning and chemical synthesis of DNA, we were able to produce bacterially a reasonably large polypeptide, human growth hormone, in a nonprecursor form.

HUMAN GROWTH HORMONE

Human growth hormone (HGH) is synthesized in the anterior lobe of the pituitary gland. It contains 191 amino acids and has a molecular weight of approximately 21,500. The clinical usefulness of HGH in the treatment of children with hypopituitary dwarfism is well established (8,11). Additionally, HGH may be effective in the treatment of bleeding ulcers, bone fractures, muscular dystrophy, and a variety of other disorders (8,11). Unlike insulin, which is not species-specific, only GH obtained from human pituitaries is active in man. The resulting short supply of HGH has precluded the full utilization of its beneficial potential. Therefore, HGH was an obvious choice in the attempt to produce a hormone by bacteria via recombinant DNA technology.

The initial translation product of HGH mRNA is pre-HGH, in which a signal peptide is attached to the NH_2-terminus of HGH. Signal or presequences are characteristic of secreted hormones, and are apparently removed during the secretion process. The previously determined sequence of HGH cDNA (12) provided us with the information necessary to design and construct a gene coding for HGH. This gene was inserted into a specially engineered bacterial plasmid that directed the synthesis of mature HGH in *E. coli.*

HGH GENE CONSTRUCTION

The strategy used for constructing a gene coding for HGH was based on the restriction endonuclease pattern of HGH cDNA (12). Treatment of HGH cDNA with the restriction endonuclease *Hae*III gives a 551 base pair (bp) DNA fragment that codes for amino acids 24 to 191 of HGH and that contains 46 bp of noncoding DNA at the 3' end of the gene. We prepared HGH cDNA from human pituitary mRNA, isolated a 551 bp *Hae*III fragment, and cloned it into the plasmid pBR322 (1), giving the plasmid pHGH31 (4).

The DNA coding for the remainder of HGH was prepared by the chemical synthesis approach. The synthetic plan is shown in Fig. 1. This DNA "adaptor" fragment contains an ATG initiation codon and coding sequences for amino acids 1 to 23 of HGH. The 5' ends have single-stranded cohesive termini for the *Eco*RI and *Hin*dIII restriction sites. The same *Hae*III site present in HGH cDNA is incorporated at amino acids 23 and 24 to facilitate joining with the cDNA fragment to form a synthetic-natural "hybrid" gene. When inserted into a plasmid downstream from a suitable bacterial promoter and ribosome binding site, this gene could be expected to direct the synthesis of fMet-HGH. The fact that most bacterial proteins do not contain NH_2-terminal methionines suggests that the fMet should be efficiently removed, resulting in the direct expression of mature HGH.

The twelve indicated deoxyoligonucleotides (Fig. 1) were synthesized by the improved phosphotriester method (2). The assembly and cloning of these DNA fragments to give the plasmid pHGH3 are summarized in Fig. 2.

The joining of the two separately cloned HGH DNA fragments to form the complete gene is shown in Fig. 3. A 77-bp fragment coding for amino acids 1 to 23 of HGH was isolated from pHGH3 after cleaving with *Eco*RI and *Hae*III. *Hae*III treatment of pHGH31 yielded the 551 bp fragment described

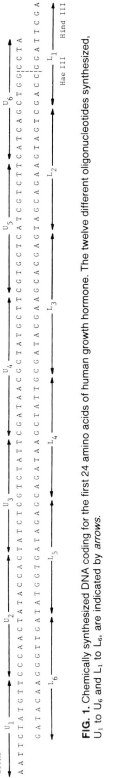

FIG. 1. Chemically synthesized DNA coding for the first 24 amino acids of human growth hormone. The twelve different oligonucleotides synthesized, U_1 to U_6 and L_1 to L_6, are indicated by *arrows*.

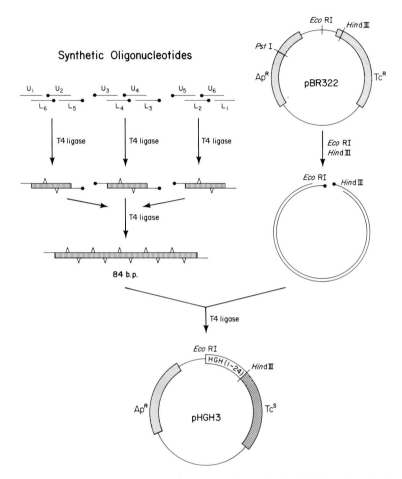

FIG. 2. Assembly and molecular cloning of chemically synthesized DNA coding for the first 24 amino acids of HGH. Oligonucleotides are indicated by *lines*, 5′ phosphate groups by *dots*. Experimental details are published elsewhere (ref. 4).

above. *Xma*I treatment of this fragment removed 39 bp of DNA from the 3′ noncoding region and gave a 512 bp fragment coding for amino acids 24 to 191 and containing one "blunt" end and one "sticky" end. Ligation of these two fragments resulted in a highly polymerized DNA mixture. Treatment with *Eco*RI and *Sma*I (which recognizes the same sequence as *Xma*I but leaves blunt ends) converted the ligation mixture to three distinct products. One of these was the desired 591 bp fragment coding for the entire HGH sequence. This fragment was cloned into the expression vector pGH6, a derivative of pBR322 containing two *lac* promoters (4). After transformation of χ1776 (3), plasmids containing HGH gene sequences were identified by the Grunstein-Hogness colony screening procedure (6) and by restriction analysis of plasmid

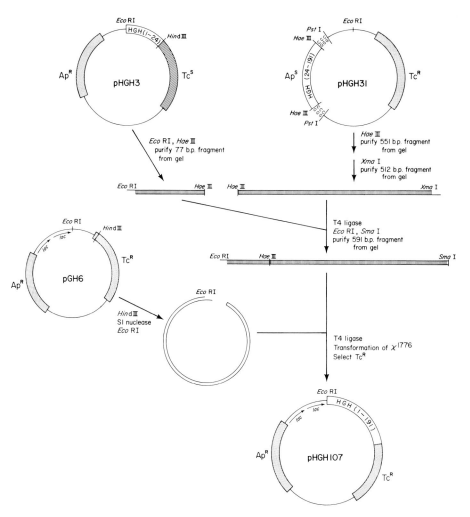

FIG. 3. Construction of plasmid (pHGH107) for the expression of HGH in *E. coli.* See text and ref. 4 for experimental details.

DNA. The HGH sequence of one of the transformants, pHGH107, was verified by the Maxam-Gilbert procedure (10).

pHGH107 contains 11 bp between the *lac* AGGA ribosome binding site (9) and the ATG translational start. In the naturally occurring *lac* system, this separation is 7 bp. To restore the exact *lac* sequence in this region, pHGH107 was cleaved with *Eco*RI, treated with S1 nuclease to digest single-strand ends, and reclosed by ligation as shown in Fig. 4. The resulting plasmid, pHGH107-1, contains an *Alu*I site instead of an *Eco*RI site and might be expected to have increased translational efficiency over pHGH107.

```
5'... A G G A A A C A G A A T T C T A T G ...
3'... T C C T T T G T C T T A A G A T A C ...
                                    Eco RI
```

```
          Eco RI
          S1 Nuclease
          T4 Ligase
```

```
5'... A G G A A A C A G C T A T G ...
3'... T C C T T T G T C G A T A C ...
                              Alu I
```

FIG. 4. Removal of *Eco*RI site from pHGH107 to restore the exact *lac* sequence in the region between AGGA ribosome binding site and ATG translation initiation codon. The resulting plasmid is pHGH107-1.

BACTERIAL EXPRESSION OF HGH

Extracts of χ1776 containing the HGH plasmids were assayed for HGH expression by radioimmunoassay (RIA). The results are shown in Table 1. Both pHGH107 and pHGH107-1 specify the synthesis of substantial amounts of radioimmunoactive HGH. However, it is somewhat surprising to find that the addition of 4 bp of DNA to the *lac* sequence between the ribosome binding site and the translational start codon increases HGH expression.

TABLE 1. *Radioimmunoassay of HGH in bacterial extracts[a]*

Strain	Cell density (cells/ml)	HGH by RIA (μg/ml)	HGH copies/cell
χ1776/pHGH107	3.6×10^8	2.4	186,000
χ1776/pHGH107–1	3.6×10^8	1.5	116,000
χ1776/pBR322	3.6×10^8	0	0
D1210/pHGH107	3.8×10^8	2×10^{-4}	15
D1210/pHGH107 (IPTG)	3.8×10^8	1.0	75,000

[a] *E. coli* strains containing the appropriate plasmid were grown to a density of $A_{550} = 1$ and harvested by centrifugation. The cell pellet was resuspended in 55 μl of 50 mM Tris-HCl (pH 8), 50 mM EDTA, 15% sucrose, 1 mg/ml lysozyme, and 0.025% lithium dodecylsulfate. After 30 min at 0°C, 10 μl of 150 mM Tris-HCl (pH 7.5), 280 mM MgCl$_2$, 4 mM CaCl$_2$ and 1 μg of DNase I were added. The mixture was centrifuged for 15 min at 12,000 × *g*. Supernatants were analyzed by radioimmunoassay with the Phadebas HGH PRIST kit (Pharmacia). Values are expressed as micrograms per milliliter of cell culture. Where indicated, isopropyl β-D-thiogalactoside (IPTG) was added to the cell culture at a concentration of 2 mM.

The plasmid phGH107 was also transformed into the *E. coli* K-12 strain D1210, a *lac* repressor overproducing derivative of HB101 (5). The HGH production of D1210/phGH107 in response to the gratuitous inducer isopropyl-β-D-thiogalactoside (IPTG) demonstrated that HGH synthesis is under *lac* promoter control (Table 1).

Extracts of χ1776/phGH107 were analyzed by SDS-polyacrylamide gel electrophoresis and by immunoprecipitation with HGH antiserum (4). In both cases the HGH produced by *E. coli* is indistinguishable from pituitary HGH. Gel filtration of the total soluble protein from extracts of χ1776/phGH107 give an HGH fraction of about 25% purity (4). Experiments are currently in progress to purify bacterially produced HGH to homogeneity so that its biological activity and amino acid sequence can be compared with natural HGH.

DISCUSSION

An *E. coli* strain was constructed that produces human growth hormone in substantial amounts. This is the first mammalian polypeptide hormone to be directly expressed in a bacteria in a mature, nonprecursor form. The unique approach of combining chemically synthesized DNA and cDNA to form a hybrid HGH gene is generally applicable for the construction of genes coding for peptide hormones and proteins. This includes polypeptides that are initially synthesized in precursor form and later processed, or for which full length cDNA transcripts are unavailable.

REFERENCES

1. Bolivar, F., Rodriguez, R. L., Greene, P. J., Betlach, M. C., Heyneker, H. L., and Boyer, H. W. (1977): Construction and characterization of new cloning vehicles. *Gene,* 2:95–113.
2. Crea, R., Kraszewski, A., Hirose, T., and Itakura, K. (1978): Chemical synthesis of genes for human insulin. *Proc. Natl. Acad. Sci. USA,* 75:5765–5769.
3. Curtiss, R., III, Pereira, D. A., Hsu, J. C., Hull, S. C., Clark, J. E., Maturin, L. J., Sr., Goldschmidt, R., Moody, R., Inoue, M., and Alexander, L. (1977): Biological containment: The subordination of *Escherichia coli* K-12. In: *Recombinant Molecules: Impact on Science and Society,* edited by R. F. Beers, Jr. and E. G. Bassett, pp. 45–56. Raven Press, New York.
4. Goeddel, D. V., Heyneker, H. L., Hozumi, T., Arentzen, R., Itakura, K., Yansura, D. G., Ross, M. J., Miozzari, G., Crea, R., and Seeburg, P. H. (1979): Direct expression in *E. coli* of a DNA sequence coding for human growth hormone. *Nature,* 281:544–548.
5. Goeddel, D. V., Kleid, D. G., Bolivar, F., Heyneker, H. L., Yansura, D. G., Crea, R., Hirose, T., Kraszewski, A., Itakura, K., and Riggs, A. D. (1979): Expression in *Escherichia coli* of chemically synthesized genes for human insulin. *Proc. Natl. Acad. Sci. USA,* 76:106–110.
6. Grunstein M., and Hogness, D. S. (1975): Colony hybridization: A method for the isolation of cloned DNAs that contain a specific gene. *Proc. Natl. Acad. Sci. USA,* 72:3961–3965.
7. Itakura, K., Hirose, T., Crea, R., Riggs, A. D., Heyneker, H. L., Bolivar, F., and Boyer, H. W. (1977): Expression in *Escherichia coli* of a chemically synthesized gene for the hormone somatostatin. *Science,* 198:1056–1063.
8. Li, C. H., editor (1975): *Hormonal Proteins and Peptides.* Academic Press, New York.
9. Maizels, N. (1974): *E. coli* lactose operon ribosome binding site. *Nature,* 249:647.
10. Maxam, A., and Gilbert, W. (1977): A new method for sequencing DNA. *Proc. Natl. Acad. Sci. USA,* 74:560–564.
11. Raiti, S., editor (1974): *Advances in Growth Hormone Research.* National Pituitary Agency, Baltimore.

12. Goodman, H. M., Seeburg, P. H., Martial, J. A., Shine, J., Ullrich, A., and Baxter, J. D. (1979): Construction and expression in bacteria of growth hormone genes. In: *Specific Eukaryotic Genes,* edited by J. Engberg, H. Klenow, and V. Leick, pp. 179–190. Munksgaard, Copenhagen.
13. Seeburg, P. H., Shine, J., Martial, J. A., Ivarie, R. D., Morris, J. A., Ullrich, A., Baxter, J. D., and Goodman, H. M. (1978): Synthesis of growth hormone by bacteria. *Nature,* 276:795–798.
14. Villa-Komaroff, L., Efstratiadis, A., Broome, S., Lomedico, P., Tizard, R., Naber, S. P., Chick, W. L. and Gilbert, W. (1978): A bacterial clone synthesizing proinsulin. *Proc. Natl. Acad. Sci. USA,* 75:3727–3731.

Polypeptide Hormones, edited by
R. F. Beers, Jr. and E. G. Bassett.
Raven Press, New York © 1980.

5. Structure and Regulation of Pituitary Hormone Genes

Peter H. Seeburg

*Department of Molecular Biology, Genentech, Inc.,
South San Francisco, California 94080*

INTRODUCTION

Of all the endocrine glands, the anterior pituitary is the most important. The peptide hormones produced there control growth, sexual development, reproduction, thyroid activity and, to a large degree, the body's response to stress, pain, and illness. It seems obvious that expression of the genes for these biologically highly active peptides is subject to stringent and complete regulation. This chapter focuses on the gene for somatotropin (growth hormone) and its expression. Growth hormone (GH) is a single-chain peptide of 191 amino acids (14) that, in humans, is closely related (85% sequence homology) to the peptide hormone chorionic somatomammotropin (15) produced solely by the placenta. GH is also related (about 30% homology) to another pituitary peptide hormone, prolactin (28), and the similarities of the three peptides suggest a common evolutionary origin (19). The genes for GH and related peptides provide an excellent system for studying the structure and regulation of related DNA sequences, the expression of which occurs in separate tissues (pituitary and placenta) and is under a different control.

MESSENGER RNAs FOR SOMATOTROPIN AND RELATED HORMONES

The mRNAs for human growth hormone (HGH), human chorionic somatomammotropin (HCS), and rat growth hormone (RGH) have been cloned into bacteria in the form of their complementary DNAs and their sequences have been determined (8,23,24,27). The mRNAs code for peptides that carry 26 additional amino acids that are mostly of a hydrophobic nature and attached to the NH_2-terminus of the mature hormones. These pre- or single peptides are enzymatically removed during the transfer of the newly synthesized secretory proteins into the lumen of the rough endoplasmic reticulum of the endocrine cells (4). Figure 1 shows the amino acid and nucleotide sequences for the signal regions of HGH, RGH, and HCS and their respective mRNAs. It is interesting to note the striking similarities among these sequences, indicating a high degree of evolutionary conservation. Included in Fig. 1 are the 18 nucleotides that precede the AUG start codon in the three mRNAs. Since these regions may serve as ribosomal binding sites (26), their sequence conservation could be expected on the basis of identical function. In Figs. 2 and 3 the same mRNAs are compared with respect to parts of their coding and 3'-noncoding regions. It is of interest that the close sequence homology between rat and human growth hormone (as seen in Fig. 2 for the coding part of the mRNAs) is not seen in the region distal to the UAG stop codon. Although the actual nucleotide sequences diverge, structural similarities of the rat and human mRNAs are present in extended regions of a truly palindromic nature (inverted repeats). Such sequences prevent the formation of secondary structures.

At a point near the -AATAAA- stretch [common to all eukaryotic mRNAs (21)] and extending to the 3'-end, the nucleotide sequence of the three hormone mRNAs again shows a high degree of homology (data not shown). Since this region corresponds to the site of transcriptional termination for RNA polymerase in the three genes, the observed sequence similarities could reflect functional constraints on nucleotide sequence divergence.

REGULATION OF THE GROWTH HORMONE GENE IN CULTURED CELLS

Several stable cell lines (GH cells), originally derived from a rat pituitary tumor (31,35), produce GH and also prolactin (PRL). The amount of each peptide hormone synthesized within the cells can be influenced by many agents, including members from several classes of hormones (6,12,32). Of these, steroid and thyroid hormones are of particular interest since they enter the nucleus of the cell, possibly influencing the rate of transcription of target genes (see below). The action of these relatively small molecules is mediated by specific binding proteins (2,3,34). In the case of thyroid hormones, the receptor proteins are an intrinsic part of chromatin that represents a subfraction of the non-histone chromosomal proteins (2).

Monitoring the production of GH and PRL, GH cells respond to thyroid hormones [e.g., triiodothyronine (T_3)] and glucocorticoids [e.g., dexamethasone (DEX)] in the following way (17): When the cells are grown in serum-containing medium (which always contains some T_3), GH is synthesized and synthesis can be increased several-fold on the addition of 10 nM T_3. PRL is also produced, but T_3 has no influence on its synthesis. The simultaneous presence of DEX (1 μM) will result in a further increase of GH synthesis (due to a synergistic action of T_3 and DEX) and a decrease in PRL production. When the cells are grown in the absence of T_3 [either in a medium containing serum obtained from a thyroidectomized calf or in a synthetic (1) medium], synthesis of GH, but not PRL, ceases and GH levels are below detectable levels after several days (Fig. 4). GH synthesis is resumed after T_3, but not DEX, addition. Thus, at least for the expression of the GH gene, the presence of T_3 is required for

```
                  -25              -20              -15              -10               -5

HGH               Met Ala Thr Gly Ser Arg Thr Ser Leu Leu Leu Ala Phe Gly Leu Leu Cys Leu Pro Trp Leu GlN Glu Gly Ser Ala
(5') ... ACAGCUCACCUAGCUGCA AUG GCU ACA GGC UCC ACG CGG UCA UCC CUC CUG GCU UUU GGC CUC CUG CUG UGC UUG CCC CUG CUU CAA GAG GGC AGU GCC

HCS               Met Ala Leu Gly Ser Arg Thr Ser Leu Leu Leu Ala Phe Ala Leu Leu Cys Leu Pro Trp Leu GlN Glu Ala Gly Ala
     ... ACAGCUCACCUAGCUGGCA AUG GCU CUA GGC UCC CGA ACG GCU UUU GCC CUC CUG GCU CUG CUC CUG UGC UUG CUC UGC CAA GAG GCU GGU GCC

RGH               Met Ala Ala Asp Ser GlN Thr Pro Trp Leu Leu Thr Phe Ser Leu Leu Cys Leu Leu Trp Pro GlN Glu Ala Gly Ala
     ... ACAGAUCACUGAGUGGCG AUG GCU GCA GAC ACU CUU CAG ACC UUC AGC CUG CUC ACC UGG CUC CUG CUG UGC CUG CUG UGG CCU CAA GAG GCU GGU GCU
```

FIG. 1. Pre-sequences of HGH, HCS, RGH, and their mRNAs. Nucleotide sequences were determined from cDNAs cloned into bacterial plasmids (23,24), using the method developed by Maxam and Gilbert (18). Amino acid sequences were deduced from DNA sequence data.

```
       24                                                  30
HGH    Ala Phe Asp Thr Tyr Gln Glu Phe Glu Glu Ala Tyr Ile Pro Lys Glu Gln Lys Tyr Ser Phe Leu Gln Asn Pro
(5')   GCC UUU GAC ACC UAC CAG GAG UUU GAA GAA GCC UAU AUC CCA AAG GAG CAG AAG UAU UCA UUC CUG CAG AAC CCC

HCS    Ala Ile Asp Thr Tyr Gln Glu Phe Glu Glu Thr Tyr Ile Pro Lys Asp Gln Lys Tyr Ser Phe Leu His Asp Ser
       GCC AUU GAC ACC UAC CAG GAG UUU GAA GAA ACC UAU AUC CCA AAG GAC CAG AAG UAU UCG UUC CUG CAU GAC UCC

RGH    Ala Ala Asp Thr Tyr Lys Glu Phe Glu Arg Ala Tyr Ile Pro Glu Gly Gln Arg Tyr Ser  -   Ile Gln Asn Ala
       GCU GCU GAC ACC UAC AAA GAG UUC GAG CGU GCC UAC AUU CCC GAG GGA CAG CGC UAU UCC  -   AUU CAG AAU GCC


       50                                             60                                 70
HGH    Gln Thr Ser Leu Cys Phe Ser Glu Ser Ile Pro Thr Pro Ser Asn Arg Glu Glu Thr Gln Gln Lys Ser Asn Leu Glu Leu
       CAG ACC UCC CUC UGU UUC UCA GAG UCU AUU CCG ACA CCC UCC AAC AGG GAG GAA ACA CAA CAG AAA UCC AAC CUA GAG CUG

HCS    Gln Thr Ser Phe Cys Phe Ser Asp Ser Ile Pro Thr Pro Ser Asn Met Glu Glu Thr Gln Gln Lys Ser Asn Leu Glu Leu
       CAG ACC UCC UUC UGC UUC UCA GAC UCU AUU CCG ACA CCC UCC AAC AUG GAG GAA ACG CAA CAG AAA UCC AAU CUA GAG CUG

RGH    Gln Ala Ala Phe Cys Phe Ser Glu Thr Ile Pro Ala Pro Thr Gly Lys Glu Glu Ala Gln Gln Arg Thr Asp Met Glu Leu
       CAG GCU GCG UUC UGC UUC UCA GAG ACC AUC CCA GCC CCC ACC GGC AAG GAG GAG GCC CAG CAG AGA ACU GAC AUG GAA UUG


       80                                             90                                 100
HGH    Leu Arg Ile Ser Leu Leu Leu Ile Gln Ser Trp Leu Glu Pro Val Gln Phe Leu Arg Ser Val Phe Ala Asn Ser Leu Val
       CUC CGC AUC UCC CUG CUG CUC AUC CAG AGC UGG CUC GAG CCC GUG CAG UUC CUC AGG AGU GUC UUC GCC AAC AGC CUG GUG

HCS    Leu Arg Ile Ser Leu Leu Leu Ile Glu Ser Trp Leu Glu Pro Val Arg Phe Leu Arg Ser Met Phe Ala Asn Asn Leu Val
       CUC CGC AUC UCC CUG CUG CUC AUC GAG UCG UGG CUC GAG CCC GUG AGG UUC CUC AGG AGU CUC AUG UUC GCC AAC AAC CUC GUG

RGH    Leu Arg Phe Ser Leu Leu Leu Ile Gln Ser Trp Leu Gly Pro Val Gln Phe Leu Ser Arg Ile Phe Thr Asn Ser Leu Met
       CUU CGC UUC UCG CUG CUG CUC AUC CAG AGC UCA UGG CUG GGG CUC UCA CUC AGC ACG AUU ACC AAC AGC CUG AUG
```

FIG. 2. Sequence comparison of the mRNAs for HGH, HCS, and RGH in a region coding for the mature hormones.

HGH (5')   . . . UAG CUGCCCGGGUGGCAUCCC<u>UGUGACCCC</u>UCCCCAGUG</u>CCUCUCCUGGCC . . . (3')

HCS   . . . UAG GUGCCCGAGUAGCAUC–<u>CUGUGACCCCUCCCC</u>AGUGCCUCUCCUGGCC . . .

RGH   . . . UAG GCACACACUGGUGUCU–CUGCGGC<u>ACUCCCCC</u>GUU<u>ACCCCCC</u>UGUACU . . .

FIG. 3. Palindromic sequences in the mRNAs for HGH, HCS, and RGH distal to the termination codon UAG.

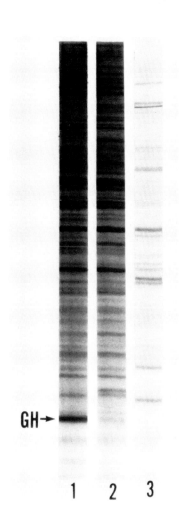

FIG. 4. Deinduction of growth hormone (GH) synthesis in rat pituitary tumor cells grown in a medium containing serum obtained from a thyroidectomized calf. ^{35}S-methionine pulse-labeled cellular proteins were resolved by sodium dodecyl sulfate polyacrylamide gel electrophoresis and the dried gel exposed to X-ray film. **Lane 1:** Cells grown in presence of thyroid hormone. **Lane 2:** Cells grown for 4 days in hypothyroid medium. **Lane 3:** Molecular weight markers.

GH→

1   2   3

glucocorticoids to exert their stimulatory influence. The repressive action of DEX on production of PRL does not seem to be T_3-dependent. It is not clear at this point whether the hormonal effects described determine the primary nuclear activity or reflect the influence of other functions. It is interesting, in this respect, to note that the strict T_3 dependence of DEX stimulation of GH production is somewhat alleviated when GH cells are grown in a synthetic medium devoid of the pancreatic hormone, insulin (2,10).

To study the complexity of the response of GH cells to thyroid and glucocorticoid hormones, pulse-labeled proteins extracted from GH cells grown under various conditions were subjected to two-dimensional gel electrophoresis (20). In this way, approximately 10% of the expressed gene products can be resolved

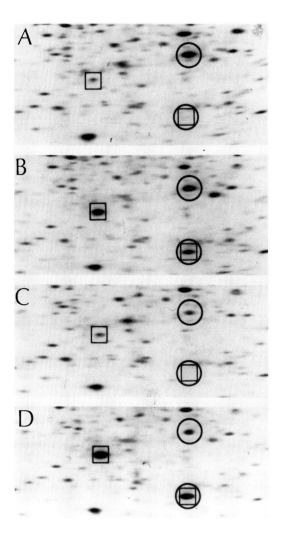

FIG. 5. Changes in the rate of synthesis of GH and PRL in rat pituitary tumor cells in response to thyroid and glucocorticoid hormones, as visualized by two-dimensional gel electrophoresis. From top to bottom, the four panels show autoradiographs of gel-resolved ^{35}S-methionine pulse-labeled proteins of cells grown A: in the absence of hormones, B: in the presence of 10 mM triiodothyromine, C: in the presence of 1 μM dexamethasone, and D: in the presence of both hormones. Squares and circles mark the position of GH and PRL, respectively. (Data from ref. 31.)

and the influence of hormones on their rates of synthesis can be determined (11). An example of such an experiment is shown in Fig. 5. Analyses suggested that in addition to GH and PRL, the synthesis of only a few other proteins is hormonally influenced, making the cellular response a very specific one. Also, proteins were found wherein T_3 does not control the ability of DEX to induce their sythesis (2,10). Since this method focuses on protein synthesis, it aids the examination of events far removed from the primary activity of hormones. The hormonal response of the cells in GH production parallels the levels of GH mRNA when the latter are monitored with a GH-specific cDNA probe (16). This indicates, although far from establishes, that T_3 and DEX influence transcription of the gene. Such an action is reminiscent of specific inducer or repressor functions well-characterized in prokaryotic systems. A detailed analysis involving the isolation and characterization of the GH gene as well as functional studies of sections of this gene will be needed to yield insight into the molecular mechanisms of hormonal control of gene expression.

STRUCTURE OF THE GENE FOR HUMAN GROWTH HORMONE

In this section, the term "GH gene" will be applied to genomic DNA pieces that hybridize to a radiolabeled DNA probe that was originally derived from GH mRNA (8). Due to the extensive sequence homology (>90%) between the mRNA of HGH and HCS, this probe can be used for the simultaneous detection of the two related genes. A distinction between them is observed by using restriction endonucleases known to cleave exclusively either the one (*Bgl*II for HGH) or the other (*Xba*I for HCS) gene within that portion hybridizing to the cDNA probe (8,27). A Southern analysis (30) of DNA from human placental tissue after *Eco*RI endonuclease cleavage revealed two DNA fragments (2.9 and 2.6 kb in length) annealed to the probe (Fig. 6). The presence of one *Xba*I site in the larger DNA fragment and one *Bgl*II site in the smaller suggested that these genomic DNA fragments contained gene sequences for HCS and HGH, respectively, and are termed "core genes." This was subsequently confirmed by DNA sequence analysis on these fragments cloned by the use of bacteriophage λ (7).

To obtain information on the sequences surrounding the core genes, a human gene bank was screened with the same probe. This bank was constructed by T. Maniatis and co-workers by cloning, into the bacteriophage vector Charon 4A, random human genomic DNA pieces of an average size of 16 kb (13). Preliminary analysis of several independent isolates from this gene bank yielded the following information on the structure of the HGH gene:

1. The 2.6 kb DNA fragment cleaved from human genomic DNA by *Eco*RI endonuclease contains most, and maybe all, of the sequence corresponding to HGH mRNA. This sequence is in the core gene that is interrupted at no less than three locations by stretches of DNA several hundred base pairs in length

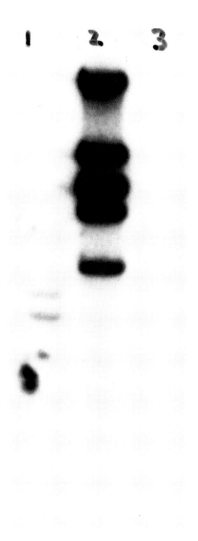

FIG. 6. Autoradiograph of a Southern blot (30) of human placental DNA cleaved by restriction endonucleases. The blotted gel was probed for GH gene sequences with ³²P-dCMP-labeled, cloned HGH cDNA (7). **Lane 1:** *Eco*RI-cleaved DNA. **Lane 2:** *Eco*RI-cleaved, ³²P-labeled λDNA as size marker (bands from top to bottom represent 21, 7.2, 5.6, 4.6, and 3 kb). **Lane 3:** *Pvu*II-cleaved DNA.

(7). Such interruptions by intervening sequences or "introns" have been found in all genes isolated to date from the genomes of higher animals (5). The introns in the HGH gene occur at sites corresponding to the codons for amino acids 31 and 71 of the peptide hormone and for the fourth amino acid of the signal peptide. Figure 7 shows the nucleotide sequence determination near the 3' end of this latter intron; a physical map of the HGH core gene is presented in Fig. 8. It is not known yet whether the 2.6 kb DNA fragment contains the region corresponding to the 5' end of HGH mRNA.

2. At least two HGH core gene isolates which differ in nucleotide sequence, but carry their introns in the same locations, were obtained. They show different

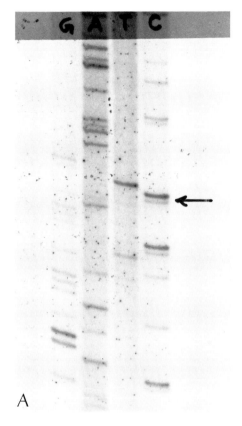

A

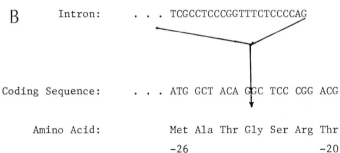

B   Intron: . . . TCGCCTCCCGGTTTCTCCCCAG

Coding Sequence: . . . ATG GCT ACA GGC TCC CGG ACG

Amino Acid: Met Ala Thr Gly Ser Arg Thr
                    -26   -20

FIG. 7. A: Nucleotide sequence determination at the 3' insertion site of an intervening sequence located in the HGH gene in a region that codes for the signal sequence of the peptide hormone. Linearized plasmid pBR322 DNA containing the HGH core gene was treated with *E. coli* exonuclease III (29) and used as a template for sequencing by the chain termination method (22) with a cloned HGH cDNA fragment (containing part of the coding sequences for the signal region) of 109 bp as primer. ^{32}P-labeled DNA products were resolved on 8% acrylamide 7 M urea gels and the dried gels exposed to X-ray film. The band pattern in the autoradiograph corresponds to the non-coding strand of the gene. The arrow marks the position of the 3' insertion site of the intron. **B:** Nucleotide sequence of the coding strand and one possible insertion scheme.

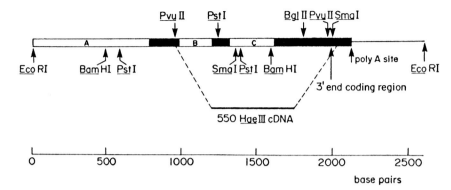

FIG. 8. A physical map of the HGH core gene. Coding sequences are shaded and intervening sequences are labeled A, B, and C.

fragment patterns when cleaved with endonucleases *Hae*III and *Bam*HI. The gene with an additional site for *Bam*HI and carrying a codon for Leu (CTG)—in place of the Pro[32](CCA) seen in HGH mRNA—was termed "variant HGH gene." Whether these isolates represent alleles and the variant is expressed, to some degree, cannot be decided at present.

3. Suggesting the presence of non-allelic HGH genes, the 2.6-kb genomic DNA piece is embedded in at least two different sequence locations. This observation stems from analysis of cloned DNA from the human gene bank (25). Most importantly, in at least one location in the genome, the gene sequences for HGH and HCS are in close proximity (see Fig. 9), and separated by no more than 7 kb. In the clone which carries both core genes, the 2.6-kb DNA fragment contains the variant, as discerned by digestion with endonucleases *Hae*III and *Bam*HI.

DISCUSSION

The genes for GH and related peptides provide an excellent system for elucidating the molecular mechanisms involved in the control of gene expression by thyroid and steroid hormones. Thus, the issue of whether defined sequence elements are present in hormonally-regulated genes (permitting the involvement of hormone-receptor complexes) can be approached by a characterization of the isolated genes. The anatomy of the HGH and HCS genes in the parts detected by a cDNA probe provides nothing exceptional. Similar to other genes, the coding sequences are interrupted in several locations by a core gene that is about 1000 base pairs larger than that predicted from the size of HGH mRNA. Since sites of interaction with hormone receptors could be located in any part of the gene and since their structure cannot be anticipated, knowledge of the nucleotide sequence of the entire gene has to be complemented by a functional analysis of the various parts of the gene. Such an analysis can be approached

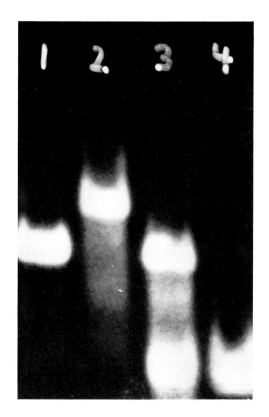

FIG. 9. Autoradiograph of a Southern blot (30) of bacteriophage λ4A DNA containing pieces of human genomic DNA with HGH and/or HCS gene sequences. The DNA was cleaved with restriction endonucleases *EcoRI* and *Xbal* prior to agarose gel electrophoresis. The blotted gel was probed with ^{32}P-dCMP-labeled HGH cDNA. Lanes contain DNA from independent phage isolates. Bands correspond to 2.6-kb HGH core gene **(Lane 1)**, nonallelic HGH and/or HCS gene sequences **(Lane 2)**, HGH core gene and *Xbal*-cleaved HCS core gene **(Lane 3)**, and *Xbal*-cleaved HCS core gene **(Lane 4)**. The presence of both HGH and HCS core genes in cloned human DNA (see **Lane 3**) indicates proximity of these genes in at least one location of the genome.

by employing newly-developed techniques of gene transfer into cells of higher animals, using either the isolated gene itself (33) or the gene linked to viral vectors (9) for cellular transformations. Proof that a cloned genome DNA fragment contains the whole GH gene will be demonstrated if (a) it directs the production of GH in the recipient cell and, (b) this production can simulate *in vivo* hormonal control. As to hormone receptors, the high copy number of SV40 DNA in the nuclei of permissive cells and the small size of the molecule makes SV40 an attractive vector to probe for proteins that specifically bind to various portions of the GH gene inserted into the viral DNA.

It is hoped that the structural and functional characterization of the isolated genes for HGH and HCS will shed light on the mechanisms governing the tissue-specific expression of highly homologous DNA sequences. Since both genes have been found to be in close proximity in at least one site of the genome, the simplest model for determining tissue specificity would assume the presence of another such genomic locus: one being expressed in the pituitary, the other in the placenta. In this model, the isolated DNA piece would have placental expression, since the HGH core gene is of a variant type. Experiments are under way to explore this and other possible models.

ACKNOWLEDGMENTS

The author thanks his colleagues J. Shine, J. C. Fiddes, J. A. Martial, J. D. Baxter, and A. Ullrich for many fruitful collaborations. This work was supported in part by Grant 19997 from the National Institutes of Health.

REFERENCES

1. Bauer, R. F., Arthur, L. O., and Fine, D. L. (1976): Propagation of mouse mammary tumor cell lines and production of mouse mammary tumor virus in a serum-free medium. *In Vitro,* 12:558–563.
2. Baxter, J. D., Eberhardt, N. L., Apriletti, J. W., Johnson, L. K., Ivarie, R. D., Schachter, B. S., Morris, J. A., Seeburg, P. H., Goodman, H. M., Latham, K. R., Polansky, J. R., and Martial, J. A. (1979): Thyroid hormone receptors and responses. *Recent Prog. Horm. Res.,* 35:97–147.
3. Baxter, J. D., and Ivarie, R. D. (1978): Regulation of gene expression by glucocorticoid hormones: Studies of receptors and responses in cultured cells. In: *Receptors and Hormone Action, Vol. 2,* edited by B. W. O'Malley and L. Birnbaumer, pp. 251–296. Academic Press, New York.
4. Blobel, G., and Dobberstein, B. (1975): Transfer of proteins across membranes: I. Presence of proteolytically processed and unprocessed nascent immunoglobulin light chains on membrane-bound ribosomes of murine myeloma. *J. Cell Biol.,* 67:835–851.
5. Crick, F. (1979): Split genes and RNA splicing. *Science,* 204:264–271.
6. Dannies, P. S., and Tashjian, A. J., Jr. (1973): Growth hormone and prolactin from rat pituitary tumor cells. In: *Tissue Culture: Methods and Applications,* edited by P. F. Kruse, Jr., and M. K. Patterson, Jr., pp. 561–569. Academic Press, New York.
7. Fiddes, J. C., Seeburg, P. H., DeNoto, F. M., Hallewell, R. A., Baxter, J. D., and Goodman, H. M. (1979): Structure of genes for human growth hormone and chorionic somatomammotropin. *Proc. Natl. Acad. Sci. USA,* 76:4294–4298.
8. Goodman, H. M., Seeburg, P. H., Martial, J. A., Shine, J., Ullrich, A., and Baxter, J. D. (1979): Structure and expression in bacteria of growth hormone genes. In: *Alfred Benson Symposium, 13.* Munksgaard, Copenhagen.
9. Hamer, D. H., and Leder, P. (1979): Expression of the chromosomal mouse β^{maj}-globin gene cloned in SV40. *Nature,* 281:35–40.
10. Ivarie, R. D., Baxter, J. D., and Morris, J. A. (1979): Hormonal domains of response in rat pituitary tumor cells: Dependent and independent action of thyroid hormone, glucocorticoids, and insulin in changing specific gene expression in GH_3 cells in culture *(submitted for publication).*
11. Ivarie, R. D., and O'Farrell, P. H. (1976): The glucocorticoid domain: Steroid-mediated changes in the rate of synthesis of rat hepatoma proteins. *Cell,* 13:41–55.
12. Kohler, P. O., Frohman, L. A., Briolson, W. E., Vanha-Perttula, T., and Hammond, J. M. (1969): Cortisol induction of growth hormone synthesis in a cloned line of rat pituitary cells in culture. *Science,* 166:633–634.
13. Lawn, R. M., Fritsch, E. F., Parker, R. C., Blake, G., and Maniatis, T. (1978): The isolation and characterization of linked δ- and β-globin genes from cloned library of human DNA. *Cell,* 15:1157–1174.
14. Li, C. H. (1972): Hormones of the adenohypophysis. *Proc. Am. Philos. Soc.,* 116:365–382.
15. Li, C. H., Dixon, J. S., and Chung, D. (1973): Amino acid sequence of human chorionic somatomammotropin. *Arch. Biochem. Biophys.,* 155:95–110.
16. Martial, J. A., Baxter, J. D., Goodman, H. M., and Seeburg, P. H. (1977): Regulation of growth hormone messenger RNA by thyroid and glucocorticoid hormones. *Proc. Natl. Acad. Sci. USA,* 74:1816–1820.
17. Martial, J. A., Seeburg, P. H., Guenzi, D., Goodman, H. M., and Baxter, J. D. (1977): Regulation of growth hormone gene expression: Synergistic effects of thyroid and glucocorticoid hormones. *Proc. Natl. Acad. Sci. USA,* 74:4293–4295.
18. Maxam, A., and Gilbert, W. (1977): A new method for sequencing DNA. *Proc. Natl. Acad. Sci. USA,* 74:560–564.
19. Niall, H. D., Hogan, M. L., Sauer, R., Rosenblum, I. Y., and Greenwood, F. C. (1971): Sequences

of pituitary and placental lactogenic and growth hormones: Evolution from a primordial peptide by gene reduplication. *Proc. Natl. Acad. Sci. USA,* 68:866–869.

20. O'Farrell, P. H. (1975): High resolution two-dimensional electrophoresis of proteins. *J. Biol. Chem.,* 250:4007–4021.

21. Proudfoot, N. J., and Brownlee, G. G. (1976): 3' Non-coding region sequences in eucaryotic messenger RNA. *Nature,* 263:211–214.

22. Sanger, F., Nicklen, S., and Coulson, A. R. (1977): DNA sequencing with chain-terminating inhibitors. *Proc. Natl. Acad. Sci. USA,* 74:5463–5467.

23. Seeburg, P. H., Shine, J., Martial, J. A., Baxter, J. D., and Goodman, H. M. (1977): Nucleotide sequence and amplification in bacteria of the structural gene for rat growth hormone. *Nature,* 270:486–494.

24. Seeburg, P. H. (1980): A sequence comparison of several mRNAs coding for mammalian growth hormone *(manuscript in preparation).*

25. Seeburg, P. H. (1980): *Manuscript in preparation.*

26. Shine, J., and Dalgarno, L. (1974): Identical 3'-terminal octanucleotide sequence in 18S ribosomal ribonucleic acid from different eukaryotes: A proposed rule for this sequence in the recognition of terminator codons. *Biochem. J.,* 141:609–615.

27. Shine, J., Seeburg, P. H., Martial, J. A., Baxter, J. D., and Goodman, H. M. (1977): Construction and analysis of recombinant DNA for human chorionic somato-mammotropin. *Nature,* 270:494–499.

28. Shome, B., and Parlow, A. F. (1977): Human pituitary prolactin (hPRL): The entire linear amino acid sequence. *J. Clin. Endocrinol. Metab.,* 45:1112–1115.

29. Smith, A. J. H. (1979): The use of exonuclease III for preparing single-stranded DNA for use as a template in the chain terminator sequencing method. *Nucleic Acids Res.,* 6:831–848.

30. Southern, E. M. (1975): Detection of specific sequences among DNA fragments separated by gel electrophoresis. *J. Mol. Biol.,* 98:503–517.

31. Tashjian, A. H., Jr., Bancroft, F. C., and Levine, L. (1970): Production of both prolactin and growth hormone by clonal strains of rat pituitary cells: Differential effects of hydrocortisone and tissue extracts. *J. Cell Biol.,* 47:61–70.

32. Tsai, J. S., and Samules, H. H. (1974): Thyroid hormone action: Stimulation of growth hormone and inhibition of prolactin secretion in cultured GH_1 cells. *Biochem. Biophys. Res. Commun.,* 59:420–428.

33. Wigler, M., Silverstein, S., Lee, L-S., Pellicer, A., Cheng, Y-C., and Axel, R. (1977): Transfer of purified herpes virus thymidine kinase gene to cultured mouse cells. *Cell,* 11:223–232.

34. Yamamoto, K. R., and Alberts, B. M. (1976): Steroid receptors: Elements for modulation of eukaryotic transcription. *Annu. Rev. Biochem.,* 45:721–746.

35. Yasumura, Y., Tashjian, A. H., Jr., and Sato, G. H. (1966): Establishment of four functional, clonal strains of animal cells in culture. *Science,* 154:1186–1189.

Polypeptide Hormones, edited by
R. F. Beers, Jr. and E. G. Bassett.
Raven Press, New York © 1980.

6. Human Interferon: The Messenger RNA and the Proteins

Sidney Pestka, Marian Evinger, Russell McCandliss, Alan Sloma, and Menachem Rubinstein

Roche Institute of Molecular Biology, Nutley, New Jersey 07110

STUDIES WITH INTERFERON mRNA

Our studies on interferon first centered on isolation and translation of mRNA (Fig. 1). Interferon mRNA from human cells was translated in cell-free extracts (19–21) as well as in frog oocytes (3–5). Biologically active interferon was synthesized in both the extracts and oocytes. Cell-free extracts that synthesized interferon included the ascites extracts (19–21) as well as wheat germ and reticulocyte lysates. That the activity was indeed human interferon was demonstrated by its species and antigenic specificity as well as additional characteristics of the interferons (3–5,19–21). These studies with interferon mRNA provided a number of useful insights. Since our cell-free extracts were not capable of synthesizing carbohydrates *de novo* (29), we speculated that the carbohydrate moiety was not essential for activity of the interferons (12).

Because the cell-free extracts required several micrograms of mRNA for each assay, it was difficult to accumulate for purification sufficient mRNA from induced cells. The cell-free assays consumed most of the mRNA so that after purification little remained for other studies. Thus, we turned to the use of frog oocytes (3) to conserve mRNA from induced cells. Gurdon and colleagues (9,18) demonstrated the synthesis of proteins programmed by mRNA injected into *Xenopus laevis* oocytes. Injected globin mRNA served as a template for both α and β chains. They estimated that the oocyte required about 1/1,000 of the amount of mRNA required for cell-free translation for comparable synthesis. A number of studies subsequently showed that oocytes were capable of performing secondary modifications such as cleavage of polypeptides (14,15,17), acetylation (2), glycosylation (13), and assembly (28). With the use of oocytes, we and others (3,22,26) showed that *Xenopus* oocytes could synthesize biologically active interferon.

Using *Xenopus* oocytes, we were able to show we could assay 1 ng of unfractionated mRNA from induced fibroblasts (3). The synthesis of interferon as a function of mRNA concentration, time, and temperature in *Xenopus* oocytes was determined (Fig. 2).

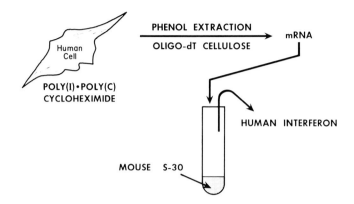

FIG. 1. Cell-free interferon synthesis. Schematic illustration of the procedures involved in the experiments. Human FS-4 fibroblast monolayers were induced to synthesize interferon by poly(I)·poly(C) in the presence of cycloheximide (20,21). RNA was extracted from the induced cells and the poly(A)-containing mRNA was isolated from the total cellular RNA by fractionation on oligo(dT)-cellulose. Translation of the mRNA was performed in an Ehrlich ascites cell-free extract. The products of translation were assayed directly for interferon activity.

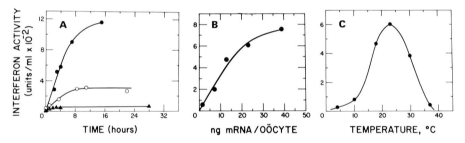

FIG. 2. A: Interferon synthesis as a function of time. Three different concentrations of injected fibroblast mRNA were used: 1.3 (▲), 7 (○), and 39 (●) ng per oocyte. Each point represents the combined yields of 10 oocytes. Incubations were performed at 23°C for the times indicated on the *abscissa*. **B:** Interferon synthesis as a function of the quantity of fibroblast mRNA injected. Each point represents yields from 10 oocytes. Incubations were performed at 23°C for 6 hr. **C:** Interferon synthesis as a function of temperature. Each point represents yields from 10 oocytes, each of which was injected with 27 ng of fibroblast mRNA. Incubations were performed at the indicated temperatures for 6 hr. (Data from ref. 3.)

SEPARATE GENES FOR HUMAN LEUKOCYTE AND FIBROBLAST INTERFERONS

Human leukocyte and fibroblast interferons have a number of distinct properties. For example, antisera produced by immunization with fibroblast interferon failed to neutralize leukocyte interferon (1,11). Leukocyte interferon exerts a high degree of activity on bovine or porcine cells, whereas fibroblast interferon is hardly active on these cells (8). In addition, leukocyte and fibroblast interferons exhibit differences in size, in their stability toward various inactivating treatments, and in their binding to lectin columns.

Differences between human leukocyte and fibroblast interferons could originate in at least two ways. There may be two separate structural genes for interferon, each coding for a protein with a unique primary sequence. Alternatively, if there were a single structural gene for interferon, differences might result from distinctive posttranslational modifications (or possibly even posttranscriptional modifications, *see below*), carried out by lymphoid or nonlymphoid cells (e.g., glycosylation, proteolytic cleavages, etc.). In this case, the same polypeptide sequence would be synthesized, but processed differently into the final active product in the different types of cells. To distinguish between these alternatives, we isolated mRNA from human lymphoblast and fibroblast cultures induced to produce their characteristic interferon and injected the mRNA into *Xenopus laevis* oocytes (3). Because the secondary modifications produced by the oocytes would be expected to be the same for a single translational product, any differences observed in the interferon produced by the oocytes should represent differences in their mRNA sequences.

Interferon synthesized when fibroblast mRNA was injected into oocytes was neutralized by antiserum to fibroblast interferon, but not by antiserum to leukocyte interferon (Fig. 3). Interferons synthesized when lymphoblastoid mRNA was injected were either not neutralized or were only partially neutralized by either antiserum alone (Fig. 3). A mixture of both antisera was required for complete neutralization. Interferons produced in intact fibroblasts or Namalva lymphoblastoid cell cultures showed the same neutralization patterns as the corresponding oocyte products. Thus, the oocyte products resemble the products of the cells from which the mRNA was derived. The fact that complete neutralization of lymphoblastoid cellular interferon required a mixture of anti-leukocyte and anti-fibroblast interferon sera suggested that lymphoblastoid interferon as well as the oocyte product synthesized after injection with mRNA from lymphoblastoid cells contained a mixture of leukocyte and fibroblast interferons (3).

The cellular specificity of interferons produced by oocytes injected with the

SOURCE OF INTERFERON or mRNA	NEUTRALIZATION WITH ANTISERA		
	ANTI-LEUKOCYTE	ANTI-FIBROBLAST	BOTH ANTISERA
FIBROBLASTS			
CELLS	○	●	
OOCYTES	○	●	
LYMPHOBLASTS			
CELLS	◖	◖	●
OOCYTES	◖	◖	●
LEUKOCYTES	●	○	

FIG. 3. Antigenic specificity of human interferons synthesized in cultured cells or in oocytes. Negative result (○) indicates lack of neutralization with antiserum diluted 1:32 (final dilution); positive result (●) indicates that the interferon activity was neutralized by the respective antiserum at a final dilution of 1:32 (or higher dilution). When a mixture of two antisera was used, the final dilution of each serum was 1:32. The symbol (◖) indicates a variable result ranging from complete lack of neutralization to only partial neutralization by antiserum. Neutralization assays were performed as described (12). (Data from ref 3.)

TABLE 1. Comparison of antiviral activities of various human interferons in cultures of human (FS-7 and GM-258) and bovine (MDBK) cells[a]

Source of interferon	Interferon titer in cultures			Ratio of interferon titers		
	FS-7	GM-258	MDBK	FS-7/MDBK	GM-258/FS-7	GM-258/MDBK
FS-4 cultures	12,288	65,536	32	384	5	2,048
	1,024,000	4,096,000	2,048	500	4	2,000
Primary leukocyte cultures	196,000	2,048,000	98,000	2	10	21
Lymphoblastoid (Namalva) cell cultures	1,536	16,384	768	2	11	21
Oocytes injected with FS-4 mRNA	1,024	4,096	<16	>64	4	>256
Oocytes injected with Namalva mRNA	32	256	16	2	8	16
mRNA	512	3,072	128	4	6	24

[a]Where two values are presented, they denote independent preparations. The higher values for Namalva mRNA represent poly(A)-containing mRNA fractionated on a sucrose gradient. The high titer FS-4 interferon was concentrated and partially purified by ultrafiltration. The interferon titers are actual titers (not corrected to a reference standard). The values for Namalva interferon represent a preparation supplied by Mr. Charles Buckler.
Data from ref. 3.

various messages (Table 1) resembled the cellular specificity of the interferon preparations produced by those same cells (3).

Thus, we concluded that lymphoblastoid interferon is a mixture of two types of interferon: leukocyte and fibroblast interferon and that the preparations of lymphoblastoid mRNA injected into oocytes contained mRNA for both types of interferon since the oocytes synthesized both interferons. These results indicate that human interferons produced in oocytes with mRNA preparations extracted from fibroblast or lymphoblastoid cells showed the same characteristic molecular weights, antigenic properties, and cellular specificities as the products of the intact cells from which the mRNA was derived. These findings support the conclusions that the mRNAs are different, and, therefore, the amino acid sequences of the interferons synthesized on these mRNA templates must be different. Accordingly, this work provides evidence for the existence of two human interferon genes, *ifnLe* and *ifnF*. Both of these genes are expressed in induced lymphoblastoid cells, but only one of these genes appears to function in the fibroblast. It also is conceivable that the genes may be overlapping and that the individual mRNAs for leukocyte and fibroblast interferons are the result of distinct splicing mechanisms characteristic of the cells from which the mRNAs are derived.

INDUCTION AND DEGRADATION OF INTERFERON mRNA

Our assay for interferon mRNA was used to distinguish between various hypotheses relating to interferon induction and biosynthesis (4). The data demonstrated that on induction with poly(I)·poly(C) human fibroblasts accumulate interferon mRNA for 1 to 1.5 hr, after which time the mRNA is rapidly degraded with a half-life of 18 min (Fig. 4, Table 2). Treatment of cells with cycloheximide prolongs the period of accumulation to 3 hr and decreases the rate of mRNA inactivation to a half-life of 49 min. Treatment with actinomycin D decreases the rate of inactivation still further with a half-life of 68 min. A comparison of cellular interferon synthesis with the relative amounts of interferon mRNA after simple induction or induction in the presence of the inhibitors (superinduction) indicates a general correlation.

The data are consistent with the following events of interferon induction. Poly(I)·poly(C) induces transcription of interferon mRNA for a period of about 1.4 to 1.5 hr. Degradation of mRNA follows exponential kinetics and proceeds at the rates designated by the half-lives (Table 2) under the various conditions. Thus, starting from about 1.5 hr, interferon mRNA is inactivated and interferon synthesis is rapidly shut off. Cycloheximide treatment prolongs the period of transcription to 3 hr and decreases the rate of mRNA degradation. Actinomycin D decreases the rate of inactivation of mRNA still further. The action of actinomycin D cannot be ascribed to increased transcription, since the concentration of actinomycin D used inhibits total RNA synthesis greater than 95%. Reduced inactivation of mRNA may be a consequence of reduced synthesis of mRNA

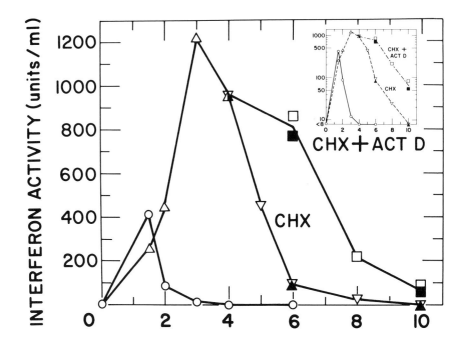

FIG. 4. Translatable interferon mRNA in cells induced with poly(I)·poly(C), poly(I)·poly(C) + cycloheximide (CHX), poly(I)·poly(C) + CHX + actinomycin D (ACT D) as a function of time. Cultures were induced at time zero with poly(I)·poly(C) (5 μg/ml) (○) or with poly(I)·poly(C) in the presence of CHX (50 μg/ml) (△, ▽, ▲, □, ■). In addition, some of these cultures were also treated with ACT-D (1 μg/ml) from 4–5 hr (□, ■). The inducing medium with CHX (and ACT D, if applicable) was removed at 5 hr; the cells were thoroughly washed and further incubated in the absence of inducer or in inhibitor-free medium. At the times indicated, the medium was removed, the cell monolayers were washed, and the cells were harvested. Poly(A)-containing mRNA was prepared from each cell pellet and injected into oocytes. Experimental values represent interferon yields obtained with 25 ng of mRNA injected per oocyte. Each point represents the mean of four interferon titrations. The zero time point represents results from numerous experiments showing that no interferon-specific mRNA was detectable in uninduced fibroblasts. The zero points on the graph represent interferon titers of <8, the lowest value that was measured. **Inset:** A logarithmic plot of the same data. (From ref. 4.)

or protein. Steinberg et al. (27) have shown that the apparent superinduction of tyrosine aminotransferase is due to decreased degradation of both tyrosine aminotransferase and its mRNA, analogous to our findings with interferon. Accordingly, decreased degradation of interferon in the presence of actinomycin D could explain the large increase in its production beyond that expected from the increase in mRNA half-life alone. In addition, the observation that the quantity of translatable interferon mRNA at 6 hr after induction with poly(I)·poly(C) was much higher in cells superinduced with 5,6-dichloro-1-β-

TABLE 2. *Comparison of interferon mRNA half-lives and total amounts of interferon and interferon mRNA*

Induction conditions for fibroblasts used as source of mRNA	mRNA half-life (min)	Relative integrated amount of interferon mRNA	Total interferon production by cells (ref. units/ml)
Poly(I)·poly(C)	18	100	1,500
Poly(I)·poly(C) + CHX	49	695	5,000
Poly(I)·poly(C) + CHX + Act-D	68	1093	30,000

The half-lives ($t_{1/2}$) for interferon-specific mRNA were calculated from the data of Fig. 4. The relative total amount of interferon-specific mRNA was determined by integrating the appropriate curves of Fig. 4. CHX, cycloheximide; Act-D, actinomycin D.

Data from ref. 3.

D-ribofuranosylbenzimidazole, an inhibitor of RNA synthesis, than in control cells (26) agrees with our data. Similar results were reported by Greene et al. (7).

In summary, on induction, the genes for interferon are activated to produce a transcript for a short time. The superinducing treatments prolong the period of accumulation and decrease the rate of degradation of this transcript.

The ability to isolate and translate interferon mRNAs makes it possible to purify them and to prepare recombinants containing the interferon sequences. Such experiments are in progress in our laboratory as well as in others.

PURIFICATION OF HUMAN LEUKOCYTE INTERFERON

Recently, interferon research has generated great interest because of promising clinical studies indicating antiviral and antitumor activities. Because no pure preparations of interferon were available for these studies, it is not yet clear that both these activities reside in the same molecular species. Complete physical and chemical characterization of the molecules depends on obtaining homogeneous interferon in sufficient amounts for characterization. To purify interferon, high resolution chromatography of proteins was developed and coupled with a high sensitivity monitoring system based on fluorescamine (see S. Stein, *this volume*). This combination of high resolution and sensitivity enabled for the first time the isolation and chemical characterization of pure human leukocyte interferon. Details of the purification and initial characterization, including amino acid analysis, of the homogeneous species have been described (23,25). As can be seen in Fig. 5, a single protein band of molecular weight 17,500 was obtained on staining with Coomassie blue on sodium dodecyl sulfate-polyacrylamide slab gel electrophoresis. After staining, the gel was cut into 1-mm slices and each fraction was assayed for interferon activity. A single peak of activity coincided with the protein band.

This purification was achieved by the procedures described in detail elsewhere (25). A summary of the procedures are outlined in Table 3 and Fig. 6. We

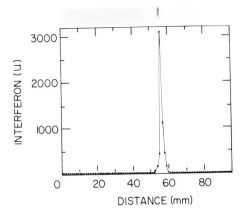

FIG. 5. Sodium dodecyl sulfate-polyacryl-amide slab gel electrophoresis of human leukocyte interferon. After electrophoresis and staining with Coomassie blue, one strip of the polyacrylamide gel was cut into 1-mm slices, the interferon eluted, and assayed for interferon activity. Interferon titers on the ordinate are expressed in terms of reference units of interferon per milliliter. (From ref. 23.)

chose to induce interferon biosynthesis in serum-free medium containing casein. The omission of serum simplified the purification and the insolubility of casein at low pH values enabled us to obtain high initial specific activity. Crude interferon contains proteins secreted by the leukocytes, some proteins from disrupted cells, and fragments of casein. Like many other purification schemes, the first stages were selective precipitation to remove the bulk of the protein and to reduce the volume (Table 3). Neither ammonium sulfate nor organic solvent fractionation provided any purification because interferon tends to coprecipitate with other proteins. We have studied this phenomenon and found that detergents can prevent it. Thus, we concluded that coprecipitation is the result of hydrophobic interactions. Fractionation under acidic conditions in the presence of Triton X-100 gave the best results.

Gel filtration at various pH values produced a broad distribution of activity and resulted in poor recovery. Only under denaturing conditions (4 M urea) did gel filtration provide an excellent yield and a relatively narrow distribution of activity. Ion exchange chromatography, hydrophobic chromatography on octyl sepharose, and chromatography on poly(U)-sepharose were found to be unsatisfactory.

The application of Lichrosorb RP-8 (octyl groups bound to silica microparticles) columns to protein fractionation was a major factor in the success of the purification procedure (Fig. 6A, C, and D; Table 3). In addition, Lichrosorb Diol, which is chemically similar to glycophase resins that have been used for exclusion chromatography of proteins, was introduced as a support for normal partition chromatography of proteins (Fig. 6B, Table 3). High recoveries of interferon activity were obtained from each chromatographic step.

Both bioassay data and the protein band corresponded to a molecular weight of 17,500. When a sample of interferon was treated with periodic acid, then subjected to electrophoresis, it was converted to a broad doublet but no appreciable reduction in molecular weight was observed (25). If this species of interferon is a glycoprotein, then the degree of glycosylation is not great or the glycosydic residues have only a small effect on mobility.

TABLE 3. *Purification of human leukocyte interferon*[a]

Step	Units recovered $\times 10^{-6}$	Protein recovered (mg)	Relative specific activity (units/mg)	Degree of purification	Recovery range per step (%)
1. Incubation medium	50	10,000	5×10^3	1	—
2. pH 4 Supernatant	50	2,000	2.5×10^4	5	100
3. 1.5% Trichloroacetic acid precipitate	40	1,000	4×10^4	8	80–100
4. Triton X-100/acetic acid supernatant	40	250	1.6×10^5	32	70–100
5. 4% Trichloroacetic acid precipitate	35	175	2×10^5	40	80–90
6. Sephadex G-100	32	57	5.6×10^5	112	70–90
7. Lichrosorb RP-8 (pH 7.5)	28	11	2.5×10^6	500	80–100
8. Lichrosorb Diol					
Peak α	11	1.1	1×10^7	5,000	
Peak β	2.5	N.D.[b]	N.D.	N.D.	70–90
Peak γ	12.5	0.21	6×10^7	12,000	
9. Lichrosorb RP-8 (pH 4)	1.6	0.0064	3×10^8	60,000	40–60
10. Lichrosorb RP-8 (pH 4)	8.2	0.021	4×10^8	80,000	40–60

[a] For determination of protein recovered in each fraction, bovine serum albumin was used as a standard. The absolute specific activity determined by amino acid analysis of the homogeneous peak of step 10 was found to be 2×10^8 units/mg calibrated against the reference standard for human leukocyte interferon (G-023–901–527). Step 9 was performed on the γ peak of step 8. Step 10 was performed on pooled material from several preparations.

[b] Not determined.

Data from ref. 25.

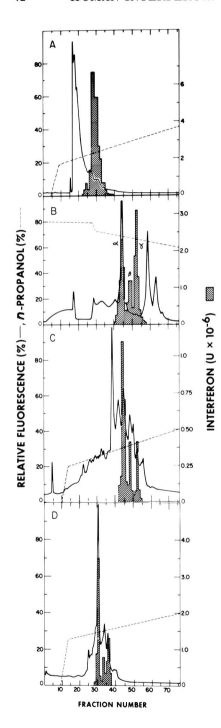

FIG. 6. High performance liquid chromatography of interferon. **A:** Chromatography on Lichrosorb RP-8 at pH 7.5. **B:** Chromatography on Lichrosorb Diol at pH 7.5. **C:** Chromatography on Lichrosorb RP-8 at pH 4. **D:** Rechromatography on Lichrosorb RP-8 at pH 4. (From ref. 25.)

On the basis of amino acid analysis of native and carboxymethylated interferon, we conclude interferon contains one disulfide bridge and one or two free sulfhydryl groups. From these data, a minimum molecular weight of 18,000 was calculated. This value is in good agreement with that obtained on gel electrophoresis.

It should be noted that only one species of interferon was purified to homogeneity and characterized. However, other species of interferon were observed and these require purification and characterization. The precise relationship of these species to one another, to the secreted material, and to the primary gene product is of major interest.

COMPARISON OF LEUKOCYTE INTERFERON FROM NORMAL AND LEUKEMIC CELLS

So far, most of the interferon used for clinical studies was produced by induction of leukocytes obtained from blood donors. Other sources of human interferon include lymphoblastoid cell cultures and fibroblast cells. Leukemic patients with high leukocyte counts could serve as a rich source of white blood cells. Leukocytes can be selectively removed from such patients by leukapheresis. By this method, an amount of leukocytes equivalent to that obtained from 100 to 300 units of blood can be obtained from a single patient with a count of 10^5 leukocytes/μl or greater.

Initially, leukocytes from various sources were tested for their ability to produce interferon on induction with viruses. We found that leukocytes obtained from patients with chronic myelogenous leukemia (CML) produced higher levels of interferon than leukocytes from patients with chronic lymphocytic leukemia or the acute leukemias as previously reported by Lee et al. (16) and Hadházy et al. (10).

Interferon produced by leukocytes from CML patients was compared with that produced by leukocytes from normal donors (24). The elution patterns from the various high performance liquid chromatographic (HPLC) columns were highly reproducible and therefore could serve as an analytical tool for comparing interferon preparations. The first HPLC step, performed on Lichrosorb RP-8 at pH 7.5, yielded almost identical patterns of proteins and activity (Fig. 7A). The second HPLC step, performed on fractions from a Lichrosorb RP-8 column applied to Lichrosorb Diol, yielded three major peaks of activity labeled α, β, and γ (Fig. 7B). As can be seen, the protein patterns were almost identical. The activity patterns are very similar except that the level of peak α was lower in preparations from leukemic cells than from normal leukocytes. Peak γ of the Diol columns was further chromatographed on Lichrosorb RP-8 at pH 4.0 (Fig. 7C). Several peaks of antiviral activity were detected. Fraction 44 from each chromatography contained homogeneous interferon and was used for amino acid analysis (Table 4). Amino acid analysis was performed with a fluorescamine analyzer on 2 μg of pure interferon. Interferons from normal

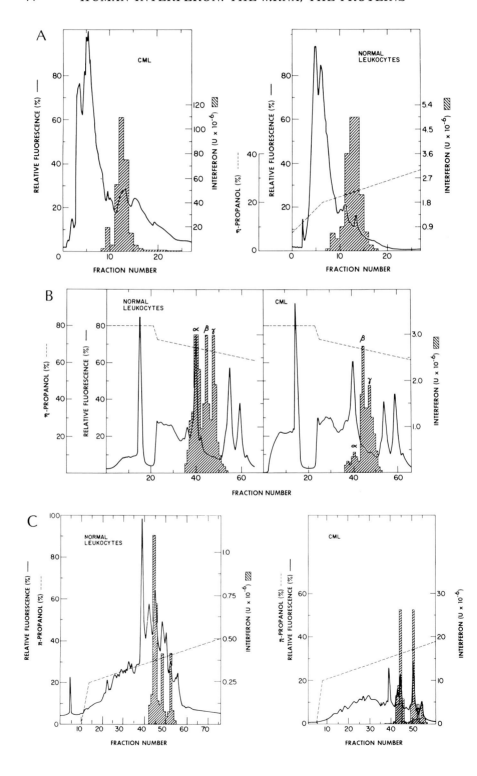

TABLE 4. *Amino acid composition of human leukocyte interferons*

	Interferon source	
Amino acid	Normal leukocytes	CML leukocytes
Asx	15	13
Ser	8	9
Thr	8	8
Glx	24	24
Pro	6	5
Gly	5	5
Ala	8	8
Val	8	8
Met	4	4
Ile	9	8
Leu	22	21
Tyr	5	5
Phe	9	9
His	3	3
Lys	12	11
Arg	7	8
Cys	3	3

From ref. 24.

and leukemic cells did not show any significant differences in amino acid composition (24).

Thus, a new practical source of human leukocyte interferon was established. It was found that interferon obtained from leukemic leukocytes exhibits the same elution characteristics on various HPLC columns and the same amino acid composition as that from normal leukocytes. We, therefore, conclude that these two interferons are essentially identical.

COMPARISON OF ANTIVIRAL AND ANTIGROWTH ACTIVITY

Interferons have been reported to have a large number of effects such as antiviral and antitumor effects, growth inhibition, and immunosuppression. Because most of these assays were performed with relatively crude preparations, less than 1% of which was human interferon, the results could have been due to components other than interferon. The availability of pure interferon now makes it possible to resolve these uncertainties.

FIG. 7. A: Chromatography of human leukocyte interferon from normal and leukemic leukocytes on Lichrosorb RP-8 at pH 7.5. CML refers to chronic myelogenous leukemia. A gradient of *n*-propanol in 1 M sodium acetate was used. (From ref. 24.) **B:** Chromatography of human leukocyte interferon on Lichrosorb Diol. A gradient of decreasing *n*-propanol concentration in 0.1 M sodium acetate was used. **C:** Chromatography of human leukocyte interferon (peak γ) on Lichrosorb (RP-8) at pH 4. A gradient of *n*-propanol in pyridine (1 M)-formic acid (2 M) was used.

TABLE 5. *Growth inhibitory activity of human leukocyte interferon[a]*

Addition to culture medium	Growth (% of control)
Unfractionated interferon	15
Homogeneous leukocyte interferon	12
No additions	100

[a] Unfractionated human leukocyte interferon was added to lymphoblastoid (Daudi) cell cultures to a final concentration of 25 and 50 units/ml. Homogeneous human leukocyte interferon was added to cultures to a final concentration of 36 units/ml. Growth of cells are expressed as a percentage of the growth of control cells after 3 days. Details of the procedures are described elsewhere (6).

To determine whether the homogeneous interferon exhibited antigrowth activity as well as antiviral activity, the effect of the homogeneous material on lymphoblastoid (Daudi) cells was examined (6). It was shown that the homogeneous human leukocyte interferon exhibited antigrowth activity as well as antiviral activity (Table 5). Thus, we conclude that the antigrowth activity is an intrinsic property of the interferon molecule.

EXPECTATIONS

The foundations for study of interferon, its mRNA, and genes have been built over the past two decades through work of many laboratories. The techniques for obtaining pure interferons are available. Despite these achievements, substantial quantities of the homogeneous interferon proteins are not readily available. The use of sensitive detection techniques for amino acids and peptides has allowed us to purify interferon and determine its amino acid composition. Advances in microsequencing methodology will be useful to obtain the total sequence of the proteins. When the recombinant DNA plasmids (or viruses) for the various interferons are available, their DNA sequences will aid determination of the protein structures. Nevertheless, it will still be necessary to determine the amino acid sequences of the proteins. Isolation of the specific interferon genes and cDNAs will permit clear definition of the genes and the chromosomal assignments corresponding to the various interferons. There will probably be a few surprises awaiting us on elucidation of the structures of these genes and their chromosomal assignments. With these foundations, it is not overoptimistic to say that we shall see the human interferons synthesized in *Escherichia coli* in the not-too-distant future.

ACKNOWLEDGMENTS

The early studies of interferon mRNA were performed in collaboration with Jan Vilček, James McInnes, Edward Havell, and Ralph Cavalieri (3,4,20,21).

Our studies on leukocyte interferon were performed with the assistance of Philip Familletti, Sara Rubinstein, and Mitchell Gross.

REFERENCES

1. Berg, K., Ogburn, C. A., Paucker, K., Mogensen, K. E., and Cantell, K. (1975): Affinity chromatography of human leukocyte and diploid cell interferons on Sepharose-bound antibodies. *J. Immunol.,* 114:640–644.
2. Berns, A. J. M., Van Kraaikamp, M., Bloemendal, H., and Lane, C. D. (1972): Calf crystallin synthesis in frog oocytes: The translation of lens-cell 14S RNA in oocytes. *Proc. Natl. Acad. Sci. USA,* 69:1606–1609.
3. Cavalieri, R. L., Havell, E. A., Vilček, J., and Pestka, S. (1977): Synthesis of human interferon by *Xenopus laevis* oocytes: Two structural genes for interferons in human cells. *Proc. Natl. Acad. Sci. USA,* 74:3287–3291.
4. Cavalieri, R. L., Havell, E. A., Vilček, J., and Pestka, S. (1977): Induction and decay of human fibroblast interferon messenger RNA. *Proc. Natl. Acad. Sci. USA,* 74:4415–4419.
5. Cavalieri, R. L., and Pestka, S. (1977): Synthesis of interferon in heterologous cells, cell-free extracts, and *Xenopus laevis* oocytes. *Tex. Rep. Biol. Med.,* 35:117–125.
6. Evinger, M., Rubinstein, M., and Pestka, S. (1980): Growth inhibition and antiviral activity of purified human leukocyte interferon. *Ann. N.Y. Acad. Sci. (in press).*
7. Greene, J. J., Dieffenbach, C. W., and Ts'o, P. O. P. (1978): Inactivation of interferon mRNA in the shutoff of human interferon synthesis. *Nature,* 271:81–83.
8. Gresser, I., Bandu, M. T., Brouty-Boye, D., and Tovey, M. (1974): Pronounced antiviral activity of human interferon on bovine or porcine cells. *Nature,* 251:543–545.
9. Gurdon, J. B., Lane, C. D., Woodland, H. R., and Marbaix, G. (1971): Use of frog eggs and oocytes for the study of messenger RNA and its translation in living cells. *Nature,* 233:177–182.
10. Hadházy, Gy., Gergely, L., Tóth, F. E., and Szegedi, Gy. (1967): Comparative study on interferon production by leukocytes of healthy and leukemic subjects. *Acta Microbiol. Acad. Sci. Hung.,* 14:391–397.
11. Havell, E. A., Berman, B., Ogburn, C. A., Berg, K., Paucker, K., and Vilček, J. (1975): Two antigenically distinct species of human interferon. *Proc. Natl. Acad. Sci. USA,* 72:2185–2187.
12. Havell, E. A., Vilček, J., Falcoff, E., and Berman, B. (1975): Suppression of human interferon production by inhibitors of glycosylation. *Virology,* 63:475–483.
13. Jilka, R. L., Cavalieri, R. L., Yaffe, L., and Pestka, S. (1977): Synthesis and glycosylation of the MOPC-46B immunoglobulin kappa chain in *Xenopus laevis* oocytes. *Biochem. Biophys. Res. Commun.,* 79:625–630.
14. Jilka, R. L., Familletti, P., and Pestka, S. (1979): Synthesis and processing of the mouse MOPC-321 κ chain in *Xenopus laevis* oocytes. *Arch. Biochem. Biophys.,* 192:290–295.
15. Laskey, R. A., Gurdon, J. B., and Crawford, L. V. (1972): Translation of encephalomyocarditis viral RNA in oocytes by *Xenopus laevis. Proc. Natl. Acad. Sci. USA,* 69:3665–3669.
16. Lee, S. H. S., van Rooyen, C. E., and Ozere, R. L. (1969): Additional studies of interferon production by human leukemic leukocytes *in vitro. Cancer Res.,* 29:645–652.
17. Mach, B., Faust, C., and Vassalli, P. (1973): Purification of 14S messenger RNA of immunoglobulin light chain that codes for a possible light-chain precursor. *Proc. Natl. Acad. Sci. USA,* 70:451–455.
18. Moar, V. A., Gurdon, J. B., Lane, C. D., and Marbaix, G. (1971): Translation capacity of living frog eggs and oocytes, as judged by messenger RNA injection. *J. Biol. Chem.,* 61:93–103.
19. Pestka, S. (1978): Human interferon: The proteins, the mRNA, the genes, the future. In: *Dimensions in Health Research—Search for the Medicines of Tomorrow,* edited by H. Weissbach, pp. 29–56. Academic Press, New York.
20. Pestka, S., McInnes, J., Havell, E. A., and Vilček, J. (1975): Cell-free synthesis of human interferon. *Proc. Natl. Acad. Sci. USA,* 72:3898–3901.
21. Pestka, S., McInnes, J., Weiss, D., Havell, E. A., and Vilček, J. (1977): *De novo* cell-free synthesis of human interferon. *Ann. N.Y. Acad. Sci.,* 284:697–702.
22. Reynolds, F. H. Jr., Premkumar, E., and Pitha, P. M. (1975): Interferon activity produced

by translation of human interferon messenger RNA in cell-free ribosomal systems and in *Xenopus* oocytes. *Proc. Natl. Acad. Sci. USA,* 72:4881–4885.

23. Rubinstein, M., Rubinstein, S., Familletti, P. C., Gross, M. S., Miller, R. S., Waldman, A. A., and Pestka, S. (1978): Human leukocyte interferon purified to homogeneity. *Science,* 202:1289–1290.

24. Rubinstein, M., Rubinstein, S., Familletti, P. C., Hershberg, R. D., Brink, L. D., Gutterman, J., Hester, J., and Pestka, S. (1979): Human leukocyte interferon: Production and purification to homogeneity by HPLC. In: *Proteins: Structure and Biological Function,* edited by E. Gross and J. Meienhofer, pp. 99–103. Pierce Chemical, Rockford, Ill.

25. Rubinstein, M., Rubinstein, S., Familletti, P. C., Miller, R. S., Waldman, A. A., and Pestka, S. (1979): Human leukocyte interferon: Production, purification to homogeneity, and initial characterization. *Proc. Natl. Acad. Sci. USA,* 76:640–644.

26. Sehgal, P. B., Dobberstein, B., and Tamm, I. (1977): Interferon messenger RNA content of human fibroblasts during induction, shut-off, and superinduction of interferon production. *Proc. Natl. Acad. Sci. USA,* 74:3409–3413.

27. Steinberg, R. A., Levinson, B. B., and Tomkins, G. M. (1975): Superinduction of tyrosine aminotransferase by actinomycin D: A reevaluation. *Cell,* 5:29–35.

28. Stevens, R. H., and Williamson, A. R. (1972): Specific IgG mRNA molecules from myeloma cells in heterogenous nuclear and cytoplasmic RNA containing poly-A. *Nature,* 239:143–146.

29. Tucker, P., and Pestka, S. (1977): *De novo* synthesis and glycosylation of the MOPC-46B mouse immunoglobulin light chain in cell-free extracts. *J. Biol. Chem.,* 252:4474–4486.

Polypeptide Hormones, edited by
R. F. Beers, Jr. and E. G. Bassett.
Raven Press, New York © 1980.

7. Synthesis of Proinsulin in Bacteria

Lydia Villa-Komaroff, *Stephen P. Naber, **Stephanie Broome,
†Argiris Efstratiadis, **Peter Lomedico, **Richard Tizard,
*William L. Chick, **Walter Gilbert

*Department of Microbiology, University of Massachusetts Medical School, Worcester,
Massachusetts 01605; *Elliott P. Joslin Research Laboratory, Harvard Medical School
and Peter Bent Brigham Hospital, Boston, Massachusetts 02115; **The Biological
Laboratories, Harvard University, Cambridge, Massachusetts 02138; and †Department
of Biological Chemistry, Harvard Medical School, Boston, Massachusetts 02115*

INTRODUCTION

The study of eukaryotic genes has been greatly facilitated by the ability to
isolate and amplify individual eukaryotic genes or segments of genes in bacteria.
It has become apparent that in some cases the bacterial cell can also synthesize
the protein encoded by the inserted eukaryotic DNA (12,18,22,28,33,37,40,45).
Because the coding region of many eukaryotic genes is interrupted by introns
(4,5,15,23,24,43), double-stranded DNA copies of mRNA or synthetic sequences
are the materials of choice when the production of an eukaryotic protein in
bacterial cells is the goal. In this chapter cloning of sequences encoding proinsulin
is described as an example of the use of recombinant DNA technology to produce
medically useful proteins.

We chose insulin for our studies not only because it is a protein that can
be identified by immunological and biological means, but also because it is a
protein that has been used therapeutically for a long period of time.

Although mature insulin consists of two polypeptide chains, A and B, it is
initially synthesized as a single polypeptide called preproinsulin. The 23 amino
acids at the NH_2-terminus of the nascent polypeptide chain are cleaved off,
presumably as the molecule moves through the endoplasmic reticulum (2,9),
producing the proinsulin molecule. Three disulfide bonds are formed, two between the A and B chains, one within the A chain, and the "connecting peptide"
(C peptide) is then cleaved from the middle of the folded molecule (39). Two
distinct insulin polypeptides encoded by separate genes are made in the rat
(14).

Ullrich et al. (44) cloned double-stranded DNA copies (ds-cDNA) of rat
preproinsulin mRNA isolated from pancreatic islets and determined sequences
covering much of these two genes. We made double-stranded DNA copies of
mRNA from a rat transplantable insulinoma and cloned them in the *Pst*I restric-

tion endonuclease site of the plasmid pBR322 (45). The *Pst*I site lies within the penicillinase gene encoded by the plasmid (41).

The *Escherichia coli* enzyme penicillinase is a periplasmic protein, the gene for which has been sequenced (1,41). Penicillinase is synthesized as a preprotein with a 23-amino acid leader sequence (41) that presumably serves as a signal to direct the secretion of the protein to the periplasmic space. Insertion of the structural information for insulin into the penicillinase gene should result in the expression of the insulin sequence as part of a hybrid protein.

CONSTRUCTION OF HYBRID DNA MOLECULES

Construction of the recombinant DNA molecules is illustrated in Fig. 1. We isolated poly(A) containing RNA from an X-ray induced, transplantable rat β cell tumor (13). This preparation directed the synthesis, in a cell-free system, of a product precipitable with anti-insulin antibody (see Table 1). Since the mRNA encoding insulin was a minor component of the poly(A) containing RNA, we used the oligo(dT)-cellulose-bound RNA without further purification as template for reverse transcription.

After the first strand was synthesized, the RNA template was destroyed with alkali. DNA polymerase was used to synthesize the second (complementary)

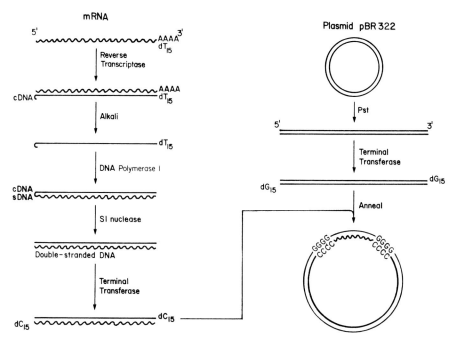

FIG. 1. Schematic illustration of the synthesis of double-stranded cDNA and the construction of the recombinant molecules. See text for additional details.

TABLE 1. *Hybrid-arrested translation and immunoprecipitation of the cell-free products*[a]

Source of arresting DNA	TCA-insoluble	Immunoprecipitable		% Immunoprecipitable[b]
		−Insulin	+Insulin	
Control I (−DNA, −RNA)[c]	2,570			
Control II (−DNA, +RNA)[d]	35,700	12,300	310	36.2
pBR322	28,800	7,850	245	29.0
Clone 3	15,100	3,630	264	26.9
13	19,600	5,190	350	28.4
15	18,600	4,850	252	28.7
16	29,200	8,830	247	32.2
17	24,000	6,700	316	30.0
18	15,900	3,690	251	25.8
19	8,650	587	277	5.0
20	15,100	4,070	231	30.6
21	21,100	5,170	223	26.7

[a] Plasmid DNA (approximately 3 μg) was digested with *Pst*I, ethanol precipitated, and dissolved directly into 20 μl deionized formamide. After heating for 1 min at 95°C each sample was placed on ice. After the addition of 1.5 μg oligo (dT)-cellulose-bound RNA, PIPES pH 6.4 to 10 mM and NaCl to 0.4 M, the mixtures were incubated for 2 hr at 50°C. (26). They were then diluted by the addition of 75 μl H$_2$O and ethanol precipitated in the presence of 10 μg wheat germ tRNA, washed with 70% ethanol, dissolved in H$_2$O, and added to a wheat germ cell-free translation mixture (35) containing 10 μCi ³H-leucine (60 Ci/mmole). Reaction mixtures of 50 μl were incubated at 23°C for 3 hr and then duplicate 2-μl aliquots were removed for trichloroacetic acid precipitation. From the remainder, two 20-μl aliquots were treated with ribonuclease, diluted with immunoassay buffer, and analyzed for the synthesis of immunoreactive preproinsulin by means of a double-antibody immunoprecipitation (35) in the absence or presence of 10 μg of bovine insulin. The washed immunoprecipitates were dissolved in 1 ml of NCS (Amersham) and counted in 10 μl of Omnifluor (New England Nuclear) by liquid scintillation.
[b] Calculated by means of the formula: (immunoprecipitable radioactivity in the absence of insulin) − (immunoprecipitable radioactivity in the presence of insulin)/(TCA-insoluble radioactivity) − (TCA-insoluble radioactivity of Control I).
[c] Reaction mixture incubated in the absence of added RNA.
[d] F cell-free translation by the direct addition of oligo (dT)-cellulose-bound RNA into the reaction mixture.
From ref. 45.

strand of DNA. This second DNA strand is covalently attached to the first strand, presumably because the enzyme utilizes the 3′ end of the first strand as a primer to begin synthesis of the second strand. The covalent linkage can be broken by treating the double-stranded product with S1 nuclease, an enzyme that hydrolyzes single-stranded DNA or RNA (16).

The double-stranded cDNA can be joined to a bacterial plasmid by using the enzyme terminal transferase to extend the 3′ ends of the DNA with a homopolymer and then annealing the DNA to linearized plasmid DNA to which has been added a complementary homopolymer (25). We used the plasmid pBR322 (3), which has been sequenced in its entirety (42). It encodes resistance to both ampicillin and tetracycline and contains several unique restriction endo-

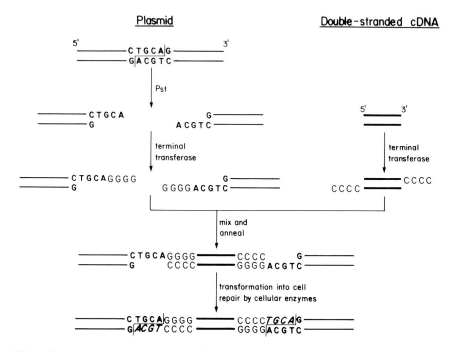

FIG. 2. The regeneration of the recognition site for the restriction endonuclease *Pst*I. The plasmid pBR322 has a single recognition site for *Pst*I. This enzyme recognizes the hexanucleotide sequence shown and cleaves the molecule so as to leave a 3′ terminal extension that lacks the last dG of the *Pst*I recognition sequence (38). Since the enzyme terminal transferase will attach homopolymer blocks to the 3′ terminus of DNA if it is given a single deoxyribonucleoside triphosphate as a substrate (11), it can be used to replace the dG at the 3′ ends. The dG-tailed plasmid can then be annealed to dC-tailed ds-cDNA, regenerating a circular DNA molecule. This molecule can be used to transform a bacterial cell. Bacterial enzymes will then fill in the gaps in the DNA molecule and ligate the ds-cDNA to the plasmid. Replication of the recombinant molecule will result in multiple copies of the initial molecule. (From ref. 46.)

nuclease sites that can be used for cloning. We used the *Pst*I site, which lies in the gene encoding penicillinase. As shown in Fig. 2, extending the 3′ ends of the ds-cDNA with d(C) and the 3′ ends of the *Pst*I-cut plasmid with d(G) results in a circular recombinant DNA molecule in which the *Pst*I recognition sequence has been reconstructed on both sides of the inserted DNA (3).

The recombinant generated by this procedure was then used to transform *E. coli* strain χ1776.

TRANSFORMATION AND IDENTIFICATION OF CLONES

At the time these experiments were performed, the NIH guidelines (30) required that mammalian DNA be cloned in a disabled bacterial host under P3 containment conditions. We therefore transformed *E. coli* strain χ1776 (an EK2 host), using pBR322 (an EK2 vector) in a biological safety cabinet in a P3 physical containment facility. More recent experiments have been done under

P2 physical containment with an EK2 host in compliance with the revised NIH guidelines.

E. coli cells can be rendered competent to take up exogenous DNA by treatment with calcium (27). If the exogenous DNA encodes resistance to an antibiotic, the cells that took up the added DNA can be detected by plating in the presence of the antibiotic. χ1776 must be treated with a modification of the standard procedure (17,45) in order to obtain efficient transformation. We obtained 2,355 transformants from 0.25 μg of double-stranded cDNA annealed to 2 μg of linearized pBR322.

The most straightforward method to identify clones containing a specific sequence is to hybridize RNA (or cDNA) to DNA in the bacterial colonies (20). However, as indicated earlier, the sequences encoding insulin represented a minor part of the RNA sequences that were used to generate the ds-cDNA that was cloned. We therefore could not use the mRNA as a probe for any specific sequence. Ullrich et al. (44) had suggested that an 80-nucleotide long fragment containing primarily insulin sequences could be obtained by treating cDNA with the restriction endonuclease *Hae*III, one of the few restriction enzymes that can cleave single-stranded DNA (21). We prepared radiolabeled cDNA, treated it with *Hae*III, isolated a 80-nucleotide fragment, and used it to screen approximately one-third of the transformants (Fig. 3A). Approximately 20%

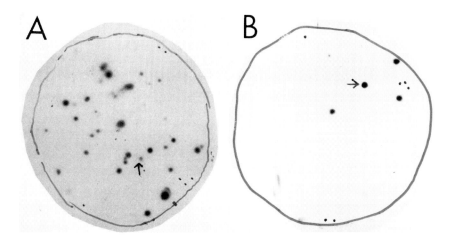

FIG. 3. Filter-hybridization analysis of colonies obtained after transformation of *E. coli* χ1776 with recombinant DNA molecules. χ1776 was transformed as described (45) and the transformed cells were plated on nitrocellulose filters overlaying agar plates containing tetracycline. The plates were incubated 48 hr at 37°C. Replicas of the filters were made as described (45). The replica filters were incubated at 37°C for 48 hr. The colonies on the first filter were screened by the filter hybridization assay (20). In this assay, the cells are broken *in situ* and the DNA is denatured by treatment with alkali. The DNA is fixed to the nitrocellulose filter and can be hybridized to radiolabeled probe. **A:** Colonies containing sequences homologous to an 80-nucleotide fragment derived from cDNA made to total mRNA and digested with the restriction endonuclease *Hae*III. **B:** Colonies containing sequences homologous to the inserted DNA in pI19.

```
                                                                              -21
                             TrpMetArgPheLeuProLeuLeuLeuAlaLeuLeuValLeuTrpGluProLysProAlaGlnAla  -1↑
      (C)TGCAGGGGGGGGGGGGGGCCCCCCCCCCCCCCACCTACGCAGGAGGAGGGGACGACGGGGACCGGGAGCCCAAGCCTGCCCAGGCT
      (G)ACGTCCCCCCCCCCCCCCGGGATGGCGCTTCCTGCCCTGCTGCCTCGTCGTCCTCTGGGAGCCCTCGGGTTCGGACGCGGGTCCGA  -1
        Pst              HhaI         HhaI                                          HaeIII
```

```
  1
  PheValLysGlnHisLeuCysGlyProHisLeuValGluAlaLeuTyrLeuValCysGlyGluArgGlyPhePheTyrThrProLysSerArgArgGlu  33
      TTTGTCAAACAGCACCTTTGTGTCCTCACCTGGTGGAGGCTCTGTACCTGGTGTGTGGGGAACGGTGGTTTTTCTTACACACCCCAAGTCCCGTGTGAA
  1   AAACAGTTTGTCGTGGAAACACCAGGAGTGGACCACCTCCGAGACATGGACCACACACCCCCTTGCCACCAAAGAAGATGTGTGGGTTCAGGCAGCACTT  99
               AvaII                                                                MboII
```

```
  34
  ValGluAspProGlnValProGlnLeuGluLeuGlyGlyGlyProGluAlaAlaGlyAspLeuGlnThrLeuAlaLeuGluValAlaAlaArgGlnLysArgGly  66
      GTGGAGGACCCGCAAGTGCCACAACTGCCAGAGCTGGGTGGAGGCCCGGAGGCCGCTGGAGGTTGCCGGCCAGAAGCGTGGC
  100 CACCTCCTGGGCGTTCACGGTGTTGACGGTCTCGACCCTGGGCCTCCGGCGACCTCCGGCGACCTCCAACGGGCCGTCTTCGCACCG  198
               AvaII          AluI               HaeIII HaeIII MboII                  HpaII
                                                HpaII  HpaII
```

```
  67
  IleValAspGlnCysCysThrSerIleCysSerLeuTyrGlnLeuGluAsnTyrCysAsn  86↓
      ATTGTGGATCAGTGCTGCACCAGCATCTGCTCCCTCTACCAACTGGAGAACTACTGCAACTGAGTCCACCACTCCCCGCCCC·····
  199 TAACACCTAGTCACGACGTGGTCGTAGACGAGGAGATGGTTGACCTCTTGATGACGTTGACTCAGGTGGTGAGGGGCGGGGG·····
                                          Hinf
```

FIG. 4. DNA sequence of the insertion in clone pI19. Nucleotides are numbered beginning with the first base of the sequence encoding proinsulin. Nucleotides in the 5' direction from position 1 in the message strand were identified by negative numbers, beginning with −1. Amino acids are numbered beginning with the first amino acid of proinsulin, while the last amino acid of the leader sequence (preregion) is numbered as −1. Restriction endonuclease cleavage sites experimentally verified are underlined and identified. The *arrows* indicate, in order, the ends of the leader sequence, and the peptides B, C, and A. (From ref. 45.)

of the clones were positive. We purified DNA from several of the colonies that hybridized most strongly with the 80-nucleotide fragment and digested it with several restriction endonucleases. When we compared the pattern of fragments obtained with each enzyme with the pattern predicted by the sequence data of Ullrich et al. (44), none of the DNAs contained any of the predicted fragments. This result indicated that none of the clones examined contained insulin sequences. We concluded that the major component of the 80-base pair fragment did not correspond to insulin sequences and we rescreened some of the positive clones by using hybrid-arrested, cell-free translation (32).

Translation of a mixture of mRNAs *in vitro* will result in synthesis of all of the proteins encoded by the mRNAs. Synthesis of a specific protein can be detected by precipitating that protein with antibody directed against it. The hybrid-arrested translation method is based on the principle that mRNA in the form of an RNA:DNA hybrid does not direct cell-free protein synthesis. We therefore incubated aliquots of oligo(dT)-bound RNA with linearized plasmid DNA from several clones under conditions favoring DNA:RNA hybridization (7), added them to cell-free translation systems, and assayed for specific inhibition of insulin synthesis. One of the plasmids tested, pI19, inhibited the synthesis of material precipitable with anti-insulin antibody, as shown in Table 1. When DNA from pI19 was digested with several restriction endonucleases, the sizes of the fragments obtained were consistent with those predicted by the published sequence information (44).

Direct sequence analysis of this DNA confirmed the presence of DNA encoding insulin. The sequence of pI19 is shown in Fig. 4. It corresponds to rat insulin I and encodes the entire preproinsulin chain with the exception of the first two amino acids of the reported preregion (9).

We used the inserted DNA in pI19 to screen the rest of the transformants (Fig. 3B). Approximately 2.5% (48/1745) of the clones hybridized strongly to this probe. We also used this DNA to measure the amount of insulin mRNA present in the oligo(dT)-bound RNA used to generate these clones. This hybridization analysis indicated that 0.3% of the RNA used as template for double-stranded cDNA synthesis encoded insulin.

EXPRESSION

As mentioned earlier, the ds-cDNA was inserted into the gene encoding penicillinase, a protein of 286 amino acid residues. The *Pst*I site in this gene lies between the codons for amino acids 182 and 183 (20) of penicillinase. The result of inserting ds-cDNA into the *Pst*I site is illustrated in Fig. 5. If the inserted DNA is in the correct orientation and in phase, that is, the coding strand of the inserted DNA is joined to the coding strand of the plasmid by a d(G)-d(C) linker that is a multiple of 3, we might expect the production of a hybrid protein. This protein would consist of the NH_2-terminal portion of penicillinase joined to a portion of preproinsulin by a group of glycine residues.

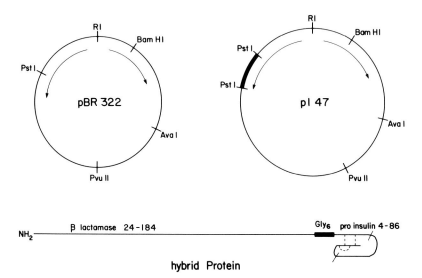

FIG. 5. Schematic diagram of a hybrid protein produced by insertion of ds-cDNA into the *Pst*I site of pBR322. **Left:** pBR322, showing the position of several endonuclease sites (3,42). The *arrow* to the right of the RI site indicates the position and the direction of transcription of the genes encoding tetracycline resistance. The *arrow* to the left of the RI site indicates the position and direction of transcription of the genes encoding β-lactamase, the enzyme that confers penicillin resistance. **Right:** Structure of pI47, a clone containing inserted DNA encoding insulin I. The insertion lies between two *Pst*I sites regenerated as illustrated in Fig. 2. The *arrow* to the left of the RI site indicates the hybrid protein that would result from the transcription of the β-lactamase gene through the inserted DNA. The scheme assumes the inserted DNA has a termination codon (see Fig. 9). **Bottom:** Structure of the hybrid protein; the *dotted lines* indicate the disulfide bonds present in insulin and the *small solid lines* indicate the boundaries of the C peptide. (From ref. 46.)

Since the insulin moiety is at the end of the molecule, we might expect it to fold into its proper shape, exposing antigenic determinants of native insulin. In our initial experiments (45) we found that almost two-thirds of the clones carrying inserts were ampicillin-resistant. We interpreted this datum to mean that the hybrid protein contained the active site of penicillinase. However, as shown in Fig. 6, this resistance is more likely due to the loss of the inserted sequence and the regeneration of an intact β-lactamase gene. We nevertheless screened colonies of the 48 clones containing insulin in sequences for the presence of insulin antigenic determinants, using a solid-phase radioimmunoassay (RIA) (6).

This assay utilizes the fact that antibody molecules bind very tightly to plastics such as polyvinyl or polystyrene (8). Polyvinyl sheets coated with antibody are exposed to lysed bacteria; if the antigen is present in the bacteria, it will bind to the antibody. The immobilized antigen can then be detected by exposing the coated polyvinyl sheet (and the antigen–antibody complex bound to it) to radioiodinated antibody. The antigen will then be sandwiched between the anti-

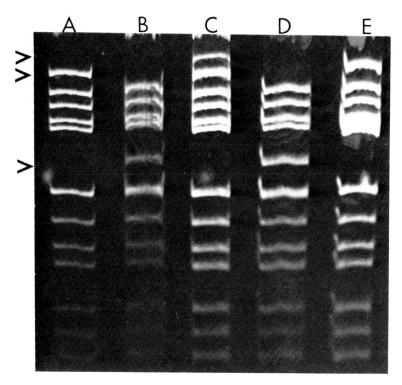

FIG. 6. Loss of DNA segments inserted into the *Pst*I site of pBR322. Bacterial cells containing pl47 were spread on a rich agar plate containing 50µg/ml ampicillin. A single colony was selected, grown in the presence of tetracycline, and plasmid DNA was prepared. The DNA was cleaved with the restriction endonucleases *Hae*III or *Hae*III + *Pst*I and run on a 6% native polyacrylamide gel. The DNA bonds were visualized by staining the gel with ethidium bromide and photographing the gel illuminated with ultraviolet light. The large DNA bonds do not resolve and are excluded from the figure. The *arrowheads* indicate, from top to bottom, the position of a *Hae*III band containing insulin sequence in pl47 and pl19; the *Hae*III band of pBR322 that contains the unique *Pst*I site; the position of one of the bonds resulting from the double digestion of pBR322 DNA with *Hae*III and *Pst*I (the second band is not resolved on this gel). **A:** pBR322 DNA digested with *Hae*III. **B:** pBR322 DNA digested with *Hae*III and *Pst*I. **C:** pl47 DNA digested with *Hae*III. **D:** pl47 DNA digested with *Hae*III and *Pst*I. **E:** pl19 DNA digested with *Hae*III.

bodies attached to the plastic sheet and those carrying the radioactive label. Autoradiography will show the position of the colonies containing the antigen. This method is particularly suited for detecting a hybrid protein, since the polyvinyl disk can be coated with antibodies directed against one protein (e.g., penicillinase) and the immobilized antigen can be labeled with ^{125}I-antibodies directed against another protein (e.g., insulin).

We coated plastic disks with anti-insulin antibody and used ^{125}I-anti-insulin to detect solely insulin antigenic determinants. Disks coated with anti-penicillin-ase antibody and exposed to ^{125}I-anti-insulin detect the presence of a fused

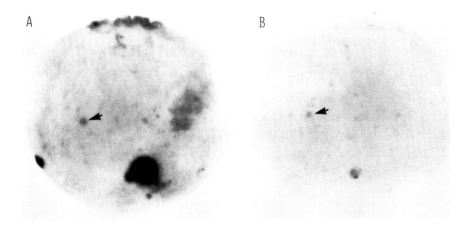

FIG. 7. Initial detection of penicillinase-insulin hybrid polypeptides in an insulin cDNA clone. Cells from colonies of the 48 insulin cDNA clones and from control colonies, χ1776 and χ1776-pBR322, were applied to an agarose/lysozyme/EDTA plate. Positive controls (1μl of wash buffer containing 5 ng of insulin and 1 μl of wash buffer containing 5 ng of penicillinase) also were spotted on plate. Antigen was absorbed to an IgG-coated polyvinyl disk during a 1-hr incubation at 4°C. Immobilized antigen was labeled by setting the plastic disk on a solution containing radioiodinated anti-insulin IgG. The autoradiographs are of disks precoated **A:** with anti-insulin IgG, or **B:** with anti-penicillinase IgG, exposed on Kodak X-OMAT R film, using a DuPont Cronex Lighting Plus intensifying screen for 12 hr at −70°C. *Arrows* indicate the signal generated by clone pI47. The large exposed area in the lower right of **A** is the positive control for insulin detection (From ref. 45.)

protein, as do disks coated with anti-insulin and exposed to radioiodinated anti-penicillinase. A representative result is shown in Fig. 7. One clone, pI47, gave a positive response with all of the combinations described above; this indicates the presence of a penicillinase-insulin hybrid polypeptide.

To determine whether this fused protein is secreted, we grew clone pI47 in liquid culture and extracted the proteins by osmotic shock, a method that does not lyse bacteria (31). Figure 8 shows that the insulin antigen is found in the periplasmic space, indicating that the fused protein is secreted.

We sequenced pI47 to determine the sequence around the junctions. Figure 9 shows that a proinsulin I cDNA lies in the *Pst*I site in the correct orientation and in phase. Amino acid residue 182 of penicillinase is connected by six glycine residues to the fourth amino acid of rat proinsulin. The structure of this hybrid polypeptide is shown in Fig. 5.

BIOLOGICAL ACTIVITY

Although detection of insulin antigenic determinants in the hybrid protein suggests that the proinsulin portion of the molecule has assumed its correct tertiary structure, immunoreactivity does not necessarily imply biological activity. To investigate biological activity of the insulin produced by the bacteria, we utilized the rat epididymal fat pad assay (40). This assay measures the conver-

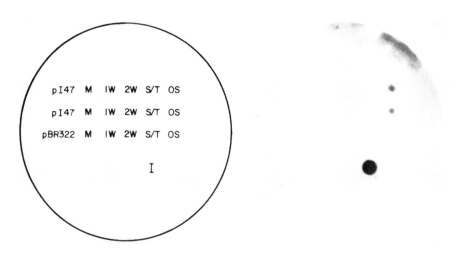

FIG. 8. Release of insulin antigen from χ1776-pl47 cells by osmotic shock. One liter of χ1776-pl47 cells growing at 37°C in M9 medium (29) supplemented with diaminopimelic acid, thymidine, and 0.2% glucose were harvested at a density of 5 × 10⁷ cells/ml and washed twice in 10 ml of cold 30 mᴍ NaCl/10 mᴍ Tris-HCl. The cells were then osmotically shocked (30) by resuspending the final wash pellet in 10 ml of 20% sucrose/30 mᴍ Tris-HCl, pH 8, at room temperature, made 1 mᴍ in EDTA, shaken at room temperature for 10 min, pelleted, resuspended in 10 ml of cold distilled water, shaken in an ice bath for 10 min, and again pelleted. The resulting supernatant fluid was termed the "water wash." As a control, 1 liter of α1776-pBR322 was grown and treated in a similar manner. Aliquots of 1 µl of each fraction to be assayed for the presence of insulin antigen were applied to the surface of a 1.5% agar plate. **A:** Positions of each fraction on the plate. M, Medium; 1W, first wash supernatant; 2W, second wash supernatant; S/T, sucrose/Tris supernatant; OS, distilled water wash. **B:** Autoradiograph showing results of a two-site radioimmuno assay (RIA) of these fractions. Antigen was absorbed to a polyvinyl disk and labeled using anti-insulin IgG. The large exposed area on the film marks the position of a positive RIA control, 5 ng of insulin. X-OMAT R film was exposed, using a Du Pont Cronex Lighting Plus screen for 12 hr at −70°C. A spectrophotometric assay for β-galactosidase (29) indicated that no more than 4% of cells lyse during this procedure. (From ref. 45.)

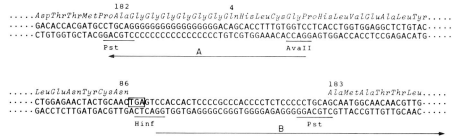

FIG. 9. Partial DNA sequence of the insertion in clone pl47. Clone pl47 was digested with *Hinf* and two fragments, H1 and H2 (approximately 1,700 and 280 base pairs long, respectively) were isolated. H1 contains the NH₂-terminal portion of the penicillinase gene and the bulk of the cDNA insert. H1 was digested with *Ava* II, end labeled and digested again with *Pst*I. A fragment 39 nucleotides long (fragment A, *arrow*) was isolated and sequenced. Fragment H2 was end labeled and digested with *Alu* I (which cuts at the region corresponding to amino acid 200 of penicillinase). A fragment 88 base pairs long (fragment B, *arrow*) was isolated and sequenced. The termination sequence TGA is boxed. (From ref. 45.)

sion of I-^{14}C-glucose to $^{14}CO_2$, a process that is stimulated by insulin. Because proinsulin generally has much less biological activity than insulin (36), we treated the material obtained by osmotic shock of χ1776-pI47 with trypsin under conditions known to convert porcine proinsulin to monoarginine and dealanated insulin (10,36). Table 2 shows that a trypsinized osmotic extract from χ1776-pI47 stimulated the conversion of glucose to CO_2 to a greater extent than did the trypsinized extract from χ1776-pBR322. The addition of anti-insulin antibodies to the trypsinized extracts had no effect on the stimulation caused by χ1776-pBR322 extracts, but abolished the additional stimulation seen with χ1776-pI47 extracts. We conclude that at least 18% of the insulin detected immunologically can be converted to a biologically active form. Because a variety of biological materials can either nonspecifically stimulate or inhibit this bioassay (19,34),

TABLE 2. *Biological activity of insulin synthesized in bacterial cells*[a]

Material assayed	Tissue (cpm/mg)	Immunoreactive insulin concentration (μU/ml)	Biologically active insulin (μU/ml)
None	40	—	—
pI47 Osmotic wash	194	597	—
pI47 Osmotic wash + anti-insulin serum	115	—	—
pBR322 Osmotic wash	109	0	—
pBR322 Osmotic wash + anti-insulin serum	106	—	—
pI47-[pI47 + AIS]	79	—	115 (19%)
Porcine insulin, no addition	20	25	—
Porcine insulin, no addition	100	150	—

[a] Cells from cultures of χ1776-pI47 and χ1776-pBR322 were grown and treated as described in the legend to Fig. 8. To maintain a ratio of substrate protein:trypsin:trypsin inhibitor of 100:1:100, protein concentrations of osmotic extracts which were less than 1 mg/ml were adjusted to that value by the addition of human serum albumin. The protein concentrations in this reaction ranged from 1.0 to 2.97 mg/ml. The pH of the osmotic extracts varied from 6.9 to 7.4 before trypsinization. To 10 volumes of osmotic extract (3.25–6.20 ml) prewarmed to 37°C, 0.25 volume of freshly prepared TPCK-trypsin (400 μg/ml) was added. Incubation was continued for 10 min at 37°C. The reaction was stopped by addition of 0.25 volume of freshly prepared soybean trypsin inhibitor (40 mg/ml). The hydrolysates were distributed in either 0.5 or 1.0 ml portions into the 10-ml flasks used in the fat pad bioassay, quick-frozen, and lyophilized overnight.

Biological activity of bacterial osmotic extracts was determined in triplicate by using a standard rat epididymal fat pad bioassay (34). The triplicate lyophilized samples were reconstituted with either 0.5 or 1.0 ml of Krebs-Ringer bicarbonate buffer containing the following additives: gelatin (1 mg/ml), D-glucose (3.0 mg/ml), 1-^{14}C-glucose (2 μCi/ml of medium), and where appropriate, 5 or 10 μl of guinea pig antiporcine insulin serum. The flasks containing medium were weighed to the nearest 0.1 mg and a single, small (15–30 mg) piece of epididymal fat pad from one of three 100 to 150 g Wistar Lewis male rats was added to each flask (34). The flasks containing the tissue were reweighed and gassed with humidified 95% O_2: 5% CO_2 for 5 min. Incubation of the flasks was continued for 2 hr at 37°C with constant shaking.

Carbon dioxide was liberated by the addition of 0.1 ml of 10 N H_2SO_4 to the medium and was trapped in 0.4 ml of hyamine hydroxide contained in a cup suspended from the flask stopper. This incubation was continued at room temperature for 70 min with constant shaking. The cup containing the hyamine was placed into 10 ml of liquid scintillation fluid and the $^{14}CO_2$ level determined. One unit = 48 μg of porcine insulin.

we are currently purifying the hybrid protein in an attempt to determine more accurately the biological activity of the protein synthesized in bacterial cells.

DISCUSSION

By using cDNA cloning technology, and an extremely sensitive assay to detect expression, we were able to construct a derivative of *E. coli* strain χ1776 that synthesizes and secretes into the periplasmic space a fused protein carrying antigenic determinants of both insulin and penicillinase. This was accomplished by inserting double-stranded cDNA carrying the structural information for insulin into a restriction site within the penicillinase structural gene. The fused DNA sequence is expressed as a polypeptide folded so as to reveal insulin antigenic shapes. Trypsinization of the fused protein results in a product that has some insulin biological activity. The exact structure of the trypsinization product of the fused protein is not known. We assume that after the release of the C peptide, the A chain of the product is identical to that of rat insulin I; however, the B chain lacks the COOH-terminal Ser and has a minimum of 12 extra amino acids at the NH_2-terminus (amino acids 177–182 of penicillinase and six connecting Gly residues). It is possible that the trypsinization product of the fused protein might be less active biologically because of its altered B chain. However, it is equally likely that bacterial components from the periplasmic space interfere with the biological assay. Studies are underway to purify and test the biological activity of the hybrid protein.

ACKNOWLEDGMENTS

This work was supported by National Institutes of Health grants AM 21240 and GM 09541–17 to Walter Gilbert, and grant AM 15398 to William L. Chick. We thank Leslie Delong for help with the figures and Jeannine Gallagher for preparing the manuscript.

REFERENCES

1. Ambler, R. P., and Scott, G. K. (1978): Partial amino acid sequence of penicillinase coded by *Escherichia coli* plasmid RGK. *Proc. Natl. Acad. Sci. USA*, 75:3732–3736.
2. Blobel, G., and Dobberstein, B. (1975): Transfer of proteins across membranes. 1. The presence of proteolytically processed and unprocessed nascent immunoglobulin light chains on membrane-bound ribosomes of murine myeloma. *J. Cell Biol.*, 67:835–851.
3. Bolivar, F., Rodriquez, R. L., Greene, P. J., Betlach, M. C., Heyneker, H. L., and Boyer, H. W. (1977): Construction and characterization of new cloning vehicles. II. A multipurpose cloning system. *Gene*, 2:95–113.
4. Brack, C., and Tonegawa, S. (1977): Variable and constant parts of the immunoglobulin light chain gene of a mouse myeloma cell are 1250 nontranslated bases apart. *Proc. Natl. Acad. Sci. USA*, 74:5652–5656.
5. Breathnach, R., Mandel, J. L., and Chambon, P. (1977): Ovalbumin gene is split in chicken DNA. *Nature*, 270:314–319.
6. Broome, S., and Gilbert, W. (1978): Immunological screening method to detect specific translation products. *Proc. Natl. Acad. Sci. USA*, 75:2746–2749.

7. Casey, J., and Davidson, H. (1977): Rates of formation and thermal stabilities of RNA:DNA duplexes at high concentrations of formamide. *Nucleic Acids Res.,* 4:1539–1552.
8. Catt, K., and Tregear, G. W. (1967): Solid-phase radioimmunoassay in antibody coated tubes. *Science,* 158:1570–1571.
9. Chan, S. J., Keim, P., and Steiner, D. F. (1976): Cell-free synthesis of rat preproinsulins: Characterization and partial amino acid sequence determination. *Proc. Natl. Acad. Sci. USA,* 73:1964–1968.
10. Chance, R. E., Ellis, R. M., and Bromer, W. W. (1968): Porcine proinsulin: Characterization and amino acid sequence. *Science,* 161:165–167.
11. Chang, L. M. S., and Bollum, F. J. (1971): Enzymatic synthesis of oligodeoxynucleotides. *Biochemistry,* 10:536–542.
12. Chang, A. C. Y., Nunberg, J. H., Kaufman, R. J., Erlich, H. A., Schmike, R. T., Cohen, S. N. (1978): Phenotypic expression in *E. coli* of a DNA sequence coding for mouse dihydrofolate reductase. *Nature,* 275:614–624.
13. Chick, W. L., Warren, S., Chute, R. N., Like, A., Lauris, V., and Kitchen, K. C. (1977): A transplantable insulinoma in the rat. *Proc. Natl. Acad. Sci. USA,* 74:628–632.
14. Clark, J. L., and Steiner, D. F. (1969): Insulin biosynthesis in the rat: Demonstration of two proinsulins. *Proc. Natl. Acad. Sci. USA,* 62:278–285.
15. Efstratiadis, A., Lomedico, P., Rosenthal, N., Kolodner, R., Tizard, R., Perler, F., Villa-Komaroff, L., Naber, S., Chick, W., Broome, S., and Gilbert, W. (1979): The structure and transcription of rat proinsulin genes. In: *Eukaryotic Gene Regulation, (ICN-UCLA Symposium on Molecular and Cellular Biology, Vol. XIV)* edited by T. Maniatis, R. Axel, and C. F. Fox, pp. 301–315. Academic Press, New York.
16. Efstratiadis, A., and Villa-Komaroff, L. (1979): Cloning of double-stranded cDNA. In: *Genetic Engineering: Principles and Methods, Vol. 1,* edited by A. Hollaender and J. Setlow, pp. 15–36. Plenum Press, New York.
17. Enea, V., Vovis, G. F., and Zinder, N. D. (1975): Genetic studies with heteroduplexes DNA of bacteriophage f1. Asymmetric segregation, base correction, and implications for the mechanism of genetic recombination. *J. Mol. Biol.,* 96:495–509.
18. Fraser, T. H., and Bruce, B. J. (1978): Chicken ovalbumin is synthesized and secreted by *Escherichia coli. Proc. Natl. Acad. Sci. USA,* 75:5936–5940.
19. Goldberg, A. L., and St. John, A. C. (1976): Intracellular protein degradation in mammalian and bacterial cells. II. *Annu. Rev. Biochem.,* 45:747–803.
20. Grunstein, M., and Hogness, D. S. (1975): Colony hybridization: A method for the isolation of cloned DNAs that contain a specific gene. *Proc. Natl. Acad. Sci. USA,* 72:3961–2965.
21. Horiuchi, K., and Zinder, N. D. (1975): Site specific cleavage of single-stranded DNA by a *Hemophilus* restriction enzyme. *Proc. Natl. Acad. Sci. USA,* 72:2555–2558.
22. Itakura, K., Hirose, T., Crea, R., Riggs, A. D., Heyneker, H. L., Bolivar, F., and Boyer, H. W. (1977): Expression in *Escherichia coli* of a chemically synthesized gene for the hormone somatostatin. *Science,* 198:1056–1063.
23. Jeffreys, A. J., and Flavell, R. N. (1977): The rabbit β-globin gene contains a large insert in the coding sequence. *Cell,* 12:1097–1108.
24. Lai, E. C., Woo, S. L. C., Dugaiczyk, A., Catterall, J. F., and O'Malley, B. W. (1978): The ovalbumin gene: Structural sequences in native chicken DNA are not continuous. *Proc. Natl. Acad. Sci. USA,* 75:2205–2209.
25. Lobban, P. E., and Kaiser, A. D. (1973): Enzymatic end-to-end joining of DNA molecules. *J. Mol. Biol.,* 78:453–471.
26. Lomedico, P. T., and Saunders, G. F. (1976): Preparation of pancreatic mRNA: Cell-free translation of an insulin-immunoreactive polypeptide. *Nucleic Acids Res.,* 3:381–391.
27. Mandel, M., and Higa, A. (1970): Calcium-dependent bacteriophage DNA infection. *J. Mol. Biol.,* 53:159.
28. Merecereau-Puijalon, O., Royal, A., Cami, B., Garapin, A., Krust, A., Gannon, G., and Kourilsky, P. (1978): Synthesis of an ovalbumin-like protein by *Escherichia coli* K12 harbouring a recombinant plasmid. *Nature,* 275:505–510.
29. Miller, J. H. (1972): *Experiments in Molecular Genetics.* Cold Spring Harbor Laboratories, New York.
30. National Institutes of Health (1976): Recombinant DNA research guidelines. *Federal Register,* 41:27,902–27,943.

31. Neu, H. C., and Heppel, L. A. (1965): The release of enzymes from *Escherichia coli* by osmotic shock and during the formation of spheroplasts. *J. Biol., Chem.,* 240:3685–3692.
32. Paterson, B. M., Roberts, B. E., and Kuff, E. L. (1977): Structural gene identification and mapping by DNA-mRNA hybrid arrested cell-free translation. *Proc. Natl. Acad. Sci. USA,* 74:4370–4379.
33. Ratzkin, B., and Carbon, J. (1977): Functional expression of cloned yeast DNA in Escherichia coli. *Proc. Natl. Acad. Sci. USA,* 74:487–491.
34. Renold, A. E., Martin, D. R., Dagenais, Y. M., Steinke, J., Nickerson, R. J., and Sheps, M. S. (1960): Measurement of small quantities of insulin-like activity using rat adipose tissue. 1. A proposed procedure. *J. Clin. Invest.,* 39:1487–1498.
35. Roberts, B. E., and Paterson, B. M. (1973): Efficient translation of tobacco mosaic virus RNA and rabbit globin 9S RNA in a cell-free system from commercial wheat germ. *Proc. Natl. Acad. Sci. USA,* 70:2330–2334.
36. Rubenstein, A. H., Melani, F., and Steiner, D. R. (1972): Circulating proinsulin: Immunology, measurement, and biological activity. In: *Handbook of Physiology, Vol. 1,* edited by R. O. Greep, E. B. Astwood, D. F. Steiner, N. Freinkel, and S. R. Greiger, pp. 515–534. American Physiological Society, Washington, D.C.
37. Seeburg, P. H., Shine, J., Martial, J. A., Ivarie, R. D., Morris, J. A., Ullrich, A., Baxter, J. D., and Goodman, H. M. (1978): Synthesis of growth hormone by bacteria. *Nature,* 276:795–798.
38. Smith, R., Blattner, R. F., and Davis, A. (1976): The isolation and partial characterization of a new restriction endonuclease from *Providencia stuartii. Nucleic Acids Res. Commun.,* 3:343–353.
39. Steiner, D. F., Kemmler, W., Clark, J. L., Oyer, P. E., and Rubenstein, A. H. (1972): The biosynthesis of insulin. In: *Handbook of Physiology, Vol. 1,* edited by R. O. Greep, E. B. Astwood, D. F. Steiner, N. Freinkel, and S. R. Greiger, pp. 175–198. American Physiology Society, Washington, D.C.
40. Struhl, K., Cameron, J. R., and Davis, R. D. (1976): Functional genetic expression of eukaryotic DNA in *Escherichia coli. Proc. Natl. Acad. Sci. USA,* 73:1471–1475.
41. Sutcliffe, J. G. (1978): Nucleotide sequence of the ampicillin resistance gene of *Escherichia coli* plasmid pBR322. *Proc. Natl. Acad. Sci. USA,* 75:3737–3741.
42. Sutcliffe, J. G. (1978): *Nucleotide Sequence of pBR322.* Doctoral Dissertation, Harvard University, Cambridge, Mass.
43. Tilghman, S. M., Tiemeier, D. C., Seidman, J. G., Peterlin, B. M., Sullivan, M., Maizel, J. V., and Leder, P. (1978): Intervening sequence of DNA identified in the structural portion of a mouse β-globin gene. *Proc. Natl. Acad. Sci. USA,* 75:725–729.
44. Ullrich, A., Shine, J., Chirgwin, J., Pictet, R., Tischer, E., Rutter, W. J., and Goodman, H. M. (1977): Rat insulin genes: Construction of plasmids containing the coding sequences. *Science,* 196:1313–1319.
45. Villa-Komaroff, L., Efstratiadis, A., Broome, S., Lomedico, P., Tizard, R., Naber, S. P., Chick, W. L., and Gilbert, W. (1978): A bacterial clone synthesizing proinsulin. *Proc. Natl. Acad. Sci. USA,* 75:3727–3731.
46. Villa-Komaroff, L., Broome, S., Naber, S., Efstratiadis, A., Lomedico, P., Tizard, R., Chick, W. L., and Gilbert, W. (1980): The synthesis of insulin in bacteria: A model for the production of medically useful proteins. In: *Second International Symposium on Enzyme Therapy in Genetic Diseases,* edited by R. Desnick. The National Foundation *(in press).*

Polypeptide Hormones, edited by
R. F. Beers, Jr. and E. G. Bassett.
Raven Press, New York © 1980.

8. Discussion

Moderator: Christian B. Anfinsen

P. H. Seeburg: Dr. Komaroff, what about cell resistance?

L. Villa-Komaroff: Yes, I forgot that. Strain 1776 is not a recombination-minus strain, as you probably know. It is the bacterial host that is required, at present, for use in experiments involving primate or mammalian DNAs.

The use of tailing, plus the restriction site, generate both a direct repeat and an inverted repeat at two ends of the insert. What we were seeing, when we examined more closely the phenomenon, was that the insert was being eliminated in such a way that the *Pst* site was being regenerated. This resulted in an intact β-lactamase that conferred β-ampicillin resistance on the cells.

We have now seen that phenomenon several times, as have other labs. It appears not to occur as frequently in a recombination-minus host, but these numbers are very tentative so that I can't be more specific than that.

C. B. Anfinsen: Dr. Pestka, do you feel that it would be possible, eventually, to use the direct translation of message as a feasible method for making quantities of interferon?

S. Pestka: The problem is, where would you get large amounts of message? I don't think there is any way to generate the large amounts of message that would make commercial use feasible.

C. B. Anfinsen: Is the problem one of purification, or simply getting enough crude mRNA?

S. Pestka: Simply getting enough message.

C. B. Anfinsen: In the case of lymphoblastoid cells, which we now grow in 200 to 300 liter batches—and probably will scale up to much larger batches fairly soon in collaboration with the Fort Detrick group—we hope to get kilos of cells. Might this offer a possibility if there were a way of preparing sufficiently pure message? Is the translation system available if you have large enough quantities of messenger?

S. Pestka: Yes, it is available; if you have enough message to use it, I think you have a unique way of labeling the interferon. Furthermore, using a cell-free system or the oocyte system, you could then probably generate additional homogeneous message.

P. H. Seeburg: May I raise a point? When you translate message *in vitro*, you would presumably obtain the precursor of interferon; it would also not be glycosylated.

Do you have any idea of the relative activities of cell-produced interferon as compared with the *in vitro* product? The same question would hold for material from bacterial clones.

S. Pestka: We don't have a comparison of the nonglycosylated and glycosylated interferons. We know that the nonglycosylated is active. I think an answer to that question might come from work in Dr. Anfinsen's lab.

C. B. Anfinsen: If one specifically removes the carbohydrate side chains (how completely we are not sure—there may still be a few residues of sugar left per molecule, but certainly 80 or 90% has been removed), the activity is the same.

It was interesting to find that on injecting this into rats, survival time in the circulation was about 50% higher than with the normal glycosylated material. Not only is it active but it persists for a longer time.

If carbohydrate were required, it is obvious that the peptide chemists should retire from the field because one doesn't have methods for the chemical addition of carbohydrates.

D. V. Goeddel: Do you feel that you have isolated the same interferon as Dr. Pestka? You report one methionine residue; he reports four.

S. Pestka: That is right. We find four methionines.

D. V. Goeddel: That is right.

C. B. Anfinsen: Amino acid composition is, unfortunately, a very coarse screen. We might easily have two methionines. This residue is more difficult than most to estimate.

I think Michel Revel, at the Weizmann Institute, using incorporation of labeled methionine during message translation, observes something like four to six.

In the case of Michel Revel's studies, the extra methionines may include an initiation methionine plus, perhaps, additional residues in a precursor section.

S. Pestka: That is possible. I think Revel's message source is fibroblast cells. There may well be some difference between the fibroblast and leucocyte interferons.

Tan reported less than two methionines. I would have to check on that.

L. Villa-Komaroff: Dr. Geoddel, do you have any other constructions in which the relative locations of the promoter and the ribosome binding site have been modified?

D. V. Goeddel: No, that is the first time we have done it. The growth hormone system turns out to be an easy system in which to study production, because the assay is so sensitive.

D. H. Gelfand: I would like to inquire about what I believe might have been a misstatement of fact. David Goeddel indicated that it wasn't possible, using DNA and message, to get biologically active, nonhybrid proteins.

The first biologically active, eukaryotic, mammalian gene product was obtained, in Stanley Cohen's lab during collaboration with others at Stanford, with mouse dihydrofolic reductase. This is not a hybrid protein.

D. V. Goeddel: I said polypeptide hormone. I didn't say protein for that reason.

B. W. Erickson: I am very curious about the slide you showed in which the oocyte was being impaled on a small silver needle. I wonder what the efficiency of production of peptide or protein from an impaled, single oocyte is. If Chris Anfinsen or Sid Pestka were able to make 1,000-gallon batches and isolate the messenger RNA, would they require hundreds of people injecting oocytes to get the product?

S. Pestka: Actually, with a fair amount of message, it is quite feasible to make picomole amounts of interferon by the injection of these oocytes. That is certainly sufficient for radiolabeling the product. In fact, we have already injected message into these oocytes for the synthesis of other proteins to pave the way for our interferon work, and we had a couple of surprises: one of them, when we injected the Kappa 46-B message, which is for an immunoglobulin μ chain, into the oocyte. It virtually took over the entire oocyte and it was the major protein made. Very surprising.

In addition, we were able to label it sufficiently with radioactive amino acids in the oocyte system to actually sequence the protein and to show that, in fact, the oocyte cleaves the polypeptide chain in the same way as does the mouse cell from which that message was obtained.

We also showed that the oocyte adds the carbohydrate to that chain on the same amino acid position as does the mouse cell; although we haven't determined the structure of the carbohydrate, we have tentatively concluded that its structure differs from the one added in the mouse cell, but is attached to the same amino acid.

I think what this tells us is that the oocyte and the recognition signals for cleavage and carbohydrate addition have remained stable for many millions of years during evolution. I have elaborated on your question, but I believe it is quite feasible for one person to make huge amounts of interferon by this technique.

C. B. Anfinsen: What about using soluble wheat germ-type systems?

S. Pestka: The efficiency of the message is approximately one-thousandth in the wheat germ system compared with the oocyte.

L. Villa-Komaroff: Sid, have you used the oocyte homogenate as a cell-free system?

S. Pestka: Yes, we have. We haven't explored this in detail, although it looked extremely promising. We gave it up because the intact oocyte works so well that we decided not to bother with the homogenate.

Once you get used to using this oocyte and to making your own micropipettes, it is rather efficient. It looks extremely laborious at first. One can easily inject about 100 oocytes in a couple of hours. There is, of course, no one in the laboratory doing this all day long. They would go out of their minds.

D. S. Blackman: Dr. Pestka, when you plotted the amount of interferon produced as a function of the amount of messenger RNA added, you got a curve that looked very much like a Michaelis-Menten curve as it rose linearly and then began to level off.

For those of us who are enzyme chemists, I wonder if you could comment on the shape of that curve? Why did it level off?

S. Pestka: The curve levels off because we have saturated the oocyte. We have seen this with Kappa 46-B and globin as well. All the messages, whether they are pure messages or unfractionated messenger RNA preparations, level off at about 20 to 30 ng per oocyte. You simply saturate the oocyte and get no additional synthesis from added message. The oocyte has only so many ribosomes that are able to add additional mRNA.

K. A. Folkers: I had the impression, before this current era of great progress of interferons, that there were innumerable interferons and that species specificity was perhaps something of concern. In any case, I think your technique of purification by HPLC allows comparisons. Do you predict that there will be few interferons or many of them?

S. Pestka: Do I predict there will be more than one human interferon?

K. A. Folkers: I thought there were innumerable interferons.

S. Pestka: Between the species?

K. A. Folkers: Yes. Has that concept changed?

S. Pestka: It has changed quite a bit, although the original concept still persists. Each interferon that has been isolated has specificity on different cell types. But the concept that was originally suggested—that interferon was virtually totally species-specific—is not correct as the result of the extensive studies that have been carried out in the last few years.

For example, it was first thought that the human interferons were only active on human cells and not on cells of other species. But, in fact, human *fibroblast* interferon is the most species specific of the human interferons. It is not, however, as active on other cell types as is the human leukocyte interferon.

To give you some numbers: taking 100% of the activity of interferon on human cells, its activity on bovine cells would be approximately 0.25%. However, human leukocyte interferon, tested on certain bovine cells, would exhibit anywhere from 50 to 200% the activity it shows on human cells.

This is also true of the animal interferons. Bill Carter, and his colleagues at Roswell Park, showed that if you study bovine and porcine leukocyte interferon, these cross-react with human cells, cat cells, and others.

I think a part of your question, if I remember it correctly, was: Are the interferons from different species different chemically? Was that also part of your question?

K. A. Folkers: To some extent, yes.

S. Pestka: We have very little knowledge on this because insufficient quantities of the various interferons have been purified to an extent where significant chemical characterizations can be made. There are available amino acid analyses on mouse interferon and on two human interferons and there appears to be remarkable similarity. But of course this doesn't tell us very much about the chemical structures of material that has not been purified too much. I am reminded of some experiments that we did with Havell and Vilček some years ago, in which the fibroblast material that was being used as the source of interferon some days would produce almost only leukocyte type and some days fibroblast type, at least in terms of antibody cross reactivity. Perhaps there is some regulation mechanism that we don't know about that one type of cell makes several kinds in different proportions depending on how they feel that day.

That is for the future, obviously.

A. W. Goldstein: Dr. Pestka, you indicated a note of caution in that most, in fact all, of the clinical trials, at least in terms of tumor studies, have been done with crude interferon preparations that are about 10% pure. There is, therefore, the possibility that the antitumor effects are due to some other lymphokines and there is some evidence from animal models that there are certain other lymphokines having potent anti-tumor effects.

But you also indicated that there is evidence now that the purified interferon has antigrowth properties. Were those studies done *in vitro,* or what is the evidence that purified interferon preparation has antitumor properties, *in vivo,* in animal models?

S. Pestka: Pure human interferon has not, to my knowledge, been used in any animal model. The only *animal* model that one can use with human tumors is, of course, the human variety, and possibly the nude mouse bearing human tumors. Studies like this are now in progress in collaborative work with Nate Kaplan and Gordon Sato at San Diego.

We plan to use homogeneous material to test whether the interferon can inhibit human tumors in a nude mouse. Preliminary studies were carried out with human tumor cells and the interferon does inhibit their growth.

A. W. Goldstein: In vitro, though.

S. Pestka: Yes, *in vitro.*

A. W. Goldstein: Is there any study that you know of using an animal interferon, purified or almost purified to study *in vivo* activity?

S. Pestka: Yes, there are actually quite a large number of studies with mouse interferon in mice, in combination with other chemotherapeutic reagents, or without them, that show that interferon is active.

However, in those studies, interferon preparations that were still relatively impure were used. There would still be the same problems in interpretation.

A. W. Goldstein: I am aware of those studies. Perhaps Dr. Anfinsen can answer whether there have been animal studies to show antitumor properties *in vivo* with a purified interferon? Is it still an open question that, in terms of antitumor activity, we are really dealing with some other lymphokines?

C. B. Anfinsen: I think the purest material that has been used in quantity is that obtained from Finland, from leukocytes. I doubt if it is more than a few percent pure.

I think Carter has recently done some experiments, perhaps not on tumors— possibly on herpes zoster—with some more highly purified interferon. Is that right, Sidney?

S. Pestka: I can elaborate on that. I think the Finnish material has a specific activity of about 10^6 units per milligram, which would put it in the range of

1% purity—perhaps a little under that. It varies slightly from preparation to preparation.

As Chris said, interferon has been used clinically in a highly purified form. The fibroblast interferon prepared by Bill Carter is, I imagine, in the range of 3 to 7% purity. This has been injected directly into malignant melanoma nodules in human patients with promising results. The nodules that were injected disappeared, whereas the control nodules elsewhere on the skin remained.

However, the bulk of protein present is not interferon, even in those preparations.

J. Francis: Dr. Pestka, have you characterized, in terms of size or activity, the α, β, and γ peaks of your HPLC effluent?

I noticed that, in the purification table, the β component didn't seem to have been assayed or its purification determined.

S. Pestka: We only purified the gamma peak. (You can compare the leukemic with the normal cell.) The reason for that is that this peak was in most abundance. At this time, Dr. Rubenstein is in the process of trying to purify all the other peaks.

C. B. Anfinsen: Could I ask the insulin producers here at the discussion table, how far along they are toward producing, say, a cupful of insulin by recombinant techniques?

L. Villa-Komaroff: Olé!

There are proteins that are being produced in bacteria at quite high levels; for example, you have heard David Goeddel discuss growth hormone.

For reasons that relate possibly to the proteolytic sensitivity of insulin and possibly to the construction of the hybrid proteins, the levels in our hands reach, perhaps, 5,000 micro units from a liter of bacterial cells; that is not a lot.

D. V. Goeddel: The insulin we have made by the approach of producing the A chain in one bacterial strain and the B chain in another and recombining them yields on the order of 200,000 molecules per cell. The limiting factor to producing a cupful is still the current guideline on growing 10 liters or more.

L. Villa-Komaroff: I know you have made radioimmune insulin that is positive by radioimmunoassay from these studies. Has that material been tested in a biologic assay?

D. V. Goeddel: We get this question all the time. It is being done now. The project—at least this part of it—has been taken over by Eli Lilly. We are not set up to do biological assays. The latest we have heard is that they are doing such assays this month.

M. Mevarech: As I understood from the lectures, the main obstacle of using recombinant DNA techniques is methods for screening the colonies.

I would like to ask Dr. Pestka how he can approach, more easily, the problem of screening recombinants once he has sequence of the protein.

S. Pestka: I think these techniques have been established by a number of laboratories.

In essence, once the sequence of interferon is available, theoretically one can synthesize the entire gene. This has been done by the triester technique that Le Ron pioneered and Coron successfully used with Boyer and their colleagues to clone and make the insulin; as a matter of fact, synthesize the insulin as well as the somatastatin.

Human leukocyte interferon, is, we estimate, 154 amino acids. Having the sequence, one can relatively easily synthesize a DNA primer that represents a portion of that sequence. This can be used as a primer for making cDNA, either in the first or second strand, or in fact the sequence can be used as a probe.

One has to keep in mind that there is a degeneracy in the code but, by appropriately and intelligently selecting the sequences that one will make, one can limit this and make very useful probes and primers.

K. A. Folkers: Can you imagine the possibility of using a double basic amino acid sequence such as Arg-Arg or Lys-Lys, where you don't have that double basic pair in the peptide hormone itself, and then employ some rather specific enzyme that would cleave at the double base pair? One might also consider three or four adjacent basic amino acids. Is that a reasonable possibility?

D. V. Goeddel: We have actually used that procedure to produce the insulin A chain. We made synthetic proinsulin containing the "connecting peptide" but introduced two basic residues preceding the A chain. By cleaving with trypsin, we obtained A chain that was chemically identical to the natural form.

B. W. Erickson: I would like to mention some comments that Dr. Edward Rike of the Rockefeller University gave on Monday in Toronto. He was presenting a lecture on a symposium devoted to insulin.

He proposed that an enzyme he has been working on for about 5 years actually may be the one that carves out insulin from the pro-hormone *in vivo*. Specifically, he thinks that plasminogen activator may be a candidate. It evidently has, or he believes it has, a high specificity for double basic residues.

So it may be that the tryspin is not the molecule of choice in performing the enzymatic part of genetic engineering, but that there are much more specific enzymes of a serine-protease nature. It would be much more selective and might not give internal splits in proteins.

S. G. Mizroch: Aside from the obvious clinical implications of insulin, weren't there any smaller or easier-to-work-hormones that you might have pursued before tackling insulin?

L. Villa-Komaroff: There are. The group in California has done both growth hormone and somatastatin. I am sure they are working on others—David may wish to comment.

D. V. Goeddel: Somatastatin was actually done before insulin. Then we did the insulin—both chains.

As far as the application of the guidelines, all of these studies have been done on a small scale.

D. E. Gelfand: Peter, I was really fascinated by the sequence conservation at the 5' ends of rat and human growth hormone with the lack of sequence conservation at the 3' nontranslated region.

Could you comment on that? Do you have any models?

C. B. Anfinsen: Would you please repeat the question?

P. H. Seeburg: He is astonished at the extent of sequence conservation in the messenger RNA for growth hormone in rat and human. You expect some sequence conservation because of the 60% homology in amino acid sequences. But you do not expect to find high homology in the nontranslated portions of the messages. You do see a very high degree of homology in the 5', untranslated portion, namely, in the region where translation starts. I assume the ribosomes are similar in rats and humans.

M. Wilchek: I would like to ask, as an organic chemist, whether it would be possible to use your methods for getting modified hormones, like hormones that contain D-amino acid residues or that are more stable than regular hormones, or modified ones containing nitrotyrosine, or should you always aim for the native compound? In essence, can the methods that were described today be utilized to make abnormal proteins—analogs of the normal proteins, and so forth, that would have different properties, stability, and species characteristics?

D. V. Goeddel: The intact cell will not incorporate D-amino acid, except very rarely, so I doubt that these techniques can be used effectively to make them. But a number of tricks *can* be used.

In cell-free extracts, D-amino acids are incorporated, if they are put on tRNA. Sidney Hecht at MIT has worked out an elegant technique for putting virtually any amino acid he wants onto tRNA molecules and, with combinations of such technology, using the recombinant DNA techniques and messenger RNA, one can generate a huge number of analogs.

We have had some discussions with Sidney Hecht about making some types of such compounds.

K. Itakura: Dr. Anfinsen, you have already made purified interferon. How about its sequence?

C. B. Anfinsen: The first person to purify interferon convincingly was, I think, Dr. Ernest Knight of DuPont, who is here in the audience. This was actually 3 or 4 years ago. The specific activity was around 2 to 5×10^8 units/mg.

The material that Sid Pestka's group and we are making seems to have about the same level of activity.

Sequencing has just begun but the first data are at a stage where they are not sufficiently solid to talk about.

I know that Dr. Knight has a certain number of residues from the NH_2-terminus in his fibroblast preparation, and we have perhaps not quite as many in the lymphoblastoid system; that is where it stands at the moment. There is perhaps enough to start adding the COOH-terminal amino acid to a solid phase resin for peptide synthesis.

K. Itakura: Dr. Anfinsen, you are interested in making interferon by peptide synthesis. Can you hope to join 154 residues in this manner? How long would it take to make such a large peptide, compared with using recombinant techniques?

C. B. Anfinsen: You first have to be a very good chemist. Then you either have to work for the government, where you can hopefully get enough money to buy monomers, or else get a big grant. Lastly, you hire 30 Ph.D.s and get a whip. In about a year you have a kilo. . . .

Polypeptide Hormones, edited by
R. F. Beers, Jr. and E. G. Bassett.
Raven Press, New York © 1980.

9. Introduction to Section B: Chemistry of Peptide Hormones

Karl Folkers

Institute for Biomedical Research, University of Texas, Austin, Texas 78712

When a chemist thinks about the chemistry of an identified natural product, he generally thinks in terms of the three phases of the investigation: isolation, structure, and synthesis. The semantics is a little different when the peptide chemist thinks about the chemistry of a peptide hormone in terms of isolation, sequencing, and synthesis. Sequencing is limited structural elucidation, because one is frequently establishing the linkage between known units. Synthesis of a peptide hormone is also limited, because one is generally achieving the linkage between known units. Solid-phase synthesis of peptides has emerged as a great step forward. The users of solid-phase synthesis generally praise the technique for what it has accomplished. It seems that the non-users are the most critical of the technique, possibly because they are focusing on the disadvantages rather than the advantages. The disadvantages, also acknowledged by the users, are diminishing as the technique is continuously improved as is the case for nearly all breakthroughs in experimental chemistry.

We are fortunate to have a chapter on one of the most advanced ultramicro procedures for isolation, and then an account of the advances in sequencing. The two chapters concluding this section will inform us about the best protected amino acids and how to use them in the best automated solid-phase synthesis.

Polypeptide Hormones, edited by
R. F. Beers, Jr. and E. G. Bassett.
Raven Press, New York © 1980.

10. Ultramicro Isolation and Analysis of Peptides and Proteins

Stanley Stein

Roche Institute of Molecular Biology, Nutley, New Jersey 07110

INTRODUCTION

High-performance liquid chromatography (HPLC) with a bioassay, radio-immunoassay, or radioreceptor assay has been used for the identification and quantitation of specific peptides, as well as for their isolation in pure form. A sensitive fluorometric detection system for amino acids, peptides, and proteins has enabled the chemical analysis of small quantities of these purified peptides. A brief description of the instrumentation used for HPLC and fluorescent detection will be presented, followed by representative applications to the opioid peptides, concluding with some general suggestions on the use of HPLC for the separation of peptides and proteins.

INSTRUMENTATION AND METHODS

The advantage of HPLC over conventional chromatography is that the individual components remain in narrow bands while eluting from the column. Therefore, components with minor structural differences may be completely separated in one or two chromatographic runs. Column effluents may be monitored with the reagent fluorescamine, which reacts with primary amines to form highly fluorescent adducts (22). Fluorescamine is ideally suited for analysis of the effluent of HPLC columns, since the reaction is completed within seconds, thereby minimizing post-column band spreading. Since fluorescamine and its hydrolysis by-products are nonfluorescent, the reagent may be added in a continuous fashion to the column effluent. However, in order to further utilize the peptide it is necessary to split the stream (1) so that one portion of the column effluent is allowed to react with fluorescamine, while the remainder goes to a fraction collector (Fig. 1). For purely analytical applications, such as amino acid analysis, all of the column effluent may be allowed to react with fluorescamine (4,20). The limit of detection with currently available instrumentation is 10 to 100 pmoles. It is, therefore, possible to carry out the isolation of a peptide or protein on the nanomole scale and use only a small percentage of the peptide for column monitoring. Detection of peptide fragments, generated as a first step in sequence analysis, and amino acid analysis are both possible at the picomole level. However, the main limiting factors so far have been amine contamination

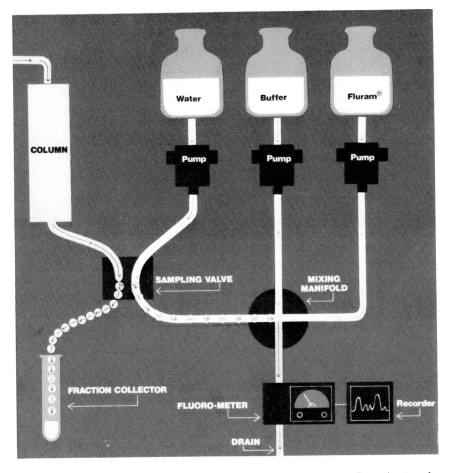

FIG. 1. Schematic illustration of the column monitoring system. The sampling valve transfers aliquots of column effluent at a pre-determined rate into the detection system. The aliquots are picked up by a stream of water, mixed with borate buffer (pH 9.3) and fluorescamine (Fluram®) in acetone, and the generated fluorescence is measured in a flow-cell and recorded. The ratio of column effluent collected to that used for fluorescence assay is readily adjustable from less than 1% to essentially 100%.

in the buffers and solvents, as well as loss of peptide encountered at these low levels. The steps taken to deal with these problems are discussed in a later section. HPLC has also been used with sensitive ultraviolet absorption at short wavelengths (200–215 nm) (6,15), but this technique is inherently nonspecific. The highly specific fluorometric method is more versatile and practical.

APPLICATIONS

Isolation and Structural Analysis of Opioid Peptides

Biologically active peptides and proteins are usually present at low concentrations and investigators have required tissues from large numbers of large animals for their isolations. The sensitivity of the present methodology allows the isolation of active peptides from laboratory animals commonly used for physiological and pharmacological studies. This is important, since minor differences in the primary structure of the same active peptide may occur between species and these same differences can have profound effects on radioimmunoassays or bioassays. For this reason, we have isolated and characterized the opioid peptides from the rat.

The first two opioid peptides were isolated by Hughes and co-workers (7) from pig brain. These peptides, which mimic morphine in two different bioassays, have the structures Tyr-Gly-Gly-Phe-Met (Met-enkephalin) and Try-Gly-Gly-Phe-Leu (Leu-enkephalin). Larger peptides, that is, the endorphins, containing the Met-enkephalin sequence within their structures were subsequently isolated from pituitary tissue (12,13). The structure of β-lipotropin, which contains within it the sequences of β-, γ-, and α-endorphin, as well as Met-enkephalin, is shown in Fig. 2.

With the aid of a radioreceptor assay for opiates (5) we isolated 2 nmoles of rat β-lipotropin (10,000 daltons) from 40 anterior pituitaries (16). We determined that the amino acid composition of rat β-lipotropin differs from those of human and ovine β-lipotropins. Rat β-endorphin (3,500 daltons) was isolated from 200 rat pituitaries with a yield of 6 nmoles (17). Its amino acid composition was found to be the same as that of ovine and camel β-endorphin. Comparative

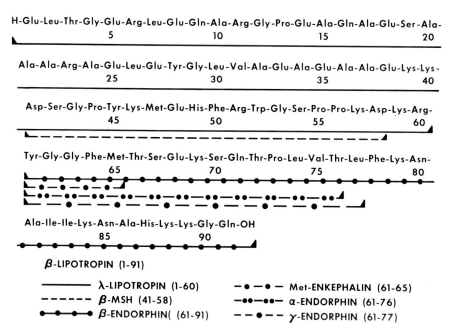

FIG. 2. Primary structure of sheep β-lipotropin. Fragments containing the Met-enkephalin sequence at the NH₂-termini are active in the opioid radioreceptor assay.

tryptic peptide mapping using HPLC with fluorescent detection indicated that the sequences of rat and camel (and ovine) β-endorphin are identical (17).

During these studies on the rat pituitary, we detected a protein (ca. 30,000 daltons) that appeared to be the precursor of β-lipotropin (16,18). Chemical analysis was used to establish this point in the following manner. When β-lipotropin (or β-, γ-, or α-endorphin) is digested with trypsin, only one of the fragments, β-lipotropin 61–69, contains the enkephalin sequence (see Fig. 2) and is active in the radioreceptor assay. Tryptic digestion of the partially purified protein from the rat pituitary similarly yielded only one active peptide fragment, which eluted at the same position from an HPLC column as the nonapeptide β-lipotropin 61–69. An identical precursor protein was found by Mains and co-workers (14) in a line of mouse pituitary tumor cells and was shown to be a common precursor to β-lipotropin and corticotropin. We have succeeded in purifying this protein, which we named pro-opiocortin, to homogeneity from a single camel pituitary and it has been partially characterized (8).

Stimulated by immunocytochemical observations (19) we used our methodology to investigate the opioid peptides in the adrenal medulla. Granules were isolated from bovine adrenal medulla and lysed with a dilute acid solution. The released peptides and proteins were separated by gel filtration and by HPLC (11,21). Both Met-enkephalin and Leu-enkephalin were found to be present in approximately the same concentration and relative proportions as in brain striatal tissue. However, a previously unknown series of opioid peptides and putative enkephalin precursors was discovered (11,21). One peptide, approximately the size of β-endorphin, differed from β-endorphin and eluted from the HPLC column at a position differing from any of the known opioid peptides. Another large peptide, approximately the size of β-lipotropin, was digested with trypsin. The fragment possessing opioid activity did not elute at the same position on HPLC as the nonapeptide β-lipotropin 61–69, demonstrating that the present peptide was not β-lipotropin. One of these peptides has been isolated. Amino acid analysis of this peptide indicates that it is an intermediate in the biosynthesis of Met-enkephalin (21) and furthermore, that the biosynthetic pathway for the enkephalins does not involve β-endorphin as as intermediate.

Identification and Quantitation of Opioid Peptides

Since slaughterhouse or autopsy tissue is usually not processed until hours or days after death, the possibility of nonspecific proteolysis must be considered. This can lead to degradative loss of the physiologically active components and to artifactual generation of components with *in vitro* biological activity. When working with laboratory animals it is possible to remove the tissues of interest within minutes after sacrifice. Tissues can be immediately frozen or homogenized in cold, dilute acid (pH 2) in the presence of protease inhibitors. During the work on the low molecular weight opioid peptides in rat pituitary (16), we were able to identify Met-enkephalin, β-endorphin, and α-endorphin, but there was no opioid activity detectable at the elution positon of γ-endorphin. Whether

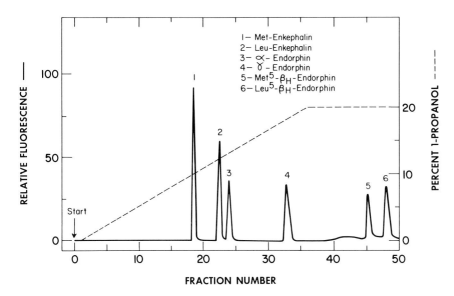

FIG. 3. Separation of synthetic opioid peptides. A Lichrosorb RP-18 column was run at room temperature at 40 ml/hr. Initial and final eluants both contained 0.5 M formic acid adjusted to pH 4.0 with pyridine. The sample containing 2 nmoles of each endorphin and 10 nmoles of each enkephalin, was injected in 1 ml of the initial buffer and 6% of the effluent was monitored.

γ-endorphin is absent from the rat due to a peculiarity of that species or is a degradative artifact in other species remains to be determined.

In an analytical application, Met-enkephalin and Leu-enkephalin were measured in different regions of mouse brain (10). For this procedure the tritiated forms of both enkephalins were obtained from commercial sources and purified by HPLC. An aliquot of each, equivalent to a few thousand counts per minute and representing a fraction of a picomole was added and an internal standard to the homogenate of each brain region. After removal of proteins by precipitation with trichloroacetic acid, each extract was chromatographed on the HPLC column. A typical separation of opioid peptides is shown in Fig. 3. Elution conditions had been optimized for the separation of the enkephalins in a rapid fashion (9) and samples were processed at the rate of one per hour. An aliquot of the fraction from every run corresponding to each enkephalin was taken for quantitation by the radioreceptor assay and another aliquot was taken for counting radioactivity in order to determine recovery through the procedure. The HPLC provided the specificity and the radioreceptor assay provided the quantitation.

GUIDELINES FOR HIGH PERFORMANCE LIQUID CHROMATOGRAPHY

Sample Handling

Volatile solvents and buffers are used as eluants whenever possible to facilitate the recovery of sample after column chromatography. The fluorescent detection system does not allow the use of amine containing buffers. Furthermore, commercially available chemicals typically contain amine contaminants, which must be removed by distillation over ninhydrin.

Peptides and proteins in low concentrations may irreversibly bind to glass and other surfaces. To avoid such losses, it is advisable to allow solutions of the peptide to come in contact only with polypropylene tubes or pipet tips. Lyophilization of proteins can result in large losses and near the end of an isolation it may be preferable to concentrate samples *in vacuo* rather than take them to dryness. Similarly, ultrafiltration or dialysis may have to be avoided.

The peptides and proteins studied in this laboratory to date have all been stable with respect to their biological activity. In fact, pro-opiocortin must be digested with trypsin in order to release the peptide that is active in the radioreceptor binding assay. The HPLC of enzymes has been performed with gel permeation and ion exchange (2,3). The problems of enzyme denaturation on the reverse-phase column are now being studied in this laboratory.

Tissues are usually homogenized and extracted under conditions that inhibit proteolytic activity. Initial fractionation is often by size on Sephadex columns. However, for the isolation or analysis of low molecular weight peptides, removal of proteins by trichloroacetic acid precipitation or boiling is preferable. Large volumes of the sample solution can be pumped onto the column (provided the component of interest is not eluted by the sample diluent) without loss of resolution. In this way the HPLC column can be used to concentrate the peptides in the sample, obviating the need for lyophilization. Milligram amounts of peptides may be applied to a standard (25 × 0.46 cm) HPLC column without a significant loss of resolution. However, the effect of concentration of material at the top of the resin bed can be deleterious with some peptides that tend to aggregate or precipitate. One result of this problem is a memory effect, in which only a portion of the material injected into the column elutes during the initial run and the remainder elutes at the same position in later runs. Another result is a loss of resolution.

Selection of Chromatography Conditions

Reverse-phase chromatography has proven to be most useful for the separation of peptides. In this technique, the solute partitions between the mobile phase and a hydrophobic stationary phase bonded to a silica matrix. A gradient of increasing concentration of 1-propanol in buffer has been used for both small and large peptides, but a weaker eluant such as methanol may be used for small, more hydrophilic peptides. For the best resolution the column is typically run at an acidic pH with formic acid and pyridine in the eluant. By varying the pH (e.g., from 3 to 5.5) it is possible to change the separation pattern. The selectivity is such that a change of only 2% in the propanol content of the eluant can determine whether a component is strongly retarded or rapidly eluted from the column (Fig. 4). Therefore, resolution may be optimized by

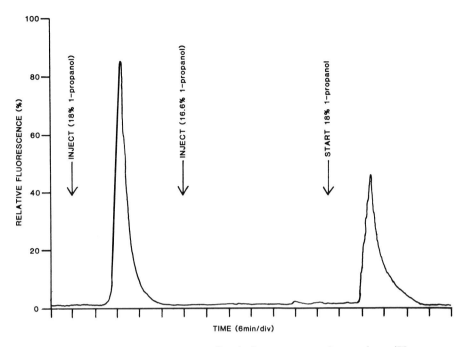

FIG. 4. Isocratic elution of bovine serum albumin from a reverse-phase column (50 nm pore, C_8). The protein (100 μg) eluted between 1 and 2 column volumes of 18% propanol. However, reinjection of sample and elution with several column volumes of 16.6% propanol was not sufficient; the protein was then eluted with 18% propanol.

using very shallow gradients for elution. Several resins, containing the functional groups C_{18}, C_8, CN, and phenyl can be used in the reverse-phase mode. The selectivity of each resin is slightly different (Fig. 5) and the sequential use of two resin types with the same gradient can achieve great purification.

HPLC of proteins requires special considerations. Proteins above 40,000 daltons may be excluded from the 6 or 10 nm pores of the standard commercial resins. Fifty-nanometer pore C_8 and CN resins have been prepared in this laboratory (R. Lewis, *in preparation*) and used for the chromatography of proteins as large as collagen chains (95,000 daltons) and tyrosinase (128,000 daltons). The use of a low eluant flow rate is also important in order to obtain the best resolution from an HPLC column. A flow rate of 15 ml/hr with a 25 × 0.46 cm column approaches the optimal efficiency of several hundred theoretical plates for the chromatography of a protein (as opposed to up to several thousand for small peptides). High recoveries (70–90%) are typically obtained from the reverse-phase column even for the chromatography of a few micrograms of protein. However, poor recoveries have been found with reverse-phase and other columns produced by some manufacturers. It is recommended that columns not described in the references from this laboratory be tested for recovery.

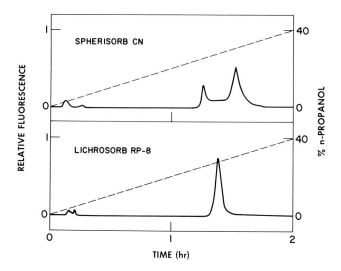

FIG. 5. Comparison of two different reverse-phase resins. A sample of pro-opiocortin appeared to be nearly homogeneous on the RP-8 column. However, chromatography of the same sample under identical elution conditions on the CN column showed it to be heterogeneous.

CONCLUSIONS

It is apparent that HPLC has become a standard research technique. The procedures described in this chapter, and given in more detail in the publications from this laboratory, have been developed in accordance with the design of the fluorescent detection system. This combination allows for the isolation and characterization of peptides and proteins in a rapid fashion and on a scale requiring far less starting material than by conventional chromatographic procedures. The basic procedures outlined here, however, are applicable to HPLC separations of peptides and proteins with any detection system. HPLC is also a valuable technique when used in conjunction with a radioimmunoassay or bioassay for quantitative analysis, since it provides an important criterion of specificity.

ACKNOWLEDGMENTS

Thanks are due to Drs. R. V. Lewis and S. Kimura for providing chromatograms describing recent advances in the HPLC of proteins.

REFERENCES

1. Böhlen, P., Stein, S., Stone, J., and Udenfriend, S. (1975): Automatic monitoring of primary amines in preparative column effluents with fluorescamine. *Anal. Biochem.,* 67:438–445.
2. Chang, S. H., Gooding, K. M., and Regnier, F. E. (1976): High-performance liquid chromatography of proteins. *J. Chromatogr.,* 125:103–114.

3. Chang, S. H., Noel, R., and Regnier, F. E. (1976): High speed ion exchange chromatography of proteins. *Anal. Chem.,* 48:1839–1845.
4. Felix, A. M., and Terkelsen, G. (1973): Total fluorometric amino acid analysis using fluorescamine. *Arch. Biochem. Biophys.,* 157:177–182.
5. Gerber, L. D., Stein, S., Rubinstein, M., Wideman, J., and Udenfriend, S. (1978): Binding assay for opioid peptides with neuroblastoma X glioma hybrid cells: Specificity of the binding site. *Brain Res.,* 151:117–126.
6. Hancock, W. S., Bishop, C. A., Prestidge, R. L., Harding, D. R. K., and Hearn, M. T. W. (1978): High-pressure liquid chromatography of peptides and proteins. II. The use of phosphoric acid in the analysis of underivatised peptides by reverse-phase high-pressure liquid chromatography. *J. Chromatogr.,* 153:391–398.
7. Hughes, J., Smith, T. W., Kosterlitz, H. W., Fothergill, L. A., Morgan, B. A., and Morris, H. R. (1975): Identification of two related pentapeptides from the brain with potent opiate agonist activity. *Nature,* 258:577–579.
8. Kimura, S., Lewis, R. V., Gerber, L. D., Brink, L., Rubinstein, M., Stein, S., and Udenfriend, S. (1979): Purification to homogeneity of camel pituitary pro-opiocortin, the common precursor of opioid peptides and corticotropin. *Proc. Natl. Acad. Sci. USA,* 76:1756–1759.
9. Lewis, R. V., Stein, S., and Udenfriend, S. (1979): Separation of opioid peptides utilizing high performance liquid chromatography. *Int. J. Pept. Protein Res.,* 13:493–497.
10. Lewis, R. V., Stern, A. S., Gerber, L. D., Stein, S., and Udenfriend, S. (1979): Separation of all known naturally occurring opioid peptides on a single column high performance liquid chromatography. *Fed. Proc.,* 38:373 (Abstr. 762).
11. Lewis, R. V., Stern, A., Rossier, J., Stein, S., and Udenfriend, S. (1979): Putative enkephalin precursors in bovine adrenal medulla. *Biochem. Biophys. Res. Commun.,* 89:822–829.
12. Li, C. H., and Chung, D. (1976): Isolation and structure of an untriakontapeptide with opiate activity from camel pituitary glands. *Proc. Natl. Acad. Sci. USA,* 73:1145–1148.
13. Ling, N., Burgus, R., and Guillemin, R. (1976): Isolation, primary structure, and synthesis of alpha-endorphin and gamma-endorphin, two peptides of hypothalamic-hypophysial origin with morphinomimetic activity. *Proc. Natl. Acad. Sci. USA,* 73:3942–3946.
14. Mains, R. E., Eipper, B. A., and Ling, N. (1977): Common precursor to corticotropins and endorphins. *Proc. Natl. Acad. Sci. USA,* 74:3014–3018.
15. Rivier, J. E. (1978): Use of trialkyl ammonium phosphate (TAAP) buffers in reverse-phase HPLC for high resolution and high recovery of peptides and proteins. *J. Liquid Chromatogr.,* 1:343–366.
16. Rubinstein, M., Stein, S., Gerber, L., and Udenfriend, S. (1977): Isolation and characterization of the opioid peptides from rat pituitary: β-Lipotropin. *Proc. Natl. Acad. Sci. USA,* 74:3052–3055.
17. Rubinstein, M., Stein, S., and Udenfriend, S. (1977): Isolation and characterization of the opioid peptides from rat pituitary: β-Endorphin. *Proc. Natl. Acad. Sci. USA,* 74:4969–4972.
18. Rubinstein, M., Stein, S., and Udenfriend, S. (1978): Characterization of pro-opiocortin, a precursor to opioid peptides and corticotropin. *Proc. Natl. Acad. Sci. USA,* 75:669–671.
19. Schultzberg, M., Lundberg, J. M., Hökfelt, T., Terenius, L., Brand, J., Elde, R. P., and Goldstein, M. (1978): Enkephalin-like immunoreactivity in gland cells and nerve terminals of adrenal-medulla. *Neuroscience,* 3:1169–1186.
20. Stein, S., Böhlen, P., Stone, J., Dairman, W., and Udenfriend, S. (1973): Amino acid analysis with fluorescamine at the picomole level. *Arch. Biochem. Biophys.,* 155:202–212.
21. Stern, A., Lewis, R. V., Kimura, S., Rossier, J., Gerber, L. D., Brink, L., Stein, S., and Udenfriend, S. (1979): Isolation of the opioid heptapeptide Met-enkephalin[Arg[6]-Phe[7]] from bovine adrenal medullary granules and striatum. *Proc. Natl. Acad. Sci. USA,* 76:6680–6683.
22. Udenfriend, S., Stein, S., Böhlen, P., Dairman, W., Leimgruber, W., and Weigele, M. (1972): Fluorescamine: A reagent for assay of amino acids, peptides, proteins, and primary amines in the picomole range. *Science,* 178:871–872.

Polypeptide Hormones, edited by
R. F. Beers, Jr. and E. G. Bassett.
Raven Press, New York © 1980.

11. Current Advances in Sequencing as Applied to the Structure Determination of Ribosomal Proteins

Brigitte Wittmann-Liebold

Max-Planck-Institute for Molecular Genetics, D-1000 Berlin-Dahlem 33, West Germany

INTRODUCTION

Knowledge of the primary structure of proteins is a prerequisite for understanding their functions and how they participate in biological processes at a molecular level. However, the sequence analysis of the proteins is still rather time-consuming and limitations in the techniques as well as in the isolation of the proteins can cause problems.

We have undertaken the task of determining the primary structures of the proteins derived from the *Escherichia coli* ribosome. This is essential for understanding the mechanism of protein biosynthesis. However, severe problems encountered in sequencing these proteins such as their limited yields and solubility, the high content of some amino acids (e.g., alanine, leucine, or lysine), the clustering of certain amino acids in some regions of the chains, the extremely basic character of some of them, and the occasional occurrence of unusual amino acids forced us to select new strategies and more sensitive sequencing techniques suitable for routine protein analysis.

The current advances made during the investigations on the ribosomal proteins are presented in this chapter and the advantages of the new techniques are briefly discussed. The recent results on the structures of the ribosomal proteins are also summarized.

NUMBER OF RIBOSOMAL PROTEINS

The number of ribosomal proteins has been found to be 50 to 60 in bacterial ribosomes and 70 to 80 in cytoplasmic ribosomes of eukaryotes. When the protein mixture extracted from *E. coli* ribosomes is separated by two-dimensional polyacrylamide gel electrophoresis, 21 spots (S1–S21) from the small and 34 spots (L1–34) from the large ribosomal subunit are detected (54). In the small subunit, the number of spots corresponds to the number of individual proteins (102), whereas in the large subunit the spot L8 was shown to consist of a complex of three proteins: L7/L12 and L10 (74). Furthermore, it was revealed by biochemical and immunological studies (85) that protein L26 from the large subunit is identical to protein S20 from the small subunit. It is likely that this protein is distributed between the two subunits when the 70S ribosome dissociates into its two subunits. Therefore, there are 32 individual proteins in the large subunit of the *E. coli* ribosome. Although one of them (L7) differs only in the presence of an acetyl group at its NH_2-terminus from L12 (93), we continue to regard L7 and L12 as two individual proteins.

PROTEIN ISOLATION

All *E. coli* ribosomal proteins have been isolated and characterized by chemical, physical, and immunological techniques. The first method of isolation was extraction of the proteins with 67% acetic acid from the ribosome and then separation by column chromatography on cellulose exchangers and by gel filtration in the presence of 6 M urea (100). A purification scheme is presented in Table 1. The proteins isolated in this way have been used mainly for molecular weight determinations and for immunological and biochemical studies (100,102). For these purposes this isolation method is superior to other procedures, such as the ones described below, as this method yields water-soluble protein samples that are completely salt free. They are more suitable for enzymatic digestions as higher cleavage rates can be obtained with soluble proteins. Furthermore, thin-layer techniques can be directly applied in the separation of the peptides, whereas traces of salts remaining after salt extractions of proteins interfere with migration of peptides on thin-layer plates. In our experience, a given protein may behave differently depending on the purification procedure chosen. Thus, precipitation or lyophilization may influence the subsequent behavior of the

TABLE 1. *Purification scheme of ribosomal proteins*

E. coli cells 100 g $\hat{=}$ 1.8 g 70S ribosomes		
1. Zonal centrifugation → subunits (sucrose gradients 7–38%)	30S + 50S ~300 mg 600 mg	
2. Separation RNA/proteins (66% acetic acid)	100 mg S-proteins, 200 mg L-proteins	
3. CM-cellulose column chromatography (6 M urea, pyridine acetate gradients)		
4. Gel filtration on Sephadex (15% acetic acid)		
5. Desalting on Biogel (15% acetic acid)		
6. Dialysis and storage (−20°C) (in 2% acetic acid)	S-proteins 1–3 mg L-proteins <2 mg	

protein and hence the sequence analysis even if the protein is desalted carefully. For instance, remaining traces of ammonium sulfate decrease the efficiency of an automated Edman degradation.

For physical studies of the ribosomal proteins, for example, circular dichroism (CD), nuclear magnetic resonance (NMR), shape determination, and crystallization (which require the maximal conservation of the native structure), a procedure has been developed that completely avoids the use of acetic acid, urea, and lyophilization (36). By washing ribosomal subunits with increasing concentrations of salts, for example, LiCl or NaCl, groups of proteins were removed and further fractionated by CM-Sephadex chromatography and gel filtration on Sephadex G-75 in buffers of high ionic concentrations but without urea. These proteins show a reversed solubility to those isolated by the acid-urea conditions (48) and are soluble at high salt concentrations and less soluble at low salt concentrations. This enables experiments to be performed under reconstitutive conditions (0.35 M salt) without the problems of protein precipitation. Many of the physical studies described below have been performed with proteins isolated by this gentler procedure. Furthermore, comparative studies have also been made with proteins isolated by the different methods.

The isolation of ribosomal proteins that are active in the reconstitution assay and in functional tests has recently been described (122). The isolation procedure consists of three steps: first, prefractionation by washing of 50S subunits with high concentrations of salt; second, gel filtration on Sephadex; and third, column chromatography on carboxymethyl cellulose in the presence of 6 M urea.

PRIMARY STRUCTURE OF *E. Coli* WILD TYPE RIBOSOMAL PROTEINS

The biochemical studies of ribosomal proteins until 1974 have been reviewed in some detail (102). Until then only the proteins S4 and L7/L12 had been sequenced completely.

The primary structures of 19 proteins from the small and of 29 proteins from the large subunit of the *E. coli* ribosome have now been determined (Table 2). In addition, the sequences of proteins L4 and L17 have been completed (Kimura et al., *unpublished results*). Elucidation of the remaining four proteins, namely, S1 and S2 from the small and L2 from the large subunit, is in progress. Determination of their sequences, with the possible exception of protein S1, can be expected in the very near future.

In addition to the 50 *E. coli* ribosomal proteins, the complete primary structure has been determined for the initiation factors IF-1 and IF-3 as well as for two proteins, NS1 and NS2, which tightly bind to native 30S subunits (Table 2). The latter two proteins are indistinguishable (91) from the proteins HU (83) and HD (7), which have been identified as DNA binding proteins.

The amino acid sequence analysis of the ribosomal proteins has been rendered more difficult by the occurrence of a number of modified amino acids in several of these proteins. Acetylation of the NH_2-terminus was identified in proteins

TABLE 2. E. coli ribosomal and related proteins whose primary structures have been determined

Protein	Amino acids	MW	References Wild type	Protein	Amino acid	MW	References Wild type
S3	232	25,852	13	L12	120	12,178	93
S4	203	23,137	84	L13	142	16,019	65
S5	166	17,515	112	L14	120	13,227	70
S6	135	15,704	49	L15	144	14,981	44
S7K	177	19,732	78	L16	136	15,296	20
S7B	153	17,131	78	L18	117	12,770	21
S8	129	13,996	2	L19	114	13,002	19
S9	128	14,569	24	L20	117	13,366	121
S10	(103)	(11,736)	127	L21	103	11,565	47
S11	128	13,728	28	L22	110	12,226	104
S12	123	13,606	43	L23	99	11,013	113
S13	117	12,968	59	L24	103	11,185	105
S14	(97)	(11,063)	126	L25	94	10,694	9,38
S15	87	10,001	69	L26	86	9,553	a
S16	82	9,191	96	L27	84	8,993	29
S17	83	9,573	124	L28	77	8,875	116
S18	74	8,896	123	L29	63	7,273	8
S19	91	10,299	125	L30	58	6,411	80
S20	86	9,553	117	L31	62	6,971	18
S21	70	8,369	95	L32	56	6,315	114
L1	233	24,599	12	L33	54	6,255	118
L3	209	22,258	71	L34	46	5,381	23
L5	178	20,171	27	IF-1	71	8,119	75
L6	176	18,832	25	IF-3	181	20,695	14
L7	120	12,206	93	NS1	90	9,225	66
L10	165	17,736	39,45	NS2	90	9,535	66
L11	141	14,874	37				

[a] Same as S20.

S5 (112), S18 (123), and L7 (93). Because of the blocked NH_2-termini, use of the sequenator was not possible for studies of the NH_2-terminal regions of these proteins and hence delayed the elucidation of their primary structure. The terminal amino acids of other proteins, namely, S11, L11, L16, L33, and IF-3, were found to be modified by methylation (Table 3).

Protein L11 is the most heavily methylated *E. coli* ribosomal protein. It contains nine methyl groups, namely, three at the NH_2-terminal amino acid, trimethylalanine, and six at the two internal trimethyllysines in positions 3 and 39, respectively (37). The occurrence of modified amino acids not at the NH_2-terminus but in the internal regions of the protein has also been demonstrated in several other proteins—namely, S12, L3, L7/L12, and L16 (Table 3). The modified amino acid in position 88 of S12 (43) is likely to be a derivative of aspartic acid, since the product of the Edman degradation step (22) gave a mass ion identical to that of aspartic acid, although it does not comigrate with this component in thin-layer chromatography. Furthermore, determination of the DNA sequence of this region revealed a triplet corresponding to aspartic acid as M. Nomura *(personal communication)* has reported. In some of the S12 mutants, an aspartic acid residue has been found in position 88 (43). The enzyme system modifying the aspartic acid residue in position 88 of the wild-type S12 protein apparently has become inactive in these mutants.

Since the DNA sequence has recently been determined for several genes of *E. coli* ribosomal proteins (76,77), it now is possible to compare the nucleotide sequences with the previously published amino acid sequences. There is complete agreement for most of the studied proteins, namely, L1, L7/L12, L11, L14, S11, and S12, whereas a few discrepancies remain for proteins S17 and L10. The sequence Arg-Pro-Cys in positions 63-65 of S17 differs from Cys-Arg-Pro, which was deduced from the DNA sequence. The sequence proposed for protein

TABLE 3. *Occurrence of modified amino acids in* E. coli *ribosomal proteins*

Protein	Position	Modified amino acid	Reference
S5	1	*N*-Acetylalanine	112
S11	1	*N*-Monomethylalanine	26,28
S12	88	Derivative of Asp	43[a]
S18	1	*N*-Acetylalanine	123
L3	150	N^5-Monomethylglutamine	71
L7	1	*N*-Acetylserine	93
L7/L12	81	N^ϵ-Monomethyllysine	93
L11	1	*N*-Trimethylalanine	37
L11	3	N^ϵ-Trimethyllysine	37
L11	39	Trimethyllysine	37
L16	1	*N*-Monomethylmethionine	20,26
L16	81	Derivative of Arg	20
L33	1	*N*-Monomethylalanine	26,118
IF-3	1	*N*-Monomethylmethionine	14

[a] See text.

L10 is in agreement with that of Heiland et al. (45), except that the glutamine in position 116 of L10 (which should be glutamic acid according to the DNA sequence) and the arginine residue in position 84 of L10 [which has independently been determined by two protein sequencing groups (39,45)] has not been found to correspond to a triplet in the DNA. Studies to resolve these discrepancies are in progress.

SEQUENCE DETERMINATION

The rapid progress in the elucidation of the primary structure of the ribosomal proteins was made possible by a number of improvements in the techniques for amino acid sequence analysis. Several major advances enable one to sequence proteins and peptides more quickly, more reliably, and with less material. These advances were:

(a) technical improvements of the Beckman liquid-phase sequencer (103,110), including the construction of an automated conversion device (111);

(b) improvements in the solid-phase sequencing technique (56,106,115);

(c) the application of mass spectrometry and high pressure liquid chromatography (89,128) to the identification of phenyl-thiohydantoin amino acids (PTH-amino acids);

(d) availability of more sensitive amino acid analyzers;

(e) isolation of peptides by thin-layer techniques and micro column procedures (30,49);

(f) introduction of a new reagent, namely, 4-N,N-dimethylaminoazobenzene-4'-isothiocyanate (DABITC) (22), for the manually performed Edman degradation method. Using the latter method, an amount of 2 to 8 nmoles of peptide or protein is enough to sequence 20 to 30 amino acid residues. This results in a 10- to 20-fold higher sensitivity as compared to previous techniques. Whereas 5 to 10 years ago elucidation of the primary structure required 50 to 200 mg of material, this can now be achieved with only a few milligrams.

LIQUID—PHASE EDMAN DEGRADATION

The spinning cup sequencing principle developed by Edman and Begg (34) is now widely used in sequence analysis of proteins and polypeptide fragments, and has become of major importance in sequencing laboratories. The advantages of automated liquid-phase degradations as compared with manual methods are obvious:

(a) the film technique, allowing higher repetitive yields;

(b) permanent nitrogen atmosphere;

(c) constant delivery of reagents and solvents;

(d) almost identical drying processes;

(e) less destruction of released amino acid derivatives; and

(f) full use of time after normal working hours.

In spite of these benefits, there are still some problems with this technique: the chemical and sequence specific limitations. More important, however, is inadequate technical design of the main parts of the sequencer. The following disadvantages have to be considered.

Disadvantages of the Beckman Sequencer

Sample Wash-out from the Sequencer Cup

Proteins and mainly peptides are extracted during the solvent washes. Therefore, the amounts of benzene and ethyl acetate delivered should be kept as low as possible. The optimal volume can be found easily by monitoring the pH of the effluent during the washes after the coupling stage. In our modified sequencer *(see below)*, 5 ml each of both solvents suffices to extract the residues of the reagent and of the quadrol. Furthermore, mechanical losses of protein occur during the drying of the film, when the change from one drying stage to another (restricted to rough, or rough to fine vacuum, respectively) is made too rapidly, caused by different efficiencies of the pumps.

Oxygen Penetration

Frequently leaks in the cup compartment or at the vacuum connections and valves (e.g., the bimba valve) allow the entry of oxygen, especially at the high vacuum stages. Further, the many inlets at the cup compartment (e.g., delivery lines, scoop, and thermistor) can be the source of problems. Future sequencers should be designed to minimize the number of such connections.

Constant Drying Processes

Constant drying processes can be achieved only if a prolonged, stable vacuum is provided. A means for preservation of the vacuum is a prerequisite for this stability. An accumulation of semi-volatile substances in the cup compartment or in vacuum lines and valves causes a lowering of repetitive degradative yields and an increase of by-product contamination of the amino acid derivatives.

Salt Formation

Cross-contamination of reagents and solvents and their leakage into the reaction chamber result in increasing contamination and thickness of the protein film thereby affecting the quality of the degradation.

Lack of Automated Conversion

The anilinothiazolinones are very oxygen-sensitive and their exposure to strong acids (together with traces of water)—as in the cleavage or conversion—causes destructive losses and deamidations. Therefore, it is necessary that the conversion and degradation occur simultaneously; this is possible if an automated device connected to the sequencer is used. However, this capability is lacking in the liquid-phase sequencer.

IMPROVEMENTS TO THE BECKMAN SEQUENCER

A standard Model 890 Beckman sequencer equipped with a normal cup (not undercut) was extensively modified (103,110,111) as summarized in the following:

(a) *The vacuum system* was redesigned completely. The restricted, rough, and fine vacuum functions of the Beckman 890, having three different outlets, two pumps, and three different vacuum valves (which are operated successively) were replaced by a two-stage vacuum drawn by a single pump (Alkatel 2030C). Only one outlet was kept, namely, the opening to the fine site, which leads directly to a newly-designed aluminum casing (Fig. 1). Two solenoid valves (Leybold-Heraeus) were placed in parallel in the branched lines; the one controlling the restricted vacuum connects the cup compartment and the vacuum source through a restriction of 0.5 mm × 1 cm (this is our "rough" vacuum, function 28). The second solenoid valve was mounted in the larger diameter line ("fine" vacuum, function 29). Further, two sensors to measure the difference in the vacuum at the cup and the pump site were installed on the casing, thus allowing the tightness of the casing and cup chamber to be tested. Drying of the protein film is achieved by (a) actuating the "rough" valve while delivering 1-sec pulses of nitrogen (function 26), every 30 sec for a total of 100 sec; (b) actuating only the "rough" valve for 100 to 200 sec; and (c) by actuating the "rough" and "fine" valves simultaneously (function 28 + 29) for 100 to 150 sec. The advantage of this vacuum system is that the complete cleaning of the vacuum casing and the vacuum lines is possible. The pulses of nitrogen are governed by a timer correlated with the free function 27.

The vacuum line includes a removable cooling trap made from glass that is connected to the vacuum lines by means of a stainless steel adapter, as shown in Fig. 2. The trap is immersed in a stainless steel liquid nitrogen dewar. It is emptied every 4 days (during the coupling reaction or at the end of a degradation cycle) and the casing is cleaned every month. The vacuum lines and connections are fabricated from stainless steel tubing having standard flanges (Leybold-Heraeus) that are tightened with special vitron-Teflon O-rings (Jaeger, Bietigheim). A second pump provides the vacuum for the fraction collector and the conversion device. The efficiency of the vacuum in the cup compartment during all degradation cycles is monitored on a chart recorder described previously (103). The vacuum values obtained at the end of every degradation cycle are usually at 2.7 or less Pa (20 millitorr) even if long runs are performed.

This improved vacuum system has reduced oxidative losses in the sequencer, eliminated the buildup of condensed material in the vacuum lines, and considera-

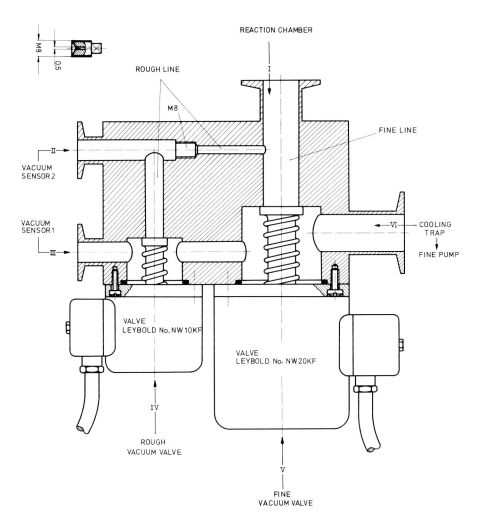

FIG. 1. Vacuum casing as installed in an improved Beckman sequencer. See text for details.

bly decreased the contaminations of the PTH-amino acids with by-products. The pulses of nitrogen during the first vacuum stages preserve the film and the released thiazolinones when it is still in liquid form. As a result, we think that this method of film preservation is superior to the nitrogen-feeding at the fine vacuum stage installed in the newer Beckman models.

(b) *A double-walled cup cover* (vacuum-tight up to 2.7 Pa) made from glass was installed. The constant temperature of 55°C for the cup compartment is provided by thermostated water that flows through the wall. At the top of this cover a Kel F adapter was inserted (Fig. 3). It contains three inlets for (a) a single delivery line *(see below)*, (b) the nitrogen line (N_2I, function 26) pressurizing the cup chamber, and (c) the scoop, fabricated from gold (Degussa,

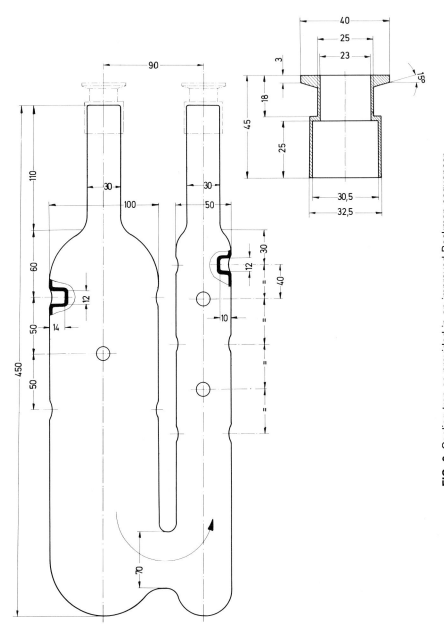

FIG. 2. Cooling trap as provided in an improved Beckman sequencer.

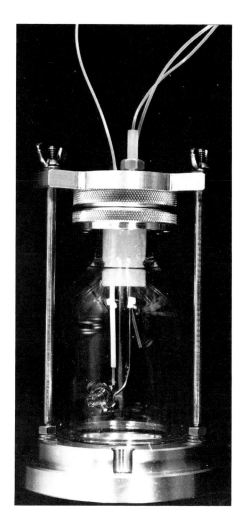

FIG. 3. A double-walled cup cover constructed to tighten the cup compartment in a Beckman sequencer. See text for details.

quality 999.9). The scoop is fixed in the vertical position and can be adjusted for positioning in the groove by turning. The heating system for the cup compartment provided in the Beckman unit is used as an additional heater.

(c) *Dead-volume free delivery valves* were installed to replace the Beckman reagent, solvent, nitrogen, waste, and collect valves in addition to the corresponding pilot valves. They are diaphragm valves (Fig. 4) and constructed from a Teflon manifold. This manifold contains a central zigzag bore with a single outlet for all reagents and solvents delivered into the cup. The various inlet lines from the bottles into the manifold are arranged in the following sequence: R3 (heptafluoric butyric acid, HFB), S3 (dichloroethane/benzene, 1:1), R1 (PITC, phenylisothiocyanate in heptane), R2 (quadrol-buffer), S1 (benzene), S2 (ethyl acetate), and N_2II (nitrogen, function 41). This nitrogen is situated

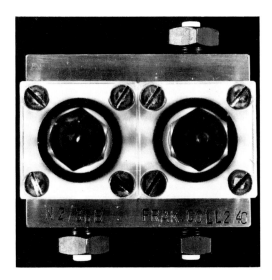

FIG. 4. Dead-volume free delivery valves (Type II) as constructed for an improved Beckman sequencer.

at the last position of this series and its valve is opened after every delivery of a reagent or solvent to empty the inner zigzag bore and the outer delivery line to the cup. The Teflon diaphragm valves are actuated pneumatically by means of three-way universal solenoid valves (Festo) connected to a 9×10^5 Pa compressed air supply to keep the membranes closed and a coarse vacuum to open them.

These diaphragm valves are the second type of valves designed and constructed in our laboratory. The first type, installed in our Beckman sequencer 7 years ago, was used for the NH_2-terminal studies on many of the ribosomal L-proteins (102,103). The earlier valves were also of a manifold arrangement but fabricated from Kel F. To close the delivery valves, small Teflon adapters were pushed into the delivery position (Fig. 5) by means of compressed air. The first type of valves required repolishing after several months use, as their movement caused slight surface abrasions. The newer style of valves have been service-free for three years, occupy much less space than the original Beckman valves, and are very inexpensive—as only Teflon and aluminum (used as a frame to maintain the manifold's shape) are needed. These valves are resistant to corrosive chemicals over long periods of time, remain free of abrasion, and can be used for all types of sequenators, synthesizers, or such.

(d) *The automated device* for the conversion of the anilinothiazolinones to the PTH-amino acids has been a component of our Beckman sequenator since 1972. It was initially used for the studies on the ribosomal S-proteins (103) and has remained unchanged; it is described in detail elsewhere (111). Positions 36 to 42 on the Beckman programmer were re-wired to relays to control the

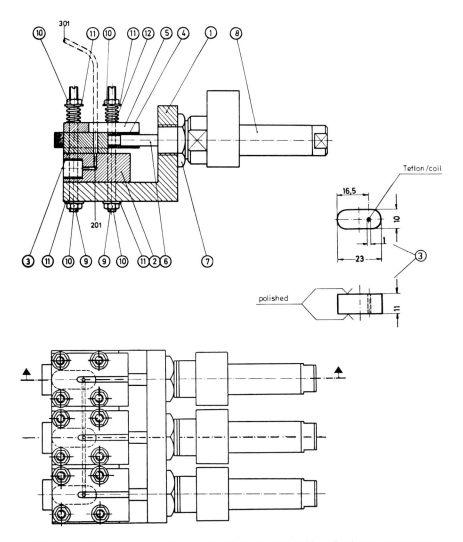

FIG. 5. Dead-volume free delivery valves (Type I) provided in a Beckman sequencer.

functions needed for the automated conversion. The delivery of the conversion medium R4 (20% aqueous trifluoric acid) and of the solvent R5 (dichloroethane/methanol, 7:3) (which dissolves the PTH amino acids and delivers them into the fraction collector) is made by diaphragm valves identical to those described above and arranged in series, namely, R4, R5, and N_2III (for nitrogen purging of the delivery line into the converter).

This device, especially constructed for the Beckman sequencer, has the advantage that the acid resulting from the conversion reaction can be quickly removed by means of a nitrogen purge (N_2IV). The optimal conversion time at 55°C in 20% TFA is 25 to 30 min, including the drying time. Normally, both S3 washes are collected and are used for the conversion. PTH-glutamine and PTH-asparagine free of desamidation and in good yields are obtainable under these conditions. Further, PTH-arginine and PTH-histidine need no special treatment prior to subsequent identification (without ethylacetate extraction).

SOLID-PHASE SEQUENCING

Polypeptide sequencing using this technique was introduced by R. A. Laursen (56). The peptide or protein is covalently bound to a resin that is then loaded into a micro column and the reagents and solvents used in the Edman degradation are rinsed through it. The advantages of this method can be summarized as follows:

(a) no wash-out of peptides;
(b) reagents and solvents are of analytical grade (sequenator grade not required);
(c) no problems of system leakage and decreased efficiency of pumps;
(d) inexpensively constructed equipment;
(e) low maintainance costs;
(f) easily operated by untrained personnel.

In 1970, we built the apparatus used for studies of the diverse peptides of the ribosomal proteins from plans of the original machine designed by Dr. Laursen because this type of sequencer was not available commercially. This machine still operates well and has not required modifications, although a dual column system capable of processing two peptides simultaneously was added. For test runs, comparative studies, and time saving, this accessory proved to be very beneficial. Temperature of the columns is maintained at 45°C by placing them in a block of aluminum.

After repeated solid-phase sequencing of ribosomal peptides, we have observed the following:

(a) The limitations of these techniques reside mainly in the attachment of the peptides to the resin.

(b) Selection of the optimal resin and method of attachment are very important. Peptides with a COOH-terminal lysine are best attached to an aminopolystyrene resin with p-phenylene-diisothiocyanate (DITC) at pH 8.5 to 9.5, the first method Laursen (56) described. All other peptides having a maximal length of 20 to 30 residues were attached at their COOH-terminal carboxyl group to aminopolystyrene by means of a water-soluble carbodiimide, [1-ethyl-3-(3-dimethylaminopropyl)-carbodiimide (EDC)] at pH 5.0 (106,115). The peptides used in this method were not protected and must be free of traces of acids. If the attachment is performed under relatively mild conditions (1 to 2 hr at 30°C), the COOH-terminal carboxyl groups react more quickly than those on the side chain. Unfortunately, a lower yield (30 to 50%) of released PTH-glutamic acid and aspartic acid is obtained. Additionally, introducing protecting groups onto small quantities (30 to 50 nanomoles) of starting peptide is not possible as by-products formed under this treatment interfere with the degradation. Peptides with more than 30 residues are better linked to porous glass supports, namely the DITC-glass prepared from CPG-10 glass (Serva: 220–400 mesh, 40–80 μm, pore size 75 Å) or from CPG-100 (Pierce: uncoated, 200–400 mesh, 37–74 μm) as described by Wachter et al. (98). For cyanogen bromide fragments, a method using TETA-resin (triethylenetetramine-polystyrene) has been successfully employed (57). Additional details of the various methods for attachment of peptides to a solid support are given elsewhere (57).

(c) The solubility of a certain peptide under the selected attachment conditions strongly influences the final yield. For instance, basic peptides that tend to precipitate at pH 8 to 9 are less firmly attached at this pH. To avoid this, the tryptic lysine-peptides of ribosomal proteins are frequently bound with EDC to the resin at a low pH. Further, salt contamination decreases the solubility of peptides and hence their attachment yield.

(d) During the cleavage stage of a resin-bound peptide, exposure to the acid (in most cases TFA is used) is a critical step. If short cleavage times (about 3 min) are employed, severe overlapping, caused by bulky amino acid residues, can result. During long exposures (about 10–15 min), the cleavage is almost complete and no significant overlapping is observed. However, in addition to the partial destruction of labile anilinothiazolinones, the peptide-resin linkage, the resin Si-O bonds, or an acid labile peptide bond (e.g., Asp-Pro) may be affected by the acid and, as a consequence, the yield of released amino acid derivative is significantly decreased. Most of our studies used a medium cleavage time of 8 min.

(e) Various buffer solutions employed in the coupling with PITC have also been used to degrade the resin-bound peptides. Lacking a proper swelling of the resin under the conditions used, poor degradation usually occurs. Instead of the morpholine/pyridine buffers used earlier, 2.5% triethanolamine in dimethylformamide, as proposed by E. Wachter *(personal communication),* was found to be superior as a coupling buffer in the apparatus.

CHEMICAL AND SEQUENCE-SPECIFIC PROBLEMS IN EDMAN DEGRADATIONS

The major problems of the chemistry of the Edman degradation can be summarized as follows:

(a) oxidative desulfuration of the phenylthiocarbamyl peptides resulting in the formation of a phenylcarbamyl peptide;

(b) incomplete reactions cause overlapping of amino acids with bulky side chains;

(c) increased background interference by random, acid-catalysed cleavage of peptide bonds;

(d) formation of aniline caused by water contamination of the PITC reagent and formation of thiourea and dithiourea derivatives;

(e) partial blocking of the free NH_2-terminal groups by contaminating anhydrides;

(f) aldehyde and peroxide contaminations of the reagents;

(g) destruction of the anilinothiazolinones and PTH-amino acids, thereby complicating quantitation of the degradations;

(h) problems of identification of the PTH-amino acids; and

(i) separation of the peptide or protein from by-products and residual reagents during degradation.

A number of sequence-specific difficulties resulting in a significant decrease in yield after degradation have been observed during analysis of the following sequences:

(a) Hydrophobic areas or repetitive sequence regions in which bulky residues occur strongly influence the degradation. As an example, the sequence Ala-Ala-Ala-Ala-Val-Ala-Val-Ala-Ala (positions 34 to 42) of the ribosomal protein L12 is cited. Another example of this type was the sequence found in the histone H_1 from sperm of the sea urchin *Parechinus angulosus* (90) (mainly alanine and lysine residues) that created background problems.

(b) Proline-proline sequences or proline adjacent to isoleucine or valine drastically decreases the yields of repetitive degradation as reported by Brandt et al. (11). Further examples occur in the partial sequences of ribosomal protein L11 (37): Pro-Ser-Pro-Pro-Val-Gly-Pro (positions 19–25), Leu-Pro-Ile-Pro-Val-Val-Ile-Thr-Val (positions 52–60), and Pro-Pro-Ala-Ala-Val-Val-Leu-Leu (positions 73–79).

These sequence areas can only be degraded if the cleavage step is repeated at least 3 to 4 times. Also, an arginine residue preceding a Pro-Ile or Pro-Pro sequence results in poor degradation. In the solid-phase technique, good performance can be tested by degrading bradykinin (Arg-Pro-Pro-Gly-Phe-Ser-Pro-Phe-Arg). If the cleavages are incomplete, poor yields of the third proline residue are obtained.

(c) Another problem arises when areas with a considerably high content of basic residues are analyzed. For instance, the NH_2-terminal sequence of protein L16 having the sequence Met-Leu-Gln-Pro-Lys-Arg-Thr-Lys-Phe-Arg-Lys-Met-His-Lys-Gly-Arg-Asn-Arg resulted in a much higher frequency of overlapping as compared with other ribosomal proteins. The same was observed with the NH_2-terminal sequence Met-Asp-Lys-Lys-Ser-Ala-Arg-Ile-Arg-Arg-Ala-Thr-Arg-Ala-Arg-Arg-Lys of protein L18.

(d) Similarly, the clustering of acidic residues, like Glu-Glu-Asp, affects the Edman degradation. In this case, repeated coupling has helped to overcome this problem.

MICROSEQUENCING

The minimal quantity of peptide required for this technique depends on the sensitivity of the detection methods utilized and on the quality of the degradation.

Minute amounts of peptide require a high quality performance of the sequenator in order to release the PTH-amino acids without impurities. Although the application of high-pressure liquid chromatography for the identification of the PTH-amino acids (89,128) permits their detection at picomole levels, the contaminants of the degradations are usually the limiting factors. Therefore, the need for a redesign of the sequenators so as to minimize the quantity of peptide to be sequenced became apparent.

In the future, the quantities of proteinaceous material available for sequencing studies may be limited and the routine techniques currently used for these purposes remain problematic. One remedy consists of adding polymeric carriers like Polybrene (50,55,72,92), or parvalbumin (81), or other blocked proteins during liquid-phase degradation to retain the peptide in the spinning cup. However, Polybrene itself is soluble in benzene and can be easily extracted if the quadrol program is used; in addition, Polybrene causes extra peaks in the high-pressure liquid chromatograms. The analysis of less than 10 to 30 nanomoles peptide in liquid-phase degradation is still risky and should not be considered as a simple routine analysis. On the other hand, 30 to 100 nmoles starting material can be degraded without further support if the sequencer has high performance characteristics. It is hoped that advances in sequenator design as well as increased accuracy of detection by HPLC will permit less than 30 nmoles of polypeptide to be routinely sequenced.

Microsequencing of the ribosomal peptides was recently performed manually using a double coupling: first with 4-N,N-dimethylaminoazobenzene-4'-isothiocyanate (DABITC), and followed by PITC to complete the coupling reaction (22). The advantage of this technique is that colored amino acid phenylthiohydantoin derivatives, as products, are directly visible (in the picomole range) on polyamide sheets, whereas the by-products of the degradation are only visible under ultraviolet light. The direct identification of the released derivatives permits an unambiguous recovery of the glutamines, asparagines, arginines, and histidines. Therefore, this method is a good alternative to the manually performed dansyl-Edman degradation. Furthermore, the amounts required in the newly developed technique are considerably smaller than those of the dansyl-Edman method. At present, the combined DABITC-PITC degradation technique for sequence studies on ribosomal proteins has been a routine method for more than a year.

ISOLATION OF PEPTIDES ON A MICRO SCALE

In the field of sequencing ribosomal proteins, the need for the isolation of nanomolar amounts of peptides evolved several new approaches. The strategy used in sequencing this class of proteins has been discussed in detail (106). The main advances were the development of a micro column system (see Fig. 6) for the separation of 4 to 6 mg protein hydrolysates with high resolution (2,30,45,49) and the purification of peptides by thin-layer chromatography techniques, performed one-dimensionally after gel filtrations on columns (loaded with 1 to 6 mg hydrolysate) or performed two-dimensionally on thin-layer finger-

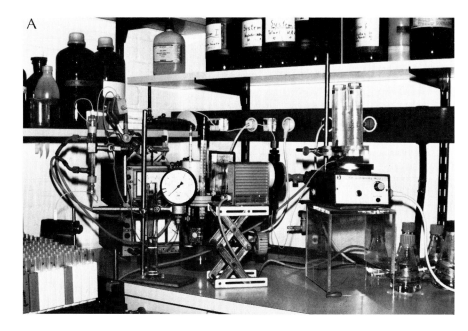

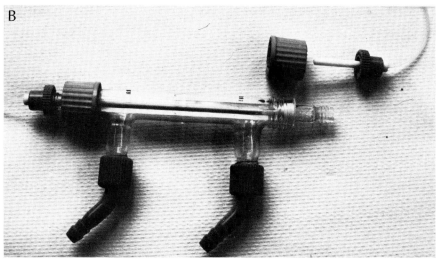

FIG. 6.A: Device for the isolation of peptides on a micro scale using Dowex 50 × 4 resin (200–400 mesh). **B:** The column (9 × 0.2 cm) for peptide separation on a micro scale.

prints after the application of 10 nmoles of protein hydrolysates (45,49). The peptides eluted from the thin-layer sheets are pure enough for further analysis (in the 1–2.5 nanomole range) on a high performance amino acid analyzer or they can directly be analyzed by manual sequencing. With the new DABITC-PITC degradation method, the quantity of peptide obtained from 3 to 5 fingerprints (5–10 nmoles) suffices for a complete sequencing of a short (15–20 residues) peptide. For solid-phase sequencing, one to two fractions of a micro column run (0.5 ml each) are enough to establish the entire sequence. These techniques helped to overcome separation problems attendant to the classic purification methods (such as paper chromatography) and further, significantly decreased the time required for sequence studies on the ribosomal proteins [for details see (106)].

COMPARISON OF THE SEQUENCE OF RIBOSOMAL PROTEINS FROM *E. Coli*

The knowledge of the primary structures of almost all proteins known to be present in the *E. coli* ribosome permits one to search for the existence of significant homologies among this set of proteins. If such homologies are observed, it would indicate that the ribosomal proteins are derived from a common ancestor. Therefore, the amino acid sequences of the *E. coli* ribosomal proteins (Table 2) were compared, using computer programs, in a search for identical regions. The numbers of identical tri-, tetra-, penta-, or hexapeptides obtained in this way were compared with the numbers obtained by performing the same comparison with completely unrelated proteins whose primary structures were taken from the literature, and also with artificial proteins that have the same amino acid compositions and lengths as the *E. coli* ribosomal proteins but whose amino acid sequences were randomly generated by a computer program. The frequency pattern of the occurrence of identical peptides was similar in all three cases: the native ribosomal proteins, their artificially generated isomers, and the unrelated proteins from the literature. Therefore, one can conclude that, with the exception of L7/L12 and S20/L26, there is no evidence of the existence of strong structural homologies among those *E. coli* ribosomal proteins studied (108), although in a few cases very weak homologies may be observed (45,96,107,117). This result is in good agreement with the conclusions drawn from immunological studies with antibodies against the individual *E. coli* ribosomal proteins, where no significant cross-reaction between any of the proteins was detected (86–88).

SEQUENCE ANALYSIS OF *E. Coli* MUTANT RIBOSOMAL PROTEINS

Many mutants of *E. coli* that have altered ribosomal proteins (as revealed by two-dimensional gel electrophoresis) have been isolated. Mutants are now available for almost all of the *E. coli* ribosomal proteins [see reviews (17) and (102)]. Most of these mutants have been isolated by techniques dependent on their temperature-sensitivity (32,33) or by their altered behavior towards antibiotics. A streptomycin-dependent strain was used in a very efficient manner for isolating ribosomal mutants from which mutations of a very large number of ribosomal proteins were obtained. In this way, mutants with alterations in each

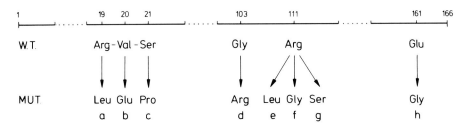

FIG. 7. Amino acid replacements in protein S5 of *E. coli* mutants. **a:** Spc[r-9]; **b:** spc[r-7]; **c:** spc[r-13]; **d:** N660; **e:** d1023 and N421; **f:** nea-314; **g:** nea-319; and **h:** 0–1 (in which the mutation resulted in a shortened peptide chain). (Data from ref. 101.)

of 50 proteins (i.e., 95% of those present in the *E. coli* ribosomes) have been isolated. There are mutants which harbor up to eight altered proteins in the same ribosome.

As reviewed (102), biochemical analyses have been carried out on 43 different mutants with alterations in proteins S4, S5, S6, S8, S12, S17, or L24 and whose amino acid replacements have been localized. Most of these studies were performed with the mutationally altered proteins S5 and S12. Figure 7 summarizes the amino acid replacements in protein S5 revealed to date. The amino acid exchanges in various spectinomycin-resistant mutants are clustered in positions 19–21 of this protein. Clustering of amino acid replacements has also been found in neamine-resistant mutants having an altered protein S5 and in erythromycin-resistant mutants bearing a protein L4 alteration. Details about these mutants appear elsewhere (101).

Figure 8 illustrates the amino acid exchange in protein S12. The following two points can be concluded from our biochemical studies:

(a) All replacements are clustered in only two short regions of protein S12, namely, in position 42 and within a region consisting of positions 85–91. No amino acid exchanges in any of the many mutants analyzed so far have been detected outside of these two short regions.

(b) The replacement of a single amino acid in protein S12 suffices to make

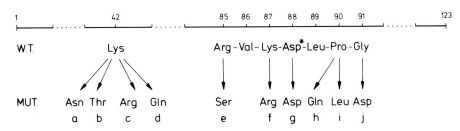

FIG. 8. Amino acid replacements in protein S12 of mutants of *E. coli*. **a:** SM-10, L44-1, L1-401; **b:** L44-2; **c:** SM-5, L11-His1; **d:** N421; **e:** d1023; **f:** SN-1, L44-4, L1-431; **g:** d1023, VT; **h:** nea-319; **i:** T776/39:3, T776/40:4, T779/25:3, nea-314; and **j:** N660. Asp* in position 88 is a derivative of aspartic acid. (Data from ref. 101.)

the ribosome streptomycin-resistant. Since it has been shown by reconstitution tests (73) that protein S12 alone confers the altered streptomycin resistance, it follows that the replacement of only one of the 8,000 amino acids present in the E. coli ribosome induces the altered ribosomal response to the antibiotic.

COMPARISONS BETWEEN THE AMINO ACID SEQUENCES OF RIBOSOMAL PROTEINS FROM E. Coli AND OTHER ORGANISMS

Compared with the approximately 50 completed sequences of ribosomal proteins from E. coli, little is known about the structure of ribosomal proteins from other organisms. The amino acid sequences of seven such proteins, namely, one from Bacillus subtilis (51,53), one from B. stearothermophilus, (Kimura et al., unpublished), three from yeast (52, and T. Itoh et al., unpublished), one from the brine shrimp Artemia salina (5), and one from rat liver ribosomes (A. Lin et al., unpublished) have been reported. Furthermore, partial sequences of ribosomal proteins are available from several bacterial species [(97) and reviewed in (63)], from yeast (3), from wheat germ (62), and from rat liver (4,109).

Three major points emerge from a number of the biochemical studies on these various proteins:

(a) The amino acid sequences of ribosomal proteins from bacterial species, e.g., E. coli and Bacillus subtilis (belonging to different families), show significant structural homologies. This is illustrated by the comparison of the complete primary structures of protein B-L9 from B. subtilis and proteins L7/L12 from E. coli (Fig. 9). More than 50% of the amino acid residues are identical in both proteins (51,53).

(b) The amino acid sequence of a ribosomal protein HL20 from the halophilic Halobacter cutirubrum resembles, in different regions, that of E. coli proteins L7/L12 and Artemia salina protein eL12 (5,63), whereas there is little homology between the E. coli and the Artemia protein (5,53). Thus, the halophile Halobacter

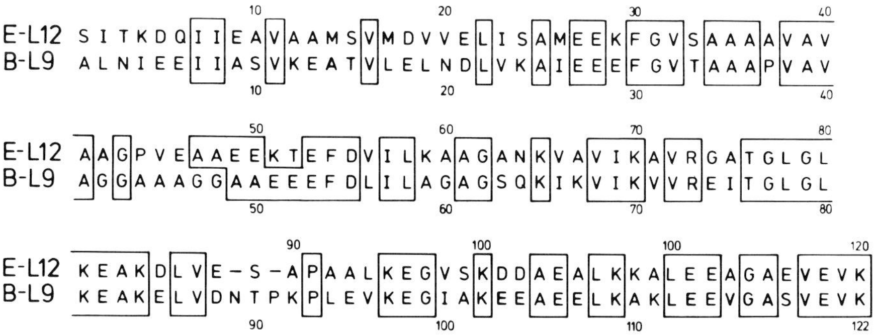

```
                    10                  20                  30                  40
E-L12  S I T K D Q I I E A V A A M S V M D V V E L I S A M E E K F G V S A A A A V A V
B-L9   A L N I E E I I A S V K E A T V L E L N D L V K A I E E E F G V T A A A P V A V
                    10                  20                  30                  40

                    50                  60                  70                  80
E-L12  A A G P V E A A E E K T E F D V I L K A A G A N K V A V I K A V R G A T G L G L
B-L9   A G G A A A G G A A E E E F D L I L A G A G S Q K I K V I K V V R E I T G L G L
                    50                  60                  70                  80

                    90                 100                 100                 120
E-L12  K E A K D L V E - S - A P A A L K E G V S K D D A E A L K K A L E E A G A E V E V K
B-L9   K E A K E L V D N T P K P L E V K E G I A K E E A E E L K A K L E E V G A S V E V K
                    90                 100                 110                 122
```

FIG. 9. Comparison of the primary structures of E. coli protein E-L12 and B. subtilis protein B-L9. Abbreviations for the amino acids are the one-letter code.

has an interesting phylogenetic position with properties of both prokaryotes and eukaryotes.

(c) The amino acid sequence of the few yeast ribosomal proteins studied to date exhibits some homologies with the sequence of other eukaryotic ribosomal proteins, e.g., from *Artemia salina* (3,5) or from rat liver (52,109). However, only a very low degree of sequence homology, if any, has been detected between ribosomal proteins from *E. coli* and those from yeast, *Artemia,* or rat (5,52, 97,109). It is possible that knowledge of the spatial structure of these proteins would show a higher degree of homology than examination of the primary structure permits. Interestingly, the phylogenetic relationship among various eukaryotic species, e.g., yeast and rat, is (at least as far as the primary structure of ribosomal proteins is concerned) greater than between a unicellular eukaryote (yeast) and a unicellular prokaryote *(E. coli).*

SECONDARY STRUCTURE

Prediction of Secondary Structure

On the basis of the known amino acid sequences, the secondary structures of ribosomal proteins have been predicted (40,41,119,120). Four different predictive methods were used to calculate the conformational states such as α-helix, extended structure, random coil, and turn or bend. An example is shown in Fig. 10. When at least three of the four prediction methods were in agreement with the conformational state of the amino acid residues, this was taken to indicate a high probability of this particular structure occurring in this region of the sequence.

The results on the prediction of the secondary structures show that each of the ribosomal proteins studied has a unique secondary structure that differs from that of all other proteins. The α-helix content of many proteins ranges between 20 and 40%. Several proteins (e.g., S20, L7/L12, and L29) have a high, while others (e.g., S12 and L27) have a low α-helix content. The values predicted for extended structure are low, i.e., less than 20%, for all proteins, whereas those for turns range between 10 and 30% for most proteins. A comparison of these predictive values with those experimentally determined is given elsewhere (101).

It is possible to construct, by the use of computer graphics, models of the

FIG. 10. Secondary structures of the homologous proteins B-L9 of *B. subtilis* **(top)** and EC-L12 of *E. coli* **(bottom),** as predicted according to four different methods. The symbols represent residues in helical (𝟃 𝟃), turn or bend (⌐⌐), extended (W), and coil (—) conformational states. The line "PRE" summarizes the secondary structure obtained when at least three out of the four predictions are in agreement. The percentage values for helix, turns, etc. symbolized in line PRE for the proteins sequenced to date are found in ref. 101. The amino acid sequence (one-letter code) of proteins BS-L9 and EC-L12 is shown at the bottom. For details see ref. 41.

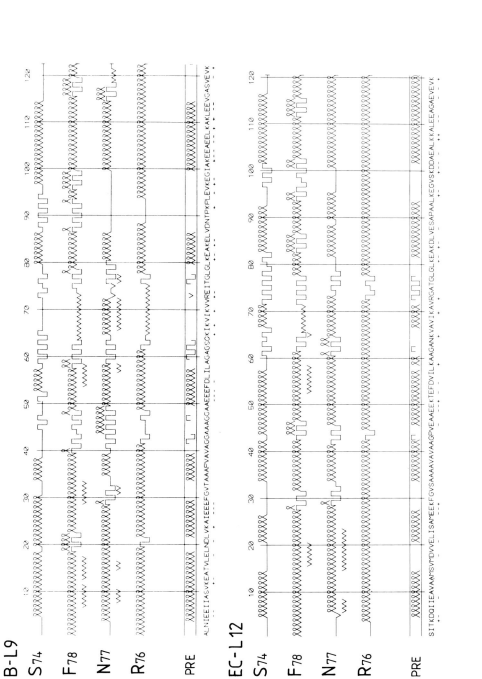

ribosomal proteins based on these prediction methods; more information, how-ever, is needed to construct a feasible three-dimensional model. This information can be obtained—in the absence of crystallographic data—from proton magnetic resonance data that could provide information as to the folding of the protein chain and from intramolecular cross-linking studies.

Circular Dichroism

Circular dichroism (CD) studies have provided information about the second-ary structure of the ribosomal proteins.

Early experiments examined a mixture of proteins and it was generally con-cluded that both in the ribosomal and in the isolated (usually by acetic acid extraction) state, the proteins contained ~25% α-helix in addition to some β-pleated sheets and random coil conformation. Similar measurements on the proteins L7/L12 have shown these values varying from 45 to 60%.

The CD spectra of proteins S3, S4, S6, S7, and S8 gave α-helix values ranging from 18% for S6 to 50% for S7, with an average of 18% β-structure. A change, resulting from alteration of structure, was observed upon heating to 42°C. Other investigators have studied S4 and reported values of 26 to 32% α-helix, little or no β-structure, and 32% α-helix; a β-structure value of 14% has been cited. Additional details are given elsewhere (101).

It has been suggested that the CD spectra of ribosomal proteins examined free in solution represent a unique conformation that is different from their conformation in the ribosome. This suggestion was prompted by subtraction of the CD spectrum of the rRNA from that of the total ribosome.

Unfortunately, in many CD measurements there is a great deal of variation in the method of preparing the ribosomal proteins. When proteins prepared with acetic acid and urea (48) were used for CD studies (46), it was found that most of them contained relatively low levels of ordered structure. In this case, it was not possible to use either the method of Rosenkranz and Scholtan (82) or that of Chen et al. (31) in order to calculate values of α-helix, β-pleated sheet, and random coil.

The CD spectra of all proteins that were prepared by the recently developed salt extraction method (35,60) show higher α-helix values than those of the urea-acetic acid extracted proteins described above (J. A. Littlechild and J. Dijk, *personal communication*). The salt extracted proteins did not show signifi-cant differences in secondary structure when changing the salt concentration over the range of 5 to 300 mM salt (potassium fluoride) in contrast to the behavior of the histone proteins [see (10)]. When the salt extracted ribosomal proteins are dialyzed with 6 M urea/methylamine at pH 7.0 and then re-dialyzed with a phosphate buffer containing 0.3 M potassium fluoride, the same CD spectra as seen before this treatment are obtained for several of the ribosomal small subunit proteins. This implies that, in these cases, exposure to urea at pH 7.0 will unfold the protein and allow refolding into the same secondary structure upon dialysis with a "reconstitution type" buffer (J. A. Littlechild and A. M. Freund, *personal communication*). It is clear from these studies that the proteins isolated by the gentler procedure contain more ordered structure than those prepared by harsher methods.

TERTIARY STRUCTURE

Information concerning the tertiary structure of the ribosomal proteins in solution was obtained by Proton Magnetic Resonance (PMR) [reviewed in (101)] and except for S4 and S16 they showed little tertiary structure. A greater number of shifted resonances (indicating more tertiary structure) were observed on examination of the salt extracted proteins. These studies have recently been extended to proteolytic-resistant "cores" of some of the proteins, as in case of protein S4 (61), which was found to retain at least some of the functions of the intact protein.

Microcalorimetry has also been used to examine the tertiary folding of these molecules during the process of heat denaturation. In addition, fluorimetric studies have been performed on some of the tryptophan-containing proteins, e.g., S4 and S7. Recent fluorescence polarization analyses of protein S1 have suggested that it contains at least two domains that can rotate independently; this is in agreement with low-angle X-ray scattering studies of S1 [reviewed in (101)].

Parallel to these investigations, great effort has been made to crystallize the ribosomal proteins. Crystals of a COOH-terminal fragment of protein L7/L12 have been reported by Liljas and co-workers (58); more recently orthorhombic crystals with a space group $P_{2_12_12}$ diffracting to a resolution of 3.5 Å have been obtained from the first intact ribosomal protein B-L17 (6). This protein is derived from *Bacillus stearothermophilus* whose proteins appear to have a "tighter" structure.

SHAPE OF RIBOSOMAL PROTEINS

Low-angle X-ray scattering, neutron scattering and sedimentation, viscosity, and diffusion studies have been employed to elucidate the structure and shape

TABLE 4. *Low angle X-ray scattering of ribosomal proteins*

Protein	$R_g{}^a$(Å)	Protein	$R_g{}^a$(Å)
S1	60–80	S16	21
S3	31	S20	27
S4	26–42	L11	34
S7	27	L7/12	36–41
S8	23	L18	26
S15	26	L25	24

[a] Radius of gyration.

TABLE 5. *Hydrodynamic studies of ribosomal proteins*

Protein	Axial ratio[a]	Protein	Axial ratio[a]	Protein	Axial ratio[a]
S1	10	S15	5.5	L6	4.6
S2	6	S17	3.8	L9	5.0
S3	5.5	S18	10	L7/12	>10
S5	7	S20	6.3	L11	4.5
S6	3.8	S21	8.7	L24	3.2
S8	2.3	L1	5.5	L25	4.0
S13	2.0	L3	5.8	L30	3.2

[a] The axial ratio in relation to unity.

of ribosomal proteins in solution. The scattering curves of many of the proteins so examined indicate that S1, S18, and L7/L12 have elongated shapes, whereas others (S8, etc.) were found to be more globular. The results obtained are summarized in Tables 4 & 5; experimental details are provided elsewhere (101).

CROSS-LINKING OF RIBOSOMAL COMPONENTS

Protein-protein cross-linking techniques have been used for a number of years establishing the topography of the *E. coli* ribosome [see reviews (15,16)]. This principle has now been extended to include the RNA-protein and RNA-RNA cross-linking within ribosomal subunits. However, it has become clear that an identification of the ribosomal components involved in the cross-linkage is no longer sufficient to provide useful structural information. The complexity of the ribosomal particles, and in particular the elongated shapes of many of the proteins, demand that the cross-linking analysis be pursued to the level of determining the specific amino acids or nucleotides that are cross-linked.

In the case of protein-protein cross-linking, this determination has been accomplished for proteins S5 and S8 that are cross-linked by dimethyl (^{14}C)-suberimidate in the 30S subunit. After its isolation, the protein pair was digested with trypsin and the two peptides involved in the cross-linkage were purified. Sequence analysis established that the lysine residue in position 166 of protein S5 was cross-linked to lysine 93 in protein S8 (1). Therefore, the distance between these two amino acids within the 30S subunit cannot exceed 8 Å, i.e., the length of the bifunctional reagent dimethyl suberimidate (Fig. 11).

The studies primarily concerned with RNA-protein cross-linking have been divided into two parts, namely, a search for suitable bifunctional reagents and the development of methodology for the detailed analysis of the cross-linking points.

This latter problem has been approached using a simple cross-linking system in which protein S7 (and no other protein) is covalently linked to 16S RNA of the 30S subunit by low doses of ultraviolet irradiation (67). To analyze the cross-linked peptide, a ^{32}P-labeled S7-oligonucleotide complex is isolated, and,

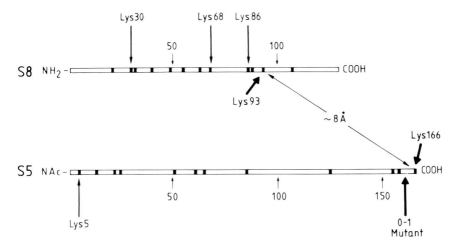

FIG. 11. Protein-protein cross-linking in the *E. coli* ribosome. Amino acid residue Lys-93 of protein S8 cross-linked by dimethylsuberimidate (length: 8 Å) to amino acid residue Lys-166 of protein S5.

after digestion with trypsin, a labeled peptide can be positively identified, followed by a determination of its amino acid content and sequence (68).

For the cross-linked oligonucleotide, a ribonucleoprotein fragment (containing the cross-linked protein) is first isolated. This RNP fragment is then applied to a special polyacrylamide gel system in the presence of a non-ionic detergent, thereby deproteinizing the fragment and at the same time separating RNA from the cross-linked RNA-protein complex. The latter can be isolated, subjected to fingerprint analysis, and its position in the 16S RNA sequence determined. The results showed an RNA region from which a single characteristic oligonucleotide was absent; this oligonucleotide was confirmed, as by direct analysis of the short oligonucleotide remaining attached to the protein as containing the site of cross-linking (129). Further studies established that the uracil residue in position 1239 of the 16S RNA is cross-linked to methionine-114 in protein S7 (130). Therefore, these two points must be in close contact within the 30S subunit (Fig. 12).

The methods just mentioned were developed for the purpose of their application to the cross-linking by bifunctional chemical reagents, where it would be expected that several proteins are simultaneously cross-linked to the RNA within the 30S particle. It is also important to note that the methodology requires that (a) the cross-linkage remain intact throughtout the analysis, and (b) therefore, reversible cross-linking reagents are of no advantage in this type of experiment. The small, symmetrical compound, *bis*-(2-chloroethyl)-amine, was found to be a suitable bifunctional reagent and led to the stable cross-linking of a number of proteins to RNA within intact 30S and 50S subunits in reasonable yield at low concentrations of reagent under physiological conditions (94). Some

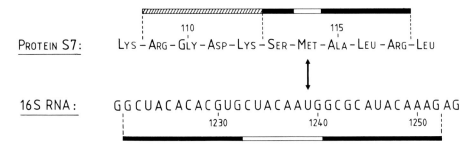

FIG. 12. RNA-protein cross-linking in the *E. coli* ribosome. Amino acid residue Met-114 of protein S7 cross-linked by ultraviolet irradiation to nucleotide U-1239 in the 16S RNA.

of these proteins have been identified on two-dimensional gels, and the stability of the cross-linkage can be demonstrated by the use of ^{32}P-labeled subunits, in which case the isolated cross-linked proteins contain a ^{32}P-label. The methodology described above is currently being applied to identify the cross-linking sites of several of these proteins (79).

Due to its symmetry, *bis*-(2-chloroethyl)-amine should also be able to form RNA-RNA cross-linkages. This has been found to be the case as demonstrated by Zwieb et al. (131) by the cross-linkage of 16S and 23S RNA within the 70S ribosome. Other reagents for both RNA-protein and RNA-RNA cross-linking are currently being developed. One of them, 1,4-phenyl-diglyoxal, has been used in the identification of an intramolecular cross-link between guanosine-2 and guanosine-112 in the stem region of the 5S RNA molecule (99).

Because the sequences of the 5S RNA and of the three proteins (L5, L18, and L25) that bind to that RNA are known (42), this RNA-protein complex is an excellent system for studying the interaction of its components. The sites at which the three proteins bind to the 5S RNA of *E. coli* and *Bacillus stearother-mophilus* have been identified. Neutron scattering analyses of the 5S RNA cross-linked to the L18 or L25 protein showed that the RNA and the protein portions of the complex are almost equally distributed and that the mass-centers of both proteins are separated by 115 Å (64). Binding of the proteins to the 5S RNA significantly alters its conformation as revealed by oligonucleotide binding studies.

CONCLUSIONS

Recently, protein chemists have become more interested in micro scale approaches for sequencing proteins. Several years ago, investigations on their primary structure were limited to cases where sufficient quantities were available. Many proteins cannot be obtained in sufficient amounts to allow the application of classic investigations on their structure or functional role.

For several years a considerable effort has been devoted to the determination of the primary structures of the *E. coli* ribosomal proteins. Because only minute amounts of them were available in purified form, initially this goal seemed to be nearly impossible. However, new techniques such as the automated degradations, the use of higher performance of amino acid analyzers, and newly developed methods for the purification of proteins and their peptides enabled such an approach to be realized. This has resulted in the complete sequence elucidation of 50 of these proteins, as well as of some related proteins, listed in Table 2.

The application of the improved techniques has also accelerated the determination of the primary structure of the ribosomal proteins from several other organisms, and has facilitated studies for which efficient and sensitive methods for sequence analysis of peptides or proteins are essential, the elucidation of the amino acid alterations in mutant proteins, the identification of cross-linkages on a molecular level, and the isolation of large protein fragments for use in antibody production.

This chapter is primarily concerned with those advances in the methodology which were found to be sensitive and practicable enough for a routine analysis of various proteins in the nanomole range. Several other methods proposed in the literature have not yet been applied or do not seem sufficiently reliable to risk the minute quantities of isolated peptide material. Further progress toward sequencing in the picomole range may be foreseen in the future.

REFERENCES

1. Allen, G., Capasso, R., and Gualerzi, C. (1979): Identification of the amino acid residues of proteins S5 and S8 adjacent to each other in the 30S ribosomal subunit of *Escherichia coli*. *J. Biol. Chem.*, 254:9800–9806.
2. Allen, G., and Wittmann-Liebold, B. (1978): The amino acid sequence of the ribosomal protein S8 of *Escherichia coli*. *Hoppe Seyler's Z. Physiol. Chem.*, 359:1509–1525.
3. Amons, R., van Agthoven, A., Pluijms, W., Möller, W., Higo, K., Itoh, T., and Osawa, S. (1977): A comparison of the amino terminal sequence of the L7/L12-type proteins of *Artemia salina* and *Saccharomyces cerevisiae*. *FEBS Lett.*, 81:308–310.
4. Amons, R., van Agthoven, A., Pluijms, W., and Möller, W. (1978): A comparison of the alanine-rich sequences of the L7/L12-ribosomal proteins from rat liver, *Artemia salina* and *Escherichia coli*, with the amino-terminal region of the alkali light chain A_1 from rabbit myosin. *FEBS Lett.*, 86:282–284.
5. Amons, R., Pluijms, W., and Möller, W. (1979): The primary structure of ribosomal protein eL12/eL12-P *from Artemia salina* 80S ribosomes. *FEBS Lett.*, 104:85–89.
6. Appelt, K., Dijk, J., and Epp, O. (1979): The crystallization of protein B-L17 from the 50S ribosomal subunit of *Bacillus stearothermophilus*. *FEBS Lett.*, 103:66–70.
7. Berthold, V., and Geider, K. (1976): Interaction of DNA with DNA-binding proteins. *Eur. J. Biochem.*, 71:443–449.
8. Bitar, K. G. (1975): The primary structure of the ribosomal protein L29 from *Escherichia coli. Biochim. Biophys. Acta*, 386:99–106.
9. Bitar, K. G., and Wittmann-Liebold, B. (1975): The primary structure of the 5S rRNA binding protein L25 of *Escherichia coli* ribosomes. *Hoppe Seyler's Z. Physiol. Chem.*, 356:1343–1352.
10. Bradbury, E. M., Hjelm, R. P., Carpenter, B. G., Baldwin, J. P., and Keale, G. G. (1977): Histone interactions and chromatin structure. In: *Nucleic Acid—Protein Recognition*, edited by H. J. Vogel, pp. 117–137. Academic Press, New York.
11. Brandt, W. F., Edman, P., Henschen, A., and von Holt, C. (1976): Abnormal behavior of proline in the isothiocyanate degradation. *Hoppe Seyler's Z. Physiol. Chem.*, 357:1505–1508.
12. Brauer, D., and Öchsner, I. (1978): The primary structure of protein L1 from the large ribosomal subunit of *Escherichia coli*. *FEBS Lett.*, 96:317–321.
13. Brauer, D., and Röming, R. (1979): The primary structure of protein S3 from the small subunit of *Escherichia coli* ribosomes. *FEBS Lett.*, 106:352–357.

14. Brauer, D., and Wittmann-Liebold, B. (1977): The primary structure of the initiation factor IF-3 from *Escherichia coli. FEBS Lett.,* 79:269–275.

15. Brimacombe, R. (1978): The structure of the bacterial ribosome. *Symp. Soc. Gen. Microbiol.,* 28:1–26.

16. Brimacombe, R., Nierhaus, K. H., Garrett, R. A., and Wittmann, H. G. (1976): The ribosome of *Escherichia coli. Progr. Nucleic Acid Res. Mol. Biol.,* 18:1–44.

17. Brimacombe, R., Stöffler, G., and Wittmann, H. G. (1978): Ribosome structure. *Annu. Rev. Biochem.,* 47:217–303.

18. Brosius, J. (1978): Primary structure of *Escherichia coli* ribosomal protein L31. *Biochemistry,* 17:501–508.

19. Brosius, J., and Arfsten, U. (1978): Primary structure of protein L19 from the large subunit of *Escherichia coli* ribosomes. *Biochemistry,* 17:508–516.

20. Brosius, J., and Chen, R. (1976): The primary structure of protein L16 located at the peptidyl-transferase center of *E. coli* ribosomes. *FEBS Lett.,* 68:105–109.

21. Brosius, J., Schiltz, E., and Chen, R. (1975): The primary structure of the 5S RNA binding protein L18 from *Escherichia coli* ribosomes. *FEBS Lett.,* 56:359–361.

22. Chang, J. Y., Brauer, D., and Wittmann-Liebold, B. (1978): Micro-sequence analysis of peptides and proteins using 4-*N,N*-dimethylaminoazobenzene-4'-isothiocyanate/phenylisothiocyanate double coupling method. *FEBS Lett.,* 93:205–214.

23. Chen, R. (1976): The sequence determination of a protein in a micro-scale: The sequence analysis of ribosomal protein L34 of *E. coli. Hoppe Seyler's Z. Physiol. Chem.,* 357:873–886.

24. Chen, R. (1977): Sequence determination of protein S9 from the *E. coli* ribosome. *Hoppe Seyler's Z. Physiol. Chem.,* 358:1415–1430.

25. Chen, R., Arfsten, U., and Chen-Schmeisser, U. (1977): The primary structure of protein L6 from the aminoacyl-tRNA binding site of the *E. coli* ribosome. *Hoppe Seyler's Z. Physiol. Chem.,* 358:531–535.

26. Chen, R., Brosius, J., Wittmann-Liebold, B., and Schäfer, D. (1977): Occurrence of methylated amino acids as N-termini of proteins from *E. coli* ribosomes. *J. Mol. Biol.,* 111:173–181.

27. Chen, R., and Ehrke, G. (1976): The primary structure of the 5S RNA binding protein L5 of *Escherichia coli* ribosomes. *FEBS Lett.,* 69:240–245.

28. Chen, R., Kamp, R., and Wittmann-Liebold, B. (1980): The primary structure of protein S11 from the small subunit of the *Escherichia coli* ribosome *(submitted).*

29. Chen, R., Mende, L., and Arfsten, U. (1975): The primary structure of protein L27 from the peptidyl-tRNA binding site of *Escherichia coli* ribosomes. *FEBS Lett.,* 59:96–99.

30. Chen, R., and Wittmann-Liebold, B. (1975): The primary structure of protein S9 from the 30S subunit of *Escherichia coli* ribosomes. *FEBS Lett.,* 52:139–140.

31. Chen, J.-H., Yang, J. T., and Martinez, H. M. (1972): Determination of the secondary structures of proteins by circular dichroism and optical rotatory dispersion. *Biochemistry,* 11:4120–4131.

32. Dabbs, E. R. (1978): Mutational alterations in 50 proteins of the *E. coli* ribosome. *Mol. Gen. Genet.,* 165:73–78.

33. Dabbs, E. R. (1978): Kasugamycin-dependent mutants of *E. coli. J. Bacteriol.,* 136:994–1001.

34. Edman, P., and Begg, G. (1977): A protein sequenator. *Eur. J. Biochem.,* 1:80–91.

35. Dijk, J., and Ackermann, I. (1980): The isolation of "native" ribosomal proteins from *Escherichia coli* under non-denaturing conditions. II. Purification of proteins from the 50S subunit. *J. Biol. Chem. (in press).*

36. Dijk, J., and Littlechild, J. (1979): Purification of ribosomal proteins from *Escherichia coli* under non-denaturing conditions. *Methods Enzymol.,* 49:481–502.

37. Dognin, M. J., and Wittmann-Liebold, B. (1977): The primary structure of L11, the most heavily methylated protein from *E. coli* ribosomes. *FEBS Lett.,* 84:342–346.

38. Dovgas, N. U., Markova, L. F., Mednikova, T. A., Vinkurov, L. M., Alakhov, Y. B., and Ovchinnikov, Y. A. (1975): The primary structure of the 5S RNA binding protein L25 from *Escherichia coli* ribosomes. *FEBS Lett.,* 53:351–354.

39. Dovgas, N. U., Vinukurov, L. M., Velmoga, I. S., Alakhov, Y. B., and Ovchinnikov, Y. A. (1976): The primary structure of protein L10 from *Escherichia coli* ribosomes. *FEBS Lett.,* 67:58–61.

40. Dzionara, M., Robinson, S. M. L., and Wittmann-Liebold, B. (1977): Prediction for secondary structures of ten proteins from the 50S subunit of the *Escherichia coli* ribosome. *J. Supramol. Struct.,* 7:191–204.

41. Dzionara, M., Robinson, S. M. L., and Wittmann-Liebold, B. (1977): Secondary structures

of proteins from the 30S subunits of the *Escherichia coli* ribosome. *Hoppe Seyler's Z. Physiol. Chem.,* 358:1003–1019.

42. Erdmann, V. A. (1976): Structure and function of 5S and 5.8S RNA. *Progr. Nucleic Acid Res. Mol. Biol.,* 18:45–90.

43. Funatsu, G., Yaguchi, M., and Wittmann-Liebold, B. (1977): Primary structure of protein S12 from the small *E. coli* ribosomal subunit. *FEBS Lett.,* 73:12–17.

44. Giorginis, S., and Chen, R. (1977): The primary structure of protein L15 located at the peptidyltransferase center of *E. coli* ribosomes. *FEBS* 84:347–350.

45. Heiland, I., Brauer, D., and Wittmann-Liebold, B. (1976): Primary structure of protein L10 from the large subunit of *E. coli* ribosomes. *Hoppe Seyler's Z. Physiol. Chem.,* 357:1751–1770.

46. Heiland, I., and Snatzke, G. (1979): CD-Spectroskopie zur Bestimmung der Sekundärstruktur ribosomaler Proteine von *E. coli. Hoppe Seyler's Z. Physiol. Chem.,* 360:279–280.

47. Heiland, I., and Wittmann-Liebold, B. (1979): The amino acid sequence of ribosomal protein L21 of *E. coli. Biochemistry,* 18:4605–4612.

48. Hindennach, I., Kaltschmidt, E., and Wittmann, H. G. (1971): Ribosomal proteins. X. Isolation of proteins from 50S ribosomal subunits of *E. coli. Eur. J. Biochem.,* 23:7–11.

49. Hitz, H., Schäfer, D., and Wittmann-Liebold, B. (1977): Determination of the complete amino acid sequence of protein S6 from the wild-type and a mutant of *E. coli. Eur. J. Biochem.,* 75:497–512.

50. Hunkapiller, M. W., and Hood, L. E. (1978): Direct microsequence analysis of polypeptides using an improved sequenator, a nonprotein carrier (Polybrene) and high pressure liquid chromatography. *Biochemistry,* 17:2124–2133.

51. Itoh, T., and Wittmann-Liebold, B. (1978): The primary structure of *Bacillus subtilis* acidic ribosomal protein B-L9 and its comparison with *E. coli* proteins L7/L12. *FEBS Lett.,* 96:392–394.

52. Itoh, T., and Wittmann-Liebold, B. (1978): The primary structure of protein 44 from the large subunit of yeast ribosomes. *FEBS Lett.,* 96:399–402.

53. Itoh, T., and Wittmann-Liebold, B. (1980): The primary structure of *Bacillus subtilis* acidic ribosomal protein B-L9. Isolation and characterization of peptides and complete amino acid sequence. *J. Biochem. (Tokyo),* 87:1185–1201.

54. Kaltschmidt, E., and Wittmann, H. G. (1970): Ribosomal proteins, XII: Number of proteins in small and large ribosomal subunits of *E. coli* as determined by two-dimensional electrophoresis. *Proc. Natl. Acad. Sci. USA,* 67:1276–1282.

55. Klapper, D. G., Wilde, C. E., and Capra, J. D. (1978): Automated amino acid sequence of small peptides utilizing Polybrene. *Anal. Biochem.,* 85:126–131.

56. Laursen, R. A. (1971): Solid-phase Edman degradation: The automatic peptide sequencer. *Eur. J. Biochem.,* 20:89–102.

57. Laursen, R. A., and Horn, M. J. (1977): Coupling methods and strategies in solid-phase sequencing. In: *Advanced Methods in Protein Sequence Determination,* edited by S. B. Needleman, pp. 21–37. Springer Verlag, Heidelberg.

58. Liljas, A., Eriksson, S., Donner, D., and Kurland, C. G. (1978): Isolation and crystallization of stable domains of the protein L7/L12 from *Escherichia coli* ribosomes. *FEBS Lett.,* 88:300–304.

59. Lindemann, H., and Wittmann-Liebold, B. (1977): Primary structure of protein S13 from the small subunit of *E. coli* ribosomes. *Hoppe Seyler's Z. Physiol. Chem.,* 358:843–863.

60. Littlechild, J. A., and Malcolm, A. L. (1978): A new method for the purification of 30S ribosomal proteins from *Escherichia coli* using non-denaturing conditions. *Biochemistry,* 17:3363–3369.

61. Littlechild, J. A., Morrison, C. A., and Bradbury, E. M. (1979): Proton magnetic resonance studies of *Escherichia coli* ribosomal protein S4 and a C-terminal fragment of this protein. *FEBS Lett.,* 104:90–94.

62. Matheson, A. T., Möller, W., Amons, R., and Yaguchi, M. (1980): Comparative studies on the structure of ribosomal proteins, with emphasis on the alanine-rich, acidic ribosomal "A" protein. In: *Ribosomes,* edited by J. E. Davies et al, pp. 297–332. University Park Press, Baltimore.

63. Matheson, A. T., Yaguchi, M., Nazar, R. N., Visentin, L. P., and Willick, G. E. (1978): The structure of ribosomes from moderate and extreme halophilic bacteria. In: *Energetics and Structure of Halophilic Microorganisms,* edited by S. R. Caplan and M. Ginzburg, pp. 481–501. Elsevier/North-Holland, Amsterdam.

64. May, R., Stöckel, P., Strell, I., Hoppe, W., Lorenz, S., Erdmann, V. A., Wittmann, H. G., Crespi, H. L., and Katz, J. J. (1978): Determination of quaternary structures of multicomponent macromolecules by the label triangulation method: Ribosomes and ribosomal partial complexes. *Abstracts of the 12th Federation of European Biochemical Societies Meeting.* Abstr. 1643.

65. Mende, L. (1978): The primary structure of protein L13 from the large subunit of the *E. coli* ribosomes. *FEBS Lett.,* 96:313–316.

66. Mende, L., Timm, B., and Subramanian, A. R. (1978): Primary structures of two homologous ribosome-associated DNA-binding proteins of *Escherichia coli. FEBS Lett.,* 96:395–398.

67. Möller, K., and Brimacombe, R. (1975): Specific cross-linking of proteins S7 and L4 to ribosomal RNA by UV-irradiation of *E. coli* ribosomal subunits. *Mol. Gen. Genet.,* 141:343–355.

68. Möller, K., Zwieb, C., and Brimacombe, R. (1978): Identification of the oligonucleotide and oligopeptide involved in an RNA-protein cross-link induced by ultraviolet irradiation of *E. coli* 30S ribosomal subunits. *J. Mol. Biol.,* 126:489–506.

69. Morinaga, T., Funatsu, G., Funatsu, M., and Wittmann, H. G. (1976): Primary structure of the 16S rRNA binding protein S15 from *E. coli* ribosomes. *FEBS Lett.,* 64:307–309.

70. Morinaga, T., Funatsu, G., Funatsu, M., Wittmann-Liebold, B., and Wittmann, H. G. (1978): Primary structure of protein L14 isolated from *E. coli* ribosomes. *FEBS Lett.,* 91:74–77.

71. Muranova, T., Muranova, A. V., Markova, L. F., and Ovchinnikov, Y. A. (1978): The primary structure of ribosomal protein L3 from *Escherichia coli* 70S ribosomes. *FEBS Lett.,* 96:301–305.

72. Niall, H. D., Jacobs, J. W., van Rietschoten, J., and Tregear, G. W. (1974): A new approach to microsequence analysis of proteins. *FEBS Lett.,* 41:62–64.

73. Ozaki, M., Mizushima, S., and Nomura, M. (1969): Identification and functional characterization of the protein controlled by the streptomycin-resistant locus in *E. coli. Nature,* 222:333–339.

74. Pettersson, I., Hardy, S. J. S., and Liljas, A. (1976): The ribosomal protein L8 is a complex of L7/L12 and L10. *FEBS Lett.,* 64:135–138.

75. Pon, C., Wittmann-Liebold, B., and Gualerzi, C. (1979): Structure-function relationships in *Escherichia coli* initiation factors. II. Elucidation of the primary structure of initiation factor IF-1. *FEBS Lett.,* 101:157–160.

76. Post, L. E., Arfsten, A. E., Reusser, F., and Nomura, M. (1978): DNA sequences of promoter regions for the str and spc ribosomal protein operons in *E. coli. Cell,* 15:215–229.

77. Post, L. E., Strycharz, G. D., Nomura, M., Lewis, H., and Dennis, P. P. (1979): Nucleotide sequence of the ribosomal gene cluster adjacent to the gene for RNA polymerase subunit β in *E. coli. Proc. Natl. Acad. Sci. USA,* 76:1967–1701.

78. Reinbolt, J., Tritsch, D., and Wittmann-Liebold, B. (1978): The primary structure of ribosomal protein S7 from *E. coli* strains K and B. *FEBS Lett.,* 91:297–301.

79. Rinke, J., Zwieb, C., Meinke, M., Ulmer, E., and Maly, P. (1979): RNA-Protein Quervernetzung innerhalb des *E. coli* Ribosomes. *Hoppe Seyler's Z. Physiol. Chem.,* 360:353.

80. Ritter, E., and Wittmann-Liebold, B. (1975): The primary structure of protein L30 from *Escherichia coli* ribosomes. *FEBS Lett.,* 60:153–155.

81. Rochat, H., Bechis, G., Kopeyan, C., Grégoire, J., and van Rietschoten, J. (1976): Use of parvalbumin as a protecting protein in the sequenator: An easy and efficient way for sequencing small amounts of peptides. *FEBS Lett.,* 64:404–408.

82. Rosenkranz, H., and Scholtan, W. (1971): Eine verbesserte Methode zur Konformationsbestimmung von helicalen Proteinen aus Messungen des Circulardichroismus. *Hoppe Seyler's Z. Physiol. Chem.,* 352:896–904.

83. Rouviere-Yaniv, J., and Gros, F. (1975): Characterization of a novel, low-molecular weight DNA-binding protein from *Escherichia coli. Proc. Natl. Acad. Sci. USA,* 72:3428–3432.

84. Schiltz, E., and Reinbolt, J. (1975): Determination of the complete amino acid sequence of protein S4 from *E. coli* ribosomes. *Eur. J. Biochem.,* 56:467–481.

85. Stöffler, G. (1974): Structure and function of the *Escherichia coli* ribosome: Immunochemical aspects. In: *Ribosomes,* edited by M. Nomura, A. Tissièves, and P. Lengyel, pp. 615–667. Cold Spring Harbor Laboratory, Cold Spring Harbor, New York.

86. Stöffler, G., and Wittmann, H. G. (1971): Sequence difference of *Escherichia coli* ribosomal proteins as determined by immunochemical methods. *Proc. Natl. Acad. Sci. USA,* 68:2283–2287.

87. Stöffler, G., and Wittmann, H. G. (1971): Ribosomal proteins. XXV. Immunological studies on *Escherichia coli* ribosomal proteins. *J. Mol. Biol.,* 62:407–409.

88. Stöffler, G., and Wittmann, H. G. (1977): Primary structure and three-dimensional arrangement of proteins within the *E. coli* ribosome. In: *Molecular Mechanisms of Protein Biosynthesis,* edited by H. Weissbach and S. Pestka, pp. 117–202. Academic Press, New York.

89. Strickland, M., Strickland, W. N., Brandt, W., von Holt, C., Wittmann-Liebold, B., and Lehmann, A. (1978): The complete amino-acid sequence of histone H2B$_{(3)}$ from sperm of the sea urchin *Parechinus angulosus. Eur. J. Biochem.,* 89:443–452.

90. Strickland, W. N., Strickland, M., Brandt, W. F., von Holt, C., Lehmann, A., and Wittmann-Liebold, B. (1980): The primary structure of histone H$_1$ from sperm of the sea urchin *Parechinus angulosus. Eur. J. Biochem.,* 104:567–578.

91. Suryanarayana, T., and Subramanian, A. R. (1978): Specific association of two homologous DNA-binding proteins to the native 30S ribosomal subunits of *Escherichia coli. Biochim. Biophys. Acta,* 520:342–357.

92. Tarr, G. E., Beecher, J. F., Bell, M., and McKean, D. J. (1978): Polyquaternary amines prevent peptide loss from sequenators. *Anal. Biochem.,* 84:622–627.

93. Terhorst, C., Möller, W., Laursen, R., and Wittmann-Liebold, B. (1973): Amino acid sequence of a 50S ribosomal protein involved in both EFG and EFT-dependent GTP-hydrolysis. *Eur. J. Biochem.,* 34:138–152.

94. Ulmer, E., Meinke, M., Ross, A., Fink, G., and Brimacombe, R. (1978): Chemical cross-linking of protein to RNA within intact ribosomal subunits from *E. coli. Mol. Gen. Genet.,* 160:183–193.

95. Vandekerckhove, J., Rombauts, W., Peeters, P., and Wittmann-Liebold, B. (1975): Determination of the complete amino acid sequence of protein S21 from *Escherichia coli* ribosomes. *Hoppe Seyler's Z. Physiol. Chem.,* 356:1955–1976.

96. Vandekerckhove, J., Rombauts, W., and Wittmann-Liebold, B. (1977): The complete amino acid sequence of protein S16 from *Escherichia coli. Hoppe Seyler's Z. Physiol. Chem.,* 358:989–1002.

97. Visentin, L. P., Yaguchi, M., and Matheson, A. T. (1979): Structural homologies in alanine-rich acidic ribosomal proteins from pro- and eucaryotes. *Can. J. Biochem.,* 57:719–726.

98. Wachter, E., Machleidt, W., Hofner, H., and Otto, J. (1973): Aminopropyl glass and its *p*-phenylene diisothiocyanate derivative, a new support in solid-phase Edman degradation of peptides and proteins. *FEBS Lett.,* 35:97–102.

99. Wagner, R., and Garrett, R. A. (1978): A new RNA–RNA cross-linking reagent and its application to ribosomal 5S RNA. *Nucleic Acids Res.,* 5:4065–4076.

100. Wittmann, H. G. (1974): Purification and identification of *Escherichia coli* ribosomal proteins. In: *Ribosomes,* edited by M. Nomura, A. Tissières, and P. Lengyel, pp. 93–114. Cold Spring Harbor Laboratory, Cold Spring Harbor, New York.

101. Wittmann, H. G., Littlechild, J., and Wittmann-Liebold, B. (1979): Structure of ribosomal proteins. In: *Ribosomes,* edited by J. E. Davies et al., pp. 51–88. University Park Press, Baltimore.

102. Wittmann, H. G., and Wittmann-Liebold, B. (1974): Chemical structure of bacterial ribosomal proteins. In: *Ribosomes,* edited by M. Nomura, A. Tissières, and P. Lengyel, pp. 115–140. Cold Spring Harbor Laboratory, Cold Spring Harbor, New York.

103. Wittmann-Liebold, B. (1973): Amino acid studies on ten ribosomal proteins of *E. coli* with an improved sequenator equipped with an automatic conversion device. *Hoppe Seyler's Z. Physiol. Chem.,* 354:1415–1431.

104. Wittmann-Liebold, B. (1980): The primary structure of protein L22 from the large subunit of the *Escherichia coli* ribosome. *FEBS Lett. (in press).*

105. Wittmann-Liebold, B. (1979): Primary structure of protein L24 from the *Escherichia coli* ribosome. *FEBS Lett.,* 108:75–80.

106. Wittmann-Liebold, B., Brauer, D., and Dognin, J. (1977): Strategy and micro methods applied in the sequencing of the ribosomal proteins and of the initiation factor IF-3 of *E. coli.* In: *Solid Phase Methods in Protein Sequence Analysis,* edited by A. Previero and M. A. Coletti-Previero, pp. 219–232, Elsevier/North-Holland, Amsterdam.

107. Wittmann-Liebold, B., and Dzionara, M. (1976): Comparison of amino acid sequences among ribosomal proteins of *E. coli. FEBS Lett.,* 61:14–19.

108. Wittmann-Liebold, B., and Dzionara, M. (1976): Studies on the significance of sequence homologies among proteins from *E. coli* ribosomes. *FEBS Lett.*, 65:281–283.
109. Wittmann-Liebold, B., Geissler, A. W., Lin, A., and Wool, I. G. (1980): The sequence of the amino-terminal region of rat liver ribosomal proteins S4, S6, S8, L6, L7a, L18, L27, L30, L37, L37a and L39. *J. Supramol. Struct. (in press)*.
110. Wittmann-Liebold, B., Geissler, A. W., and Marzinzig, E. (1975): Studies on the primary structure of 14 proteins from the large subunit of *E. coli* ribosomes with an improved protein sequenator and with mass spectrometry. *J. Supramol. Struct.*, 3:426–447.
111. Wittmann-Liebold, B., Graffunder, H., and Kohls, H. (1976): A device coupled to a modified sequenator for the automated conversion of anilinothiazolinones into PTH-amino acids. *Anal. Biochem.*, 75:621–633.
112. Wittmann-Liebold, B., and Greuer, B. (1978): The primary structure of protein S5 from the small subunit of the *E. coli* ribosome. *FEBS Lett.*, 95:91–98.
113. Wittmann-Liebold, B., and Greuer, B. (1979): The primary structure of protein L23 from the large subunit of the *Escherichia coli* ribosome. *FEBS Lett.*, 108:69–74.
114. Wittman-Liebold, B., Greuer, B., and Pannenbecker, R. (1975): The primary structure of protein L32 from the 50S subunit of *E. coli* ribosomes. *Hoppe Seyler's Z. Physiol. Chem.*, 356:1977–1979.
115. Wittmann-Liebold, B., and Lehmann, A. (1975): Comparison of various techniques applied to the amino acid sequence determination of ribosomal proteins. In: *Solid Phase Methods in Protein Sequence Analysis,* edited by R. A. Laurson, pp. 81–90. Pierce Chemical, Rockford, Illinois.
116. Wittmann-Liebold, B., and Marzinzig, E. (1977): Primary structure of protein L28 from the large subunit of the *E. coli* ribosomes. *FEBS Lett.*, 81:214–217.
117. Wittmann-Liebold, B., Marzinzig, E., and Lehmann, A. (1976): Primary structure of protein S20 from the small ribosomal subunit of *E. coli. FEBS Lett.*, 68:110–114.
118. Wittmann-Liebold, B., and Pannenbecker, R. (1976): Primary structure of protein L33 from the large subunit of the *Escherichia coli* ribosome. *FEBS Lett.*, 86:115–118.
119. Wittmann-Liebold, B., Robinson, S. M. L., and Dzionara, M. (1977): Prediction of secondary structures in proteins from the *Escherichia coli* 30S ribosomal subunit. *FEBS Lett.*, 77:301–307.
120. Wittmann-Liebold, B., Robinson, S. M. L., and Dzionara, M. (1977): Predictions for secondary structures of six proteins from the 50S subunit of *Escherichia coli* ribosome. *FEBS Lett.*, 81:204–213.
121. Wittmann-Liebold, B., and Seib, C. (1979): The primary structure of protein L20 from the large subunit of the *E. coli* ribosome. *FEBS Lett.*, 103:61–65.
122. Wystup, G., Teraoka, H., Schulze, H., Hampl, H., and Nierhaus, K. H. (1979): 50S subunit from *E. coli* ribosomes: Isolation of active ribosomal proteins and protein complexes. *Eur. J. Biochem.*, 100:101–113.
123. Yaguchi, M. (1977): Primary structure of protein S18 from the small *E. coli* ribosomal subunit. *FEBS Lett.*, 59:217–220.
124. Yaguchi, M., and Wittmann, H. G. (1978): The primary structure of protein S17 from the small ribosomal subunit of *E. coli. FEBS Lett.*, 87:37–40.
125. Yaguchi, M., and Wittmann, H. G. (1978): Primary structure of protein S19 from the small ribosomal subunit of *E. coli. FEBS Lett.*, 88:227–230.
126. Yaguchi, M., and Wittmann, H. G. (1980): The primary structure of protein S14 from the small subunit of the *Escherichia coli* ribosome *(submitted)*.
127. Yaguchi, M., and Wittmann, H. G. (1980): The primary structure of protein S10 from the small subunit of the *Escherichia coli* ribosome *(submitted)*.
128. Zimmermann, C. L., Apella, E., and Pisano, J. J. (1977): Rapid analysis of amino acid phenylthiohydantoins by high-performance liquid chromatography. *Anal. Biochem.*, 77:569–573.
129. Zwieb, C., and Brimacombe, R. (1978): RNA-protein cross-linking in *E. coli* 30S ribosomal subunits: A method for the direct analysis of the RNA regions involved in the cross-links. *Nucleic Acids Res.*, 5:1189–1206.
130. Zwieb, C., and Brimacombe, R. (1979): RNA-protein cross-linking in *E. coli* 30 ribosomal subunits. *Nucleic Acids Res.*, 6:1775–1790.
131. Zwieb, C., Ross, A., Rinke, J., Meinke, M., and Brimacombe, R. (1978): Evidence for RNA–RNA cross-link formation in *E. coli* ribosomes. *Nucleic Acids Res.*, 5:2705–2720.

Polypeptide Hormones, edited by
R. F. Beers, Jr. and E. G. Bassett.
Raven Press, New York © 1980.

12. Automated Solid-Phase Peptide Synthesis

Bruce W. Erickson, Thomas J. Lukas, and Michael B. Prystowsky

The Rockefeller University, New York, New York 10021

THE SOLID-PHASE METHOD

The chemical synthesis of peptides was greatly simplified through the introduction of solid-phase peptide synthesis by R. B. Merrifield in 1963 (18). This novel method was based on a concept that Merrifield devised in May 1959, some 20 years ago. The basic strategy involves covalent attachment of the COOH-terminal amino acid of the desired peptide to an insoluble solid support and coupling of the remaining amino acids one by one until the desired peptide is fully assembled. Then the desired peptide is cleaved from the solid support and purified in solution. This approach appeared to be a simple and quick means of obtaining relatively pure peptides in high yield.

Merrifield initially demonstrated the solid-phase method by synthesis of the simple tetrapeptide Leu-Ala-Gly-Val (18). He soon extended it to the synthesis of polypeptide hormones, such as bradykinin (19), angiotensin (17), and insulin (16). During this time, Merrifield and J. M. Stewart constructed an automated apparatus for assembling the peptide chain (20). This solid-phase synthesizer was used by Gutte and Merrifield (10,11) to achieve the first chemical synthesis of an enzyme, ribonuclease A, only 6 years after the solid-phase method was first introduced (18).

Solid-phase synthesis of peptides offers certain advantages over solution methods (1,6,18). The peptide intermediates remain covalently bound to the solid support throughout assembly of the desired peptide chain. Thus they can be efficiently separated from soluble reagents and by-products by repeated washing and filtering of the solid phase. This scheme avoids the material losses normally experienced during isolation and purification of peptide intermediates in solution. The support-bound peptide intermediates can be prepared in high yield by using the soluble reagents in excess to drive the reactions to completion. All of the chemical reactions involved in assembly of the desired peptide chain can be carried out conveniently in a single reaction vessel, which also minimizes material losses by avoiding the physical transfer of intermediates.

The increased simplicity, convenience, speed, and efficiency of solid-phase synthesis are achieved at the expense of certain potential disadvantages. Since the peptide intermediates remain covalently bound to the solid support, they are not isolated and purified after each reaction. Although soluble by-products are readily washed away, any by-products that remain bound to the support can only be removed at the end of the synthesis. Thus, the purity of the final crude peptide depends strongly on the efficiency of the chemical reactions used for chain assembly and the absence of significant side reactions. Since the stepwise assembly of a peptide from its amino acids requires the success of many consecutive reactions, each reaction must be not only highly efficient but also highly selective. Much effort has been devoted during the last decade to finding better chemical procedures for solid-phase synthesis and better methods for purification of the desired peptide (1,6).

AUTOMATED SOLID-PHASE PEPTIDE SYNTHESIS

Once the *N-tert*-butyloxycarbonyl (Boc) derivative of the first amino acid is attached to the solid support, the subsequent Boc-amino acids are added to the growing peptide chain by repetition of a *synthetic cycle* of three reactions: deprotection, neutralization, and coupling, as illustrated in Fig. 1. First, the α-amino group is deprotected by removal of the Boc protecting group with an acid. Second, the resulting protonated α-amino group is neutralized with a base. Third, the free α-amino group is coupled with an activated derivative of the next Boc-amino acid. Since these three reactions can be repeated many times in the same reaction vessel to add any of the 20 genetically coded amino acids, solid-phase assembly of the peptide chain is readily accomplished with an automatic synthesizer.

The first automated instrument for solid-phase peptide synthesis was described by Merrifield and co-workers in 1966 (21). It consisted of a reaction vessel, a liquid-handling system, and a programmable control unit. The glass reaction vessel contained a sintered-glass disc for filtration of the solid phase. The glass-and-fluorocarbon plumbing system stored and measured the reagent solutions and solvents and transferred them into and out of the reaction vessel. The electrical control unit contained a mechanical stepping drum for storing a preset program to control the timers, valves, pump, and shaker. By 1976, at least 14 different designs for automatic synthesizers had been operated successfully and five were available commercially (6).

A potential source of problems with these automatic synthesizers is the possible occurrence of side reactions due to cross-contamination between reservoirs and tubes containing different reagents and solvents. For example, a trace of acid inadvertently introduced during the coupling step could cause premature loss of the Boc protecting group, which would be followed by the undesirable coupling of a second molecule of that Boc-amino acid. This problem is marginal when the reagents and solvents are selected by accurately machined rotary valves (21). But it can be serious with the more common practice of using solenoid valves to deliver several reagents to a common manifold (5).

These synthesizers are automatic in the sense that they carry out the physical

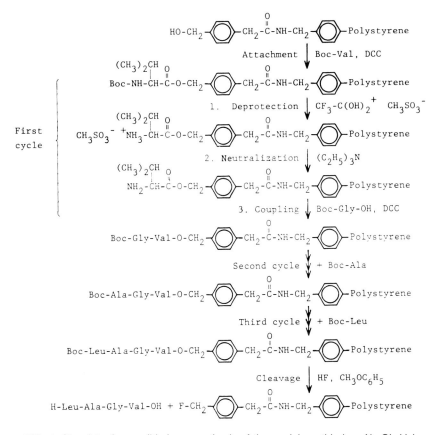

FIG. 1. Chemistry for a solid-phase synthesis of the model peptide Leu-Ala-Gly-Val.

manipulations of solid-phase synthesis according to a preset program. In the language of process control, they operate by *closed-loop* control but generally lack the capacity to deviate from the preset program. Any changes in the synthetic procedure require the intervention of the human operator while the synthesizer is under *open-loop* control, as illustrated in Fig. 2.

The control units of these synthesizers cannot vary the conditions of the individual reactions or the order of the reactions in response to the degree of completeness of the reactions. Such feedback control of the synthetic reactions is desirable not only for the savings in time, but also for the increased yield and purity of the desired peptide product. For example, if the reaction time has been set at 1 hr for a given coupling step, these automatic synthesizers cannot shorten the reaction time for a coupling already complete after 20 min or lengthen it for a coupling still incomplete after 1 hr. In the former case, the last 40 min of the preset coupling period would be time lost, but the yield and purity of the desired peptide intermediate probably would not suffer. In

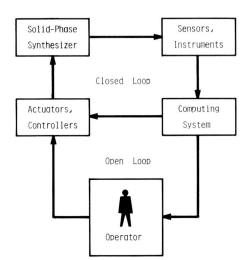

FIG. 2. Process control of a solid-phase synthesizer: open-loop versus closed-loop control.

the latter case, however, the peptide chains that failed to couple in 1 hr would normally give rise to deletion peptides lacking that amino acid. This would decrease the yield of the desired peptide and increase the amount and number of contaminating peptides present at the end of the synthesis.

REACTION MONITORING

The problem of incomplete chemical reactions can be assessed by *monitoring* the progress of the reactions (1,6). Since the neutralization reaction is a very fast process involving proton transfer, only the deprotection and coupling reactions, which involve the breaking or making of a carbon-nitrogen bond, are usually monitored. A useful monitoring method should be sensitive, accurate, rapid, and readily automated. It should be able to measure accurately at least 99.5% completion of coupling or deprotection. Monitoring methods that require destruction of a portion of the solid phase or require many hours to give a measurement of the progress of the reaction are not useful in a long synthesis.

Reaction monitoring can be used in four progressively more sophisticated ways during automated solid-phase synthesis, as outlined in Table 1. First, monitoring during execution of a preset synthetic program under closed-loop control provides a record of the course of the synthesis for subsequent assessment of the probable sources of major peptide by-products. Second, reaction monitoring during open-loop control provides a relatively rapid measurement of the completeness of the reaction in question. It gives the operator the option of taking remedial measures, such as repeating the reaction or varying the reaction conditions, before proceeding to the next reaction. Third, if the synthesizer control unit has a computing system that can use the monitoring data to determine the completeness of the reaction, reaction monitoring during closed-loop feed-

TABLE 1. *Six types of real-time process control for solid-phase synthesizers*

Type of control	Process control parameter			
	Process monitoring	Open-loop control	Sequencing control	Optimizing control
	Synthesizer control parameter			
	Presence of reaction monitoring	Need for operator decisions	Feedback of reaction completion	Modification of reaction conditions
Operator (manual)	No	Yes	No	No
Closed-loop (automatic)	No	No	No	No
Closed-loop with reaction monitoring	Yes	No	No	No
Open-loop with reaction monitoring	Yes	Yes	No	No
Closed-loop with reaction monitoring and feedback	Yes	Default	Yes	No
Closed-loop with reaction monitoring, feedback, and optimization	Yes	Default	Yes	Yes

back control can allow the control unit to choose one of several responses. For example, the control unit can decide to advance to the next reaction if a preset level of completion has been met, to repeat the reaction if this level has not been met, or to default to open-loop control and wait for the operator if a preset number of reaction attempts has failed to achieve the preset level of completion. Fourth, if the synthesizer control unit has been programmed to use more than one set of reaction conditions for a given type of reaction, the reaction conditions can be varied to maximize the completeness of reaction.

Two useful approaches for monitoring the reactions performed by a solid-phase peptide synthesizer are *discontinuous* titration of the number of free amino groups remaining in the solid phase *after* the reaction and *continuous* spectrophotometric measurement of the changing concentration of a soluble reagent or product *during* the reaction. Two solid-phase synthesizers have been described that include an automatic monitoring system for controlling the synthesis. Both of these monitoring systems discontinuously measure the total number of amino groups remaining after coupling or deprotection. In each case, the synthesis is interrupted until the appropriate monitoring operations are performed on the entire solid phase.

A flow chart showing the steps and decisions involved in operation of these monitoring systems is shown in Fig. 3. The synthesizer control unit determines the next synthetic operation and executes it. When the reaction is over, the monitoring system measures the number of free amino groups present. This

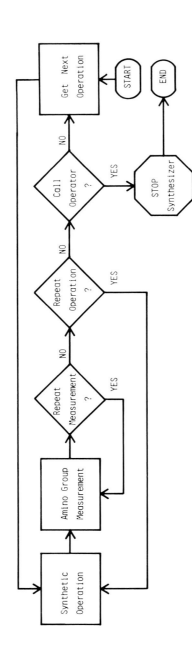

FIG. 3. Flow chart for control of solid-phase synthesizers equipped to monitor the number of free amino groups after deprotection or coupling.

information is needed to decide whether to allow the synthesizer to continue under closed-loop control to the next synthetic operation or to change to open-loop control by stopping the synthesizer and calling the operator.

Three logical decisions must be made in controlling this process. (a) Should the measurement be repeated to get a more reliable reading of a small or inherently variable result? If so, the number of free amino groups is measured again. If not, (b) should the synthetic operation be repeated to achieve a more desirable result? If so, the operation is repeated. If not, (c) should the operator be called to remedy an unacceptable result? If so, the process control loop is opened by stopping the synthesizer and summoning the operator. If not, the process control loop remains closed and the synthesizer advances to the next synthetic operation. This scheme for monitoring control of the solid-phase synthesizer requires preset limits for (a) the maximum number of times that measurement of the number of free amino groups should be repeated, (b) the maximum number of times that each synthetic operation should be repeated, and (c) the range of values that are considered acceptable for each synthetic operation.

Photometric Picrate Monitoring

Hodges and Merrifield (13) have developed a monitoring system that automatically measures the number of free amino groups present after deprotection or coupling. This monitoring system controls a Beckman Instruments Model 990 automatic peptide synthesizer and is based on the photometric picrate method of Gisin (9). After all free amino groups are temporarily converted into ammonium picrate groups, the amount of ionically bound picrate is displaced as a solution of trialkylammonium picrate and the absorbance of this solution is measured at 362 nm. Automatic picrate monitoring is directed by an electronic control unit that is independent of the punched tape control unit of the Beckman synthesizer. After the second coupling step, if the monitoring system detects the presence of an amount of picrate above a preset level, it directs the synthesizer to shut down at the end of the current synthetic cycle. This interruption of the synthesis minimizes the formation of large deletion peptides by allowing the operator either to increase the coupling efficiency by repeating the coupling step or to block the remaining peptide chains by acetylation or other chain-terminating reaction.

This picrate monitoring system has a dynamic range of about 0.4 to 4,000 μmoles with an accuracy of about 0.2% for peptides lacking histidine and about 1% for peptides containing N^{im}-2,4-dinitrophenylhistidine (13). One drawback of the photometric picrate method is the increasing background that can be observed as the length of the peptide chain increases during a long synthesis (12). But this problem can be overcome by using several large volumes of 5% dimethylformamide in dichloromethane to remove the picric acid bound nonspecifically to the resin (15).

Electrometric Perchlorate Monitoring

Brunfeldt and his colleagues (4) have developed a monitoring system that automatically measures the number of free amino groups present after coupling or deprotection by electrometric titration with perchloric acid. This monitoring system has been incorporated into the solid-phase peptide synthesizer described by Brunfeldt et al. (5), which is similar to the Schwarz Bioresearch synthesizer. A solution of 0.4% perchloric acid in 1,1,2-trichloroethane, ethanol, and water is added through a Radiometer autoburette to the synthesizer reaction vessel containing a suspension of the solid phase in dichloromethane and acetic acid. The difference in electrochemical potential between a glass pH electrode and a calomel reference electrode is recorded continuously. The volume of the perchloric acid titrant required to change the potential difference to a preset value is taken as a measure of the number of free amino groups and other titratable groups present in the solid phase.

This electrometric perchlorate monitoring procedure has also been incorporated into a solid-phase synthesizer controlled by a 16-bit Computer Automation minicomputer (27). More recently, the computer has been programmed for closed-loop feedback control of the synthesis (28). Based on the titration results, the computer can decide to repeat the titration, repeat the reaction (deprotection, coupling), or, if necessary, stop the synthesis and summon the operator, as shown in Fig. 3. This monitoring system has a dynamic range of about 2 to 400 μmoles and an accuracy of about 1% (27). One drawback of perchloric acid monitoring is the termination of growing peptide chains by acetylation, which is evidently due to the presence during the coupling step of residual acetic acid carried over from the monitoring (4).

Both of these monitoring methods suffer from the disadvantage that the synthesis must be interrupted for treatment of the solid phase with the monitoring acid (picric, perchloric). Not only is time lost but also the purity of the desired peptide may be decreased by exposure to the monitoring acid. For example, certain acid-sensitive protecting groups are not compatible with these acids. A different approach to monitoring the course of the synthetic reactions involves continuously measuring the appearance or disappearance of a chromophore.

Continuous Photometric Monitoring

Merrifield (ref. 6, p. 367) measured rates for the coupling of activated Bpoc-amino acids to aminoacyl supports by continuously recording the 255-nm absorbance of the 2-(4-biphenylyl)-2-propyloxycarbonyl (Bpoc) group. Part of the liquid in the reaction vessel of the Rockefeller synthesizer (21) was pumped through an external ultraviolet monitor as the coupling reaction proceeded.

More recently, Birr (3) measured the course of coupling of Ddz-amino acids and the subsequent removal of the Ddz group in his centrifugal solid-phase synthesizer by continuously monitoring the 280-nm absorbance of the 2-(3,5-dimethoxyphenyl)-2-propyloxycarbonyl (Ddz) group. In this case, the centrifugal reactor itself served as the pump to direct part of the reaction liquid to the ultraviolet monitor. The operator followed the recording of the absorbance to decide when to repeat the reaction or proceed to the next reaction. In addition, the neutralization reaction and even the washing operations between reactions could be monitored with this apparatus. One minor drawback of this synthetic system is that the wash solvents are added to the solid phase in several small portions, which provides a discontinuous recording of the washing efficiency. This monitoring system should be able to pass the monitoring data to a more sophisticated synthesizer controller to allow closed-loop feedback control of the completeness of the reactions.

Continuous photometric monitoring of the deprotection and coupling reactions provides a more immediate measure of the completeness of these reactions than do the discontinuous photometric picrate and electrometric perchlorate procedures. In principle, a computing system controlling a solid-phase synthesizer could use the continuous stream of photometric data to determine the extent of reaction even as the reaction proceeds and use this information to decrease or increase the preset reaction time to achieve a preset level of completion. This situation would represent closed-loop control with monitoring, feedback, and optimization of the reaction conditions (Table 1).

CONTINUOUS-FLOW SOLID-PHASE PEPTIDE SYNTHESIS

Each of the solid-phase synthesizers mentioned above operates by the addition of reagent solutions and solvents to the reaction vessel in several discrete portions. In 1970, Bayer and colleagues (2) explored the possibility of packing the solid phase in a column and passing the reagent solutions and solvents through this column in a continuous flow. Their solid support consisted of Waters Associates Biopak silica to which 1,4-bis(hydroxymethyl)benzene was covalently bound. In 1971, Scott and co-workers (25) similarly described the use of polystyrene-coated glass beads as a solid support. They used an automatic solid-phase synthesizer (26) specifically designed to continuously pass solvents and reagents through a column packed with this solid support. Both research groups demonstrated the feasibility of continuous-flow solid-phase synthesis through the assembly of model peptides. Since these exploratory studies used a special apparatus and unusual solid supports, continuous-flow synthesis has not been applied to biologically important peptides.

We have recently constructed a continuous-flow solid-phase synthesizer from the readily available components of a high-pressure liquid chromatograph (7). This synthesizer was operated successfully using conventional 1% cross-linked polystyrene rather than a solid support designed for high-pressure chromatographic separations.

Continuous-Flow Synthesizer

The synthesizer was assembled from the modular components of a Waters Associates high-pressure liquid chromatograph, as shown in Fig. 4. It consists of a high-pressure pump, a sample injector, a stainless-steel column, and an ultraviolet detector. The solid support is placed in the column and reagent solutions and solvents are pumped through the injector, column, and detector as needed. The acidic solution for deprotection, the basic solution for neutralization, or dichloromethane for washing is selected by a three-port valve on the pump. The liquid leaving the detector passes through a second three-port valve on the pump, from which it can be directed to waste, delivered to a fraction collector, or recycled back through the pump.

The several operations used to add one amino acid residue to the peptide are listed in Table 2. The acidic deprotection solution is not the commonly used 6.5 M trifluoroacetic acid in dichloromethane but 0.1 M trifluoroacetic acid containing 0.01 M methanesulfonic acid (8). The acidic species that actually removes the Boc protecting group is not the neutral trifluoroacetic acid molecule but its conjugate acid, $CF_3C(OH)_2^+ X^-$ or *protonated* trifluoroacetic acid (7). Only 0.01 M methanesulfonic acid is needed to generate approximately the same concentration of protonated trifluoroacetic acid as is formed by autoprotonation in 6.5 M trifluoroacetic acid.

During the coupling step, the Boc-amino acid is activated with *N,N'*-dicyclo-hexylcarbodiimide (DCC) to form the symmetric anhydride, which is loaded into the injector and injected into the column. To conserve the valuable Boc-amino acid reagent, the solution leaving the detector is recycled through the system, as indicated by the heavy black line in Fig. 4. At the end of the coupling reaction, the excess Boc-amino acid can be recovered by directing the coupling solution to the fraction collector.

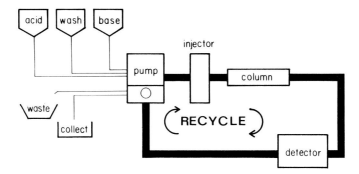

FIG. 4. Schematic diagram of a continuous-flow solid-phase synthesizer using components from a high-pressure liquid chromatographic system.

TABLE 2. *A procedure for peptide assembly with a continuous-flow solid-phase synthesizer*

Operation	Solution
Deprotection	0.01 M CH_3SO_3H and 0.10 M CF_3CO_2H in CH_2Cl_2
Washing	CH_2Cl_2
Neutralization	0.3 M Et_3N in CH_2Cl_2
Washing	CH_2Cl_2
Coupling	0.1 M Boc-amino acid symmetric anhydride in CH_2Cl_2
Washing	CH_2Cl_2

Initial Results

Our initial experiments used a solid phase consisting of a Boc-amino acid esterified to hydroxymethyl-*copoly*(styrene–1% divinylbenzene), or polysytrene for brevity. Synthesis of the model tetrapeptide Leu-Ala-Gly-Val was readily achieved with the continuous-flow synthesizer. Boc-Val-polystyrene was converted into Boc-Leu-Ala-Gly-Val-polystyrene in about 5 hr by using two 15-min couplings of each Boc-amino acid symmetric anhydride (7). The crude peptide mixture obtained on HF cleavage of the solid phase was shown, by low-pressure ion-exchange chromatography, to contain 98% of the desired peptide. Continuous-flow solid-phase synthesis furnished this model peptide in comparable purity to the product obtained from a conventional manual synthesis in a shaking glass vessel, in which the reagent solutions and solvents were added in discrete portions.

Analysis of the peptide by-products obtained from synthesis of Leu-Ala-Gly-Val can also be performed by high-pressure liquid chromatography (24). The separation of this model peptide from four deletion peptides by chromatography on a reverse-phase column is shown in Fig. 5A. This high-pressure reverse-phase separation requires only about 5% of the sample and about 5% of the time needed for the conventional low-pressure ion-exchange separation.

Recently, we also examined the use of Boc-amino acids esterified to 4-(hydroxymethyl)phenylacetamidomethyl-*copoly*(styrene–1% divinylbenzene), or Pam-polystyrene, as the solid support (24). Pam-polystyrene is about 100 times more stable than polystyrene to premature loss of peptide chains during acid deprotection of the Boc-peptide intermediates (22). In addition, this solid support minimizes the termination of growing peptide chains by trifluoroacetylation (14). Not only can Pam-polystyrene be prepared free of the hydroxymethyl sites that mediate trifluoroacetylation, but also its increased stability to acid minimizes the formation of new hydroxymethyl sites during the synthesis (14, 22,23).

The model peptide Leu-Ala-Gly-Val was assembled on Pam-polystyrene under continuous-flow conditions in 4.5 hr using two 30-min couplings for each residue (24). The chemical structure of Pam-polystyrene and the chemical reactions

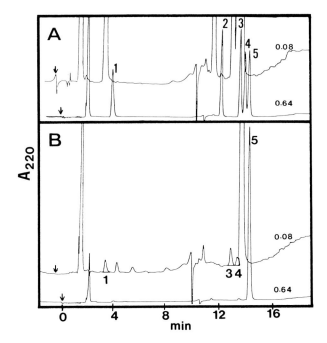

FIG. 5. Reverse-phase high-pressure liquid chromatographic separation of the model peptide Leu-Ala-Gly-Val (5) and four deletion peptides: Ala-Gly-Val (1), Leu-Val (2), Leu-Ala-Val (3), and Leu-Gly-Val (4). Peptides were eluted from a Waters Associates μBondapak C18 column using a linear gradient of 0–16% isopropanol in aqueous 5 mM triethylammonium phosphate and were monitored at 220 nm on scales of both 0.08 and 0.64 absorbance units full scale. **A:** Mixture of synthetic peptide standards (50–70 nmoles); **B:** Crude peptide mixture synthesized on 1% cross-linked polystyrene using two 30-min couplings with Boc-aminoacyl symmetric anhydride.

involved in this synthesis are shown in Fig. 1. The reverse-phase separation of the resulting product mixture is shown in Fig. 5B. The predominant product was the desired tetrapeptide (97.1%). Small amounts of three single-deletion peptides (0.9% Ala-Gly-Val, 1.5% Leu-Ala-Val, and 0.5% Leu-Gly-Val) were also present, but the double-deletion peptide Leu-Val was not detected (<0.1%).

Continuous-flow synthesis of Leu-Ala-Gly-Val followed by reverse-phase separation of the resulting peptides provides a very quick and sensitive way to measure the influence of various synthetic conditions on peptide purity. For example, a continuous-flow synthesis using two 15-min couplings for each residue required only 3 hr and gave the desired peptide in 96.5% purity. Thus two 15-min couplings are essentially as adequate as two 30-min couplings (24).

Prospects

Work is currently in progress to automate the continuous-flow synthesizer so it will operate under closed-loop control with monitoring, feedback, and optimization of the reaction conditions (Table 1). The synthesizer is ideally configured for continuous photometric monitoring of the reagents and solvents as they leave the reaction column. Preliminary monitoring results using the ultraviolet detector have shown that continuous-flow peptide synthesis requires significantly less time, reagents, and solvents than other modes of solid-phase peptide synthesis. The incorporation into the continuous-flow solid-phase synthesizer of both continuous photometric monitoring and closed-loop computer control with feedback and reaction optimization should furnish an efficient apparatus for the automated synthesis of peptides.

ACKNOWLEDGMENTS

Our work on continuous-flow synthesis was supported in part by U.S.P.H.S. grants HL 19795, AI 15301, and CA 24435, and NSF grant PCM 77-25761.

REFERENCES

1. Barany, G., and Merrifield, R. B. (1980): Solid phase peptide synthesis. In: *The Peptides: Analysis, Synthesis, and Biology, Vol. 2,* edited by E. Gross and J. Meienhofer, pp. 1–284. Academic Press, New York.
2. Bayer, E., Jung, G., Halasz, I., and Sebestian, I. (1970): A new support for polypeptide synthesis in columns. *Tet. Lett.,* 4503–4505.
3. Birr, C. (1975): The α,α-dimethyl-3,5-dimethoxybenzyloxycarbonyl (Ddz) protecting group in nonclassical peptide synthesis. Quantitative control and continuous recording in the Merrifield synthesis. In: *Peptides 1974,* edited by Y. Wolman, pp. 117–122. Wiley, New York.
4. Brunfeldt, K., Christensen, T., and Villemoes, P. (1972): Automatic monitoring of solid phase synthesis of a decapeptide. *FEBS Lett.,* 22:238–244.
5. Brunfeldt, K., Halstrom, J., and Roepstorff, P. (1969): A punched tape controlled peptide synthesizer. *Acta Chem. Scand. B,* 23:2830–2838.
6. Erickson, B. W., and Merrifield, R. B. (1976): Solid-phase peptide synthesis. In: *The Proteins, Vol. 2,* 3rd ed., edited by H. Neurath and R. L. Hill, pp. 255–527. Academic Press, New York.
7. Erickson, B. W., and Prystowsky, M. B. (1979): Continuous-flow solid-phase peptide synthesis using an HPLC system. In: *Biological/Biomedical Applications of Liquid Chromatography II,* edited by G. L. Hawk, pp. 293–305. Marcel Dekker, New York.
8. Erickson, B. W., and Wang, C. Y. (1975): Removal of the N^{α}-*tert*-butyloxycarbonyl group with dilute methanesulfonic acid. *Abstracts of the 170th Meeting of the American Chemical Society.* ORGN 081.
9. Gisin, B. F. (1972): The monitoring of reactions in solid-phase peptide synthesis with picric acid. *Anal. Chim. Acta,* 58:248–249.
10. Gutte, B., and Merrifield, R. B. (1969): The total synthesis of an enzyme with ribonuclease A activity. *J. Am. Chem. Soc.,* 91:501–502.
11. Gutte, B., and Merrifield, R. B. (1971): The synthesis of ribonuclease A. *J. Biol. Chem.,* 246:1922–1941.
12. Hancock, W. S., Battersby, J. E., and Harding, D. R. K. (1975): The use of picric acid as a simple monitoring procedure for automated peptide synthesis. *Anal. Biochem.,* 69:497–503.
13. Hodges, R. S., and Merrifield, R. B. (1975): Monitoring of solid phase peptide synthesis by an automated spectrophotometric picrate method. *Anal. Biochem.,* 65:241–272.
14. Kent, S. B. H., Mitchell, A. R., Engelhard, M., and Merrifield, R. B. (1979): Mechanisms and prevention of trifluoroacetylation in solid-phase peptide synthesis. *Proc. Natl. Acad. Sci. USA,* 76:2180–2184.
15. Krieger, D. E., Vidali, G., Erickson, B. W., Allfrey, V. G., and Merrifield, R. B. (1979): The

synthesis of diacetylated histone H4-(1-37) for studies on the mechanism of histone deacetylation. *Bioorg. Chem.,* 8:409–427.

16. Marglin, A., and Merrifield, R. B. (1966): The synthesis of bovine insulin by the solid phase method. *J. Am. Chem. Soc.,* 88:5051–5052.

17. Marshall, G. R., and Merrifield, R. B. (1965): Synthesis of angiotensin by the solid-phase method. *Biochemistry,* 4:2394–2401.

18. Merrifield, R. B. (1963): Solid phase peptide synthesis. I. The synthesis of a tetrapeptide. *J. Am. Chem. Soc.,* 85:2149–2154.

19. Merrifield, R. B. (1964): Solid phase peptide synthesis. II. The synthesis of bradykinin. *J. Am. Chem. Soc.,* 86:304.

20. Merrifield, R. B., and Stewart, J. M. (1965): Automated peptide synthesis. *Nature,* 207:522–523.

21. Merrifield, R. B., Stewart, J. M., and Jernberg, N. (1966): Instrument for automated synthesis of peptides. *Anal. Chem.,* 38:1905–1914.

22. Mitchell, A. R., Erickson, B. W., Ryabtsev, M. N., Hodges, R. S., and Merrifield, R. B. (1976): *tert*-Butoxycarbonylaminoacyl-4-(oxymethyl)phenylacetamidomethyl-resin, a more acid-resistant support for solid-phase peptide synthesis. *J. Am. Chem. Soc.,* 98:7357–7363.

23. Mitchell, A. R., Kent, S. B. H., Engelhard, M., and Merrifield, R. B. (1978): A new synthetic route to *tert*-butyloxycarbonylaminoacyl-4-(oxymethyl)phenylacetamidomethyl-resin, an improved support for solid-phase peptide synthesis. *J. Org. Chem.,* 43:2845–2852.

24. Prystowsky, M. B., Lukas, T. J., and Erickson, B. W. (1979): Continuous-flow solid-phase peptide synthesis using Pam-resins. In: *Peptides: Structure and Biological Function,* edited by E. Gross and J. Meienhofer, pp. 349–352. Pierce Chemical, Rockford, Illinois.

25. Scott, R. P. W., Chan, K. K., Kucera, P., and Zolty, S. (1971): The use of resin coated glass beads in the form of a packed bed for the solid phase synthesis of peptides. *J. Chromatogr. Sci.,* 9:577–591.

26. Scott, R. P. W., Zolty, S., and Chan, K. K. (1972): An automated apparatus for the synthesis of peptides using resin coated glass beads in the form of a packed bed. *J. Chromatogr. Sci.,* 10:385–391.

27. Villemoes, P., Christensen, T., and Brunfeldt, K. (1976): A computer-controlled peptide synthesizer. *Hoppe Seylers Z. Physiol. Chem.,* 357:713–719.

28. Villemoes, P., Christensen, T., and Brunfeldt, K. (1978): A computerized peptide synthesizer with feedback control. *Acta Chem. Scand. B,* 23:703–713.

Polypeptide Hormones, edited by
R. F. Beers, Jr. and E. G. Bassett.
Raven Press, New York © 1980.

13. Advances in and Comparison of Protective Groups for Peptide Synthesis

Wolfgang Voelter

Institute for Organic Chemistry, University of Tübingen, D-7400 Tübingen, West Germany

INTRODUCTION

In order to avoid the formation of undesirable side products in peptide coupling reactions, all reactive functional groups not involved in the formation of the desired peptide bond should be protected. One of the most fundamental problems in synthetic peptide chemistry is the development of stable, but easily and selectively removable, masking groups. As the side chain protectors should be stable during several deblocking steps, it is desirable to use α-amino protecting residues that allow the liberation of the amino group under very mildly acidic conditions. Historically, thousands of studies were devoted to the investigations of amino protecting groups of different structure and numerous publications have dealt with the problems of carboxyl, nitrogen, hydroxyl, sulfhydryl, and thioether protection of the amino acid side chains. I shall briefly discuss a few recent developments in this area. More detailed discussions appear in the excellent monographs of Wünsch (44) and of Schröder and Lübke (36).

PROTECTIVE GROUPS USED FOR SIDE CHAIN PROTECTION OF AMINO ACIDS AND PEPTIDES

Based on the differing chemical structure of amino acids, protection of functional groups utilizing nitrogen (amino, guanido, imidazole, and indole), oxygen (ω-carboxyl and hydroxyl), and sulfur (sulfhydryl and thioether) have been developed. The functional groups in the side chains of amino acids need not be protected in every case as is demonstrated by the successful synthesis of ribonuclease (18) or of ACTH (14,22) peptides. Maximal protection may reduce the quantities of undesirable by-products during synthesis of the peptide, but this strategy is often too expensive for large-scale reactions.

N Protection

The ω-amino protective groups should not be removed under the conditions used for the liberation of NH_2 functions. One of the preferred combinations is

N^{α}-Boc, N^{ω}-Z protection. However, on repetitive coupling and deblocking steps, the N^{ω}-Z group of lysine or ornithine is partially deacylated; hence, the more stable N^{ω}-4CZ or N^{ω}-2CZ groups are more commonly used. Recently the combinations Bpoc/Boc, Ddz/Boc, or Adpoc/Boc have been applied successfully (9,20,29).

Bergmann (7) was the first to attack the problem of guanido protection of arginine by employing the nitro group. In addition, acyl, arylsulfonyl, aralkylsulfonyl, and trityl residues have been used for protection. As the guanido residue is strongly basic, protonation (4) is also suitable as a protective device. Guanido protection remains, to some extent, an unsolved problem since frequently protection is incomplete and the conditions used for the liberation of the arginine side chain cause the formation of side products. The most elegant method to cleave the protective groups from the guanido residue uses HF/anisole as a reactant.

Usually it is unnecessary to protect the imidazole ring of histidine unless the histidine is COOH-terminal; N_{im}-unprotected histidine, however, has a tendency to racemize (28). Suitable N_{im}-blocking groups are benzyl (11), trityl (3), 2,4-dinitrophenyl (39), and urethan-forming groups.

Tryptophan derivatives without a protected indole are commonly used for peptide synthsis. However, during the acidic cleavage, decomposition of the indole moiety of tryptophan frequently occurs; splitting off Boc residues often causes *tert*-butylation of the indole moiety (2).

—OH Protection

The hydroxyl groups of serine, threonine, and hydroxyproline do not always need blocking to prevent side reactions; when required, suitable blocking groups are acetyl, benzyl, or *tert*-butyl residues. Of the three residues, *tert*-butyl causes

TABLE 1. *Protecting groups for —SH in cysteine and reagents used in their cleavage*

Residue	Reagents
Acetyl (Ac)	NH_3, OH^-
Benzyl (Bzl)	HF, Na/NH_3
Benzyloxycarbonyl (Z)	CF_3COOH, NH_3, OH^-
Benzoyl (Bz)	NH_3, OH^-
tert-Butyl (But)	HF
4,4'-Dimethoxydiphenylmethyl	H^+, Na/NH_3
Diphenylmethyl (Dpm)	CF_3COOH, HF, Na/NH_3
Ethylmercapto (Et)	Thiophenol, thioglycolic acid
Isobutoxymethyl (iBm)	$(SCN)_2$
p-Methoxybenzyl (Mbzl)	CF_3COOH, HF
p-Methoxybenzyloxycarbonyl [Z(OMe)]	HBr/CH_3COOH, HCl/CH_3COOH
p-Nitrobenzyl (Nbzl)	H_2
Trityl (Trt)	CF_3COOH, $HCl/CHCl_3$, Na/NH_3

minimal side reactions under the conditions of cleavage. The —OH groups in tyrosine can be protected by tosyl, benzyl, and benzoyl residues.

—S— and —SH Protection

The thioether group in methionine usually causes no difficulty in the synthesis of Met peptides. H_2O_2 oxidizes the thioether to the corresponding methionine sulfoxide, which can then be reduced by thioglycolic acid to the original thioether after the last coupling step.

Much effort has been expended on the development of protecting groups for the —SH of cysteine. A survey of the results of these efforts is shown in Table 1.

COOH- AND NH₂-TERMINAL PROTECTION OF AMINO ACIDS AND PEPTIDES

Carboxyl and Acid Amide Protection

The most effective protection of carboxyl groups is achieved by esterification and the reagents employed in the cleavage of the different esters are summarized in Table 2.

Although generally stable, amides often give rise to various side reactions: They may be converted to nitriles (41), dipeptide amides may form diketopiperazines, and asparagine peptides may form succinimides (34,40). For these reasons, several amide protecting groups such as xanthenyl (Xan) (1), benzhydryl (Dpm) (43), 4,4′-dimethylbenzhydryl (Dbh), or 4,4′-dimethoxybenzhydryl (Mbh) (25) have been investigated. These protecting groups can be cleaved in an acid medium with CF_3COOH/anisole. For the synthesis of pyroglutamylpeptides, the discovery of the transformation (26) of Nγ-4,4′-dimethoxybenzhydryl-L-glutamine

TABLE 2. *Alcohol residues used for carboxyl protection and reagents used for cleavage of their corresponding esters*

Alcohol residue	Cleavage conditions
Benzhydryl (OBzh)	CF_3COOH, H_2
Benzyl (OBzl)	HBr/CF_3COOH, HBr/CH_3COOH, Na/NH_3, OH^-
Benzyl, ring substituted by methyl	CF_3COOH, HBr/CH_3COOH
tert-Butyl (OBut)	CF_3COOH, HBr/CH_3COOH, HCl/CH_3COOH
Ethyl (OEt)	H^+, OH^-
Methyl	H^+, OH^-
p-Methoxybenzyl	CF_3COOH, HBr/CH_3COOH
Phenyl	H_2O_2
4-Picolyl	H_2, Na/NH_3, OH^-

$$Z - NH - CH - COOR$$

with the side chain:

$$CH_2 - CH_2 - C(=O) - NH - CH(H_3CO-C_6H_4)(C_6H_4-OCH_3)$$

$$\xrightarrow{CF_3COOH}$$

pyroglutamyl — COOR

Z - Gln (Mbh) - OR

FIG. 1. Synthesis of pyroglutamic acid derivatives from Z-Gln(Mbh)-OR.

into pyroglutamic acid in the presence of boiling trifluoroacetic acid (Fig. 1) proved to be of great value.

The usefulness of glutamine protection and final transformation into a pyroglutamyl group is demonstrated by a Phe^2-TRH synthesis (Fig. 2).

Amino Protecting Groups

In the last few decades, four major types of α-amino protectors for amino acids and peptides have been developed: acyl, alkyl, sulfur- and phosphorus-containing, and urethan-forming protecting groups.

As the use of N$^\alpha$-acylated amino acids results in considerable racemization, the protecting groups of the acyl type are of limited value. Figure 3 shows the structures of some selected acyl groups used for α-amino protection.

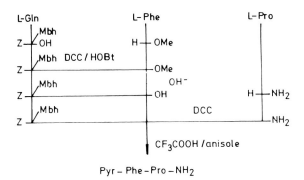

Pyr – Phe – Pro – NH$_2$

FIG. 2. Synthesis of L-Phe-L-Phe-L-Pro-NH$_2$(Phe^2-TRH). (From ref. 45.)

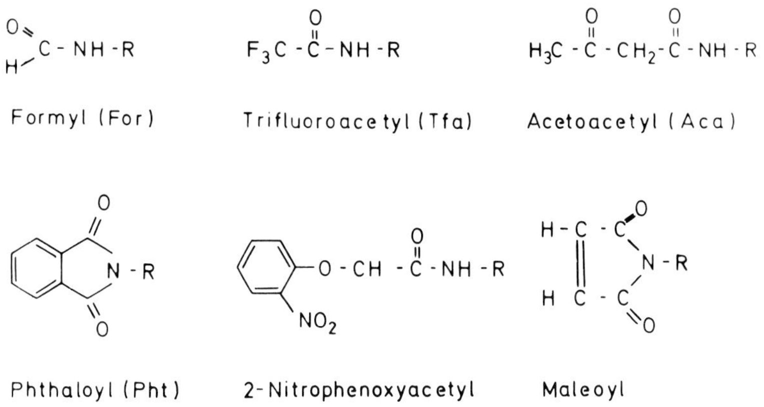

FIG. 3. Selected acyl groups used for N_α protection of amino acids.

In 1905 Fischer and Warburg (13) synthesized the first formyl amino acid. As the formyl group is relatively stable in alkali and CF_3COOH, use of it is restricted to special cases in peptide chemistry. The trifluoracetyl group is one of the few residues that is alkali labile (42) and thus has a greater utility than the For group. The acetoacetyl group (10), which is acid stable, as well as the 2-nitrophenoxyacetyl (19) and the maleoyl (23) groups, have found few synthetic applications in peptide chemistry. The phthaloyl group has received more attention since it can be introduced, by N-carbethoxyphthalimide (32) in weakly alkaline solution, into amino groups; in addition, an elegant removing method employing hydrazine (37) has been developed.

The trityl group is the only α-amino protecting group of the alkyl type that has achieved synthetic importance. It can be incorporated by means of trityl chloride (17) and is cleavable by hydrogenation or weak acids. The residue can be split off selectively even if Bpoc or Poc groups are present (33).

Of the phosphorus- and sulfur-containing protecting groups such as dibenzylphosphoryl (Dbp) (46), diphenylphosphinyl (Dpp) (24), benzylsulfonyl, tosyl (Tos) or 2-nitrophenylsulfenyl (Nps), only the Tos and Nps have received wide application.

Nitrophenylsulfenyl groups were first incorporated into amino residues in 1959 (15). The Nps residue can be removed selectively in a weakly acidic medium without cleavage of *tert*-butyl groups and, as a result, has also found wide use for the synthesis of larger peptides. The tosyl group has been used for amino protection since the early part of this century (12). Cleavage of the Tos residue can be done by Na/NH_3; unfortunately, this removal is accompanied by side reactions. Nevertheless, toluenesulfonyl blocking, due to the stability of the sulfonamide bond, is one of the best methods to protect the basic side chains or ornithine, lysine, and arginine.

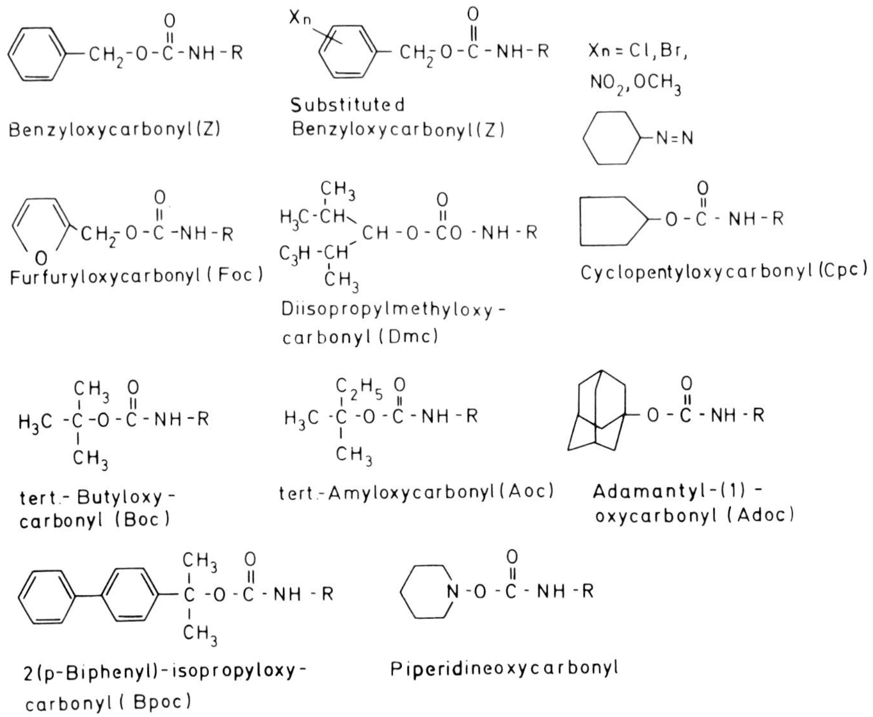

FIG. 4. Selected protective groups of the urethan type.

The development of urethan-forming protecting groups created a landmark in peptide chemistry. Ever since Bergmann and Zervas (6) introduced the benzyl-oxycarbonyl group, much effort has been expended in development of urethan-forming groups of differing structures (Fig. 4). This figure demonstrates that these compounds are derived from primary alcohols (Z and Foc), secondary alcohols (Dmc and Cpc), or tertiary alcohols (Boc, Aoc, and Bpoc). Without any doubt, Boc (30) and the Z (6) groups are those used more frequently by peptide chemists for several reasons: (a) Both groups can be incorporated into practically all the amino functions of different amino acids without any difficulty; and (b) the Z group can be split off by Pd/H$_2$ (6), Na/NH$_3$ (31), HBr/CH$_3$COOH (5), and HF (35). Differing from the Z group, the Boc residue is resistant to Pd/H$_2$ and Na/NH$_3$, thus allowing selective cleavage of one protective group in the presence of the other. As already mentioned, N$^\alpha$-Boc and N$^\omega$-Z (or, better, N$^\omega$-4CZ or N$^\omega$-2CZ) is one of the preferred combinations of protecting groups for peptide synthesis.

The excellent properties of the Boc group suggested looking for further ure-than-forming protecting groups derived from *tert*-alcohols. A search for new protective groups resulted in the development of the Bpoc (38), Ddz (8), and Azoc (27) groups, which can be cleaved under very mildly acidic conditions.

Adpoc: A NEW AMINO PROTECTING GROUP HAVING ADVANTAGEOUS PROPERTIES

Although the well-known *tert*-butyl- and benzyl-oxycarbonyl fulfill many requirements for protecting groups in straightforward peptide synthesis, it is often desirable to liberate NH_2 groups under very mildly acidic conditions so that (a) optimal protection of acid labile residues can be achieved in syntheses involving repetitive coupling and deblocking steps (solid-phase method), and (b) the indole moiety of tryptophan-containing peptides remains intact.

Despite the fact that Bpoc (see Fig. 4), Ddz [3,5-dimethoxy (α,α-dimethyl) benzyloxycarbonyl]. and Azoc (α,α-dimethyl-4-phenylazobenzyloxycarbonyl) groups cleave under the desired conditions, amino acids protected by them may decompose during storage. In addition, synthesis of Bpoc-Trp-OH is very difficult.

We (21) recently described 1-(1-adamantyl)-1-methylethoxycarbonyl (Adpoc), a protecting group lacking the above disadvantages. An intermediate in the synthesis of Adpoc amino acids is the tertiary alcohol, 2-(1-adamantyl)-2-propanol, which can be prepared from 1-adamantanecarboxylic acid via its ethyl ester as depicted in Fig. 5.

The Adpoc residue can be easily incorporated into amino acids and peptides by means of crystalline Adpoc—OPh, Adpoc—F, or Adpoc—O—N≡C (Ph,CN), the formation of which is shown in Fig. 6.

Table 3 lists the physical data and yields of pure isolated material of some Adpoc derivatives we have obtained. The Adpoc amino acids and peptides are stable for months during storage at room temperature. The Adpoc group is removed 1,000 times faster than the Boc group under very mildly acidic conditions (3% CF_3COOH in CH_2Cl_2 at 0°C for 8–10 min) and therefore allows selective cleavage. The high rates of cleavage of Adpoc from Adpoc-Trp-OH in various solvents of low acidity are shown in Table 4. Figure 7 depicts a time plot of this reaction.

The cleavage of the Adpoc group in a mildly acidic medium can easily be followed by high performance liquid chromatography (HPLC), as is demonstrated for Adpoc-Trp-OH in Fig. 8.

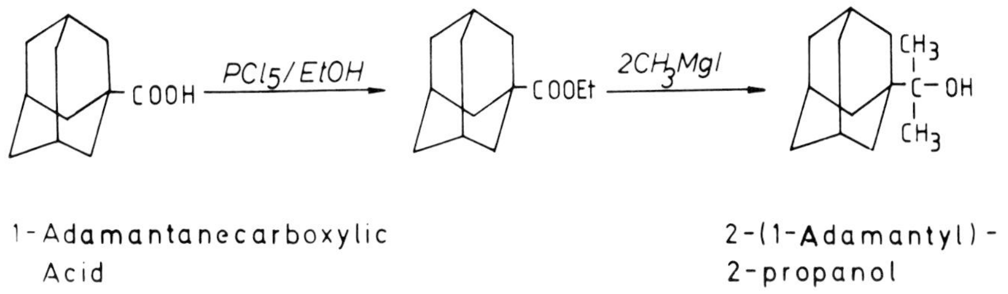

1-Adamantanecarboxylic
Acid

2-(1-Adamantyl)-
2-propanol

FIG. 5. Synthesis of 2-(1-adamantyl)-2-propanol.

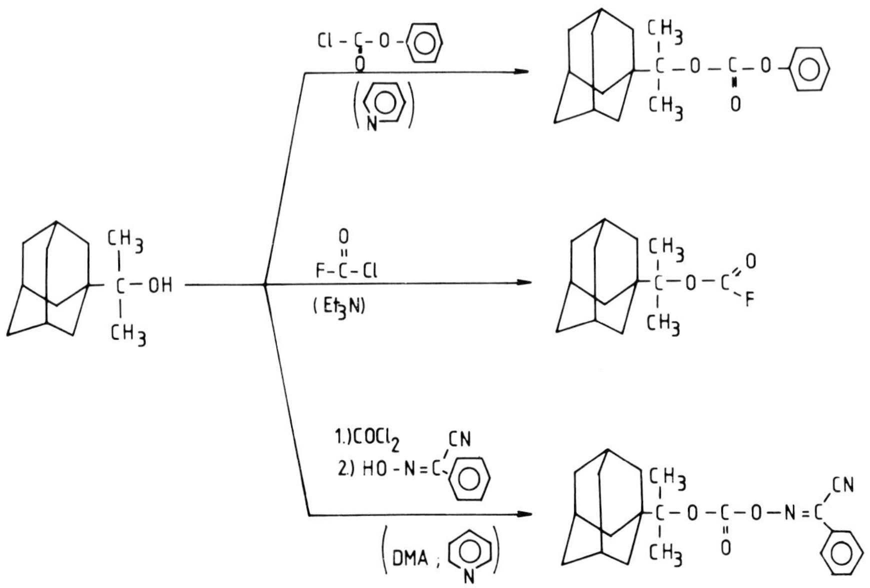

FIG. 6. Synthesis of reagents for the incorporation of the Adpoc group.

TABLE 3. *Yields and physical data of selected Adpoc derivatives*

Compound	Yield (%)	M.P. (°C)	$[\alpha]_D^{20}$ (°)
Adpoc-L-Ala·DCHA	75	155	+6.22 (c = 0.65 ETOH)
Adpoc-Gly-OH	73	178	N.D.[a]
Adpoc-L-Leu-OH	78	176	−12.8 (c = 1.2 MeOH)
Adpoc-L-Trp-OH	72	116	−6.8 (c = 1.04 MeOH)
Adpoc-L-Thr(Bzl)-OH	68	51–52	+19.8 (c = 1.02 MeOH)
Adpoc-L-Trp-L-Lys(Boc)-OH	73	134 (dec.)	−9.83 (c = 0.5 MeOH)

[a] Not determined.

TABLE 4. *Cleavage rates of Adpoc-Trp-OH in various media*

Reagent	Temperature (°C)	Cleavage		k_1 (min⁻¹)
		50% (min)	99.9% (min)	
$CF_3COOH(3\%) + CH_2Cl_2$	25	0.12	1.22	5.63
	0	1.1	11.7	0.59
$CH_3COOH + HCOOH(83\%) + H_2O$[a]	45	12.8	127	5.4×10^{-2}
$CH_3COOH (80\%)$	45	34	338	2.02×10^{-2}

[a] 7:1:2, v/v.

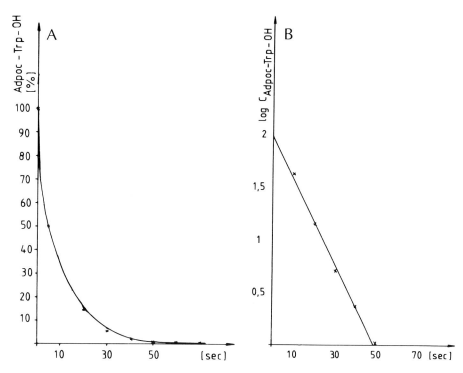

FIG. 7. Cleavage of Adpoc from Adpoc-Trp-OH in the presence of 3% TFA/CH$_2$Cl$_2$ at 25°C. **A:** % cleaved; **B:** log of concentration cleaved.

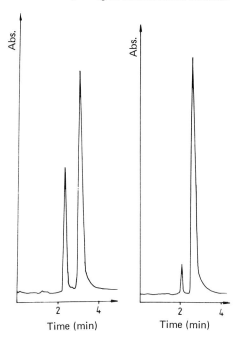

FIG. 8. HPLC chromatogram of the cleavage of Adpoc-Trp-OH. The 25 × 0.4 cm column was packed with RP8 (10 μm particle size), eluted with methanol (90%)/water (adjusted to pH 5.2 with H$_2$SO$_4$) at a flow rate of 2.5 ml/min with an inlet pressure of 12.157 MPa. Eluate monitored at 280 nm. **Left:** 20 sec; **right:** 40 sec after treatment with 3% CF$_3$COOH/CH$_2$Cl$_2$ at 25°C.

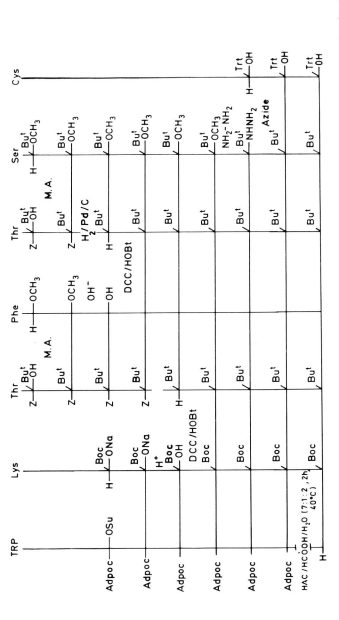

FIG. 9. Synthesis of a protected COOH-terminal heptapeptide having the natural sequence of somatostatin using Adpoc protection for the Trp residue.

Synthesis of several peptides with the natural sequence of somatostatin (Ala-Gly-Cys-Lys-Asn-Phe-Phe-Trp-Lys-Thr-Phe-Thr-Ser-Cys) reveals that the new protecting group has the following advantages:

1. Adpoc residues can be incorporated into amino groups at high yields.
2. Adpoc amino acids are crystalline compounds and stable for months at room temperature.
3. Adpoc amino acids are stable in the presence of hυ.
4. Adpoc residues are cleavable under very mild conditions.
5. Adpoc residues can be removed 1,000 times faster than Boc amino acids and permit selective cleavage.
6. Adpoc residues prevent attack of the indole ring in tryptophan.

The successful synthesis of a protected COOH-terminal heptapeptide with the natural sequence of somatostatin (16) using Adpoc protection for the tryptophan moiety demonstrates that the Adpoc residue can be selectively cleaved in a medium of low acidity $CH_3COOH/HCOOH/H_2O$ (7:1:2) at 40°C; under these conditions, the Nε-Boc group of lysine, the *tert*-butyl groups in the side chains of threonine and serine, and the trityl group of cysteine residues are not attacked (Fig. 9).

REFERENCES

1. Akabori, S., Sakakibara, S., and Shimonishi, Y. (1961): *Bull. Chem. Soc. Jpn.,* 35:1966.
2. Alakhov, Y. B., Kiryuskin, A. A., Lipkin, V. M., and Milne, G. W. A. (1970): Butylation of the tryptophan indole ring: A side reaction during the removal of t-butyloxycarbonyl and *t*-butyl protecting groups in peptide synthesis. *J. Chem. Soc. (Chem. Commun.),* 1970:406–
3. Amiard, G., Heymès, R., and Velluz, L. (1955): Sur les *N*-trityl α-amino-acides et leurs applications en synthèse peptidique. *Bull. Soc. Chim. France,* 1955:191–193.
4. Anderson, G. W. (1953): The synthesis of an arginyl peptide. *J. Am. Chem. Soc.,* 75:6081.
5. Ben Ishai, D., and Berger, A. (1952): Cleavage of *N*-carbobenzoxy groups by dry hydrogen bromide and hydrogen chloride. *J. Org. Chem.,* 17:1564–1570.
6. Bergmann, M., and Zervas, L. (1932): Über ein allgemeines Verfahren der Peptid-Synthese. *Ber. Dtsch. Chem. Gesamte,* 65:1192–1201.
7. Bergmann, M., Zervas, L., and Rinke, H. (1934): Proteolytic enzymes III.E. New process for synthesis of peptides of arginine. *Hoppe Seylers Z. Physiol. Chem.,* 224:40–44.
8. Birr, C., Lochinger, W., Stahnke, C., and Lang, P. (1972): Der α-Dimethyl-3,5-dimethoxyben-zoyloxycarbonyl (Ddz)-Rest, eine photo-und säurelabile Stickstoff-Schutzgruppe für die Peptid-chemie. *Justus Liebigs Ann. Chem.,* 763:162–172.
9. Bodansky, M., and Ondetti, M. A. (1966): *Peptide Synthesis.* Interscience, New York.
10. D'Angeli, F., Filvia, F., and Scoffone, E. (1965): The acetoacetyl group, an amino protective group of potential use in peptide synthesis. *Tet. Lett.,* 10:605–608.
11. Du Vigneaud, V., and Behrens, O. K. (1937): A method for protecting the imidazole ring of histidine during certain reactions and its application to the preparation of L-amino-*N*-methylhisti-dine. *J. Biol. Chem.,* 117:27–36.
12. Fischer, E. (1915): Reduktion der Aryl-sulfamide durch Jodwasserstoff. *Ber. Dtsch. Chem. Gesamte,* 48:93–102.
13. Fischer, E., and Warburg, O. (1905): Spaltung des Leucins in die optisch-activen Componenten mittels der Formylverbindung. *Ber. Dtsch. Chem. Gesamte,* 38:3997–4005.

14. Geiger, R., Sturm, K., and Siedel, W. (1964): Synthese eines biologisch aktiven Tricosapeptid-amids mit der Aminosäuersequenz 1-23 des Corticotropins (ACTH). *Chem. Ber.,* 97:1207–1213.

15. Goerdeler, J., and Holst, A. (1959): *N*-(*o*-Nitrobenzenesulfenyl)amino acids and -amino acid esters. *Angew Chem.,* 71:775.

16. Gupta, D., and Voelter, W. (1978): *Hypothalamic Hormones—Chemistry Physiology, and Clinical Applications.* Verlag Chemie, Weinheim.

17. Helferich, B., Moog, L., and Jünger, A. (1925): Über den Ersatz reaktionsfähiger Wasserstoffatome in Zuckern, Oxy-und Amino-säuren durch den Triphenylmethyl-Rest. *Ber. Dtsch. Chem. Gesamte,* 58:872–886.

18. Hirschmann, R., Nutt, R. F., Veber, D. F., Vitali, R. A., Varga, S. L., Jacob, T. A., Holly, F. W., and Denkewalter, R. G. (1969): Studies on the total synthesis of an enzyme. V. The preparation of enzymatically active material. *J. Am. Chem. Soc.,* 91:507–508.

19. Holley, R. W., and Holley, A. D. (1952): The removal of *N*-*o*-nitrophenoxyacetyl and *N*-chloracetyl groups from peptides. *J. Am. Chem. Soc.,* 74:3069–3074.

20. Jakubhe, H.-D., and Jeschkeit, H. (1973): *Aminosäuren, Peptide, Proteine.* Akademie-Verlag, Berlin.

21. Kalbacher, H., and Voelter, W. (1978): 1-(1-Adamantyl)-1-methylethoxycarbonyl: A new protecting group for peptide synthesis. *Angew. Chem. (Engl.),* 17:944–945.

22. Kappeler, H., and Schwyzer, R. (1961): Synthesis of a tetracosapeptide with the amino acid sequence of a highly active degradation product of β-cortocotropin (ACTH) from hog pituitary glands. *Helv. Chim. Acta,* 44:1136–1141.

23. Keller, O., and Rudinger, J. (1975): Preparation and some properties of maleimido acids and maleoyl derivatives of peptides. *Helv. Chim. Acta,* 58:531–541.

24. Kenner, G. W., Moore, G. A., and Ramage, R. (1976): Phosphinamides: New class of amino protecting groups in peptide chemistry. *Tet. Lett.,* 1976:3623–3626.

25. König, W., and Geiger, R. (1970): Eine neue Amid-Schutzgruppe. *Chem. Ber.,* 103:2041–2051.

26. König, W., and Geiger, R. (1972): Pyroglutamylpeptide. *Chem. Ber.,* 105:2872–2882.

27. Kyi, A. T., and Schwyzer, R. (1976): (*p*-Phenylazophenyl)-isopropyloxycarbonyl, a new protecting group for peptide synthesis. *Helv. Chim. Acta,* 59:1642–1646.

28. Lin, M. C., Gutte, B., Caldi, D. G., Moore, S., and Merrifield, R. B. (1972): Reactivation of des (119-124) ribonuclease A by mixture with COOH-terminal peptides: The role of phenylalanine-120. *J. Biol. Chem.,* 247:4768–4774.

29. Lübke, K., Schröder, and Kloss, G. (1975): *Chemie und Biochemie der Aminosäuren, Peptide, und Proteine, Vols. 1 & 2,* Georg Thieme, Stuttgart.

30. McKay, F. C., and Albertson, N. F. (1957): New amine-masking groups for peptide synthesis. *J. Am. Chem. Soc.,* 79:4686–4690.

31. Meienhofer, J., and Kuromizu, K. (1974): Catalytic hydrogenolysis in liquid ammonia: Stability and cleavage of some protecting groups used in peptide synthesis. *Tet. Lett.,* 37:3259–3262.

32. Nefkens, G. H., Tesser, G. I., and Nivard, R. J. (1960): Simple preparation of phthaloylamino acids via a mild phthaloylation. *Res. Trav. Chim.,* 79:688–698.

33. Riniker, B., Kamber, B., and Sieber, P. (1975): Selektive Abspaltung säurelabile Aminoschutzgruppen von Peptiden in Trifluoräthanol. *Helv. Chim. Acta,* 58:1086–1094.

34. Roeske, R. (1963): Preparation of *t*-butyl esters of free amino acids. *J. Org. Chem.,* 28:1251–1253.

35. Sakakibara, S., Shimonishi, Y., Kishida, Y., Okada, M., and Sugibara, H. (1967): Use of anhydrous hydrogen fluoride in peptide synthesis. I. Behavior of various protective groups in anhydrous hydrogen fluoride. *Bull. Chem. Soc. Jpn.,* 40:2164–2167.

36. Schröder, E., and Lübke, K. (1965): *The Peptides.* Academic Press, New York.

37. Schwyzer, R., Costopanagiotis, A., and Sieber, P. (1963): Zwei Synthesen des α-Melanotropins (α-MSH) mit Hilfe leicht entfernbarer Schutzgruppen. *Helv. Chim. Acta,* 46:870–889.

38. Sieber, P., and Iselin, B. (1968): Selektive acidolytische Spaltung von Aralkyloxycarbonyl-Aminoschutzgruppen. *Helv. Chim. Acta,* 51:614–622.

39. Siepmann, E., and Zahn, H. (1964): N_{im}-2,4-Dinitrophenyl-L-histidin. *Biochim. Biophys. Acta,* 82:412–415.

40. Sondheimer, E., and Holley, R. W. (1954): Imides from asparagine and glutamine. *J. Am. Chem. Soc.,* 76:2467–2470.

41. Stephens, C. R., Bianco, E. J., and Pilgrim, F. J. (1955): A new reagent for dehydrating primary amides under mild conditions. *J. Am. Chem. Soc.,* 77:1701–1702.

42. Weygand, F., and Czendes, E. (1952): *N*-(Trifluoracetyl)aminosäure. *Angew. Chem.*, 64:136.
43. Weygand, F., Steglich, W., Bjarnason, J., Akhtar, R., and Chytil, N. (1968): Vergleichende Untersuchungen zur Abspaltung substit. Benzylreste vom Amidstickstoff und deren Kombinations möglichkeiten mit Urethanschutzgruppen. *Chem. Ber.*, 101:3623–3641.
44. Wünsch, E. (1974): Synthese von Peptiden. In: *Methoden der Organischen Chemie, Vol. 15*, edited by E. Müller. Georg Thieme, Stuttgart.
45. Zech, K., Horn, H., and Voelter, W. (1974): Synthesis of (2-Phe)-TRH, a bioactive analog of thyroid releasing hormone (TRH). *Chem. Ztg.*, 98:209.
46. Zervas, L., and Dilaris, L. (1956): Entalkylierung und Entbenzylierung von neutralen Pyrophosphorsäureestern: Pyrophosphorylierung von Hydroxyverbindungen. *Chem. Ber.*, 89:925–933.

Polypeptide Hormones, edited by
R. F. Beers, Jr. and E. G. Bassett.
Raven Press, New York © 1980.

14. Current Advances on Biologically Active Synthetic Peptides

Karl Folkers, Johann Leban, Naoki Sakura, Georg Rampold, Elsa Lundanes, Jan Dahmen, Maria Lebek, Masahiro Ohta, and *Cyril Y. Bowers

*Institute for Biomedical Research, University of Texas, Austin, Texas 78712; and *Tulane University School of Medicine, New Orleans, Louisiana 70112*

INTRODUCTION

This chapter on current advances obviously cannot be comprehensive within the scope of this volume. I trust that each reader will find something of interest following my decision to present an overview rather than numerous facts.

THYROTROPIN-RELEASING HORMONE

The discovery of thyrotropin-releasing hormone (TRH) took place a decade ago. The role of K.F. in the elucidation of the structure and synthesis of TRH was by invitation. The final establishment of the diversified chemistry of TRH was so momentous that it stimulated all phases of research on peptide hormones probably more than any previously discovered hormone for quite some time.

Serendipity also occurred with TRH, and surprisingly opened a field of research on TRH for central nervous system (CNS) activities quite apart from the release of thyrotropin and prolactin, as exemplified by the current research of Bower et al. (4) and Nutt et al. (16) on analogs of TRH that have high neuropharmacological activity.

ENKEPHALINS AND ENDORPHINS

Probably the second most significant advance during the last decade in the peptide field has been the discovery of the enkephalins and endorphins. The amazing low molecular weight of TRH and of the enkephalins is useful for the peptide chemist having only the classic reactions at hand.

The advent of TRH stimulated some pharmaceutical companies to initiate peptide research, but this situation was enhanced to a much larger extent by studies on the enkephalins and endorphins, possibly because the industry had a greater interest in morphine than in thyrotropin.

KYOTORPHIN

The field of endocrinology quickly recovered from learning that TRH was only a peptide; thus at present there is no reluctance to accept the smallest possible peptide, a dipeptide, which shows morphine-like analgesia. Takagi et al. (21) isolated a new morphine-like substance from bovine brain with the guidance of an *in vivo* assay for analgesic activity. The new substance was identified as L-tyrosyl-L-arginine. Since these investigators made their discovery in Kyoto, and the substance is endorphin-like, they named it kyotorphin. They found that the analgesic activity of this dipeptide is approximately 4.2 times that of Met-enkephalin, and that the action is relatively long-lasting. The significance of the potent analgesic activity of an endogenous dipeptide could be another landmark in the investigations relating peptides to morphine. Schally et al. (19) reported at a recent meeting of the Endocrine Society that they had isolated the amide of this dipeptide from hypothalamic fragments, but apparently without regard to analgesia.

GENE EXPRESSION OF SYNTHETIC PEPTIDE HORMONES

The advent of expression of chemically synthesized peptide hormone genes in bacteria is also momentous. Although the previous section in this volume ("The Biological Synthesis of Peptide Hormones") surveyed this progress, the great significance of these events justifies our stating that improvements in the synthesis of oligodeoxyribonucleotides by the triester method have greatly improved the synthesis of DNA. This synthesis of DNA coupled with design and synthesis of moderately sized genes, which are incorporated into procaryotic cells for gene expression, has allowed the production of both somatostatin and the peptide chains of human insulin by *E. coli.* The production of the insulin chains by a microorganism is surely the dawn of a new era that beckons speculation and many newcomers to this important field. DNA research has recently been called "high-intensity" science.

HIGH-PRESSURE LIQUID CHROMATOGRAPHY

High-pressure liquid chromatography (HPLC) represents an almost indispensible tool in the peptide field. Probably this technique received its first widespread attention when Woodward and Eschenmoser used it so effectively in their synthesis of vitamin B_{12}. Rubenstein et al. (18) reported that they have obtained pure interferon from human leukocytes, using HPLC in the last stage of purification. They believed that this experience constituted the first example of the isolation of a pure protein by HPLC. The patterns of proteins and antiviral activity obtained with leukocytes from leukemic patients were identical to those obtained with leukocytes from normal donors. Also, the pure preparations of interferon obtained from leukemic patients and normal donors have indistinguishable amino acid compositions. This success with HPLC on reverse-phase and diol columns will surely advance knowledge on interferon and will certainly be extended to a diversity of other biologically active proteins.

HIGH-PERFORMANCE COUNTER-CURRENT DISTRIBUTION

The late Sir Robert Robinson commented that waves of chemical progress follow the discoveries of new techniques. Frequently, progress is impossible until a new technique is known. Brenner et al. (5) have uniquely advanced the art of counter-current distribution (CCD). Lyman Craig designed CCD, which advanced the objectives of chemical and biological research during World War II, while du Vigneaud featured CCD in isolating synthetic penicillin by a reaction pioneered by Stanton Harris and myself. Today, Brenner and co-workers have designed high-performance counter-current distribution, known as HPCD. They made the "stationary phase" mobile and solved the mechanical problems of mass transfer and opposing phase transports and have thereby enormously enlarged the scope of CD. The operation is said to be much simpler than the operation of the Craig apparatus. They have projected that 150 theoretical plates may be as effective as 4,000 HPLC plates. This advance of Brenner's can be expected to facilitate the isolation of new peptide hormones.

PARATHYROID HORMONE

Chemical progress is being made toward the synthesis of human parathyroid hormone, consisting of 84 amino acids. Obviously, this is a challenge for automated solid-phase synthesis. Voelter *(this volume)* has made significant contributions in the use of novel protective groups. Tregear et al. (23) have conducted two companion syntheses of hPTH$_{53-84}$, which constitutes the COOH-terminal region of the human parathyroid hormone. For one synthesis, they utilized the preformed symmetrical anhydrides of the Boc-amino acids. The purified hormone fragment, prepared by the standard method, was homogeneous and identical to the native hormone fragment. These investigators exhaustively examined the purity of the fragment by multiple analytical criteria, comparison of tryptic digests, and even sequence analysis for quantitation of contaminating deletion-containing error peptides. Interestingly, the synthetic fragment obtained by the use of the anhydride method was quite impure.

Osteoporosis is the most common metabolic bone disease in man. This disease is particularly prevalent in post-menopausal women. It has been estimated that 10 to 25% of this population over 55 years of age have this bone disease. At present there is no satisfactory therapeutic treatment, but parathyroid hormone seems to have a therapeutic potential that can be best evaluated only by further research.

NEUROTENSIN

We have been collaborating with Sune Rosell at the Karolinska Institutet on the pharmacology and chemistry of neurotensin. He is investigating both neurotensin and [Gln]⁴-neurotensin, because we had observed that synthetic [Gln]⁴-neurotensin could be converted into neurotensin under the conditions simulating the isolation of neurotensin from tissue. The conversion of Gln to Glu is known in the organic chemistry of peptides. Recent data of Rosell (17) showed that neurotensin (or possibly a metabolite of it) satisfies the rather rigid physiological criteria for the status of a true hormone. The gastrointestinal actions of the peptide are produced by administration of a very low dose. The peptide is released into the blood by a physiological stimulus such as the ingestion of food. The plasma concentration of the peptide following the ingestion of food is comparable to levels reached by exogenous neurotensin at the dosage that produces effects in the gastrointestinal tract. Neurotensin may have a physiological role as a hormone with enterogastrone-like functions.

PEPTIDE HORMONES IN REPRODUCTION

The knowledge and acceptance of the chemistry of TRH facilitated understanding the chemistry and endocrinology of luteinizing hormone-releasing hormone (LH-RH). Almost immediately there was discouragement, perhaps largely from the medicinal chemists, regarding the short half-lives of LH-RH and TRH. Medicinal chemists and the pharmaceutical industry are so accustomed to classic therapy with synthetic "non-peptides" that the clinical use of a peptide hormone such as LH-RH was not viewed with enthusiasm. The peptide chemist soon found that the substitution of a D-amino acid for glycine in position 6 of LH-RH significantly increased potency and prolonged action. A change at the COOH-terminal also improved activity. The super analogs of LH-RH have potencies up to 200 times that of the native hormone.

Today, the pendulum is swinging to a new and better use of LH-RH and its super analogs. Gutai et al. (10) studied the response to pulsatile LH-RH (GnRH). In the case of clinical hypothalamic hypogonadism as evidenced by small testes and failure to develop any secondary sex characteristics, prolonged pulsatile LH-RH was associated with a pulsatile LH response similar to the nocturnal LH peaks that are observed in normal subjects. These investigators believe that prolonged pulsatile LH-RH may provide a new therapeutic modality for the treatment of hypothalamic hypogonadism. Knobil et al. (11) administered 1 μg/min of LH-RH in hourly 6-min pulses for as long as 3 months.

Crowley et al. (8) described the chronic administration of a long-acting super analog of LH-RH, [D-Trp⁶-Pro⁹-NHEt]-LRF, in hypogonadotrophic hypogonadism and the critical nature of dosage and frequency in enhancement.

Bex and Corbin (2) have found that LH-RH and an LH-RH agonist could enhance termination of pregnancy in hypophysectomized rats and proposed, as a result of their study, an extrapituitary site of action.

Wilks et al. (25) found that [D-Phe[2]-Pro[3]-D-Phe[6]]-LH-RH, an antagonist my group designed and synthesized, altered the spontaneous preovulatory endocrine events in ovulation in the monkey. These and other studies in the nonhuman primate have given chemists in the field a sense of confidence that the future utility of the best antagonist is not to control the rat population but rather that of the human.

Studies on follicle-stimulating hormone-releasing hormone (FSH-RH) have been controversial. Some believe it exists, whereas others express doubts. The chemist and his partner for assay would be spared a difficult task if it does not exist, but the task and the controversy are not nearly as important as the hormone itself.

Lorenzen and Schwartz (13) stated that physiological data indicate that there must be a separate secretory control of FSH. Thus, the chemist has faced this goal, and is prepared for the consequences of such experimentation.

Fuchs et al. (9) recently described their continuing studies on the existence and the separation of FSH-RH from LH-RH. They used porcine hypothalamic fragments that were extracted by acetic acid, and the extractives were subsequently processed in the presence of a protease inhibitor and an antioxidant. For the chemist, evolution should have prohibited all chemically unstable peptide hormones! Gel filtration was performed by Bio-Gel P-2; subsequently, labeled LH-RH and labeled <Glu-OH were used to differentiate them from the sought FSH-RH. The data revealed a different distribution of entities that released LH and FSH in comparison to the elution behavior of labeled LH-RH and labeled <Glu-OH. An entity that released LH and FSH constituted a distinct peak in biological activity that was well separated from the peak containing labeled LH-RH. They presumed that this activity could be attributed to FSH-RH.

Lundanes and Tsuji have continued this purification with the addition of another column, CM-Sephadex, to the sequence of steps. Again, an entity that could be FSH-RH was found in one of the fractions. An alternative to FSH-RH might be that the entity is a pro-LH-RH but, in this case, the pro-hormone must be active rather than inactive.

Possible structures of pro-TRH and pro-LH-RH (Table 1) are being studied by our group. We synthesized the model [Val-Lys-Lys-Gln][1]-TRH and assayed it *in vitro*. The chemistry of this model allows cleavage and cyclization to TRH, because of the presence of Lys-Lys. This model, at a dosage of 270 ng/ml,

TABLE 1. *Possible structures of pro-TRH and pro-LH-RH*

pro-TRH	pro-LH-RH
[Peptide-Lys-Lys-Gln][1]-TRH	[Peptide-Lys-Lys-Gln][1]-LH-RH
[Peptide-Arg-Arg-Gln][1]-TRH	[Peptide-Arg-Arg-Gln][1]-LH-RH
[Peptide-Lys-Arg-Gln][1]-TRH	[Peptide-Lys-Arg-Gln][1]-LH-RH
[Peptide-Arg-Lys-Gln][1]-TRH	[Peptide-Arg-Lys-Gln][1]-LH-RH

TABLE 2. In vitro *releasing effect of* [*Val-Lys-Lys-Gln*][1]*-TRH (I) for TSH when added to pituitary incubates*[a]

Peptide	Dose (ng/ml)	Δ TSH, ng/ml Medium SE[b]	p value versus control
—	—	−430 ± 658	—
TRH	1	18,450 ± 2,023	<0.001
Analog I	90	1,609 ± 490	<0.001
Analog I	270	5,823 ± 607	<0.001

[a] Two pituitaries from 20-day old female rats were incubated in a 1-ml beaker.
[b] Mean = 9.

released one-third of the TSH that 1 ng/ml of TRH released (Table 2). We are now studying whether the activity of this model is intrinsic or due to cleavage *in vitro.*

The model [Lys-Lys-Gln][1]-LH-RH at a dosage of 50 μg per rat released, *in vivo,* just as much LH as did LH-RH at 0.1 μg per rat levels (Table 3). Again, we are now concerned whether this activity of a model of a pro-LH-RH is intrinsic or due to cleavage and cyclization. In these assays, [Val-Lys-Lys-Gln][1]-LH-RH was less active than [Lys-Lys-Gln][1]-LH-RH.

For a number of years, those studying antagonists of LH-RH generally focused on decapeptides or nonapeptides and seldom on peptides longer than 10 amino acids. Wasiak et al. (24) found that the undecapeptide [(<Glu-Pro)[1], D-Phe[2],D-Trp[3],D-Trp[6]]-LH-RH caused 100% inhibition of ovulation in rats at the low dosage of 200 μg per rat. Based on the model for the conceptual pro-LH-RH

TABLE 3. In vivo *effect of LH-RH,* [*Val-Lys-Lys-Gln*][1]*-LH-RH (II) and* [*Lys-Lys-Gln*][1]*-LH-RH (III) on release of LH in the rat*[a]

Peptide	Dose (μg/rat)	Δ LH, ng/ml Serum ± SE[b]	p value versus control
—	—	1.8 ± 0.9	—
LH-RH	0.1	39.0 ± 6.0	<0.001
Analog II	0.2	3.6 ± 1.9	NS[c]
Analog II	0.6	0.0 ± 0.03	NS
Analog II	5.0	10.0 ± 1.0	<0.001
Analog II	50.0	23.0 ± 6.0	<0.01
—	—	0.1 ± 0.3	—
LH-RH	0.1	12.0 ± 0.8	<0.001
Analog III	0.5	0.4 ± 0.2	NS
Analog III	5.0	6.0 ± 0.6	<0.001
Analog III	50.0	12.0 ± 0.9	<0.001

[a] Blood sampled before and 15 min after i.v. administration of peptide to adult male rats.
[b] Mean = 5.
[c] Not significant.

TABLE 4. *Analogs related to the "pro-hormone concept"*

Position	1	2	3		6	of	LH-RH
Ac-(Ala-Gly-Lys-Lys-)-(Gln-Pro)-D-Phe-D-Trp-Ser-Tyr-D-Trp-Leu-Arg-Pro-Gly-NH₂							
Inhibition of ovulation:		27%/750 µg/11 rats					
(<Glu-Pro)-D-Phe-D-Trp-Ser-Tyr-D-Trp-Leu-Arg-Pro-Gly-NH₂							
Inhibition of ovulation:		100%/200 µg/4 rats					
		63%/100 µg/8 rats					

From ref. 24.

that has agonist activity, the pentadecapeptide Ac-(Ala-Gly-Lys-Lys)(Gln-Pro)(D-Phe-D-Trp-Ser-Tyr-D-Trp-Leu-Arg-Pro-Gly-NH₂) was synthesized and found to inhibit ovulation in 27% of 11 rats at a dosage of 750 µg (Table 4). Irrespective of cleavage, this is remarkable potency for the first analog having as many as 15 amino acids.

Channing and co-workers (7) studied the mode of action of oocyte maturation inhibitors that are purified from porcine follicular fluid. They obtained two entities that behave like peptides and have molecular weights of about 1,000 and 2,000 daltons. Because of these findings, greater importance has been given to this aspect of reproduction.

Chang et al. (6) have reported that the synthetic COOH-terminal 45-amino acid fragment of the β-subunit of HCG, when coupled to tetanus toxoid, gives a conjugate that is immunogenic. The antisera generated to this conjugate were capable of neutralizing the biological activity of HCG during the rat uterine weight assay. More importantly, the antisera were highly specific and did not cross-react with human LH in the radioimmunoassay. We and other investigators are pursuing this approach to the control of conception.

THYMIC PEPTIDES AND IMMUNOCOMPETENCE

We shall summarize very briefly some events in the field of thymic peptides and immunocompetence that will not be included in this volume. Their importance is the primary reason for including these peptides in this chapter.

We synthesized the 49-amino acid thymopoietin II of Schlesinger and Goldstein (20), the nonapeptide FTS of Bach et al. (1), and a related dodecapeptide of our design. Bliznakov (3) has reported that the profound impairment of the humoral, hemolytic, primary immuno-response in aged mice (22 months) as compared with young mice (10 weeks) showed a partial but significant reactivation of the age-determined impairment of the immunological responsiveness. The nonapeptide and the dodecapeptide analog of FTS were perhaps a little more effective than thymopoietin II. He believed that this assay is a useful experimental model for assay of potential immunopotentiating agents. Other studies have established that the thymus is subject to age-related involution—morphological as well as functional—occurring in both animals and man.

The synthesis of the dodecapeptide, an analog of FTS, was based on the

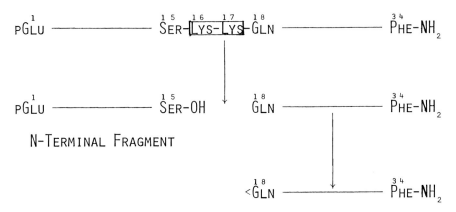

FIG. 1. Conversion of big gastrin to gastrin.

following consideration. It is rather well established that the cleavage of pro-hormones to hormones can take place at either side of a double basic dipeptide consisting of any one of the four possible combinations of lysine and arginine. Instead of a double basic pair, there may also be an adjacent three and even four basic amino acids. Of greatest relevance to this consideration is the established cleavage of big gastrin to gastrin, because it exemplifies the presence of a Gln residue adjacent to one of the basic amino acids as shown in Fig. 1. The release of [Gln][1]-gastrin allows enzymatic or nonenzymatic cyclization to the <Glu peptide, gastrin.

The same mechanism might pertain to FTS. In such a case, the structure shown in Fig. 2 may be considered. Cleavage of such a pro-FTS would yield [Gln][1]-FTS, which would then cyclize to FTS.

Interestingly, thymopoietin II has a COOH-terminal Val[47]-Lys[48]-Arg[49]. We considered the possibility that thymopoietin II and the nonapeptide may be combined in an unknown 58-amino acid peptide that could cleave between Arg[49] and Gln[50] to give thymopoietin II and Gln-FTS, which would then cyclize to FTS (Fig. 3). This conversion of Gln to Glu is exemplified by their structural formulas and is well documented in organic chemistry.

Our test of a conceptual peptide combining both thymopoietin and FTS was to synthesize the dodecapeptide depicted in Fig. 3. This dodecapeptide and FTS had comparable activity in Bliznakov's method for restoring an immune impairment in old mice. The addition of the three amino acids, Val-Lys-Arg, to FTS is a chemical novelty and that it has activity equivalent to FTS is interesting. This finding offers possible support of the concept that there is a union of thymopoietin and FTS. Evidently, in the old mouse, the dodecapeptide either has intrinsic activity or is cleaved.

$$\left[\text{PEPTIDE-BAA-BAA-GLN}\right]^1\text{-FTS}$$ **FIG. 2.** Proposed structure of a pro-FTS.

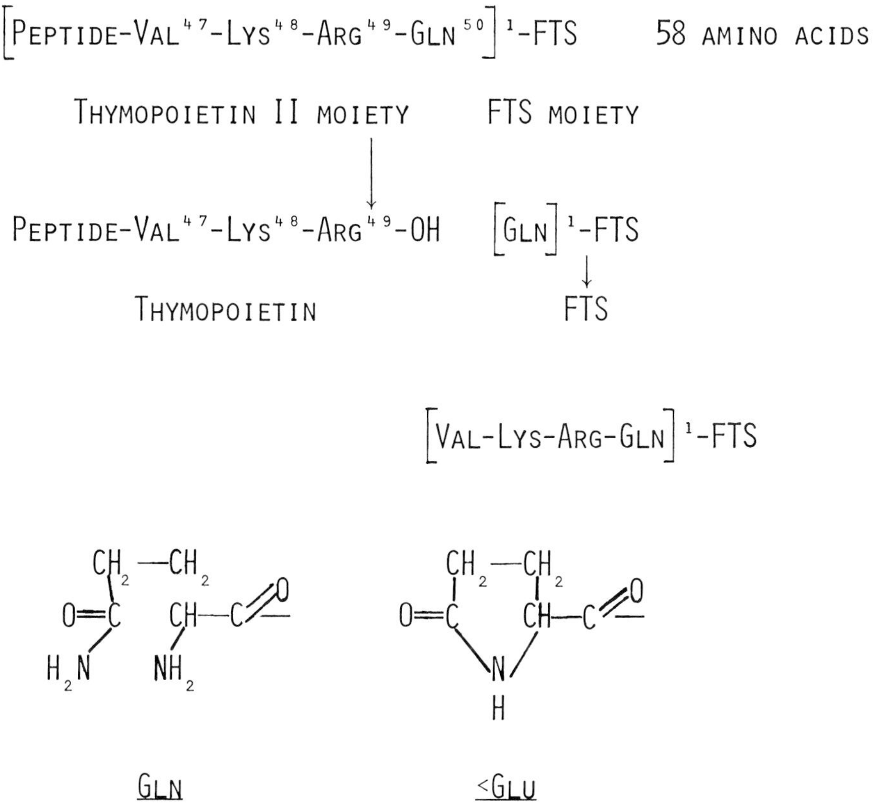

$$\Big[\text{PEPTIDE-VAL}^{47}\text{-LYS}^{48}\text{-ARG}^{49}\text{-GLN}^{50}\Big]^{1}\text{-FTS} \qquad 58 \text{ AMINO ACIDS}$$

THYMOPOIETIN II MOIETY   FTS MOIETY

PEPTIDE-VAL^{47}-LYS^{48}-ARG^{49}-OH $\Big[\text{GLN}\Big]^{1}$-FTS

THYMOPOIETIN   FTS

$$\Big[\text{VAL-LYS-ARG-GLN}\Big]^{1}\text{-FTS}$$

GLN   ≤GLU

FIG. 3. Proposal reactions of an unknown 58-amino acid peptide, and cyclization of Gln-FTS.

Martinez et al. (15) recently reported the failure of thymopoietin, ubiquitin, and synthetic FTS to restore immunocompetence in T-cell deficient mice. They considered this failure might have been due to insufficient exposure of the precursor cells to the peptides, the irrelevance of these peptides to cell maturation, or the inadequacy of a single factor to show meaningful activity to this assay.

Trainin et al. (22) have provided evidence that their THF behaves like a hormone, and we thought it would be of interest to compare some chemical characteristics of THF with those of thymosin α_1 described by Low and Goldstein (14). For this study, we synthesized thymosin α_1 by an automated solid-phase procedure. A fraction of THF, isolated by procedures published by Kook et al. (12), and our synthetic thymosin α_1 were analyzed by HPLC techniques. In this specific comparison, there was no evidence indicating that thymosin α_1 was present in the fraction of THF. After injection of 1 mg of the fraction, no thymosin α_1 peak was observed; we concluded that, within the limits of sensitivity, the content of thymosin α_1 was less than 0.1%. Earlier published analyses of these entities and our present comparison indicate that THF and thymosin α_1 are different.

Doubtless, many investigators will continue to make progress on the importance and role of one or more thymic hormones in studies of immunocompetence.

CONCLUSIONS

In final overview, the half-lives of peptide hormones are not of such concern as they were 10 years ago. Although many native hormones have multiple activities, it may be better to learn to use them effectively in medicine rather than using structurally modified hormones that could have favorable or unfavorable results. However, structural modification of peptides may lead to efficacious therapeutic agents.

The future pace of advances on peptide hormones will be lively and should yield medical treatments where they currently do not exist.

ACKNOWLEDGMENT

Appreciation is expressed to the Robert A. Welch Foundation and to Miles Laboratories, Inc. for their support of this research.

REFERENCES

1. Bach, J.-F., Dardenne, M., and Pleau, J.-M. (1977): Biochemical characterization of a serum thymic factor. *Cell,* 5:361–365.
2. Bex, F. J., and Corbin, A. (1979): LHRH or LHRH agonist-induced termination of pregnancy in hypophysectomized (HYPX) rats: Extra-pituitary site of action. In: *Abstracts of the 61st Annual Meeting of the Endocrine Society,* Abstr. 436.
3. Bliznakov, E. G., Wan, Y.-P., Chang, D., and Folkers, K. (1978): Partial reactivation of impaired immune competence in aged mice by synthetic thymus factors. *Biochem. Biophys. Res. Commun.,* 80:631–636.
4. Bower, J. D., Brewster, D., Dettmar, P. W., Metcalf, G., Morgan, B. A., and Rance, M. J. (1979): Novel TRH analogues with increased neuropharmacological activity. In: *Abstracts of the 6th American Peptide Symposium,* Abstr. 1–16.
5. Brenner, M., Müller, F., Bentz, R., Streb, B., and Walliser, H. P. (1979): High performance countercurrent distribution (HPCD). In: *Abstracts of the 6th American Peptide Symposium,* Abstr. C-V.
6. Chang, C. C., Tsong, Y. Y., Rone, J. D., Segal, S. Y., Chang, D., and Folkers, K. (1978): A highly specific antiserum to synthetic COOH-terminal peptide of human chorionic gonadotropin β-subunit. In: *Abstracts of the 34th Annual Meeting of the American Fertility Society,* Abstr.
7. Channing, C. P., Pomerantz, S. H., Stone, S. L., and Schwartz-Kripner, A. (1979): Studies on purification and mode of action of an oocyte maturation inhibitor (OMI) isolated from porcine follicular fluid (PFFI). In: *Abstracts of the 6th American Peptide Symposium,* Abstr. H-I.
8. Crowley, W., Vale, W., Beitins, I., Rivier, J., Rivier, C., and McArthur, J. (1979): Chronic administration of a long-acting LRF agonist, (D-Trp[6]-Pro[9]-NEt-LRF), in hypogonadotropic hypogonadism: The critical nature of dosage and frequency in enhancement, extinction and restoration of gonadotropin responsiveness. In: *Abstracts of the 61st Annual Meeting of the Endocrine Society,* Abstr. 16.

9. Fuchs, A., Lundanes, E., Leban, J., Folkers, K., and Bowers, C. Y. (1979): On the existence and separation of the follicle stimulating hormone releasing hormone from the luteinizing hormone releasing hormone. *Biochem. Biophys. Res. Commun.,* 88:92–96.

10. Gutai, J. P., Daneman, D., and Foley, T. P., Jr. (1979): Response to pulsatile gonadotropin releasing hormone in hypothalamic hypogonadism. In: *Abstracts of the 61st Annual Meeting of the Endocrine Society,* Abstr. 17.

11. Knobil, E., Plant, T. M., Wildt, L., and Belchetz, P. (1979): The induction of ovulatory menstrual cycles in rhesus monkeys with hypothalamic lesions by an unvarying pulsatile GnRH replacement regimen. In: *Abstracts of the 61st Annual Meeting of the Endocrine Society,* Abstr. 18.

12. Kook, A. I., Yakir, Y., and Trainin, N. (1975): Isolation and partial chemical characterization of THF, a thymus hormone involved in immune maturation of lymphoid cells. *Cell. Immunol.,* 19:151–157.

13. Lorenzen, J. R., and Schwartz, N. B. (1977): The suppression of serum FSH by a non-steroidal factor from porcine follicles: Some properties of the inhibitor "folliculostatin." In: *Novel Aspects of Reproductive Physiology,* edited by C. H. Spilman and J. W. Wilks, pp. 339–353. Halsted Press, New York.

14. Low, T. L. K., and Goldstein, A. L. (1978): The chemistry and biology of thymosin. II. Amino acid sequence analysis of thymosin α_1 and polypeptide β_1. *J. Biol. Chem.,* 254:987–995.

15. Martinez, D., Field, A. K., Schwam, H., Tytell, A. A., and Hilleman, M. R. (1978): Failure of thymopoietin, ubiquitin and synthetic serum thymic factor to restore immunocompetence in T-cell deficient mice. *Proc. Soc. Exp. Biol. Med.,* 159:195–200.

16. Nutt, R. F., Hirschmann, R., and Veber, D. F. (1979): Synthesis of <AAD-His-trans-β-methyl-TZL-NH$_2$, a TRH analog with high CNS activity. In: *Abstracts of the 6th American Peptide Symposium,* Abstr. 1–16.

17. Rosell, S., Rökaeus, Å., Mashford, M. L., Thor, K., Folkers, K. (1980): Neurotensin as a hormone. In: *Neuropeptides and Neural Transmission,* edited by C. Ajmone-Marsan and W. R. Traczyk. Raven Press, New York.

18. Rubinstein, M., Rubinstein, S., Familletti, P., Hershberg, R. D., Brink, L. D., Gutterman, J., Hester, J., and Pestka, S. (1979): Human leucocyte interferon: Production and purification to homogeneity by HPLC. In: *Abstracts of the 6th American Peptide Symposium,* Abstr. C-VI.

19. Schally, A. V., Chang, R. C. C., Huang, W. Y., Redding, T. W., Carter, W. H., Coy, D. H., and Saffran, M. (1979): Isolation, structure and biological activities of several hypothalamic peptides. In: *Abstracts of the 61st Annual Meeting of the Endocrine Society,* Abstr. 21.

20. Schlesinger, D. H., and Goldstein, G. (1975): The amino acid sequence of thymopoietin II. *Cell,* 5:361–365.

21. Takagi, H., Shiomi, H., Veda, H., and Amano, H. (1979): Morphine-like analgesia by a new dipeptide, L-tyrosyl-L-arginine (kyotorphin) and its analogue. *Eur. J. Pharmacol.,* 55:109–111.

22. Trainin, N., Small, M., Zipori, D., Umiel, T., Kook, A. I., and Rotter, V. (1975): Characteristics of THF, a thymic hormone. In: *Biological Activity of Thymic Hormones,* edited by D. W. van Bekkum and A. M. Kruisbeek, pp. 117–144. Kooyker Scientific Publications, Rotterdam.

23. Treager, G. W., Rosenblatt, M., Shepard, G. L., Tyler, G. A., Veroni, M., and Potts, J. T., Jr. (1979): Comparison of strategies for solid-phase peptide synthesis: Use of symmetrical anhydride versus standard carboiimide coupling in the synthesis of a 32-amino acid fragment of parathyroid hormone. In: *Abstracts of the 6th American Peptide Symposium,* Abstr. D-26.

24. Wasiak, T., Humphries, J., Folkers, K., and Bowers, C. Y. (1979): A new category of ovulation inhibitors: Linear LH-RH analogues having more than ten residues. *Biochem. Biophys. Res. Commun.,* 86:843–848.

25. Wilks, J. W., Folkers, K., Humphries, J., and Bowers, C. Y. (1980): Effect of [D-Phe^2,Pro^3,D-Phe^6]-luteinizing hormone releasing hormone, an antagonist, on preovulatory gonadotropin secretion in the rhesus monkey. *Biol. Reprod.* Oct. *(in press).*

Polypeptide Hormones, edited by
R. F. Beers, Jr. and E. G. Bassett.
Raven Press, New York © 1980.

15. Discussion

Moderator: Karl A. Folkers

B. W. Erickson: Dr. Folkers, do you have any evidence for the relative cleavage of two of the four dipeptide analogs? Does an Arg-Arg link adjacent to glutamine cleave more readily than any of the other analogs?

K. A. Folkers: I can't answer that question yet, but perhaps in a few weeks I could. We are just finishing the synthesis of the four models and the fourth one is still not completely purified. We would like to make such comparisons.

I have been asked for samples for testing with an enzyme that apparently has some specificity for double basic moieties; I expect to provide such samples.

B. Wittman-Liebold: Dr. Stein, how do you detect those peptides that are not stained by fluorescamine in the analytical system?

S. Stein: That is often a problem. Some peptides, for example, TRF, do not have a free amino group. So, you do miss certain peptides. It is possible, however, to collect the fractions of column effluents and hydrolyze each fraction with alkali followed by a reaction with fluorescamine or aldehyde.

B. Wittman-Liebold: We have found many peptides that do not stain very well with fluorescamine. Several other workers have also mentioned this effect. When we develop our assembly assays, we always use fluorescamine—because end code detection is better—followed by staining with anhydride to be sure that we do not miss a peptide. We find at least 10 to 20% of peptides in an assay that do not stain very well.

S. Stein: Are those prolyl peptides?

B. Wittman-Liebold: Not always. Sometimes there are lycyl peptides and glycyl peptides.

S. Stein: In the flow system, in solution, one does not have such a serious problem. Most of the NH_2-terminal amino acids, except for proline, of course, will react efficiently. On thin layer plates, however, the reaction is a little trickier.

K. A. Folkers: May I comment on Dr. Stein's remarks? In the mass spectrometry of peptides on the lowest possible scale, a clean laboratory is very essential, because there are amino acid impurities all around, when one gets down to such an almost impossible level of operation. I feel that you are working at such a low level that one should start thinking about getting rid of contaminating amino acids. I think there are times when it is really important to do these isolations on such an ultra-ultra small scale, and it is impressive to hear about using one camel or one rat. However, there are quite a few rats available, if not camels. So, tissue is not always the limiting factor. I wonder if there is not some more reasonable, low-low level at which the average investigator can operate. Maybe it is not as spectacular, but it can be more practical.

S. Stein: We found very simple procedures for purifying the buffers. The use of ninhydrin allows us to work at levels of hundreds of picomoles to 1 nanomole level without any serious problems.

The sensitivity of fluorescence can really be pushed to the picomole level or lower. Of course, you have all kinds of horrendous problems with contamination, but with fluorescent techniques one can work comfortably below the nanomole level without any problem.

H. O. J. Collier: Dr. Folkers has referred to kyotorphin. This was discussed at the recent International Narcotics Research Conference in North Falmouth. It seems that the orphin part of the name might be misleading. In fact, it doesn't bind with the active receptor as do the enkephalins, and it was suggested that it might act by releasing enkephalins. It is an analgesic, but it doesn't seem to be essentially of the endorphin type, which may be of interest.

K. A. Folkers: Presumably, "kyoto" is the most important part of the name to these people who used an *in vivo* assay to isolate this type of peptide. So, one may be inclined to forgive them the last part of the name—for the moment, anyway.

C. P. Fawcett: Dr. Folkers, several years ago I published the detection of an LHRH-like peptide that appeared to be slightly larger than LHRH, but immunologically and by bioassay, it was indistinguishable from LRH.

You have alluded a couple of times to the ease with which the pyro-Glu group is formed from larger peptides containing glutamine. What do you think of the heretical suggestion that maybe the pyro-Glu decapeptide is not the native form of LHRH?

K. A. Folkers: I think that these pro-models that we are currently working with might give us a clue to try to answer your question.

We can, you know, discuss at length whether the activity that Cyril Bowers measures is intrinsic or is due to cleavage.

I think the chemistry of the cyclization of Glu to pyro-Glu is sound. There is the example of big gastrin to gastrin, and there is a double basic pair adjacent to a Gln residue. With that example, I feel that our models are justified to make these studies.

I have shown you other examples of cleavages of pro-hormones to hormones. The β-lipotropin is a beautiful multiple model, and there is proinsulin to insulin. These peptides exemplify the same sort of cleavage. Except the gastrin, the amino acid adjacent to the double basic pair is not Gln.

Of course, we don't always have to invoke Gln in these structures, but obviously Gln sometimes occurs. So, it is conceivable that there may be a fragment larger than the decapeptide and which has some physiological significance.

E. Gross: Dr. Erickson, what quantities can you handle in your continuous solid-phase synthesizer?

B. W. Erickson: At the moment, we have been working on a scale of 0.1 to

1.0 g of resin. We are now developing an analytical scheme to prove the chemistry. We have recently purchased a Waters preparative HPLC equipped with a column that can contain 400 g of a solid support and intend, within the next year, to fill that column with a synthetic resin.

E. Gross: The reaction vessel is the column, right?

B. W. Erickson: It is the column.

D. H. Gelfand: I would like to ask Dr. Stein two questions: Is your proopiocortin analogous to the ACTH and β-lipotropin precursor? Is there additional NH_2-terminal information prior to ACTH in your precursor?

S. Stein: Yes, we call it the "pro," the endo-pro-opiocortin, because it is a precursor of β-lipotropin endorphin as well as a precursor of ACTH. It is similar to that which Mains, Eipper, and Ling described from mouse pituitary tumor cells. Interestingly enough, we discovered it as a precursor of endorphin-lipotropin and published in the same issue of *Proceedings of the National Academy of Sciences USA* as did Mains, Eipper, and Ling. So it was really a "simultaneous discovery."

We didn't realize, at the time, that it was also a common precursor to ACTH, but once we saw Mains' results, we repeated similar experiments using ACTH antibodies, and found that it was a common precursor.

D. H. Gelfand: Has reverse phase HPLC been used to purify enzymes that one normally thinks of as fairly unsteady, like restriction enzymes, DNA ligases, and so forth?

S. Stein: We have had little experience with enzymes. The few that we have dealt with, though, were quite stable.

F. E. Regnier, who has independently developed ion exchange HPLC, has been able to chromatograph LVIT and CPK isoenzymes on HPLC resins and obtains full recovery of activity.

Since he is doing ion exchange, he can do so at pH 7, and without organic solvents; so these are very mild conditions for most enzymes. So, there are ways of doing it. I am certain that HPLC will routinely be used for enzymes.

J. Ramachandran: Dr. Stein, is your bovine medullary preparation also an opiocortin? Does it have ACTH or an MSH amino acid activity?

S. Stein: We haven't checked that yet. In the first place, we don't find any proopiocortin having a molecular weight of approximately 30,000 daltons. The largest protein we do find, a precursor of opiate activity, is about 20,000 daltons. We haven't observed the equivalent pro-opiocortin β-lipotropin in the adrenal, but we plan to check these proteins using ACTH-radio-immunoassay in the near future.

M. Wilchek: Dr. Stein, is it true that fluorescamine is used only with α, and not with ϵ, amino groups? We checked polylysine as compared with polyphenylalanine and found almost the same fluorescence even though the polylysine has many amino groups.

S. Stein: No, it is not true. The ϵ amino group reacts very nicely with fluorescamine.

Perhaps with polylysine there might be some kind of inhibition phenomenon, either quenching of fluorescence, or some kind of poor reactivity, but the ϵ amino group does react very nicely. As a matter of fact, in some of the original studies, we examined a preparation in which the α amino group is blocked, and we got excellent fluorescence.

B. Wittman-Liebold: May I add another comment to that question?

We have found the same result as Dr. Stein. The ϵ amino group of the lysine reacted about the same as the NH_2-terminal amino acid group when we develop our assembly assays with fluorescamine. Also, the lysine value goes down in the amino acid analyzer when we check it, and it is comparable to the decrease of the NH_2-terminal group.

M. Wilchek: I do not say it is not reacting, but I'm saying that it doesn't fluorescence.

B. Wittman-Liebold: Yes, it is reactive with the fluorescamine.

M. Wilchek: The major color that you get, the major fluorescence that you get, is from the α amino group. The lysine contributes very little. If you take lysine by itself, you have two potentially fluorescent amino groups. When you take a peptide containing a lysine, the lysine contributes almost nothing to the color. The group which contributes is the α amino group. This we found with fluorescence.

S. Stein: No, it is fluorescent.

K. A. Folkers: Thank you for contributing to this interesting discussion period.

Polypeptide Hormones, edited by
R. F. Beers, Jr. and E. G. Bassett.
Raven Press, New York © 1980.

16. Introduction to Section C: Present Status of Hypothalamic Hormones and Their Analogs

A. V. Schally

Veterans Administration Medical Center and Tulane University School of Medicine, New Orleans, Louisiana 70146

In the 1940s, G. W. Harris, C. H. Sawyer, and others compiled anatomical, physiological, and pharmacological evidence suggesting that the anterior pituitary gland was controlled by the central nervous system (CNS). Harris indicated that this control was mediated by a neurohumoral mechanism involving the transport by hypophysial portal vessels of neurohumoral substances from the median eminence area of the hypothalamus to the anterior pituitary.

The first experimental demonstration of a hypothalamic substance foreseen by Harris, was achieved in 1955 by Saffran and Schally, and independently by Guillemin, by the discovery of a corticotropin-releasing factor (CRF). This opened the way for subsequent discoveries of other hypothalamic hormones.

In the ensuing search for other hypothalamic releasing factors during the 1960s, the groups of McCann, Guillemin, Meites, my own, and others made notable advances. The presence of at least nine hypothalamic regulators of the pituitary gland was reasonably well established. Extracts of materials were prepared that stimulated corticotropic, thyrotropic, gonadotropic, and somatotropic hormones of the pituitary, and inhibited the release of growth hormone (GH), prolactin, and melanocyte-stimulating hormone. The agents responsible for these biological activities appeared to be of such importance that research into their physiology and chemistry was vigorously pursued by several groups of investigators. However, the structure of CRF is still not established, although recently much progress on its isolation and identification has been made in my laboratory and in other laboratories.

In 1966, with my collaborators, C. Y. Bowers and T. W. Redding, I isolated thyrotropin-releasing hormone (TRH) from porcine hypothalami and determined that it contained three amino acids: glutamic acid, histidine, and proline. In 1969, we established the correct amino acid sequence of TRH and, with help from F. Enzmann, J. Boler, R. Nair, and K. Folkers, determined its structure to be (pyro)Glu-His-Pro-NH$_2$ and synthesized it. About the same time, R. Burgus and R. Guillemin independently established the structure of ovine TRH, which proved to be identical with that of porcine hormone. The chemical identification of TRH, proved the validity of Harris' "chemotransmitter hypothesis." Clinical studies rapidly established the diagnostic usefulness of TRH. This subject and clinical aspects of other hypothalamic hormones will be discussed by Dr. M. O. Thorner. Several dozen of analogs of TRH have been synthesized.

In 1971, with my collaborators A. Arimura, R. M. G. Nair, W. H. Carter, and T. W. Redding, I isolated the luteinizing hormone and follicle stimulation hormone-releasing hormone (LH-RH/FSH-RH), determined the amino acid composition, and with expert help from Y. Baba and H. Matsuo, elucidated its structure and synthesized it. Physiological and immunological studies established that LH-RH is the main link between the brain and the pituitary gland insofar as reproductive function is concerned. Various clinicians, including my collaborators A. J. Kastin, C. Gual, A. Zarate, J. Zanartu, and D. Gonzalez-Barcena, and later, others, established clinical uses of LH-RH.

Much interest was aroused by the expected medical and veterinary application of LH-RH and its derivatives for the stimulation and inhibition of fertility at the level of the brain. More than 800 stimulatory and inhibitory analogs of LH-RH have been synthesized so far. Some of these analogs were tested clinically. Dr. D. H. Coy, who has been most prolific in the synthetic field, will present an up-to-date report on analogs of LH-RH and somatostatin.

In 1973, P. Brazeau, R. Burgus, W. Vale, R. Guillemin, and collaborators isolated from sheep hypothalami and established the structure of a tetradecapeptide that they named somatostatin, which inhibited the release of GH in rats. The presence of somatostatin or growth hormone-inhibiting factor (GIF) in the hypothalamus was first observed by L. Krulich and S. M. McCann in 1968. Subsequently, we isolated porcine somatostatin and showed its primary structure to be identical with ovine somatostatin. Somatostatin was synthesized by several groups, including ours.

Studies with synthetic somatostatin demonstrated that it also inhibits the secretion of thyrotropin, insulin, glucagon, gastrin, secretin, and cholecystokinin in animals and humans. Later this hormone was found in the stomach, gut, and pancreas in addition to the brain. Somatostatin may play a role in the regulation of secretions not only of the pituitary, but also of the pancreas, stomach, and duodenum. Extensive clinical evaluation of somatostatin was carried out by Professors R. Hall, G. M. Besser, and S. Bloom in the United Kingdom in collaboration with my group, by Drs. J. Gerich and P. Forsham in the United States, and recently by Dr. R. Unger. Several dozen analogs of somatostatin have been synthesized in an attempt to obtain prolonged and selective effects. Among the most active on this topic were Drs. C. A. Meyers and D. H. Coy in my laboratory, Dr. J. Rivier at the Salk Institute, D. Sarantakis at Wyeth Laboratories, and D. F. Veber et al. at Merck Sharp & Dohme. Analogs of somatostatin may find clinical application for the control of diabetes, ulcers, acromegaly, and other diseases.

Development of antisera for TRH by R. D. Utiger and others and for LH-RH and somatostatin by Dr. A. Arimura in our laboratory and by other groups permitted the establishment of radioimmunological methods for their measurement. These methods and immunohistochemical techniques were then used to localize TRH, LH-RH, and somatostatin in various brain areas and to identify the neurons that presumably synthesize, transport, and secrete these hormones. Dr. M. Brownstein discusses the distribution of hypothalamic peptides in the brain and Dr. T. L. Donahue reports on α-MSH containing nerves.

Dr. Kastin, one of the pioneers on the extrapituitary effect of hypothalamic and other peptides, evaluates the effects of hypothalamic hormones on brain function and behavior. Dr. F. Labrie discusses the mechanism of action of hypothalamic hormones. We were very fortunate that the contributors in this section represent top authorities in the hypothalamic field.

The isolation, determination of structure, and synthesis of three hypothalamic regulatory hormones achieved in the past decade has had a great impact on endocrinology. The information gathered from animal experiments and studies in humans has led to a greater understanding of physiological processes and of many diseases. Additional hypothalamic hormones will probably be identified and synthesized during the next few years. This would in turn create still new opportunities for basic and clinical studies on hypothalamic hormones.

Polypeptide Hormones, edited by
R. F. Beers, Jr. and E. G. Bassett.
Raven Press, New York © 1980.

17. Chemistry and Physiology of Hypothalamic Hormones

A. V. Schally, T. W. Redding, R. C. C. Chang, A. Arimura,
W. Y. Huang, D. H. Coy, C. A. Meyers, E. Pedroza,
A. J. Kastin, and C. Turkelson

*Veterans Administration Medical Center and Tulane University School of Medicine,
New Orleans, Louisiana 70146*

INTRODUCTION

It is well established that the hypothalamic releasing and release-inhibiting hormones regulate the secretory activity of the anterior pituitary gland. The discovery of several of these hormones and their isolation, structural identification, and synthesis (75,79,80) established the validity of the theory of neurohumoral control of the pituitary gland suggested by Harris (35).

Some hypothalamic peptide hormones are also produced in the extra-hypothalamic brain areas and in endocrine-like cells of non-neural tissues. Thus, somatostatin is present in discrete cells of the pancreas, gastric mucosa, and duodenum, and may, through paracrine control, play an important role in the regulation of endocrine pancreas and gastrointestinal (GI) tract (3). Thyrotropin-releasing hormone has also recently been identified in the GI tract (53,58,59). In this chapter we report some of the latest biochemical, physiological, and clinical findings on hypothalamic hormones and their analogs, and especially their effects on anterior pituitary function and at other levels of the organism. The relationship between structure and activity of hypothalamic hormones, their effects on brain functions and behavior, distribution in the brain, mechanism of action, and clinical significance will be discussed by others in this volume.

CORTICOTROPIN RELEASING FACTOR

Although corticotropin releasing factor (CRF) was the first hypothalamic, hypophysiotropic hormone to be detected, attempts to isolate it in pure form were severely hampered by the complexity of assays, interference by vasopressin and ACTH-like peptides, possible need for cofactors, the loss of activity during purification, and other reasons.

Several years ago, the work on the purification of CRF was resumed in several laboratories. The results of Cooper et al. (24), Jones et al. (42), Gillies and

Lowry (31), Vale et al. (96), Gillham et al. (30), and Sayers et al. (72), together with our recent work appear to confirm the hypothesis concerning the existence of several molecules with CRF activity put forward by us more than 18 years ago (73). Our laboratory is continuing the work on isolation, sequencing, and synthesizing of peptides with CRF activity in an attempt to find the physiological CRH.

In our recent studies (78,83,89), hypothalamic extracts from nearly one-half million pig hypothalami were first separated into 14 fractions by preparative gel filtration on Sephadex G-25. Significant CRF activity was found near the void volume (fraction 2, $R_f = 0.77$), in fractions 3 and 4 ($R_f = 0.7–0.53$), in intermediate fractions (fraction 8; $R_f = 0.4$), and even in the fractions 11 and 12, which were retarded or which had low R_f (0.3) and also contained catecholamines.

CRF-active materials from Sephadex fraction No. 2 were purified by chromatography on carboxymethyl-cellulose (CMC), counter-current distribution (CCD), SE-Sephadex, gel filtration on Sephadex G-50, and partition chromatography. The results indicate that CRF activity in this fraction is due to a heptapeptide with the structure Phe-Ile-Tyr-His-Ser-Tyr-Lys (78), but the CRF activity of synthetic heptapeptide is very low. We are investigating whether the activity of this heptapeptide can be potentiated by cofactors (31).

Similar methods were used for the purification of retarded CRF from Sephadex fractions 11 and 12 with $R_f = 0.3$. After counter-current distribution, gel filtration on Sephadex G-15, and partition chromatography or ion-exchange chromatography on SE-Sephadex, more than 15 mg of a tetradecapeptide were obtained that had some CRF activity *in vitro,* but not *in vivo.* Its amino acid sequence was determined as Phe-Leu-Gly-Phe-Pro-Thr-Thr-Lys-Thr-Tyr-Phe-Pro-His-Phe (83). This tetradecapeptide was then synthesized, but subsequently it was found that this amino acid sequence is identical with residues Nos. 33–46 of the α-chain of porcine hemoglobin; it was concluded that this tetradecapeptide is most probably an artifact of extraction (83).

Fraction 8 with R_f of 0.4 from Sephadex containing CRF was purified by chromatography on CMC. Strong CRF activity was found in acidic, neutral, and basic fractions. After further purification by CCD and SE-Sephadex, the highly purified material (devoid of ACTH-like activity, but containing much lysine vasopressin) was active *in vitro* in doses of 3 ng/ml and showed an excellent dose-response relationship (78,80,89). This material was then repurified by partition chromatography. It appeared to be a decapeptide, the CRF activity of which may be potentiated by vasopressin. Its structure is being confirmed by synthesis.

The most active CRF was derived from CCD of Sephadex fraction Nos. 3 and 4 (78). It had a low contamination with lysine vasopressin (LVP) and ACTH, and was active in pituitary quarters assay and in tissue cultures of pituitary monolayer cells. On repurification on Sephadex G-25, CRF activity was completely separated from the traces of ACTH and LVP. Repurified fractions showed CRF activity *in vitro* in doses of 1 to 2 μg. CRF activity of this fraction was potentiated by LVP. This material was then repurified on SE-Sephadex. CRF activity, located in discrete fractions, stimulated ACTH release from monolayer cultures of rat pituitary cells and pituitary quarters at doses of 0.1 to 0.4 $\mu g/ml$. Its amino acid composition indicated that it may contain 16 amino acids. However, it is not yet completely pure. At this stage, this fraction was purified 90 times compared with that at the CCD stage and 50,000 times compared with the starting material. It is difficult if not impossible, at present, to interpret the finding of multiple CRF activities in hypothalamic extracts, as the CRF described above is not vasopressin and it is completely free of ACTH. It is hoped that further work will result in the isolation of various CRFs and in the determination of their physiological role.

THYROTROPIN RELEASING HORMONE

In 1966 we isolated thyrotropin releasing hormone (TRH) from porcine hypothalami and reported the correct amino acid composition of this tripeptide (77). The work in our laboratory, in collaboration with Folkers, and that of Guillemin resulted, in 1969, in the determination of structure and syntheses of porcine and ovine TRH (14,20,21,62,88).

Synthetic pyroGlu-His-Pro-NH$_2$ has been shown to stimulate thyrotropin (TSH) release in all mammals studied, including mice, rats, sheep, goats, cows, humans, and birds (75,79,80,96). TRH liberates prolactin in animals and humans (15,16,27,41,95), but it remains to be established whether this effect is physiological (34,75). TRH can also increase the synthesis of TSH and prolactin. It has been reported that TRH will stimulate colonic activity in rabbits (91). This response, which together will direct effects of TRH on the gastrointestinal tract (53,58,59) *(see below),* may explain side effects such as nausea and gastric cramps seen occasionally after administration of TRH, appears to originate in the central nervous system (CNS) and is mediated by cholinergic receptors. The possible role of TRH as a neurotransmitter in the CNS is supported by its presence at significant concentrations in the extra-hypothalamic brain areas of various classes of vertebrates examined, including rat, chicken, snake, frog, tadpole, salmon, and lamprey (40). Recently, it was demonstrated that TRH immunoreactivity is also distributed throughout the GI tract and the pancreas of the rat (53,58,59). TRH was shown to transiently inhibit tetragastrin-stimulated gastric acid secretion (59) and to enhance arginine-induced glucagon secretion (58). The generation of antibodies to TRH and the development of sensitive and specific radioimmunoassays (RIA) for this hormone (3,8,39,40,45,65) permitted also the detection of immunoreactive TRH in blood, cerebrospinal fluid, and urine of rat and man (69,96).

ANALOGS OF THYROTROPIN RELEASING HORMONE

Relatively few analogs of TRH have been synthesized, as compared with LH-RH and somatostatin, perhaps because early work (37,71) indicated that the structural requirements of this small peptide are quite stringent. Thus, most analogs have little TRH activity. However, $[(N^{3im}\text{-Me-His})^2]$-TRH has 3 to 10 times greater activity than the natural product (71,96) and $[\beta\text{-(pyrazolyl-1)-Ala}^2]$-TRH is also more active than TRH in rats and mice (26) and humans (Garcia-Centenera, Pozuelo, Coy, and Schally, *in preparation*). $[(N^{3im}\text{-Me-His})^2]$-TRH is a more potent TSH and prolactin releaser in humans than TRH (92). The activities of TRH analogs for stimulating thyrotropin release and prolactin production are quite similar (90) and a good correlation exists between binding affinity and these biological activities (96).

However, there appear to be differences between the CNS and pituitary receptors for TRH as indicated by some dissociation between TRH and CNS activity, since some analogs such as homo-pyroGlu-His-Pro-NH$_2$ and homo-pyroGlu-His-thioproline-NH$_2$ are equipotent with TRH in stimulating TSH, but have 4 to 15 times as much activity on the CNS (36).

PROLACTIN RELEASING FACTOR

Prolactin releasing factor (PRF) activity appears to be present in the hypothalami of mammals and birds (56,75). A part of the PRF activity in the hypothalamic extracts is clearly due to TRH which, under specific conditions, can greatly stimulate prolactin secretion *in vivo* and *in vitro* in various mammals, including humans (15,16,27,41,95). It has also been reported recently that administration of antisera to TRH will greatly lower prolactin levels in rats (47).

However, there is also evidence that a PRF distinct from TRH exists. Prolactin and TSH release induced by TRH can be dissociated under various physiological and clinical conditions (44). The work of several groups of investigators suggests that partially purified hypothalamic fractions, apparently different from TRH, can still stimulate the release of prolactin from rat pituitaries *in vivo* and *in vitro* (17,75,79,80,96). The search for PRF, in our own experience, has been made difficult by the presence in hypothalamic fractions of substances that increase the release of prolactin, such as TRH, and those which inhibit it, such as catecholamines (82) and γ-aminobutyric acid (87). These compounds can, under certain conditions, obscure or neutralize other PIF and PRF activities. However, we have established that several purified porcine hypothalamic fractions with physicochemical properties different from TRH, as shown by different partition coefficients on CCD, behavior on CMC, SE-Sephadex, and molecular sieving on Sephadex, can also stimulate the release of prolactin from rat pituitary fragments or from monolayer cell cultures (A. V. Schally, A. Arimura, T. W. Redding, *unpublished observations*). Natural and synthetic Tyr-Leu-Arg-Phe and Leu-Arg-Phe, which at first in several *in vivo* and *in vitro* tests appeared to have some PRF activity, were later determined to be inactive (78). Two tetrapeptides identified as Phe-Glu-His-Glu and Gly-Lys-Val-Asn and a tripeptide Lys-Phe-Tyr of natural origin had no consistent effect on PRL release in monolayer cultures of pituitary cells at doses of 1 μg/ml (78). Several dipeptides were also isolated and identified, among them Arg-Phe, Arg-Ala-NH$_2$, Tyr-Arg-NH$_2$, Phe-Tyr, Val-Trp, and Tyr-Phe (78). Large doses (1 to 10 μg/ml) of Val-Trp and Tyr-Phe were found to stimulate PRL release *in vitro* (78). Further purification and identification of other materials having PRF activity is in progress.

A variety of natural substances of CNS and extra-CNS origin, for example, melatonin, can augment prolactin release, but their effects can be explained by an action mediated via the CNS (79,80). Therefore, they do not represent the physiological PRF, the structure of which remains to be elucidated.

PROLACTIN RELEASE-INHIBITING FACTOR

Although the presence of prolactin release-inhibiting factor (PIF) activity in hypothalamic extracts was demonstrated many years ago (reviewed in refs. 56,69,75,96), the chemical nature of PIF is still unclear. Many substances are present in the brain or hypothalamic extracts that can inhibit prolactin secretion *in vitro* and *in vivo* (50,52,59,93).

It has also been demonstrated that the catecholamines influence the release of prolactin. Our recent work showed that hypothalamic catecholamines inhibit prolactin release by a direct action on the pituitary (82). When PIF activity present in acetic acid extracts of pig hypothalami was concentrated by several steps, some of the highly purified fractions that strongly suppressed the release of prolactin *in vitro* and *in vivo* were found to contain much noradrenaline and dopamine (82). The magnitude of inhibition of release of prolactin was related to noradrenaline content. Synthetic noradrenaline and dopamine powerfully inhibit the release of prolactin *in vitro* and *in vivo* (82). These results showed that catecholamines, whether synthetic or purified from hypothalamic tissue, inhibit the release of prolactin by an action exerted directly on the pituitary gland (82). Dopamine was found in the hypophysial portal blood of rats (9) and, under certain conditions, prolactin and dopamine secretion are inversely related (10). However, whether dopamine represents a physiological prolactin release inhibiting hormone remains to be elucidated.

Another hypothalamic substance with PIF activity, the effect of which, in contrast to catecholamines, cannot be blocked by perphenazine is γ-aminobutyric acid (GABA) (87). GABA was isolated by us from pig hypothalami by several purification steps. Natural and synthetic GABA inhibited prolactin release *in vitro* from isolated rat pituitary halves in doses as low as 0.1 μg/ml. The extent of inhibition was proportional to the dose; natural and synthetic GABA possessed identical PIF activity (87). Similarly, synthetic GABA suppressed prolactin release in monolayer cultures of rat pituitary cells and inhibited the TRH-stimulated prolactin secretion. GABA also had PIF activity *in vivo,* although large doses were needed for an effect (87). The results indicate that GABA can inhibit prolactin release by a direct action on the pituitary gland, but again it is not known whether this effect is physiological or pharmacological, the doses needed to obtain an effect being rather large (87). Our observation that GABA inhibits prolactin release was confirmed by recent *in vitro* work (50), *in vivo* studies (51), clinical observations (A. Guitelman et al., *in preparation*); and pharmacological investigations (61).

Other compounds (different from catecholamines and GABA, but still unidentified) with PIF activity are present in pig hypothalamic extracts. Some of them are polypeptides (A. V. Schally, T. W. Redding, and A. Arimura, *unpublished observations*). Further work is needed to identify the physiological PIF.

MELANOCYTE-STIMULATING HORMONE RELEASE-INHIBITING FACTOR

The release of melanocyte-stimulating hormone (MSH) from the pars intermedia of the pituitary gland is controlled by hypothalamic stimulating factor (MRF) and inhibitory factor (MIF), the latter having a predominant role (75,79,84). However, considerable confusion still exists as to the identity of MIF and MRF. The first prospective MIF was isolated from bovine hypothalami and identified as H-Pro-Leu-Gly-NH₂ in this laboratory (63,84). The group of Walter (23) originally observed that H-Pro-Leu-Gly-NH₂ could be formed by incubating oxytocin with an enzyme present in hypothalamic tissue and that this tripeptide inhibits MSH release in the rat.

Several analogs of MIF have been synthesized recently. These peptides include H-Pro-*N*-isobutyl-Gly-Gly-NH₂ and two stereoisomers of both H-Pro-*N*-Me-Leu-Gly-NH₂ (L,L) and (L,D) and H-Pro-*N*-Me-Leu-Ala-HN₂ (L,L,D) and (L,D,D) (29). All analogs except L,L potentated behavioral effects of L-DOPA in mice and all antagonized fluphenazine-induced catalepsy in rats. In these tests, L-Pro-*N*-Me-D-Leu-Gly-NH₂ was the most active after parenteral or oral administration; it also affected brain catecholamine turnover (29).

LUTEINIZING HORMONE- AND FOLLICLE-STIMULATING HORMONE-RELEASING HORMONE

In 1971 we isolated luteinizing hormone- and follicle-stimulating hormone-releasing hormone (LH-RH/FSH-RH), determined its structure, and synthesized it (7,54,55,74,86). Extensive physiological, biochemical, immunological, veterinary, and clinical investigations with LH-RH followed (75,85). In addition, the interest in possible medical applications of LH-RH analogs caused a tremendous activity in the field of their synthesis. These investigations are so extensive, that only the recent or key developments will be described.

Actions on the Pituitary

Porcine LH-RH corresponding in structure to pyroGlu-His-Trp-Ser-Tyr-Gly-Leu-Arg-Pro-Gly-NH₂ was first synthesized by us (54,55) and then by many other groups (96). This made the new hormone readily available for a variety of basic and clinical studies. The structure of ovine LH-RH was later shown to be identical with the porcine hormone (19) and subsequent biochemical and immunological studies indicated that bovine, human, and rat LH-RH probably have the same structure (75,85,96). Our original observations that natural porcine LH-RH and the synthetic decapeptide release both LH and FSH (74,86) have been confirmed and extended in a variety of animals, including rats, mice, rabbits, golden hamsters, mink, spotted skunk, impala, rock hyrax, dogs, cats, sheep, cattle, pigs, horses, monkeys, and humans (75,85). Ovulation can be induced in most of these species with LH-RH. Increases in sex steroid levels in blood have also been reported after administration of LH-RH (75,79,80,85). LH-RH is also active in birds, such as domestic fowl and pigeons; in some species of fish, such as rainbow trout, brown trout, and carp; and in amphibia. This indicates also that species specificity does not occur with LH-RH (79,80).

Investigations of the routes of administration in rats, humans, and other species, revealed that LH-RH and its analogs are effective not only after intravenous, subcutaneous, intramuscular, and intracarotid injection, but also after intravaginal, intrarectal, intranasal, cutaneous, and even oral administration (75,79,80). However, the dose required for suitable effects by extravascular routes are 50 to 10,000 times larger than the parenteral.

The evidence that the LH-RH decapeptide also has FSH-RH activity *in vivo* and *in vitro* is now indisputable. Our results indicate that LH-RH decapeptide represents the bulk of FSH-RH activity in the hypothalamus (76). Various immunological results *(see below)* strongly support the importance of LH-RH as the physiological FSH-releasing hormone. This view is strongly supported by the work of Cattanach et al. (22), who showed that LH-RH deficient mutant mice have a reduced pituitary and plasma content of FSH, in addition to LH, and immature primary and accessory sex organs. Recent studies by Wise et al. in Barraclough's laboratory (97), in which selective secretion of FSH was induced by infusion of small doses of LH-RH, provide further physiological evidence that LH-RH also is FSH-RH.

Immunological Studies with Luteinizing Hormone-Releasing Hormone

A large number of immunological studies has been carried out with LH-RH. Antisera to LH-RH have been produced in rats, rabbits, guinea pigs, and sheep; from these studies, several RIAs were developed (4,43,46). Passive immunization of rats with LH-RH antiserum blocked the preovulatory surge of LH and FSH and prevented ovulation (46,75). In golden hamsters, administration of antisera to LH-RH caused an arrest of follicular maturation, reduction in serum estradiol, and blockage of both LH surge and of ovulation (28). Reduction in serum FSH and LH after passive or active immunization of rats with LH-RH supports the physiological role of this decapeptide in the regulation of FSH secretion (85). LH-RH is also necessary for normal implantation of fertilized ova and maintenance of pregnancy (2,64).

The availability of antisera to LH-RH made possible various studies on localization of LH-RH by RIAs or immunocytochemical methods (69), which will be reviewed in subsequent chapters. LH-RH has been detected by bioassay and by RIA in the hypophysial portal blood of rats and monkeys and in peripheral circulation of women at mid-cycle ovulatory LH surge, and in post-menopausal women. LH-RH, like other hormones, appears to be released in pulsatile fashion (79,80).

Analogs of Luteinizing Hormone-Releasing Hormone

Since the first step in the action of LH-RH may involve binding to the pituitary plasma membrane receptors, an *in vitro* assay using highly purified pituitary cell membrane preparations was developed (66,67) in our laboratory. We have determined that the number of binding sites for LH-RH is approximately 2.36 pM/mg of protein with a high affinity constant of 7.1×10^9 M^{-1}. We have also observed that the superactive agonist [D-Trp^6]-LH-RH and the antagonist [D-Phe^2-D-Trp^3-D-Phe^6]-LH-RH compete with LH-RH for its pituitary plasma membrane receptors, displacing the ^{125}I-LH-RH more strongly than its parent hormone. Therefore, both stimulatory and inhibitory analogs of LH-RH apparently exert their action through the same pituitary plasma membrane receptors as those of LH-RH. The more potent and long-acting effect of such superactive analogs as [D-Trp^6]-LH-RH could be due to their higher ability to bind to the pituitary LH-RH receptors. Similarly, the blockade of ovulation of several inhibitory analogs of LH-RH, such as [D-Phe^2-D-Trp^3-D-Phe^6]-LH-RH can be explained by the same mechanism (66,67).

Administration of the superactive analogs [D-Ala^6-desGly-NH$_2$^{10}]-LH-RH ethylamide, [D-Leu^6-desGly-NH$_2$^{10}]-LH-RH ethylamide, [D-Ser(But)^6-desGly-NH$_2$^{10}]-LH-RH ethylamide, and [D-Trp^6]-LH-RH induces protracted stimulation of release of LH and FSH in humans lasting as long as 24 hr (85,89). Therefore, they may be more convenient and practical to use than LH-RH, which has occasionally been given three times daily for therapeutic purposes (79,80,85). These analogs can be administered not only by parenteral, but also by intranasal, intravaginal, intrarectal, and oral routes if suitable doses are given (79,80). However, therapeutic regimens for induction of ovulation in anovulatory women and treatment of oligospermia in men are not yet established. In view of paradoxical antifertility effects of large doses of LH-RH and long-acting superactive analogs, caution must be exercised in devising clinical protocols (79,80).

The inhibitory analog [D-Phe^2,D-Trp^3,D-Phe^6]-LH-RH was shown to suppress the liberation of LH and FSH in response to exogenous LH-RH in humans and lower the elevated levels of gonadotropins in patients with low or absent gonadal function (32,80). The progress being made in the area of LH-RH analogs should lead to development of new birth control methods.

GROWTH HORMONE-RELEASING FACTOR

The release of growth hormone (GH) from the anterior pituitary is regulated by a dual system of hypothalamic control: one inhibitory and one stimulatory (75,80,96). The stimulatory effect on GH release of some hypothalamic fractions (94) appears to be due to a growth hormone-releasing factor (GH-RF), first detected more than 13 years ago (75,79), that, under some conditions, might predominate over the inhibitory action of somatostatin. Despite the intense effort by several groups to isolate it and determine the structure of GH-RF, this problem is still not solved. However, using antisera to somatostatin or columns of Sepharose linked to anti-somatostatin-γ-globulin to eliminate somatostatin and its precursors, we have obtained new evidence for the existence of GH-RF. We have also purified several fractions with GH-RF activity by gel filtration on Sephadex G-25 or G-50, by CCD, by chromatography on CMC and SE-Sephadex, and on partition columns (78). Among the substances with GH-releasing factor activity purified from pig hypothalami were two peptides, Lys-Phe-Tyr and Gly-Lys-Val-Asn (78). The tetrapeptide appeared to be more active in stimulation of the release of GH in monolayer cultures of rat anterior pituitary cells, but further work is necessary to determine its physiological role. These peptides were recently synthesized. The testing of synthetic peptides, combined with purification of other materials with GH-RF activity is continuing (78,80).

SOMATOSTATIN

The presence in ovine hypothalamic extracts of a substance that inhibited the release of GH was first demonstrated by Krulich and McCann (49). Somatostatin (growth hormone release-inhibiting hormone or GH-RIH) was isolated first from ovine hypothalami by Brazeau et al. (18) and subsequently from porcine hypothalami by our group (81). The primary structure of this peptide is identical in both species: H-Ala-Gly-Cys-Lys-Asn-Phe-Phe-Trp-Lys-Thr-Phe-Thr-Ser-Cys-OH (18,81). Somatostatin was synthesized by several groups (25,70). Synthetic somatostatin was found to produce a remarkable array of actions on diverse endocrine and exocrine cells (79,80,96). These findings gained physiological significance when we found somatostatin-like immunoreactivity in high concentrations within those tissues affected by the hormone (3). Thus, in addition to the hypothalamus, somatostatin appears to be localized in other parts of the CNS, neurohypophysis, and spinal cord as well as in pancreas, stomach, and gut (3,38,80).

Larger, highly basic forms of somatostatin found in pig hypothalami are biologically and immunologically active (81). We also recognized two types of immunoreactive somatostatin in extracts from rat pancreas, stomach, and duodenum (3). Somatostatin immunoreactive peptides with higher molecular weight were also found in ovine hypothalami (57) and in porcine small intestine (68). These molecules may all represent precursors of somatostatin.

Effects on Pituitary

The inhibitory action of somatostatin on both basal and stimulated secretion of GH in a variety of *in vitro* and *in vivo* assays was shown in several animal species, including humans (12,33,34,79,80). Both the reduced (linear) and oxidized (cyclic) forms are active (96). A physiological role for somatostatin in the regulation of GH secretion is supported by our observations that passive immunization of rats with antisera to somatostatin elevates plasma GH levels and prevents the stress-induced decrease of GH (6). Somatostatin also suppresses the basal and TRH-induced secretion of TSH, but not of prolactin, and it may play a physiological role in the regulation of TSH secretion (5).

Effects on Pancreas

Somatostatin inhibits basal as well as stimulated secretion of insulin and glucagon by a direct action on the β- and α-pancreatic islet cells (1,60). Somatostatin affects the exocrine pancreas as well, suppressing pancreatic bicarbonate and protein secretion (48).

Effects on Stomach and Gut

Somatostatin inhibits basal gastrin and that released in response to food (13). In addition, somatostatin suppresses the gastric acid and pepsin response to pentagastrin, as well as the gastric acid response to food and hypoglycemia in cats with gastric fistulae (34,79,80). This demonstrates that somatostatin exerts direct action on the parietal and peptic cells of the stomach (34) and that it can affect exocrine as well as endocrine secretions. Subsequently, somatostatin has been found to inhibit the release of secretin, cholecystokinin pancreozymin, gastric inhibitory polypeptide, vasoactive intestinal polypeptide, pancreatic polypeptide, and motilin (11,48,80).

Analogs of Somatostatin

Somatostatin is of little therapeutic value since it has many actions and a short biological half-life (34,79,80). Analogs of somatostatin are being developed in order to impart them enhanced, selective, prolonged, and antagonistic activities. Some of the more promising analogs have been tested clinically in humans. Long-acting analogs with selective activities may be useful in the treatment of acromegaly, juvenile diabetes, diabetic retinopathy, peptic ulcers, acute pancreatitis, and other conditions (79,80).

SUMMARY

The present status of knowledge on hypothalamic regulatory peptide hormones was reviewed. In the last decade, the isolation, determination of structure, and synthesis of at least three hypothalamic regulatory hormones (TRH, LH-RH/FSH-RH, and somatostatin) have been achieved. Development of antisera for these hormones permitted the establishment of radioimmunological methods for their measurement. Numerous analogs of these hormones have been synthesized and evaluated biologically in an attempt to obtain peptides which would be clinically more desirable than the original hormones, including inhibitory analogs in the case of LH-RH. The work on isolation of CRF from porcine hypothalamus was resumed. Several peptides with CRF activity were identified structurally, and their physiological role is being investigated. Other purified hypothalamic peptides and non-peptide materials have been determined to have PRF, PIF, and GH-RF activities, but their physiological importance remains to be determined. Our recent results confirm and extend previous findings of high concentrations of various peptides in brain tissue, many of which contain biological activities. Further work is needed to characterize chemically the additional releasing and inhibiting hormones.

ACKNOWLEDGMENTS

Some basic studies originating in our laboratory and described in this review were supported in part by the Veterans Administration, NIH Research grants AM-07467, AM-18370, and AM-09094, and NIH contract HD-8-2819.

REFERENCES

1. Alberti, K. G. M. M., Christensen, S. E., Iverson, J., Seyer-Hansen, K., Christensen, N. J., Hansen, P. A., Lundbaek, K., and Ørskov, H. (1973): Inhibition of insulin secretion by somatostatin. *Lancet,* 2:1299–1301.
2. Arimura, A., Nishi, N., and Schally, A. V. (1976): Delayed implantation caused by administration of sheep immunogamma globulin against LH-RH in the rat. *Proc. Soc. Exp. Biol. Med.,* 152:71–75.
3. Arimura, A., Sato, H., Dupont, A., Nishi, N., and Schally, A. V. (1975): Somatostatin: Abundance of immunoreactive hormone in rat stomach and pancreas. *Science,* 189:1007–1009.
4. Arimura, A., Sato, H., Kumasaka, T., Worobec, R. B., Debeljuk, L., Dunn, J., and Schally, A. V. (1978): Production of antiserum to LH-releasing hormone (LH-RH) associated with gonadal atrophy in rabbits: Development of radioimmunoassay for LH-RH. *Endocrinology,* 93(5):1092–1103.
5. Arimura, A., and Schally, A. V. (1976): Increase in basal and thyrotrophin releasing hormone (TRH)-stimulated secretion of thyrotrophin (TSH) by passive immunization with antiserum to somatostatin in rats. *Endocrinology,* 98:1069–1072.
6. Arimura, A., Smith, W. D., and Schally, A. V. (1976): Blockade of the stress-induced decrease in blood GH by anti-somatostatin serum in rats. *Endocrinology,* 98:540–543.
7. Baba, Y., Matsuo, H., and Schally, A. V. (1971): Structure of the porcine LH- and FSH-releasing hormone. II. Confirmation of the proposed structure by conventional sequential analyses. *Biochem. Biophys. Res. Commun.,* 44:459–463.
8. Bassiri, R. M., and Utiger, R. D. (1972): The preparation and specificity of antibody to thyrotropin-releasing hormone. *Endocrinology,* 90:722–727.

9. Ben-Jonathan, N., Neill, M. A., Arbogast, L. A., Peters, L. L., and Hoefer, M. T., (1978): Dopamine in hypophysial portal blood during late pregnancy lactation and following ovariectomy (abstract). In: *Proceedings of the 60th Annual Meeting of the Endocrine Society,* p. 193.

10. Ben-Jonathan, N., Oliver, C., Weiner, R., Mical, R. S., and Porter, J. C. (1979): Dopamine in hypophysial portal plasma of the rat during the estrous cycle and throughout pregnancy. *Endocrinology,* 100(2):452–458.

11. Besser, G. M., and Mortimer, C. H. (1976): Clinical neuroendocrinology. In: *Frontiers in Endocrinology,* edited by L. Martini and W. F. Ganong, p. 227–254. Raven Press, New York.

12. Besser, G. M., Mortimer, C. H., Carr, D., Schally, A. V., Coy, D. H., Evered, D., Kastin, A. J., Tunbridge, W. M. G., Thorner, M. O., and Hall, R. (1974): Growth hormone release inhibiting hormone in acromegaly. *Br. Med. J.,* 1:352–355.

13. Bloom, S. R., Mortimer, C. H., Thorner, M. O., Besser, G. M., Hall, R., Gomez-Pan, A., Roy, V. M., Russell, R. C. G., Coy, D. H., Kastin, A. J., and Schally, A. V. (1974): Inhibition of gastrin and gastric acid secretion by growth hormone release inhibiting hormone. *Lancet,* 2:1106–1109.

14. Böler, J., Enzmann, F., Folkers, K., Bowers, C. Y., and Schally, A. V. (1969): The identity of chemical and hormonal properties of the thyrotropin releasing hormone and pyroglutamyl-histidine-proline-amide. *Biochem. Biophys. Res. Commun.,* 37:705–710.

15. Bowers, C. Y., Friesen, H., Hwang, P., Guyda, J. J., and Folkers, K. (1971): Prolactin and thyrotropin release in man by synthetic pyroglutamyl-histidyl-prolinamide. *Biochem. Biophys. Res. Commun.,* 45:1033–1041.

16. Bowers, C. Y., Weil, A., Chang, J. K., Sievertsson, H., Enzmann, F., and Folkers, K. (1970): Activity-structure relationships of thyrotropin releasing hormone. *Biochem. Biophys. Res. Commun.,* 40:683–691.

17. Boyd, A. E., Spencer, E., Jackson, I. M. D., and Reichlin, S. (1976): Prolactin-releasing factor (PRF) in porcine hypothalamic extract distinct from TRH. *Endocrinology,* 99:861–871.

18. Brazeau, P., Vale, W., Burgus, R., Ling, N., Butcher, M., Rivier, J., and Guillemin, R. (1973): Hypothalamic polypeptide that inhibits the secretion of immunoreactive pituitary growth hormone. *Science,* 179:77–79.

19. Burgus, R., Butcher, M., Amoss, M., Ling, N., Monahan, M., Rivier, J., Fellows, R., Blackwell, R., Vale, W., and Guillemin, R. (1972): Primary structure of the ovine hypothalamic luteinizing hormone releasing factor (LRF). *Proc. Natl. Acad. Sci. USA,* 69:278–282.

20. Burgus, R., Dunn, T. F., Desiderio, D., Guillemin, R. (1969): Structure moleculaire du facteur hypothalamique hypophysiotrope TRF d'origine ovine: Mise en evidence par spectrometrie de masse de la sequence PCA-His-Pro-NH₂. *C.R. Acad. Sci. [D] (Paris),* 269:1870–1873.

21. Burgus, R., Dunn, T. F., Desiderio, D., Ward, D. N., Vale, W., and Guillemin, R. (1970): Characterization of ovine hypothalamic hypophysiotropic TSH-releasing factor. *Nature,* 226:321–325.

22. Cattanach, B. M., Iddon, C. A., Charlton, H. M., Chiappa, S. A., and Fink, G. (1977): Gonadotrophin-releasing hormone deficiency in a mutant mouse with hypogonadism. *Nature,* 269:338–340.

23. Celis, M. E., Taleisnik, S., and Walter, R. (1971): Regulation of formation and proposed structure of the factor inhibiting the release of melanocyte releasing hormone. *Proc. Natl. Acad. Sci. USA,* 68:1428–1433.

24. Cooper, D. M. F., Synetos, D., Christie, R. B., and Schulster, D. (1976): Studies on the nature of corticotrophin releasing hormone and its partial purification from porcine hypothalami. *J. Endocrinol.,* 71:171–172.

25. Coy, D. H., Coy, E. J., Arimura, A., and Schally, A. V. (1973): Solid-phase synthesis of growth hormone-release inhibiting factor. *Biochem. Biophys. Res. Commun.,* 54:1267–1273.

26. Coy, D. H., Hirotsu, Y., Redding, T. W., Coy, E. J., and Schally, A. V. (1975): Synthesis and biological properties of the [2-L-β-(Pyrazolyl-1)alanine] analogs of luteinizing hormone-releasing hormone and thyrotropin-releasing hormone. *J. Med. Chem.,* 18:948–949.

27. Debeljuk, L., Redding, T. W., Arimura, A., and Schally, A. V. (1973): Effect of TRH and triiodo thyronine on prolactin release in sheep. *Proc. Soc. Exp. Biol. Med.,* 142:421–423.

28. de la Cruz, A., Arimura, A., de la Cruz, K. G., and Schally, A. V. (1976): Effect of administration of anti-serum to luteinizing hormone-releasing hormone on gonadal function during the estrous cycle in the hamster. *Endocrinology,* 98:490–497.

29. Failli, A., Sestanj, K., Immer, H. U., and Gotz, M. (1977): Synthetic MIF analogues. Part I:

Synthesis by four-component condensation (4 CC) and classical methods. *Arzneim. Forsch.,* 27:2286–2289.

30. Gillham, B., Hillhouse, E. W., and Jones, M. T. (1976): Further studies on the purification of corticotrophin releasing factor from the rat hypothalamus *in vitro. J. Endocrinology,* 71:60P–61P.

31. Gillies, G., and Lowry, P. (1979): Corticotrophin releasing factor may be modulated vasopressin. *Nature,* 278:463.

32. Gonzalez-Barcena, D., Kastin, A. J., Coy, D. H., Nikolics, K., and Schally, A. V. (1977): Suppression of gonadotropin release in man by an inhibitory analogue of LH-releasing hormone. *Lancet,* 2:997–998.

33. Hall, R., Besser, G. M., Schally, A. V., Coy, D. H., Evered, D., Goldie, D. J., Kastin, A. J., McNeilly, A. S., Mortimer, C. H., Phenekos, C., Tunbridge, W. M. G., and Weightman, D. (1973): Action of growth hormone release inhibitory hormone in men and in acromegaly. *Lancet,* 2:581–584.

34. Hall, R., and Gomez-Pan, A. (1976): The hypothalamic regulatory hormones and their clinical applications. *Adv. Clin. Chem.,* 18:173–212.

35. Harris, G. W. (1955): *Neural Control of the Pituitary Gland.* Edward Arnold, London.

36. Hirschmann, R. F. (1976): Some recent developments in the synthesis of biologically active peptides. In: *Proceedings of the Fifth International Symposium of Medicinal Chemistry,* edited by J. Matthieu. Elsevier/North-Holland, Amsterdam.

37. Hofmann, K., and Bowers, C. Y. (1970): Polypeptides. XLVII. Effect of the pyrazole-imidazole replacement on the biological activity of thyrotropin-releasing hormone. *J. Med. Chem.,* 13:1099–1101.

38. Hökfelt, T., Efendic, S., Hellerstrom, C., Johansson, O., Luft, R. and Arimura, A. (1975): Cellular localization of somatostatin in endocrine-like cells and neurons of the rat with special references to the A_1-cells of the pancreatic islets and to the hypothalamus. *Acta Endocrinol. (Suppl. 200),* 80:5–41.

39. Hökfelt, T., Fuxe, K., Johansson, O., Jeffcoate, S., and White, N. (1975): Thyrotropin-releasing hormone (TRH)-containing nerve terminals in certain brain stem nuclei and in the spinal cord. *Neurosci. Lett.,* 1:133–139.

40. Jackson, I. M. D., and Reichlin, S. (1974): Thyrotropin-releasing hormone (TRH): Distribution in hypothalamic and extrahypothalamic brain tissues of mammalian and submammalian chordates. *Endocrinology,* 95:854–862.

41. Jacobs, L., Snyder, P., Wilber, J., Utiger, R., and Daughaday, W. H. (1971): Increased serum prolactin after administration of synthetic thyrotropin releasing hormone (TRH) in man. *J. Clin. Endocrinol. Metab.,* 33:996–998.

42. Jones, M. T., Gillham, B., and Hillhouse, E. W. (1977): The nature of corticotropin releasing factor from rat hypothalamus *in vitro. Fed. Proc.,* 36:2104–2109.

43. Kerdelhué, B., Jutisz, M., Gillessen, D., and Studer, R. O. (1973): Obtention of antisera against a hypothalamic decapeptide (luteinizing hormone/follicle stimulating hormone releasing hormone) which stimulates the release of pituitary gonadotrophins and development of its radioimmunoassay. *Biochem. Biophys. Acta.,* 297:540–548.

44. Klindt, J., Davis, S. L., and Ohlson, D. (1979): Plasma concentration of thyrotropin-releasing hormone, thyrotropin, prolactin and growth hormone during five-day domestic pump infusion of thyrotropin-releasing hormone. *Endocrinology,* 104(1):45–49.

45. Koch, Y., Baram, T., and Fridkin, M. (1976): Generation of specific antiserum to thyrotropin-releasing hormone and its use in a radioimmunoassay. *FEBS Lett.,* 63:295–298.

46. Koch, Y., Ghobsieng, P., Zor, U., Fridkin, M., and Lindner, H. R. (1973): Suppression of gonadotropin secretion and prevention of ovulation in the rat by antiserum to synthetic gonadotropin-releasing hormone. *Biochem. Biophys. Res. Commun.,* 55:623–629.

47. Koch, Y., Goldhaber, G., Fireman, I., Zor, U., Shani, J., and Tal, E. (1977): Suppression of prolactin and thyrotropin secretion in the rat by antiserum to thyrotropin-releasing hormone. *Endocrinology,* 100:1476–1478.

48. Konturek, S. J., Tasler, J., Obtulowicz, W., Coy, D. H., and Schally, A. V. (1976): Effect of growth hormone-release inhibiting hormone on hormones stimulating exocrine pancreatic secretion. *J. Clin. Invest.,* 58:1–6.

49. Krulich, L., and McCann, S. M. (1969): Effect of GH-releasing factor and GH-inhibiting factor on the release and concentration of GH in pituitaries incubated *in vitro. Endocrinology,* 85:319–324.

50. Lamberts, S. W. J., and MacLeod, R. M. (1978): Studies on the mechanism of the GABA-mediated inhibition of prolactin secretion. *Proc. Soc. Exp. Biol. Med.,* 158:10–13.

51. Libertun, C., Arakelian, M. C., Larrea, G. A., and Foglia, V. G. (1979): Inhibition of prolactin secretion by GABA in female and male rats. *Proc. Soc. Exp. Biol. Med.,* 161:28–31.

52. Macleod, R. M. (1969): Influence of norepinephrine and catecholamine-depleting agents on the synthesis and release of prolactin and growth hormone. *Endocrinology,* 85:916–923.

53. Martino, E., Lernmark, A., Seo, H., Steiner, D., and Refetoff, S. (1978): High concentration of thyrotropin-releasing hormone in pancreatic islets. *Proc. Natl. Acad. Sci. USA,* 75(9):4265–4267.

54. Matsuo, H., Arimura, A., Nair, R. M. G., and Schally, A. V. (1971): Synthesis of the porcine LH- and FSH-releasing hormone by the solid-phase method. *Biochem. Biophys. Res. Commun.,* 45:822–827.

55. Matsuo, H., Nair, R. M. G., Arimura, A., and Schally, A. V. (1971): Structure of the porcine LH- and FSH-releasing hormone. I. The proposed amino acid sequence. *Biochem. Biophys. Res. Commun.,* 43:1334–1339.

56. Meites, J., and Clemens, J. A. (1972): Hypothalamic control of prolactin secretion. In: *Vitamins and Hormones,* edited by R. S. Harris, P. L. Munson, E. Diczfalusy, and J. Glover, pp. 165–221. Academic Press, New York.

57. Millar, R. P. (1978): Somatostatin immunoreactive peptides of higher molecular weight in ovine hypothalamic extracts. *J. Endocrinol.,* 77:429–430.

58. Morley, J., Levin, S. R., Pehlevanian, M., Adachi, R., Pekary, A. E., and Hershman, J. M. (1979): The effects of thyrotropin-releasing hormone on the endocrine pancreas. *Endocrinology,* 104(1):137–139.

59. Morley, J., Steinbach, J., Feldman, E. J., and Solomon, T. E. (1979): The effects of thyrotropin releasing hormone (TRH) on the gastrointestinal tract. *Life Sci.,* 24:1059–1066.

60. Mortimer, C. H., Carr, D., Lind, T., Bloom, S. R., Mallinson, C. N., Schally, A. V., Tunbridge, W. M. G., Yeomans, L., Coy, D. H., Kastin, A. J., Besser, G. M., and Hall, R. (1974): Effects of growth-hormone release-inhibiting hormone on circulatory glucagon, insulin and growth hormone in normal, diabetic, acromegalic and hypopituitary patients. *Lancet,* 1:697–701.

61. Müller, E. E., Cocchi, D., Locatelli, V., Parati, E. A., and Mantegazza, P. (1978): Neurotransmitter control of GH and prolactin secretion. In: *Central Regulation of the Endocrine System,* edited by K. Fuxe, T. Kokfelt, and R. Luft, pp. 417–456. Plenum, New York.

62. Nair, R. M. G., Barrett, J. F., Bowers, C. Y., and Schally, A. V. (1970): Structure of porcine thyrotropin-releasing hormone. *Biochemistry,* 9:1103–1106.

63. Nair, R. M. G., Kastin, A. J., and Schally, A. V. (1971): Isolation and structure of hypothalamic MSH release inhibiting hormone. *Biochem. Biophys. Res. Commun.,* 43:1376–1381.

64. Nishi, N., Arimura, A., de la Cruz, K. G., and Schally, A. V. (1976): Termination of pregnancy by sheep anti-LHRH gamma globulin in rats. *Endocrinology,* 98:1024–1030.

65. Oliver, C., Charvet, J. P., Codaccioni, J. L., Vague, J., and Porter, J. C. (1974): TRH in human CSF. *Lancet,* 1:873.

66. Pedroza, E., Vilchez-Martinez, J. A., Fishback, J., Arimura, A., and Schally, A. V. (1977): Binding capacity of luteinizing hormone-releasing hormone and its analogue for pituitary receptor sites. *Biochem. Biophys. Res. Commun.,* 79:234–238.

67. Pedroza, E., Vilchez-Martinez, J. A., Piyachaturawat, P., and Schally, A. V. (1979): Actions of stimulatory and inhibitory analogues of LH-RH on the content and binding of LH-RH in the hypothalamus and pituitary (abstract). In: *Proceedings of the 61st Annual Meeting of the Endocrine Society,* p. 182.

68. Pradayrol, L., Chayvialle, J., Carliquist, M., and Mutt, V. (1978): Isolation of a porcine intestinal peptide with C-terminal somatostatin. *Biochem. Biophys. Res. Commun.,* 85:701–708.

69. Reichlin, S., Saperstein, R., Jackson, I. M. D., Boyd, III, A. E., and Patel, Y. (1976): Hypothalamic hormones. *Annu. Rev. Physiol.,* 38:389–424.

70. Rivier, J., Brazeau, P., Vale, W., Ling, N., Burgus, N., Gilon, C., Yardley, J., and Guillemin, R. (1973): Synthese totale par phase solide d'un tetradecapeptide ayant les proprietes chimiques et biologiques de la somatostatine. *C.R. Acad. Sci. [D] (Paris),* 276:2737–2740.

71. Rivier, J., Vale, W., Monahan, M., Ling, N., and Burgus, R. (1972): Synthetic thyrotropin-releasing factor analogs. 3. Effect of replacement or modification of histidine residue on biological activity. *J. Med. Chem.,* 15:479–482.

72. Sayers, G., Hanzmann, E., and Vegh, M. (1978): A highly potent CRF from bovine hypothalami tissue (abstract). In: *Proceedings of the 60th Annual Meeting of the Endocrine Society,* p. 456.

73. Schally, A. V., Andersen, R. N., Lipscomb, H. S., Long, J. M., and Guillemin, R. (1960): Evidence for the existence of two corticotropin releasing factors, α and β. *Nature,* 188:1192–1193.

74. Schally, A. V., Arimura, A., Baba, Y., Nair, R. M. G., Matsuo, H., Redding, T. W., Debeljuk, L., and White, W. F. (1971): Isolation and properties of the FSH and LH-releasing hormone. *Biochem. Biophys. Res. Commun.,* 43:393–399.

75. Schally, A. V., Arimura, A., and Kastin, A. J. (1973): Hypothalamic regulatory hormones. *Science,* 179:341–350.

76. Schally, A. V., Arimura, A., Redding, T. W., Debeljuk, L. Carter, W., Dupont, A., and Vilchez-Martinez, J. A. (1976): Re-examination of porcine and bovine hypothalamic fractions for additional luteinizing hormone and follicle stimulating hormone-releasing activities. *Endocrinology,* 98:380–391.

77. Schally, A. V., Bowers, C. Y., Redding, T. W., and Barrett, J. F. (1966): Isolation of thyrotropin releasing factor (TRF) from porcine hypothalamus. *Biochem. Biophys. Res. Commun.,* 25:165–169.

78. Schally, A. V., Chang, R., Huang, W-Y., Redding, T. W., Carter, W., Coy, D. H., and Saffran, M. (1979): Isolation, structure and biological activities of several hypothalamic peptides (abstract). In: *Proceedings of the 61st Annual Meeting of the Endocrine Society,* p. 78.

79. Schally, A. V., Coy, D. H., and Meyers, C. A. (1978): Hypothalamic regulatory hormones. *Annu. Rev. Biochem.,* 47:89–128.

80. Schally, A. V., Coy, D. H., Meyers, C. A., and Kastin, A. J. (1979): Hypothalamic peptide hormones: Basic and clinical studies. In: *Hormonal Proteins and Peptides, Vol. 4,* edited by C. H. Li, pp. 2–55. Academic Press, New York.

81. Schally, A. V., Dupont, A., Arimura, A., Redding, T. W., Nishi, N., Linthicum, G. L., and Schlesinger, D. H. (1976): Isolation and structure of somatostatin from porcine hypothalami. *Biochemistry,* 15:509–514.

82. Schally, A. V., Dupont, A., Arimura, A., Takahara, J., Redding, T. W., Clemens, J., and Shaar, C. (1976): Purification of a catecholamine-rich fraction with prolactin release-inhibiting factor (PIF) activity from porcine hypothalami. *Acta Endocrinol. (Kbh.),* 82:1–14.

83. Schally, A. V., Huang, W. Y., Redding, T. W., Arimura, A., Coy, D. H., Chihara, K., Chang, R. C. C., Raymond, V., and Labrie, F. (1978): Isolation, structural elucidation and synthesis of a tetradecapeptide with *in vitro* ACTH-releasing activity corresponding to residues 33–46 of the α-chain of porcine hemoglobin. *Biochem. Biophys. Res. Commun.,* 82:582–588.

84. Schally, A. V., and Kastin, A. J. (1966): Purification of a bovine hypothalamic factor which elevates pituitary MSH levels in rats. *Endocrinology,* 79:768–772.

85. Schally, A. V., Kastin, A. J., and Coy, D. H. (1976): LH-releasing hormone and its analogues: Recent basic and clinical investigations. *Int. J. Fertil.,* 21:1–30.

86. Schally, A. V., Nair, R. M. G., Redding, T. W., and Arimura, A. (1971): Isolation of the luteinizing hormone and follicle-stimulating hormone-releasing hormone from porcine hypothalami. *J. Biol. Chem.,* 246:7230–7236.

87. Schally, A. V., Redding, T. W., Arimura, A., Dupont, A., and Linthicum, G. L. (1977): Isolation of gamma-amino butyric acid from pig hypothalami and demonstration of its prolactin release-inhibiting (PIF) activity *in vivo* and *in vitro*. *Endocrinology,* 100:681–691.

88. Schally, A. V., Redding, T. W., Bowers, C. Y., and Barrett, J. F. (1969): Isolation and properties of porcine thyrotropin releasing hormone. *J. Biol. Chem.,* 244:4077–4088.

89. Schally, A. V., Redding, T. W., Chihara, K., Huang, W. Y., Chang, R. C. C., Carter, W. H., Coy, D. H., and Saffran, M. (1978): Purification of several substances with corticotropin releasing activity (CRF) from pig hypothalamic extracts (abstract). In: *Proceedings of the 60th Annual Meeting of the Endocrine Society,* p. 181.

90. Sievertsson, H., Castensson, S., Lindgren, O., and Bowers, C. Y. (1974): Studies on tetrapeptides related to thyrotropin-releasing hormone and luteinizing hormone releasing hormone. *Acta Pharma. Suec.,* 11:67–76.

91. Smith, J. R., La Hann, T. R., Chestnut, R. M., Carino, M. A., and Horita, A. (1977): Thyrotropin releasing hormone: Stimulation of colonic activity following intracerebroventricular administration. *Science,* 196:660–661.

92. Sowers, J. R., Hershman, J. M., Carlson, H. E., Pekary, A. E., Reed, A. W., Nair, M. G., and Baugh, C. M. (1976): Dose-response of prolactin and thyrotropin to N^{3im}-methyl-thyrotropin releasing hormone in euthyroid men. *J. Clin. Endocrinol. Metab.,* 43:856–860.

93. Takahara, J., Arimura, A., and Schally, A. V. (1974): Suppression of prolactin release by a

purified porcine PIF preparation and catecholamines infused into a rat hypophysial portal vessel. *Endocrinology,* 95:462–465.

94. Takahara, J., Arimura, A., and Schally, A. V. (1975): Assessment of GH releasing hormone-activity in Sephadex-separated fractions of porcine hypothalamic extracts by hypophysial portal vessel infusion in the rat. *Acta Endocrinol.,* 78:428–434.

95. Tashjian, A., Barowsky, N., and Jensen, D. (1971): Thyrotropin releasing hormone: Direct evidence for stimulation of prolactin production by pituitary cells in culture. *Biochem. Biophys. Res. Commun.,* 43:516–423.

96. Vale, W., Rivier, C., and Brown, M. (1977): Regulatory peptides of the hypothalamus. *Annu. Rev. Physiol.,* 39:473–527.

97. Wise, P. M., Rance, N., Barr, G. D., and Barraclough, C. A. (1979): Further evidence that luteinizing hormone-releasing hormone also is follicle-stimulating hormone-releasing hormone. *Endocrinology,* 104(4):940–947.

Polypeptide Hormones, edited by
R. F. Beers, Jr. and E. G. Bassett.
Raven Press, New York © 1980.

18. Structure-Activity Studies on Hypothalamic Hormones: Recent Developments

David H. Coy, Imre Mezo, Escipion Pedroza, Mary V. Nekola, Andrew V. Schally, William Murphy, and Chester A. Meyers

Department of Medicine, Tulane University School of Medicine and Veterans Administration Hospital, New Orleans, Louisiana 70112

INTRODUCTION

Apart from attempts to derive compounds with increased central nervous system (CNS) activity based on the structures of thyrotropin-releasing hormone and melanotropin-release inhibiting factor, the great majority of structure-activity work is presently being carried out on luteinizing hormone-releasing hormone (LH-RH) and somatostatin. This chapter, therefore, is confined to these two hormones.

LUTEINIZING HORMONE-RELEASING HORMONE

The chemistry of LH-RH can be conveniently divided between analogs having greatly enhanced gonadotropin-releasing activities and those acting as competitive inhibitors. Many of the "superagonists" were in part a by-product of the search for antagonists and, in general they contain bulky D-amino acids in position 6 of the chain (Fig. 1), in some cases in conjunction with substitutions for Gly in position 10. At present, there is considerable interest in this class of compounds due to their unanticipated anti-fertility effects generated in part by their prolonged ability to release massive amounts of the gonadotropins. The potencies of these compounds are really as high as are needed and their chemistry has consequently remained static for a number of years.

It is with the antagonist molecules that most structure-activity work is being performed. With respect to their design, the first three residues of the LH-RH decapeptide seem to form a critical area for allowing a lowering of agonist activity while retaining binding affinity for receptors. Thus, <Glu has

<Glu-His-Trp-Ser-Tyr-Gly-Leu-Arg-Pro-Gly-NH₂
 1   2   3   4   5   6   7   8   9   10

FIG. 1. Amino acid sequence of LH-RH.

been replaced by several D-amino acids, His by D-Phe and, an even better modification, Trp by D-Trp. The presence of bulky D-amino acids in position 6, particularly D-Phe and D-Trp, which are so effective for increasing agonist activity, are also highly effective of improving inhibitory activity. Conversely, replacement of Gly[10] by alkylamides or azaglycine, beneficial where the agonists are concerned, are of little value in the inhibitors.

With respect to synthesis, methods have been reported numerous times but it should be emphasized that, with the replacement of so many residues with hydrophobic amino acids, the water solubility of the more active antagonists is quite low. This necessitates purifications in concentrated acetic acid solutions and during bioassay peptides must be injected either as propylene glycol-saline solutions or as suspensions in oil.

The inhibitory peptides are usually assayed for their blockade of ovulation effects after single injections into 4-day cycling rats given at 12 noon on the proestrous day. Three years ago, the best inhibitors were capable of producing full blockade in this system at single doses of approximately 1 mg. Among the approaches that we took to improve on this was an investigation of the properties of some dimeric (3) and semi-dimeric (6) compounds designed with the potential of binding to more than one receptor at a time.

The substitution of a functional D-amino acid such as D-Lys in position 6 allows the introduction of various groups onto the ϵ-amino group without risk of totally destroying binding affinity, since it is known that increasing the size of the side chain in this position is usually beneficial. Incorporation of *bis*-Boc-D-Lys allowed the remainder of the chain to be extended at two points to give an analog with two NH_2-termini shown in Table 1. The inhibitory activity of this branched chain analog was much higher than the straight D-Lys[6]-analog. The peptide with three NH_2-termini, prepared via incorporation of *bis*-Boc-D-Lys-D-Lys, had much diminished activity. Likewise, with a partial NH_2-terminus or COOH-terminus branching, activity was lost so that the effect is due to the presence of the whole extra NH_2-terminus and is not simply due to a side chain size phenomenon.

TABLE 1. N^{ϵ}-compounds [D-Phe^2,D-Trp^3,D-Lys^6]-LH-RH: blockade of ovulation in the rat

	X	
	|	
	pGlu-D-Phe-D-Trp-Ser-Tyr-D-Lys-Leu-Arg-Pro-Gly-NH$_2$	

Peptide, X=	Dose (mg)	Blockade (%)
H	1.5	0
pGlu-D-Phe-D-Trp-Ser-Tyr	1	73
(pGlu-D-Phe-D-Trp-Ser-Tyr)$_2$Lys	1	22
pGlu-His	1	10
Succ-Leu-Arg-Pro-Gly-NH$_2$	1	11
Succ-D-*p*-Cl-Phe-Leu-Arg-Pro-Gly-NH$_2$	1	0

TABLE 2. N^{ϕ}-compounds of [D-Phe^2,D-Trp^3,D-p-NH$_2$-Phe^6]-LH-RH: blockade of ovulation in the rat

pGlu-D-Phe-D-Trp-Ser-Tyr-D-p-NH$_2$-Phe-Leu-Arg-Pro-Gly-NH$_2$

Peptide, X=	Dose (mg)	Blockade (%)
H	1	56
pGlu-D-Phe-D-Trp-Ser-Tyr	1	91
	0.5	57

Aromatic D-amino acids in position 6 are much more effective than D-Lys for improving inhibitory activity—the linear D-p-NH$_2$-Phe^6-analog shown in Table 2 giving significant blockade of ovulation at a 1 mg dose. The branched chain derivative was indeed substantially more active than its Lys counterpart.

These results encouraged us to investigate the properties of full dimers and again we began with the D-Lys^6-analog, which could be readily dimerized by reaction with dicarboxylic acid pentafluorophenyl esters. All the dimeric derivatives (Table 3) had considerably increased activity and the best of them, the succinoyl and isophthaloyl compounds, were more active than the branched chain peptides. Again, however, where more than two chains were involved, such as the trimesoyl trimer, activity was lost, presumably due to steric problems.

A more recent modification reported by Rivier et al. (5) for increasing inhibitory activity is replacement of <Glu in position 1 by its D-isomer. Table 4 depicts more D-Lys dimers containing this substitution and, for instance, with the isophthaloyl derivative, D-<Glu almost tripled inhibitory activity. Since increased activity was observed in going from D-Lys to D-p-NH$_2$-Phe in the branched chain peptides, the study was extended to D-p-NH$_2$-Phe^6 dimers (Table

TABLE 3. N^{ϵ}-dimeric compounds of the [D-Phe^2,D-Trp^3,D-Lys^6]-LH-RH: blockade of ovulation in the rat

pGlu-D-Phe-D-Trp-Ser-Tyr-D-Lys-Leu-Arg-Pro-Gly-NH$_2$
|
X
|
pGlu-D-Phe-D-Trp-Ser-Tyr-D-Lys-Leu-Arg-Pro-Gly-NH$_2$

Peptide, X=	Dose (mg)	Blockade (%)
Succinoyl	1	80
	0.5	40
Terephthaloyl	1	89
	0.5	0
Isophthaloyl	1	100
	0.5	60
Trimesoyl (trimer)	1	0

TABLE 4. N^ϵ-dimeric compounds of [D-pGlu¹,D-Phe²,D-Trp³,D-Lys⁶]-LH-RH: blockade of ovulation in the rat

D-pGlu-D-Phe-D-Trp-Ser-Tyr-D-Lys-Leu-Arg-Pro-Gly-NH₂
|
X
|
D-pGlu-D-Phe-D-Trp-Ser-Tyr-D-Lys-Leu-Arg-Pro-Gly-NH₂

Peptide, X=	Dose (mg)	Blockade (%)
Isophthaloyl	0.25	100
	0.125	30
Suberyl	0.5	90
	0.25	11
Boc-aspartyl	0.5	50

5). In this case, our extrapolations did not work out as planned because both the D- and L-<Glu compounds were really not much more effective than the analogous D-Lys dimers. In this series, the D-<Glu¹-modification also had a less beneficial effect than it did in some less active analogs.

In parallel with these polymer studies, we had also begun to look more closely at position 2, particularly the effect of various substituents on the benzene ring of the D-Phe residue. Beattie et al. (1) reported some modest increases in antagonism with D-*p*-F-Phe in this position; however, the observation had never been extended to some of the new compounds. We examined D-*p*-Cl-, D-*p*-F-, and D-*p*-Br-Phe² in several situations (Table 6) and, overall, the *p*-Cl compounds appeared to have slightly improved properties. For instance, the isophthaloyl dimer of [D-<Glu¹,D-*p*-Cl-Phe²,D-Trp³,D-Lys⁶]-LH-RH showed a distinct trend toward higher activity when compared with the corresponding D-Phe²-peptide. The D-*p*-F-Phe² followed by the D-*p*-Br-Phe²-analogs were less effective. In addition to the D-<Glu¹-modification, Channabasaviah and Stewart (2) found that several other D-amino acids in position 1 were also yielding promising results, particularly when acylated. We examined some D-Phe¹-analogs containing halogenated D-Phe in position 2, several of which are shown in Table 7. As expected,

TABLE 5. Dimeric N^ϕ-Ala-D-*p*-NH₂-Phe⁶-antagonists

LH-RH analog	Dose (mg)	Blockade of ovulation (%)
D-Phe²,D-Trp³,N-Ala-D-*p*-NH₂-Phe⁶-	1.0	20
D-pGlu-D-Phe²,D-Trp³,N-Ala-D-*p*-NH₂-Phe⁶-	0.5	30
Isophthaloyl-*bis*(D-Phe²,D-Trp³,N-Ala-D-*p*-NH₂-Phe⁶-LH-RH)	0.25	40
	0.125	0
Isophthaloyl-*bis*-(D-pGlu¹,D-Phe²,D-Trp³,N-Ala-D-*p*-NH₂Phe⁶-LH-RH)	0.25	80
	0.125	33

TABLE 6. *Antagonists containing D-pGlu¹ and p-halogeno-D-Phe²*

Peptide	Dose (mg)	Blockade of ovulation (%)
D-pGlu¹,D-Phe²,D-Trp³,D-Lys⁶-LH-RH	1.5	100
	0.5	25
Isophthaloyl dimer of above	0.25	100
	0.125	30
D-pGlu¹,D-*p*-Cl-Phe²,D-Trp³,D-Lys⁶-LH-RH	1	60
Isophthaloyl dimer of above	0.25	100
	0.125	53
	0.063	30
D-pGlu¹,D-*p*-F-Phe²,D-Trp³,D-Lys⁶-LH-RH	1	60
D-pGlu¹,D-*p*-Br-Phe²,D-Trp³,D-Lys⁶-LH-RH	1	0
D-pGlu¹,D-*p*-Cl-Phe²,D-Trp³,D-Lys⁶-LH-RH	0.25	30

the nonacylated version of [D-Phe¹,D-Phe²,D-Trp³,D-Phe⁶]-LH-RH had no activity even at moderate doses; however, to our surprise, replacement of D-Phe² by D-*p*-Cl-Phe dramatically increased antiovulatory activity so that complete blockade was obtained with 0.25 mg. The D-*p*-Br-Phe²-analog was less active and the F-derivative inactive at the same dose. This was the reverse of the situation existing when D-<Glu is in the first position. As soon as the D-*p*-Cl-Phe²-analog was acylated at its free NH₂-terminus, activity was greatly increased. Succinylation more than doubled activity; however, the choice of acyl groups was critical; for instance, activity was lost when an electron-withdrawing trifluoroacetyl group was incorporated.

In the last two analogs in Table 7, D-Phe in position 6 was replaced by D-Trp which is recognized to be a slightly better modification. The activity of the free amino peptide was not improved, but the *N*-acetyl derivative gave excellent blockade of ovulation at doses as low as 30 μg. Given as a suspension in

TABLE 7. *D-Phe¹-antagonists*

Peptide	Dose (mg)	Blockade of ovulation (%)
D-Phe¹,D-Phe²,D-Trp³,D-Phe⁶-LH-RH	1	0
D-Phe¹,D-*p*-Cl-Phe²,D-Trp³,D-Phe⁶-LH-RH	0.25	82
	0.125	11
D-Phe¹,D-*p*-Br-Phe²,D-Trp³,D-Phe⁶-LH-RH	0.25	50
D-Phe¹,D-*p*-F-Phe²,D-Trp³,D-Phe⁶-LH-RH	0.25	10
Succ-D-Phe¹,D-*p*-Cl-Phe²,D-Trp³,D-Phe⁶-LH-RH	0.125	80
	0.062	50
TFA-D-Phe¹,D-*p*-Cl-Phe²,D-Trp³,D-Phe⁶-LH-RH	1	0
D-Phe¹,D-*p*-Cl-Phe²,D-Trp³,D-Trp⁶-LH-RH	0.125	0
Ac-D-Phe¹,D-*p*-Cl-Phe²,D-Trp³,D-Trp⁶-LH-RH	0.062	100
	0.031	64

corn oil (which tends to increase the activity of several of the monomeric peptides), an 80% blockade of ovulation was observed at a dose of 20 μg per animal. The Cl-modification appears to increase inhibitory activity by about a factor of 7. Comparing the contrasting results exhibited by the D-p-Cl-Phe²-analogs of the D-<Glu¹ and D-Phe¹ series, it is possible that the favorable results with the latter are due to interactions between the aromatic side chains. Whether these are primarily steric or electronic in character should be clarified by looking at the effects of various substituents in various places on both rings in studies presently in progress.

In a space of 3 years we have gone from analogs such as [D-Phe²,D-Trp³, D-Phe⁶]-LH-RH to the Cl-analog described here with a 30-fold increase in inhibitory activity. In clinical tests (4) a number of years ago, [D-Phe²,D-Trp³, D-Phe⁶]-LH-RH began to produce inhibition of gonadotropin release at 90 mg per person, an enormous dose. By extrapolation, the new analog could be effective in the range of 3 to 5 mg and its potency should make possible many critical biological studies.

SOMATOSTATIN

As has been pointed out, somatostatin (Fig. 2) has an amazing array of endocrine and gastrointestinal activities that seriously complicate the bioassays necessary for structure-activity experiments. Thus, unlike the situation with LH-RH, the rate-controlling step in the study of somatostatin analogs is often the ability to assay rather than synthesize them. Nevertheless, excellent progress has been made in discovering peptides with more selective activities and, more recently, prolonged activity. Studies on active conformations of the molecule by the synthesis of conformationally restricted analogs carried out by Veber et al. (8) has enabled that group in particular to pursue a more logical approach to analog design. Reports on glucagon release-specific D-Cys¹⁴-analogs are no longer quite as exciting as they had previously been since it seems that assays utilizing arginine-stimulated insulin and glucagon release in the rat may not reflect too well the effects of analogs on untreated animals (7).

One very important aspect of somatostatin analog research must be the design of peptides with prolonged activity and this aspect pertains to a series of position 4 analogs that we have been examining (Table 8). Lys in position 4 of the chain is a critical area of the molecule and as soon as one shifts from basic substitutions, activity drops severely. The most curious observation, however, is the large increase in activity when Lys is replaced by Phe. [Phe⁴]-somatostatin was over twice as active as the parent peptide for *in vitro* inhibition of GH

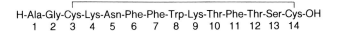

H-Ala-Gly-Cys-Lys-Asn-Phe-Phe-Trp-Lys-Thr-Phe-Thr-Ser-Cys-OH
  1   2   3   4   5   6   7   8   9   10 11 12 13 14

FIG. 2. Amino acid sequence of somatostatin.

TABLE 8. *Inhibitory activities of position 4 somatostatin analogs*

Analog	Inhibition of release (%)		
	GH[a]	GH[b]	Gastric acid[b]
Des-Lys[4]	3	—	1
Glu[4]	5	—	1
Thr[4]	1	—	1
Phe[4]	200	370	80
Phe[4],D-Trp[8]	—	460	—

[a] *In vitro.*
[b] *In vivo.*

release and on nembutal-stimulated GH release *in vivo* in the rat, the activity was even greater. Normally, D-Trp in position 8 increases the activity of somatostatin *in vivo* by about a factor of 5; however, [Phe[4],D-Trp[8]]-somatostatin was only slightly more active than the Phe[4]-peptide, suggesting that perhaps these alterations are having the same conformational effect on the molecule. It is also interesting that the Phe[4]-analog is more active *in vivo* than *in vitro,* one explanation being increased biological stability. Indeed, in preliminary experiments the peptide was considerably longer acting than somatostatin itself for inhibition of *in vivo* GH release. It should also be noted that effects on *in vivo* gastric acid release are substantially less, so that there appears to be some dissociation of activity. Whether this modification can be incorporated into some of the other analogs of interest, such as those with other dissociated activities, in order to increase and prolong their activity remains to be seen.

ACKNOWLEDGMENTS

This work was supported by NICHD Contract HD-8-2819, NIH grant AM-18370, and the Veterans Administration.

REFERENCES

1. Beattie, C. W., Corbin, A., Foell, T. J., Garsky, V., McKinley, W. A., Rees, R. W. A., Sarantakis, D., and Yardley, J. P. (1975): Luteinizing hormone-releasing hormone. Antiovulatory activity of analogs substituted in positions 2 and 6. *J. Med. Chem.,* 18:1247–1250.
2. Channabasavaiah, K., and Stewart, J. (1979): New analogs of luliberin which inhibit ovulation in the rat. *Biochem. Biophys. Res. Commun.,* 86:1266–1273.
3. Coy, D. H., Seprodi, J., Vilchez-Martinez, J. A., Pedroza, E., Gardner, J., and Schally, A. V. (1979): Structure-function studies and prediction of conformational requirements for LH-RH. In: *Central Nervous System Effects of Hypothalamic Hormones and Other Peptides,* edited by R. Collu, A. Barbeau, J. R. Ducharme, and J.-G. Rochefort, pp. 317–323. Raven Press, New York.
4. Gonzalez-Barcena, D., Kastin, A. J., Coy, D. H., Nikolics, K., and Schally, A. V. (1977): Suppression of gonadotropin release in man by an inhibitory analog of LH-releasing hormone. *Lancet,* 2:997–998.

5. Rivier, J. E., and Vale, W. (1978): [D-pGlu^1,D-Phe^2,D-Trp^{3,6}]-LRF. A potent luteinizing hormone releasing factor antagonist *in vitro* and inhibitor of ovulation in the rat. *Life Sci.,* 23:869–873.
6. Seprodi, J., Coy, D. H., Vilchez-Martinez, J. A., Pedroza, E., and Schally, A. V. (1978): Branched chain analogues of luteinizing hormone releasing hormone. *J. Med. Chem.,* 21:276–280.
7. Tarborsky, G. J., Smith, P. H., and Porte, D. (1979): Differential effects of somatostatin analogs on α- and β-cells of the pancreas. *Am. J. Physiol.,* 236:E123–E128.
8. Veber, D. F., Holly, F. W., Paleveda, W. J., Nutt, R. F., Bergstrand, S. J., Torchiana, M., Glitzer, M. S., Saperstein, R., and Hirschmann, R. (1978): Conformationally restricted bicyclic analogs of somatostatin. *Proc. Natl. Acad. Sci. USA,* 75:2636–2640.

Polypeptide Hormones, edited by
R. F. Beers, Jr. and E. G. Bassett.
Raven Press, New York © 1980.

19. Distribution of Hypothalamic Peptides

Michael J. Brownstein

Unit on Neuroendocrinology, Laboratory of Clinical Science, National Institute of Mental Health, Bethesda, Maryland 20205

INTRODUCTION

Three peptide hormones are discussed in this chapter: luteinizing hormone-releasing hormone (LH-RH), thyrotropin-releasing hormone (TRH), and growth hormone release-inhibiting hormone (somatostatin). These were isolated from hypothalamic extracts and have been assumed to be made by small, anatomically discrete populations of neurons whose processes travel to the median eminence. The isolation of the hypothalamic hormones and the development of sensitive assays for measuring them and immunohistochemical techniques for visualizing them have produced surprising results. It is becoming more and more obvious that "hypothalamic peptides" are not confined to the hypothalamus and that they must have functions unrelated to the actions that facilitated their discoveries.

ASSAYING HYPOTHALAMIC PEPTIDES

Two types of assay techniques have been used to measure the concentrations of hypothalamic peptides in tissue extracts: bioassays and radioimmunoassays (RIAs). Bioassays are often (but not invariably) difficult to perform, time consuming, and relatively insensitive. Furthermore, many structurally unrelated agents can stimulate or attenuate biological responses. Consequently, bioassays are not necessarily specific. On the other hand, intact cells do distinguish between agonists and antagonists.

Radioimmunoassays are fast and convenient. They are quite sensitive and, when done well, specific for *functional groups that react with the antibodies being used.* This is not to say, however, that RIAs are absolutely specific for the peptides that they measure. It is becoming more and more clear that most, if not all, neuropeptides are synthesized as parts of larger precursor molecules. These precursors are broken down by proteases into smaller, active agents. The precursors themselves and intermediates (i.e., "big" forms of the active peptides) may react in RIAs. Completely unrelated molecules may react as well. For example, an antibody that reacts with the NH_2-terminal end of thyrotropin releasing hormone (pyroglutamyl-histidyl-prolineamide) could be expected to react with pyroglutamyl-histidyl-glycine, a tripeptide that has recently been isolated from the urine of patients with anorexia nervosa (58).

More and more workers are using chromatographic techniques to aid in the validation of their RIAs. High-performance liquid chromatography (HPLC) is a particularly popular method for separating peptides from one another. Many similar peptides can be resolved using reverse-phase HPLC. Unfortunately, there is no guarantee that any given unknown peptide will be separated from a structurally similar standard by this or any other chromatographic procedure. In the final analysis of biologically active, immunologically reactive, chromatographically "identified" peptide still has to be sequenced to be characterized. Microsequencing techniques (especially mass spectrographic methods) are being developed that should allow a few picomoles of pure peptide to be analyzed (D. Hunt, *personal communication*).

VISUALIZING HYPOTHALAMIC PEPTIDES

The immunocytochemical techniques that have been developed for visualizing peptides at the light and electron microscopic levels depend for their specificities on the antigen-antibody reaction. Thus, these techniques cannot be any more specific than the antibodies themselves are; and, at worst, immunochemical staining is considerably less specific than the antigen-antibody reaction detected *in vitro*. In addition to false positive staining, the inability to stain structures (especially perikarya) has been a problem. This may be due in part to an inability of certain antibodies to react with peptide precursors, in part to peptide losses encountered during fixation and staining, and in part to a reduction in immunogenicity of the peptides associated with the fixation process.

Despite the problems enumerated above, the immunohistological approach has yielded very important information about the cellular and subcellular localization of peptides. This information cannot be obtained in any other way. Often immunocytochemical results can be validated by studying the effects of lesions in one part of the brain on peptide levels elsewhere. The use of more than one experimental approach should be encouraged.

STUDIES OF PEPTIDE BIOSYNTHESIS

As stated earlier, many neuropeptides are probably synthesized in neuronal perikarya by a ribosomal mechanism as parts of larger molecules. Therefore, it should be possible to demonstrate *de novo* synthesis of a peptide by the perikarya in which it seems to be present. In this way, studies of peptide biosynthesis can be used to provide the ultimate validation of inferences based on anatomical data. Recent studies of the hypothalamo-neurohypophysial system illustrate this point (13,20,21,55). Neurons in the supraoptic nucleus have been shown immunohistochemically to contain vasopressin, oxytocin, and neurophysins. These neurons have been proven to incorporate radiolabeled cysteine rapidly into two 20,000 M.W. proteins. One of these (propressophysin), a glycoprotein, contains both vasopressin and its associated neurophysin. The other (prooxyphysin), which does not appear to be glycosylated, contains oxytocin and its neurophysin. Thus, cells that are known to contain vasopressin, oxytocin, and their respective neurophysins have now also been shown to make these hormones.

Similarly, arcuate nucleus neurons in which α-MSH, ACTH, and endorphin have been visualized have now been shown to synthesize the 31,000 M.W. precursor of these hormones (41).

There is evidence that somatostatin and LH-RH are synthesized from larger precursors; TRH may or may not be. Since studies of the biosynthesis of the "hypothalamic peptides" are in their infancy, it is not yet possible to determine whether neurons that seem to contain one of these peptides can indeed manufacture it.

DISTRIBUTION OF HYPOTHALAMIC PEPTIDES

Information about hypothalamic peptides in the brain is presented below. The authors of the studies cited have relied on assays of tissue extracts and on histochemistry. The limitations of these methods should be borne in mind.

Luteinizing Hormone Releasing Hormone

In 1960 McCann showed that the rat hypothalamus contains a substance that releases luteinizing hormone (LH) from the anterior pituitary (43). Using a bioassay, he localized this material more precisely. He assayed extracts of the stalk-median eminence, ventral hypothalamus, dorsal hypothalamus, and suprachiasmatic nucleus. Most of the LH-releasing activity was in the stalk and median eminence; a small amount of activity was detected in the basal hypothalamus. Next, McCann and co-workers measured releasing activity in serial sections of the preoptic area and hypothalamus (42). They found it in a region extending from the preoptic area through the suprachiasmatic area to the median eminence and arcuate nucleus. Subsequently, Wheaton et al. assayed LH-RH in brain slices by means of RIA and confirmed the earlier bioassay data (63).

Palkovits and collaborators assayed LH-RH in samples of discrete hypothalamic nuclei that were punched out (48) of frozen serial sections of the rat hypothalamus (49). The amount of LH-RH in each tissue homogenate was determined by radioimmunoassay. A very high concentration of it was found in the median eminence, moderate levels were detected in the arcuate nucleus, and small amounts were present in the suprachiasmatic and preoptic regions. In the preoptic area, the bulk of the LH-RH is in the supraoptic crest, a vascular structure that forms part of the rostral tip of the third ventricle (32). The supraoptic crest and the other circumventricular organs are quite rich in LH-RH. The hormone present in these organs may be taken up from the cerebrospinal fluid and disposed of, or it may be secreted into the cerebrospinal fluid to act on diverse areas of the brain.

LH-RH-containing neural structures have been visualized in many species. Two principal groups of cells seem to manufacture LH-RH. One of these is found in the anterior hypothalamus, preoptic area, and septum; the other is located more posteriorly in the infundibular region. The former group of cells is especially prominent in rodents, whereas the latter predominates in primates.

The LH-RH containing neuronal system has been studied more extensively in the guinea pig (4,7,8,40) and the rat (1,4,9,22,26,31,36,44–46,52,56,57) than in other rodents. It is unusual to find LH-RH positive perikarya in normal untreated animals of either species. After treatment with pharmacological agents, LH-RH has been detected in preoptic and septal neurons in the guinea pig. The tuberal region also has LH-RH-containing cells, and LH-RH is present in axons and terminals in the median eminence and supraoptic crest. These axons can rarely be traced back to cell bodies in the arcuate region. In fact, the number of LH-RH rich axons in the infundibular region drops after electrolytic lesions are made just caudal to the septum and preoptic areas. Therefore, the majority of these tuberal axons may originate from cells that are over or rostral to the chiasm.

The results of immunocytochemical studies in the rat are more difficult to interpret than those in the guinea pig. A number of workers have succeeded in staining preterminal and terminal axons in the rat. These are found in the median eminence, supraoptic crest, septum, preoptic area, perifornical region, and stria terminalis. In spite of this, many people have been unable to visualize LH-RH in rat neuronal perikarya. Others, such as Weindl (61) and co-workers, have seen LH-RH-positive cells in the dorsal preoptic and anterior hypothalamic regions. [This is consistent with the finding that total medial basal hypothalamic deafferentations or frontal deafferentations cause marked decreases in LH-RH in the median eminence and arcuate nucleus without affecting LH-RH in the supraoptic crest (12,62)]. Still others, such as Naik (45,46) and Hoffman (22), have visualized LH-RH in cells extending from the suprachiasmatic region to the premammillary region. Obviously, more studies of the distribution of the LH-RH-containing neurons and processes in the rat are required.

In primates, most LH-RH-positive cell bodies have been found in the medial basal part of the tuber cinereum, especially in the infundibular and premammillary nuclei (6,22). There are also scattered cells in the septum and preoptic area. Although medial basal hypothalamic deafferentation in rats blocks ovulation, complete surgical isolation of the same region in monkeys does not interfere with either tonic or cyclic release of gonadotropic hormones (37). Presumably the rostrally located, LH-RH-containing neurons (those that project in primates and rodents alike to the supraoptic crest, the medial habenula, the mesencephalon, and the telencephalon) in primates (5) have other roles besides regulation of anterior pituitary function. One of these may be to orchestrate behavioral and endocrine changes.

Somatostatin

Somatostatin is found in both the central nervous system (CNS) and in the periphery, where it is present in the stomach, duodenum, jejunum, and pancreas (3,54). It has been detected in the brains of several mammals, pigeons, frogs, catfish, and hagfish (59).

Using bioassays and RIAs, a number of workers have shown that somatostatin is concentrated in the hypothalamus of the rat where its level is especially high in the median eminence (11,34). Several hypothalamic nuclei contain substantial amounts of somatostatin too: the arcuate, ventromedial, ventral premammillary, periventricular, and medial preoptic nuclei (11,34). Of these, the ventromedial nucleus is unique in being devoid of a growth hormone release-inhibiting activity (60). This nucleus may be particularly rich in a growth hormone releasing hormone.

The median eminence is not the only circumventricular organ that contains somatostatin. It is present in the supraoptic crest, the subfornical organ, the subcommissural organ, and the area postrema (50).

Outside of the hypothalamus, a number of structures in addition to the circumventricular organs have somatostatin. In fact, only about one-third of the brain's somatostatin is found in the hypothalamus. The septum, preoptic area, and thalamus have moderately high somatostatin concentrations and contribute another 30% to the total (11). The extrahypothalamic somatostatin has recently been characterized by J. Speiss and W. Vale *(personal communication)*. It appears to have the same amino acid composition as the material that was originally isolated from the hypothalamus.

Because somatostatin was found in the medial hypothalamus and outside of it, the locations of the neurons that provide the median eminence its release inhibiting hormone were not immediately obvious. Complete medial basal hypothalamic deafferentation and frontal deafferentation caused marked decreases in somatostatin in the median eminence, but did not depress somatostatin levels elsewhere (10). Therefore, cells in the tuberal area must not supply the remainder of the regions of the CNS their somatostatin. [In fact, cultured dissociated cerebral cortical neurons have recently been shown to produce their own somatostatin (S. Reichlin, *personal communication*)]. Furthermore, it seems likely that the medial basal hypothalamus must receive the bulk of its somatostatin from an area rostral to it.

Somatostatin-containing cell bodies have been visualized in the rat brain (2, 17,28). These cell bodies are located in the anterior periventricular area. When lesions were made in this area 80 to 90% decreases in somatostatin were measured in the median eminence (18). No changes in the level of the hormone were detected in the ventro-medial nucleus; presumably this nucleus has a somatostatinergic input separate from that of the median eminence.

In addition to the dense plexuses of somatostatin-containing fibers that have been observed in the median eminence, arcuate nucleus, and ventromedial nucleus (28,51,53), other fiber systems have been seen. Moderately dense fiber systems (which may arise from cells in the magnocellular hypothalamic nuclei) have been visualized in the posterior pituitary (25) and in the supraoptic crest, subfornical organ, the substantia gelatinosa, and the dorsal horn of the spinal cord. Neuronal perikarya in the spinal ganglia of the rat have been reported to contain somatostatin (23–25); some somatostatin-containing cells were found in the trigeminal ganglion, too. The somatostatin-positive nerve fibers in the lamina propria of the intestines near the ganglion cells of the myenteric plexus may belong to the spinal ganglion cells mentioned above (25,28). Somatostatin is also present in cells in the thyroid, stomach (25), and islets of Langerhans (in D cells) (16). In the pancreas, somatostatin seems to inhibit insulin and glucagon release (19,35).

Thyrotropin-Releasing Hormone

By measuring TSH release from pituitary explants, Krulich and co-workers showed that TRH is present in the median eminence, dorsomedial hypothalamus, and preoptic area of the rat (38). In discrete hypothalamic nuclei radioimmunoassayed for TRH, the peptide was found to be concentrated in the median eminence (14); in the cow, however, it was restricted to the middle portion of the zona externa (33). It was present in moderate amounts in the ventromedial, arcuate, dorsomedial, and periventricular nuclei. Modest amounts of TRH were found in the remainder of the hypothalamus, the preoptic area, and the septum pellucidum.

Several investigators have reported that immunoassayable TRH is widely distributed in the central nervous system (29,47,64). The TRH-like material in extracts of extrahypothalamic brain has been shown to have gel filtration and electrophoretic properties similar to those of TRH, and it seems to be biologically active. In spite of this, the TRH-like substance(s) found outside of the hypothalamus may not all be pyroglutamyl-histidyl-prolineamide. Jeffcoate and White have found that extracts of sheep, rat, and rabbit cerebral cortices contain an immunoassayable material that differs chromatographically from synthetic TRH (30). Kubek and colleagues have shown that human brain extracts have less TSH releasing activity than TRH immunoreactivity (39). Finally, Youngblood has stated that molecular species other than TRH are present in extra-hypothalamic brain that are capable of reacting in a "crude" TRH RIA (65). Among the substances that interfere in the radioimmunoassay for TRH are brain lipids that can be removed from samples with ether. Only the hypothalamus, septum, and preoptic area could be shown to contain authentic TRH.

Given the apparent lack of specificity of the antibodies that have been employed to measure TRH, it is not unlikely that this tripeptide has been artifactually localized by means of immunocytochemistry, especially outside of the hypothalamus, preoptic area, and septum (27). Within these three regions, TRH has been visualized in the external zone of the median eminence and in dense axonal systems of the dorsomedial nucleus, in the paraventricular nucleus, and in the perifornical region. Lower numbers of TRH-positive fibers were found in the ventromedial nuclei, periventricular nuclei, and zona incerta, and sparse networks of fibers elsewhere in the hypothalamus (24). The supraoptic crest has a fairly dense collection of TRH-containing processes; the interstitial nucleus of the stria terminalis and the lateral septal nucleus have moderate numbers of positive processes. These immunocytochemical findings agree reasonably well with RIA and bioassay data.

The locations of neurons the axons of which supply TRH to the hypothalamus are unknown. Complete deafferentation of the medial basal hypothalamus causes a substantial fall in TRH levels in this region, as does frontal deafferentiation (15). Thus, part of the TRH in the tuberal region must come from extratuberal cells. Some of these cells may reside in the periventricular area or supraoptic area (T. Hökfelt, *personal communication*).

CONCLUSIONS

The hypothalamic peptides have been detected in the hypothalamus, in extra-hypothalamic regions, and outside of the brain. In the hypothalamus, the highest levels are found in the median eminence, the axons and axon terminals of which are rich in peptides. Outside of the hypothalamus, the structures of the substances that react in peptide assays have not been rigorously determined. Moreover, there is some controversy as to the localization of the neuronal perikarya that synthesize hypothalamic peptides in a variety of species. These problems should ultimately be resolved as existing methods are refined and new methods are developed.

REFERENCES

1. Alpert, L. C., Brawer, J. R., Jackson, J. M. D., and Patel, Y. C. (1975): Somatostatin and LRH: Immunohistochemical evidence for distinct hypothalamic distribution. *Fed. Proc.,* 34:239(Abstr. 114).
2. Alpert, L. C., Brawer, J. R., Patel, Y. C., and Reichlin, S. (1976): Somatostatinergic neurons in anterior hypothalamus: Immunohistochemical localization. *Endocrinology,* 98:255–258.
3. Arimura, A., Sato, H., Dupont, A., Nishi, N., and Schally, A. V. (1975): Somatostatin: Abundance of immunoreactive hormone in rat stomach and pancreas. *Science,* 189:1007–1009.
4. Baker, B. L., Dermody, W. C., and Reel, J. R. (1974): Localization of luteinizing hormone-releasing hormone in the mammalian hypothalamus. *Am. J. Anat.,* 139:129–134.
5. Barry, J. (1978): Septo-epithalamo-habenular LRF reactive neurons in monkeys. *Brain Res..* 151:183–187.
6. Barry, J., and Carette, B. (1975): Immunofluorescence study of LRF neurons in primates. *Cell Tissue Res.,* 164:163–178.
7. Barry, J., Dubois, M. P., and Carette, B. (1974): Immunofluorescence study of the preoptico-infundibular LRF neurosecretory pathway in the normal, castrated, or testosterone-treated male guinea pig. *Endocrinology,* 95:1416–1423.
8. Barry, J., Dubois, M. P., and Poulain, P. (1973): LH-RH producing cells of the mammalian hypothalamus. *Z. Zellforsch. Microsk. Anat.,* 146:351–366.

9. Barry, J., Dubois, M. P., Poulain, P., and Leonardelli, J. (1973): Characterisation et topographie de neurones hypothalamiques immunoreactifs avec des anticorps anti-LRF de synthèse. *C.R. Acad. Sci.* [*D*] *(Paris),* 276:3191–3193.

10. Brownstein, M. J., Arimura, A., Fernandez-Durango, R., Schally, A. V., Palkovits, M., and Kizer, J. S. (1977): The effect of hypothalamic deafferentation on somatostatin in the rat brain. *Endocrinology,* 100:246–249.

11. Brownstein, M., Arimura, A., Sato, H., Schally, A. V., and Kizer, J. S. (1975): The regional distribution of somatostatin in the rat brain. *Endocrinology,* 96:1456–1461.

12. Brownstein, M. J., Arimura, A., Schally, A. V., Palkovits, M., and Kizer, J. S. (1976): The effect of surgical isolation of the hypothalamus on its luteinizing hormone-releasing hormone content. *Endocrinology,* 98:662–665.

13. Brownstein, M., and Gainer, H. (1977): Neurophysin biosynthesis in normal rats and in rats with hereditary diabetes insipidus. *Proc. Natl. Acad. Sci. USA,* 74:4046–4049.

14. Brownstein, M. J., Palkovits, M., Saavedra, J., Bassiri, R., and Utiger, R. D. (1974): Thyrotropin-releasing hormone in specific nuclei of rat brain. *Science,* 185:267–269.

15. Brownstein, M. J., Utiger, R. D., Palkovits, M., and Kizer, J. S. (1975): Effect of hypothalamic deafferentation on thyrotropin releasing hormone levels in rat brain. *Proc. Natl. Acad. Sci. USA,* 72:4177–4179.

16. Dubois, P. M., Paulin, C., Assan, R., and Dubois, M. P. (1975): Evidence for immunoreactive somatostatin in the endocrine cells of human foetal pancreas. *Nature,* 256:731–732.

17. Elde, R. P., and Parsons, J. A. (1975): Immunocytochemical localization of somatostatin in cell bodies of the rat hypothalamus. *Am. J. Anat.,* 144:541–548.

18. Epelbaum, J., Willoughby, J. O., Brazeau, P., and Martin, J. B. (1977): Effects of lesions and hypothalamic deafferentation on somatostatin distribution in the brain. *Endocrinology,* 101:1495–1502.

19. Fugimoto, W. Y., Ensinck, J. W., and Williams, R. W. (1974): Somatostatin inhibits insulin and glucagon release by monolayer cell cultures of rat endocrine pancreas. *Life Sci.,* 15:1999–2004.

20. Gainer, H., Sarne, Y., and Brownstein, M. (1977): Neurophysin biosynthesis: Conversion of a putative precursor during axonal transport. *Science,* 195:1354–1356.

21. Gainer, H., Sarne, Y., and Brownstein, M. (1977): Biosynthesis and axonal transport of rat neurohypophyseal proteins and peptides. *J. Cell Biol.* 73:366–381.

22. Hoffman, G. E. (1976): Immunocytochemical localization of luteinizing hormone-releasing hormone (LHRH) in murine and primate brain. *Anat. Rec.,* 184:429–430.

23. Hökfelt, T., Efendic, S., Hellerstrom, D., Johansson, O., Luft, R., and Arimura, A. (1975): Cellular localization of somatostatin in endocrine-like cells and neurons of the rat with special references to the A₁-cells of the pancreatic islets and to the hypothalamus. *Acta Endocrinol.* [*Suppl.*] *(Kbh.),* 80(200):5–41.

24. Hökfelt, T., Elde, R., Johansson, O., Luft, R., and Arimura, A. (1975): Immunohistochemical evidence for the presence of somatostatin, a powerful inhibitory peptide, in some primary sensory neurons. *Neurosci. Lett.,* 1:231–235.

25. Hökfelt, T., Elde, R., Johansson, O., Luft, R., Nilsson, G., and Arimura, A. (1976): Immunohistochemical evidence for separate populations of somatostatin-containing and substance P-containing primary afferent neurons in the rat. *Neuroscience,* 1:131–136.

26. Hökfelt, T., Fuxe, K., Goldstein, M., Johansson, O., Fraser, H., and Jeffcoate, S. L. (1975): Immunofluorescence mapping of central monoamine and releasing hormone (LRH) systems. In: *Anatomical Neuroendocrinology,* edited by W. E. Stumpf and L. D. Grant, pp. 381–392. Karger, Basel.

27. Hökfelt, T., Fuxe, K., Johansson, O., Jeffcoate, S., and White, N. (1975): Thyrotropin releasing hormone (TRH)-containing nerve terminals in certain brain stem nuclei and in the spinal cord. *Neurosci. Lett.,* 1:133–139.

28. Hökfelt, T., Johansson, O., Fuxe, K., Löfström, A., Goldstein, M., Park, D., Ebstein, R., Fraser, H., Jeffcoate, S., Efendic, S., Luft, R., and Arimura, A. (1975): Mapping and relationship of hypothalamic neurotransmitters and hypothalamic hormones. In: *Proceedings 6th International Congress of Pharmacology, Vol. 3, Central Nervous System and Behavioral Pharmacology,* edited by M. Airakginen, pp. 93–110. Pergamon Press, New York.

29. Jackson, I. M. D., and Reichlin, S. (1974): Thyrotropin-releasing hormone (TRH): Distribution in hypothalamic and extrahypothalamic brain tissues of mammalian and sub-mammalian chordates. *Endocrinology,* 95:854–862.

30. Jeffcoate, S. L., and White, N. (1975): Is there any thyrotropin releasing hormone in mammalian extra-hypothalamic brain tissue? *J. Endocrinol.,* 67:42P–43P.
31. King, J. C., Parsons, J. A., Erlandsen, S. L., and Williams, T. H. (1974): Luteinizing hormone-releasing hormone (LH-RH) pathway of the rat hypothalamus revealed by the unlabeled antibody peroxidase-antiperoxidase method. *Cell Tissue Res.,* 153:211–217.
32. Kizer, J. S., Palkovits, M., and Brownstein, M. (1976): Releasing factors in the circumventricular organs of the rat brain. *Endocrinology,* 98:309–315.
33. Kizer, J. S., Palkovits, M., Tappaz, M., Kebabian, J., and Brownstein, M. (1976): Distribution of releasing factors, biogenic amines, and related enzymes in the bovine median eminence. *Endocrinology,* 98:649–659.
34. Kobayashi, R., Brown, M., and Vale, W. (1977): Regional distribution of neurotensin and somatostatin in rat brain. *Brain Res.,* 126:584–588.
35. Koerker, D. J., Ruch, W., Chideckel, E., Palmer, J., Goodner, C. J., Ensinck, J., and Gale, C. C. (1974): Somatostatin: Hypothalamic inhibitor of the endocrine pancreas. *Science,* 184:482–484.
36. Kordon, C., Kerdelhué, B., Pattou, E., and Jutisz, M. (1974): Immunocytochemical localization of LHRH in axons and nerve terminals of the rat median eminence. *Proc. Soc. Exp. Biol. Med.,* 147:122–127.
37. Krey, L. C., Butler, W. R., and Knobil, E. (1975): Surgical disconnection of the medial basal hypothalamus and pituitary function in the rhesus monkey. I. Gonadotropin secretion. *Endocrinology,* 96:1073–1087.
38. Krulich, L., Quijada, M., Hefco, E., and Sundberg, D. K. (1974): Localization of thyrotropin-releasing factor (TRF) in the hypothalamus of the rat. *Endocrinology,* 95:9–17.
39. Kubek, M. J., Lorincz, M. A., and Wilber, J. F. (1977): The identification of thyrotropin releasing hormone (TRH) in hypothalamic and extrahypothalamic loci of the human nervous system. *Brain Res.,* 126:196–200.
40. Leonardelli, J., Barry, J., and Dubois, M. P. (1973): Mise en évidence par immunofluorescence d'un constituent immunologiquement apparenté au LH-RF dan l'hypothalamus et l'éminence mediane chez les mammiferes. *C. R. Acad. Sci.* [*D*] *(Paris),* 276:2043–2048.
41. Liotta, A. S., Gildersleeve, D., Brownstein, M. J., and Krieger, D. T. (1979): Biosynthesis *in vitro* of immunoreactive 31,000-dalton corticotropin/β-endorphin-like material by bovine hypothalamus. *Proc. Natl. Acad. Sci. USA,* 76:1448–1452.
42. McCann, S. M. (1962): A hypothalamic luteinizing-hormone-releasing-factor. *Am. J. Physiol.,* 202:395–400.
43. McCann, S. M., Taleisnik, S., and Friedman, H. M. (1960): LH-releasing activity in hypothalamic extracts. *Proc. Soc. Exp. Biol. Med.,* 104:432–434.
44. Naik, D. V. (1974): Immunohistochemical and immunofluorescent localization of LH-RF neurons in the hypothalamus of rat. *Anat. Rec.,* 178:424.
45. Naik, D. V. (1975): Immunoreactive LH-RH neurons in the hypothalamus identified by light and fluorescent microscopy. *Cell Tissue Res.,* 157:423–436.
46. Naik, D. V. (1975): Immuno-electron microscopic localization of luteinizing hormone-releasing hormone in the arcuate nuclei and median eminence of the rat. *Cell Tissue Res.,* 157:437–455.
47. Oliver, C., Eskay, R. L., Ben-Jonathan, N., and Porter, J. C. (1974): Distribution and concentration of TRH in the rat brain. *Endocrinology,* 95:540–553.
48. Palkovits, M. (1973): Isolated removal of hypothalamic or other brain nuclei of the rat. *Brain Res.,* 59:449–450.
49. Palkovits, M., Arimura, A., Brownstein, M. J., Schally, A. V., and Saavedra, J. M. (1974): Luteinizing hormone-releasing hormone (LH-RH) content of the hypothalamic nuclei in rat. *Endocrinology,* 96:554–558.
50. Palkovits, M., Brownstein, M., Arimura, A., Sato, H., Schally, A. V., and Kizer, J. S. (1976): Somatostatin content of the hypothalamic ventromedial and arcuate nuclei and the circumventricular organs in the rat. *Brain Res.,* 109:430–434.
51. Pelletier, G., Labrie, F., Arimura, A., and Schally, A. V. (1974): Electron microscopic immunohistochemical localization of growth hormone-release inhibiting hormone (somatostatin) in the rat median eminence. *Am. J. Anat.,* 140:445–450.
52. Pelletier, G., Labrie, F., Puviani, R., Arimura, A., and Schally, A. V. (1974): Electron microscopic localization of luteinizing hormone-releasing hormone in rat median eminence. *Endocrinology,* 95:314–315.

53. Pelletier, G., LeClare, R., Dube, D., Labrie, F., Puviani, R., Arimura, A., and Schally, A. V. (1975): Localization of growth hormone-release inhibiting hormone (somatostatin) in the rat brain. *Am. J. Anat.,* 142:397–400.

54. Reichlin, S., Saperstein, R., Jackson, I. M. D., Boyd, III, A. E., and Patel, Y. (1976): Hypothalamic hormones. *Annu. Rev. Physiol.,* 38:389–424.

55. Russell, J., Brownstein, M. J., and Gainer, H. (1980): Biosynthesis of the common precursors of vasopressin, oxytocin, and their respective neurophysins. In: *The Role of Peptides in Neuronal Function,* edited by J. Barker and T. Smith. Marcel Dekker, New York.

56. Setalo, G. (1975): LH-RH-containing neural elements in the rat hypothalamus. *Endocrinology,* 96:135–142.

52. Setalo, G., Vigh, S., Schally, A. V., Arimura, A., and Flerko, B. (1975): LH-RH containing neural elements in the rat hypothalamus. *Endocrinology,* 96:135–142.

58. Trygstad, O. E., Foss, I., Edminson, P. D., Johansen, J. H., and Reichelt, K. L. (1978): Humoral control of appetite: A urinary anorexigenic peptide. Chromatographic patterns of urinary peptides in anorexia nervosa. *Acta Endocrinol.,* 89:196–208.

59. Vale, W., Ling, N., Rivier, C., Rivier, J., Villarreal, J., and Brown, M. (1976): Anatomic and phylogenetic distribution of somatostatin. *Metabolism,* 25:1491–1494.

60. Vale, W., Rivier, C., Palkovits, M., Saavedra, J. M., and Brownstein, M. J. (1974): Ubiquitous brain distribution of inhibitors of adenohypophyseal secretion. *Endocrinology,* 94:A128.

61. Weindl, A., Sofroniev, M. V., and Schinko, I. (1976): The distribution of vasopressin, oxytocin, neurophysin, somatostatin, and luteinizing hormone releasing hormone producing neurons, In: *Evolutionary Aspects of Neuroendocrinology,* edited by A. L. Polenov, W. Bargmann, and B. Scharrer, pp. 172–183. Springer Verlag, Heidelberg.

62. Weiner, R. I., Pattou, E., Kerdelhue, B., and Kordon, C. (1975): Differential effects of hypothalamic deafferentation upon luteinizing hormone-releasing hormone in the median eminence and organum vasculosum of the lamina terminalis. *Endocrinology,* 97:1597–1600.

63. Wheaton, J. E., Krulich, L., and McCann, S. M. (1975): Localization of luteinizing hormone-releasing hormone in the preoptic area and hypothalamus of the rat using radioimmunoassay. *Endocrinology,* 97:30–38.

64. Winokur, A., and Utiger, R. D. (1974): Thyrotropin-releasing hormone: Regional distribution in rat brain. *Science,* 185:265–267.

65. Youngblood, W. W., Lipton, M. A., and Kizer, J. S. (1978): TRH-like immunoreactivity in urine, serum, and extrahypothalamic brain: Nonidentity with synthetic pyroGlu-Hist-Pro-(NH$_2$) (TRH). *Brain Res.,* 151:99–116.

Polypeptide Hormones, edited by
R. F. Beers, Jr. and E. G. Bassett.
Raven Press, New York © 1980.

20. Studies on α-Melanotropin in the Central Nervous System

*Thomas L. O'Donohue and David M. Jacobowitz

*Laboratory of Clinical Science, National Institute of Mental Health, National Institutes of Health, Bethesda, Maryland 20205; and *Department of Pharmacology, Howard University, Washington, D.C. 20059*

INTRODUCTION

α-Melanotropin or α-melanocyte-stimulating hormone (α-MSH) was originally isolated and identified as an acetyl tridecapeptideamide originating in the intermediate lobe of the pituitary gland (19). The sole function of α-MSH was thought to be regulation of pigmentary changes, particularly in poikilotherms (54). Recently, however, extrapigmentary influences of α-MSH have been described. Among these actions are potent central nervous system (CNS) effects that include facilitated arousal, motivation, attention, memory, and learning in both laboratory animals and man (10,22,30,62). Furthermore, melanotropic bioactivity is known to be present in the vertebrate brain and cerebrospinal fluid (2,18,25,41,45–47,49,64). These findings stimulated the investigation of the role of α-MSH in CNS function. Recent studies have demonstrated an extensive system of α-MSH-containing neurons in the brain (9,11,21,34,40). The presence of α-melanotropinergic neurons in the rat brain combined with the potent CNS effects of α-MSH administration suggests a possible neurotransmitter or neuromodulator role for this peptide. The purpose of this chapter is to summarize our current knowledge of the α-melanotropinergic system and its role in the CNS.

OBSERVATIONS AND DISCUSSION

Identification and Characterization of α-MSH in the Brain and Pituitary Gland

α-MSH-like immunoreactivity was identified and characterized in rat and human brain and rat pituitary by combining high-pressure liquid chromatography (HPLC) with radioimmunoassay (RIA) (34). Antibodies to α-MSH were raised against synthetic α-MSH conjugated to bovine serum albumin via carbodimide in our laboratory and also by Drs. M. C. Tonon and H. Vaudry (Laboratoire d'Endocrinologie, Mont-Saint-Aignan, France). The specificity of the antibodies was similar, as determined by HPLC or by tests of cross-reactivity with synthetic peptides. The antibodies have little or no cross-reactivity with human, monkey, or porcine β-MSH, ovine β-lipotropin, porcine ACTH or the synthetic ACTH fragments ACTH 1–16, ACTH 1–24, ACTH 1–19, ACTH 1–10, ACTH 4–11, ACTH 17–39, ACTH 11–19, ACTH 1–13, or deamidated α-MSH. All antibodies investigated cross-reacted with NH_2-terminal deacetylated α-MSH. The α-MSH RIA procedure has been described previously (34).

The characterization of immunoreactivity in rat pituitary and rat and human brain was performed by a combination of HPLC and RIA. α-MSH-like immunoreactive material in tissues was extracted by boiling in 2 N acetic acid for 10 min. Samples were then centrifuged at 8,000 × g for 5 min and aliquots of the supernatant fluid were removed and lyophilized. Lyophilates were resuspended in 40% acetonitrile and water and chromatographed. The combination of reverse phase (μBondapak C_{18}) HPLC and RIA uncovered a heterogeneity

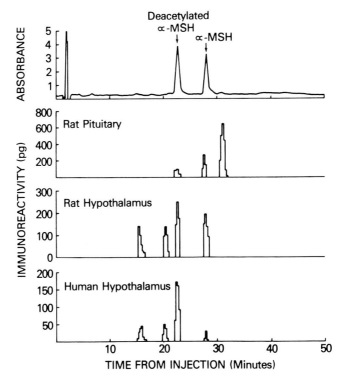

FIG. 1. High-pressure liquid chromatograms of immunoreactivity in α-MSH picogram equivalents, in extracts of rat hypothalamus, human hypothalamus, and rat pituitary. Reverse-phase chromatography was performed on a μBondapak C_{18} column. The retention times of deacetylated α-MSH and α-MSH were determined by absorbance at 254 nm **(top panel).** Fractions from tissue chromatographs were radioimmunoassayed for α-MSH. The delay time between detector and collection valve is corrected for on these plots.

of immunoreactive material in rat pituitary and human and rat hypothalamus (Fig. 1). Pituitary extracts contained three peaks of α-MSH-like immunoreactive material. The first two immunoreactive compounds, eluting at approximately 22 and 28 min, coelute precisely with standard α-MSH and deacetylated α-MSH (Peninsula Labs, California), respectively. This is consistent with the previous description of these compounds in camel pituitary (26). The identity of the third immunoreactive compound remains unknown. This peptide was present in all four pituitaries assayed, but the ratio of concentrations of immunoreactive material in peak 3 versus peak 2 (α-MSH) varied from 1:1 to 4:1. When an antibody that recognizes deacetylated α-MSH (peak 1) and α-MSH (peak 2) equally was used (Fig. 1), concentrations of α-MSH in pituitary were greater than the deacetylated α-MSH.

Human and rat hypothalamus both contain four immunoreactive compounds. Again, two peaks of immunoreactive material elute with identical retention times as standard α-MSH and deacetylated α-MSH, thus demonstrating the presence of these two peptides in rat and human brain. Whether the deacetylated compound is a precursor or metabolic product of the α-MSH remains to be determined. The first two immunoreactive peaks in rat and human hypothalamus are, as yet, unidentified but are probably closely related to α-MSH and deacetylated α-MSH in structure and function as (a) they have similar immunoreactivity, (b) similar reverse phase HPLC retention times, and (c) they are contained in the same neurons with α-MSH and deacetylated α-MSH *(see below)*.

Distribution of α-MSH in the Brain

The regional distribution of α-MSH in the rat brain was determined qualitatively by immunocytochemical techniques as well as quantitatively by a microdissection technique combined with RIA (21,34). For immunocytochemistry, the indirect procedure of Coons (8) was used with minor modifications as described previously (21). Paraformaldehyde-fixed brain sections were incubated with α-MSH antiserum (1:75 dilution) or diluted α-MSH antiserum that had been preincubated overnight with 0.1 to 1.0 μg/50 μl of standard α-MSH, monkey β-MSH, ACTH, or ACTH 1–10. Addition of 1 or 0.01 μg of α-MSH completely blocked the immunoreactivity in rat brain, while no other peptide used as a preabsorbant resulted in a decrease in immunoreactivity.

For quantitation of immunoreactivity, regions of the rat brain or cat brain were microdissected as described previously (34,38). Micropunches were delivered into 100 μl of 2 N acetic acid at 4°C. Samples were subsequently boiled for 10 min and homogenized by sonication. A 10 to 20 μl aliquot was removed for protein determination (28). Samples were then centrifuged at 8000 × g for 5 min and aliquots of supernatant were removed and lyophilized in 12 × 75 mm borosilicate glass test tubes. RIA was performed as described previously (34).

An extensive system of discrete, varicose beaded nerve fibers containing α-MSH immunoreactivity appeared to extend throughout the rat brain. Neuronal perikarya containing α-MSH-like immunoreactivity were only faintly visible in the arcuate nucleus of the hypothalamus (Fig. 2A,C) and the mitral cell layer of the olfactory bulb (Fig. 2B). Intraventricular administration of vinblastine, which destroys microtubules and therefore prevents axonal flow, causes a buildup of α-MSH in these perikarya, resulting in increased fluorescence intensity (Fig. 2A,B). Surgical formation of a hypothalamic island containing the arcuate nucleus also resulted in an increased perikaryon fluorescence intensity (Fig. 2C) and depleted extrahypothalamic α-MSH neuronal fibers.

The concentration of α-MSH in discrete brain regions is presented in Table 1. There is a good correlation between the density of immunoreactive fibers (21,34) and the concentration of α-MSH in each region. The highest concentrations of α-MSH were observed in the hypothalamic nuclei. A dense population of α-MSH-containing fibers was observed in the medial preoptic nucleus, median eminence, and the periventricular, dorsomedial (Fig. 3A), and anterior hypothalamic nuclei. Moderate concentrations and numbers of fibers were observed in the lateral preoptic, paraventricular, and posterior hypothalamic nuclei. There is, in fact, a greater than 10-fold range between the lowest and highest hypothalamic α-MSH concentrations. A 70- to 100-fold difference exists when comparing the lowest values of α-MSH in the brain with the highest values detected in the hypothalamus.

Extra-hypothalamic forebrain regions also contained significant α-MSH concentrations. In the septal region, a moderate number of α-MSH immunoreactive fibers coursed medial to the nucleus accumbens in the septohypothalamic tract and the diagonal band, and appeared to terminate in the lateral septal nucleus (Fig. 3B) and the interstitial nucleus of the stria terminalis (Fig. 3C). Numerous fibers also appeared to project from the stria terminalis to innervate the amygdala. In the thalamus, a particularly heavy distribution of α-MSH fibers and a particularly high α-MSH concentration were observed in the thalamic periventricular nucleus.

α-MSH immunoreactivity was also noted in the midbrain and hindbrain. Many α-MSH fibers were observed in the mesencephalic central gray. In the pons, moderate concentrations and numbers of fibers were observed in the dorsal lateral tegmental nucleus, dorsal parabrachial nucleus, nucleus of the tractus mesencephalicus, and the superior cerebellar peduncle. In the medulla, a moderate number of fibers were located in the nucleus of the solitary tract and only a few fibers were noted in the reticular formation. No fibers were seen in the spinal cord.

FIG. 2. A: α-MSH-containing perikaryon and axon *(arrows)* in the arcuate nucleus after intraventricular vinblastine (20 μg, 2 days); ×408. **B:** Perikarya containing α-MSH immunoreactivity in the mitral cell layer of the olfactory bulb after intraventricular vinblastine (20 μg, 2 days); ×320. **C:** α-MSH positive perikarya *(arrows)* in the arcuate nucleus of a hypothalamus island (4 days); ×280.

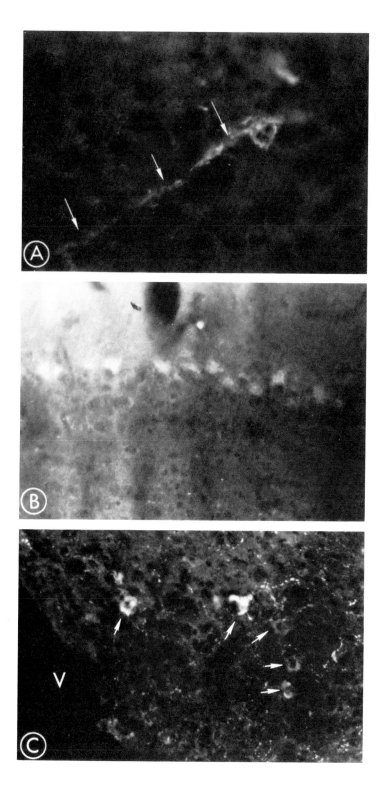

TABLE 1. Regional distribution of immunoreactive α-MSH in discrete regions of rat, cat, and human brain

Region	Rat	Cat	Subject 1	Subject 2	Subject 3
Cortex					
Pyriform cortex	0.2 ± 0.09[a]	ND[b]	—	—	—
Cingulate cortex	ND	0.17 ± 0.10	—	—	—
Hippocampus	0.25 ± 0.05	0.02 ± 0.01	ND	—	ND
Striatum					
Caudate nucleus	0.13 ± 0.03	ND	ND	—	—
Globus pallidus	0.39 ± 0.15	ND	—	—	—
Septal area					
Nucleus accumbans	0.33 ± 0.05	0.93 ± 0.35	1.46	—	—
Septum dorsalis	0.15 ± 0.07	—	—	—	—
Septum lateralis	1.29 ± 0.16	—	15.28	—	—
Interstitial nucleus of the stria terminalis, dorsal	1.43 ± 0.27	—	—	—	—
Interstitial nucleus of the stria terminalis, ventral	4.52 ± 0.41	—	—	—	—
Olfactory tubercle	0.20 ± 0.03	ND	—	—	—
Nucleus tractus diagonalis	1.04 ± 0.32	—	—	—	—
Hypothalamus and preoptic area					
Medial preoptic nucleus	3.75 ± 0.32	10.73 ± 5.69	5.51	—	0.31
Lateral preoptic nucleus	0.97 ± 0.06	0.15 ± 0.06	0	—	0.06
Suprachiasmatic nucleus	1.01 ± 0.23	27.75 ± 8.93	—	—	—
Anterior hypothalamic nucleus	3.49 ± 0.55	6.45 ± 0.54	3.75	1.61	0.36
Periventricular nucleus	7.19 ± 0.73	15.3 ± 2.95	—	—	0.09
Supraoptic nucleus	1.95 ± 0.41	1.16 ± 0.43	9.34	0.36	0.06
Paraventricular nucleus	5.75 ± 0.35	—	15.72	2.5	ND
Arcuate nucleus	8.72 ± 1.33	24.89 ± 3.65	6.97	1.63	—
Median eminence	11.02 ± 1.60	46.33 ± 8.02	16.10	2.03	0.44
Ventromedial nucleus	3.32 ± 0.63	8.72 ± 2.13	5.71	2.39	0.01
Dorsomedial nucleus	8.95 ± 0.65	—	5.95	1.7	0.006
Posterior hypothalamic nucleus	4.32 ± 0.56	0.30 ± 0.09	3.92	2.76	ND
Ansa lenticularis	3.83 ± 0.56	—	—	—	—
Medial forebrain bundle, rostral	2.34 ± 0.37	0.45 ± 0.18	—	—	—
Medial forebrain bundle, caudal	3.99 ± 0.72	—	—	—	—

Thalamus					
Anterior ventral thalamic nucleus	0.47 ± 0.18	0.16 ± 0.10	—	—	—
Ventral thalamic nucleus	0.65 ± 0.11	—	—	—	—
Rhomboid nucleus	4.56 ± 0.60	—	—	—	—
Periventricular nucleus	7.19 ± 0.73	13.34 ± 4.78	20.24	0.42	—
Parafascicular nucleus	1.34 ± 0.25	—	—	—	—
Amygdala					
Medial amygdaloid nucleus	0.90 ± 0.13	ND	ND	ND	ND
Cortical amygdaloid nucleus	1.13 ± 0.30	0.45 ± 0.28	—	—	—
Central amygdaloid nucleus	1.93 ± 0.19	0.85 ± 0.53	—	—	—
Basal amygdaloid nucleus	1.73 ± 0.16	0.51 ± 0.28	—	—	—
Midbrain					
Central gray, rostral	0.48 ± 0.09	1.17 ± 0.30	0.42	0.21	—
Central gray, caudal	3.44 ± 0.67	4.25 ± 1.56	—	—	—
Supramammilary decussation	0.36 ± 0.07	—	—	—	—
Medial geniculate body	ND	ND	—	—	—
Substantia nigra, reticular part	ND	ND	—	—	—
Superior colliculus	0.23 ± 0.10	0.01 ± 0.005	—	—	—
Inferior colliculus	0.31 ± 0.09	0.02 ± 0.01	—	—	—
Interpeduncular nucleus	0.19 ± 0.10	1.77 ± 0.92	—	—	—
Cuneiform nucleus	1.27 ± 0.26	—	—	—	—
Dorsal raphe	4.15 ± 0.87	3.48 ± 1.59	—	—	—
Medial raphe	1.96 ± 0.33	4.48 ± 2.40	—	—	—
Hindbrain					
Locus coerulus	ND	—	—	—	—
Lateral dorsal tegmental nucleus	1.49 ± 0.27	—	—	—	—
Nucleus tractus solitarus	1.07 ± 0.27	—	—	—	—
Pineal gland	2.40 ± 0.24	—	—	—	—

[a] Values in pg/μg protein ± SE.
[b] Not determined.

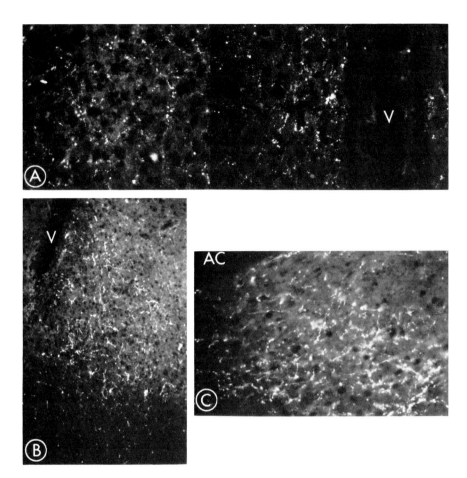

FIG. 3. α-MSH immunoreactive varicose fibers in **A:** dorsomedial nucleus along the third ventricle (V), ×211; **B:** septal area medial to the lateral ventricle (V), ×89; and **C:** interstitial nucleus of the stria terminalis ventral to the anterior commissure (AC); ×254.

Immunocytochemical α-MSH distribution studies of rat brain by Dube et al. (11) in general show good agreement with the results described here with the exception that they did not report α-MSH positive olfactory bulb perikarya. In contrast, Swaab and Fisser (51) have reported the presence of an α-MSH-like immunoreactive peptide with a distribution distinctly different from the results reported here or by Dube et al. In this regard, it is interesting to note that Loh and Gainer (27) have described the presence of MSH-like bioactivity in rat brain that is distinct from α-MSH. It is therefore possible that there is another neural system in brain that contains a peptide similar to, but not identical with, α-MSH. α-MSH was present in human brain, which is consistent with recent reports of Parker and Porter (39) and Désy and Pelletier (9).

The regional distribution of α-MSH immunoreactivity in the cat (33) and human brain was also determined by combining the micropunch technique with RIA. The qualitative, and to some extent, the quantitative distribution of the neurohormone is similar in the three species studied. Immunoreactivity has also been identified in the frog brain (56). In general, α-MSH concentrations in the cat hypothalamic nuclei seem to be somewhat greater than in the rat. Concentrations in the suprachiasmatic nucleus, however, were much higher in the cat than in the rat.

The postmortem human specimens were obtained from subject 1 (25-year-old female, cause of death—cystic fibrosis, specimens obtained 15 hr postmortem), subject 2 (33-year-old male, melanoma, 14 hr), and subject 3 (62-year-old female, cardiopulmonary arrest and adrenocarcinoma of the pancreas, 9 hr postmortem). The distribution of α-MSH in these three human brains was qualitatively similar but quantitatively different, with concentrations in subject 1 generally being greater than in subject 2, which were greater than in subject 3. The correlation of age at the time of death and brain α-MSH concentrations is currently being investigated.

Source of α-Melanocyte-Stimulating Hormone in the Brain

Two likely sources of α-MSH in the brain are the pituitary, which contains over 99% of the α-MSH in the body (57), or the numerous α-MSH-containing perikarya of the arcuate nucleus in the hypothalamus. To determine which group contributed the brain α-MSH, concentrations of α-MSH in brain were determined after hypophysectomy and after lesion of the arcuate nucleus.

The effect of hypophysectomy on both the numbers of α-MSH nerves and the concentration of α-MSH in discrete regions of the brain was investigated. Using an immunocytochemical approach, no decrease in the number of α-MSH-containing nerves was observed at 2 weeks after hypophysectomy (34). With extended periods of time, however, decreased concentrations of α-MSH are found in α-MSH terminal regions but not in the cell body region, the arcuate nucleus (32), as shown in Table 2. These data indicate that brain α-MSH is not derived from the pituitary gland but is related to pituitary function and are consistent with the findings of Oliver and Porter (37) and Vaudry et al. (57).

An arcuate nucleus origin for α-MSH nerves in brain was investigated with both radiofrequency lesions of the arcuate nucleus and hypothalamic islands containing the arcuate nucleus. Hypothalamic islands contain arcuate nuclei perikarya with increased fluorescence intensity (Fig. 2C), indicating disruption of extra-hypothalamic α-MSH afferents emanating from these cell bodies. After arcuate nucleus lesions, all major α-MSH terminal regions were markedly depleted compared to control animals (Table 3). The arcuate nucleus therefore appears to be the major source of α-MSH in the brain. These results have recently been confirmed by Eskay et al., using hypothalamic islands (14) and

TABLE 2. α-MSH concentrations in discrete brain regions of sham operated and hypophysectomized rats[a]

	Sham operated	Hypophysectomized		
Area		2 Weeks	3 Weeks	4 Weeks
α-MSH terminal regions				
Nucleus interstitialis stria	9.86 ± 3.97[b]	7.80 ± 1.62 (−21)[c]	4.0 ± 2.67 (−59)	3.33 ± 0.86[d] (−66)
Medial preoptic nucleus	10.00 ± 2.40	6.67 ± 1.64 (−33)	7.67 ± 2.78 (−23)	4.90 ± 0.96[d] (−51)
Anterior hypothalamic nucleus	9.00 ± 1.59	6.63 ± 1.14 (−30)	7.25 ± 1.86 (−19)	4.50 ± 0.90[d] (−50)
Paraventricular nucleus	11.56 ± 3.34	6.67 ± 1.28[d] (−42)	7.75 ± 4.38 (−32)	3.56 ± 1.00[e] (−69)
Paraventricular nucleus (thalamus)	13.30 ± 1.69	6.87 ± 0.73[d] (−48)	10.25 ± 3.55 (−21)	4.89 ± 0.87[e] (−63)
Median eminence	11.67 ± 2.74	11.25 ± 2.51 (−4)	10.50 ± 2.50 (−10)	6.63 ± 1.85 (−43)
Dorsomedial nucleus	8.56 ± 2.56	6.80 ± 1.53 (−20)	8.00 ± 2.02 (−7)	4.90 ± 1.75 (−42)
Amygdala	5.11 ± 0.32	5.00 ± 1.03 (−2)	4.50 ± 2.40 (−11)	3.13 ± 1.10 (−38)
α-MSH perikarya region				
Arcuate nucleus	13.38 ± 4.21	12.13 ± 4.86 (−9)	13.00 ± 4.95 (−3)	13.36 ± 2.75 (0)

[a] Number of samples: sham operated, 7–10; treatment, 2 weeks, 5–9; 3 weeks, 3–4; 4 weeks, 8–11.
[b] pg/μg protein ± SE.
[c] Parenthetic values indicate percent change from sham operated.
[d] $p < 0.05$.
[e] $p < 0.01$.

TABLE 3. Effects of arcuate lesions on the regional distribution of α-MSH

	α-MSH level[a]	
Region	Control	Lesion
Lateral septum	1.20 ± 0.30	0.16 ± 0.16[b]
Nucleus tractus diagonalis	0.76 ± 0.13	0.09 ± 0.09[b]
Interstitial nucleus of stria terminalis, dorsal and ventral	1.86 ± 0.25	0.15 ± 0.15[b]
Medial preoptic nucleus	4.17 ± 0.50	ND
Hypothalamic periventricular nucleus	7.23 ± 0.49	0.25 ± 0.25[b]
Thalamic periventricular nucleus	6.98 ± 0.75	0.17 ± 0.17[b]
Anterior hypothalamic nucleus	4.65 ± 0.75	0.27 ± 0.27[b]
Paraventricular nucleus	4.93 ± 0.35	ND
Amygdala	3.55 ± 0.53	0.03 ± 0.03[b]
Central gray (caudal)	3.44 ± 0.67	0.40 ± 0.18[b]
Pineal gland	0.58 ± 0.23	0.37 ± 0.08

[a] Values in pg/μg protein ± SE.
[b] $p < 0.01$ versus control and not significantly different from 0.0 pg α-MSH.

lesions of the arcuate nucleus region neonatally produced by the neurotoxin, monosodium glutamate (13). Consistent with the demonstration of α-MSH-containing perikarya in the mitral cells of the olfactory bulb (Fig. 2A), no decrease in the α-MSH content of the olfactory bulb was found. Whether the olfactory bulb projects α-MSH afferents into the brain is unknown at the present time.

Recent results by J. F. McKelvy and D. T. Krieger *(personal communication)* support the concept of biosynthesis of α-MSH in rat hypothalamic tissue, as tritiated amino acids can be incorporated into hypothalamic α-MSH *in vitro.* This is also likely to be the case in human brain, as Désy and Pelletier (9) have identified α-MSH-containing perikarya in the arcuate nucleus of human postmortem tissue. Furthermore, Bloch et al. (6) have shown that the cells of the human arcuate nucleus (or infundibular nucleus) contain not only α-MSH, but also β-MSH, α-endorphin, β-endorphin, ACTH 17–39, ACTH 1–24, and β-LPH. These data suggest that the brain may synthesize α-MSH and related peptides from a pro-opiocortin-like precursor, as has been demonstrated in pituitary.

Identification, Quantitation, and Characterization of α-MSH-Like Compounds in Rat and Human Cerebrospinal Fluid

Rat ventricular cerebrospinal fluid (CSF) and human lumbar CSF were collected for measurement of α-MSH. Rat ventricular CSF was obtained by cannulating the lateral ventricle of chloralose-urethane anesthetized rats and perfusing the ventricular system with artificial CSF. The perfusate was drained and collected from the cisterna magna at 20-min intervals. Human lumbar tap CSF was collected from a random group of patients at the National Institutes of

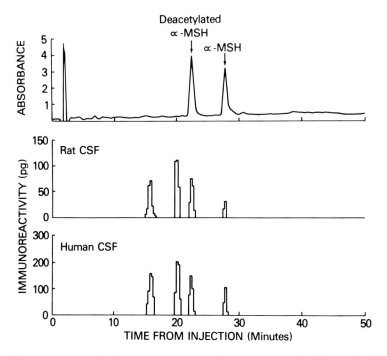

FIG. 4. High-pressure liquid chromatograms of standard deacetylated α-MSH and α-MSH and α-MSH-like immunoreactivity in human and rat cerebrospinal fluid.

Health. CSF was then lyophylized and radioimmunoassayed for α-MSH-like material either directly or after fractionation by HPLC.

Chromatographs of immunoreactive material in rat and human CSF are shown in Fig. 4. Both rat and human CSF contain four peaks of immunoreactive material. The retention times of these four peaks are identical to the four compounds in rat and human brain. Again, peak 3 and peak 4 have identical retention times as standard deacetylated α-MSH and α-MSH, respectively. Furthermore, in CSF of both rat and man, the relative heights of the four peaks of immunoreactive material are nearly identical. In both cases, peak 3, deacetylated α-MSH, is greater in magnitude than peak 4, α-MSH. The concentrations of peak 1 and peak 2, the unknowns, are greater than of peak 3 or peak 4. It is also possible that these peaks could have less affinity for the α-MSH antibody and may therefore be in much higher concentrations than deacetylated α-MSH or α-MSH. Concentrations of immunoreactive α-MSH in human lumbar tap CSF of 23 patients ranged from 4.0 to 73.3 pg/ml, with a mean of 22.9 pg/ml.

In an attempt to measure the *in vivo* release of α-MSH into the CSF, rat ventricular CSF was collected at intervals over 5 hr. Approximately 180 pg of α-MSH-like immunoreactivity per 20-min intervals was detected. As rats hypophysectomized for 2 to 3 weeks had CSF α-MSH concentrations similar to controls, immunoreactivity in rat ventricular CSF may represent neural release of α-MSH-like compounds. A further indication of a neural source of CSF α-MSH is that the four immunoreactive CSF peaks are identical to those in brain but not in pituitary.

In Vitro Release of α-MSH from Hypothalamus

An *in vitro* model for studying α-MSH release has been developed (20). In brief, approximately 225-μm slices of rat hypothalamus are resuspended in a modified Krebs-bicarbonate buffer maintained at pH 7.4 to 7.6. Samples are briefly centrifuged and the supernatant is removed and analyzed for α-MSH by RIA. Slices are resuspended in buffer and the process is repeated at 2-min intervals. Different ions or stimuli can be tested by adding these compounds to subsequent buffer changes.

As shown in Fig. 5, stimulation with 50 mM potassium results in a marked increase (250%) in α-MSH release from the slices. Potassium stimulation in the absence of calcium, with 1mM EDTA, also resulted in α-MSH release but was significantly attenuated compared to potassium stimulation in the presence of 5 mM Ca^{2+}. Veratridine (100 μM), a depolarizing agent, also markedly stimulated α-MSH release (380%). Once again, this release was significantly depressed in the absence of Ca^{2+}, demonstrating a calcium-dependent α-MSH

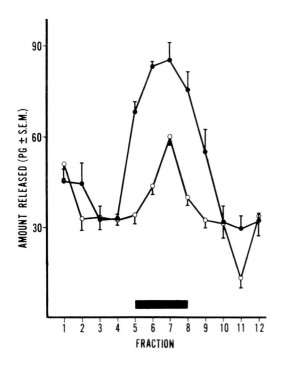

FIG. 5. Potassium-stimulated *(black horizontal bar)* release of α-MSH immunoreactivity for an hypothalamic slices in the presence *(filled circles)* and absence *(open circles)* of calcium.

release from neurons in the rat hypothalamus. Furthermore, it has been demonstrated that α-MSH immunoreactivity is located in and released from synaptic vesicles of nerve endings (3,4,58). These studies provide further evidence for a neurotransmitter or neuromodulator role for α-MSH in brain.

Circadian Rhythms of α-MSH in Rat Brain and Pineal Gland

In the first study of the physiological role of α-MSH in brain function, the presence of a diurnal variation in α-MSH concentrations in the brain and pineal gland was investigated (35,36). A diurnal variation in brain and pineal concentrations of α-MSH seemed likely as

(a) A role in attention and arousal processes has been suggested for α-MSH (10,22,62).

(b) An interaction with melatonin, a pineal hormone demonstrating a circadian variation, via a pineal-hypothalamic-pituitary loop has been suggested (23,24).

(c) There is a diurnal secretion of MSH from the pituitary gland (12,53,55).

As shown in Fig. 6, there is a significant diurnal variation of α-MSH concentration in the pineal gland and in all brain regions studied (35,36). In all cases, highest α-MSH concentrations occurred during the day and lowest levels occurred at night. In the brain, a temporal-spatial relationship seems to exist between the time of peak a-MSH concentrations in each region and the proximity of the region to the arcuate nucleus, the source of α-MSH in the brain. The arcuate nucleus and adjacent regions, the median eminence and dorsomedial nucleus, all have peaks in α-MSH concentration at 0900 hr. Regions within 1 to 2 mm of the center of the arcuate, the paraventricular and anterior hypothalamic nuclei, peak in concentrations 4 hr later, at 1300. At 1700, 8 hr after the initial peak in the arcuate nucleus, the α-MSH fibers in the medial preoptic nucleus (which are located 2 to 3 mm from their perikarya in the arcuate) reach peak α-MSH concentrations. However, the thalamic periventricular nucleus, located furthest from the arcuate nucleus, peaks in α-MSH concentrations at 0900, the same time as the arcuate nucleus. The distance between the arcuate and the periventricular nuclei may be 6 to 8 mm if fibers pass rostrally from the arcuate to the preoptic area, where they ascend along the third ventricle and pass caudally into the thalamic periventricular nucleus, as suggested by immunocytochemical studies (21). Perhaps this paradox could be explained if the α-MSH peak in the periventricular nucleus occurs 24 hr after the initial peak α-MSH concentration in the arcuate nucleus. As there is no evidence for protein synthesis outside of neuronal perikarya (5), it is significant that the arcuate nucleus achieves peak α-MSH concentrations first, since other brain regions must derive their α-MSH from the arcuate nucleus by axonal flow. Another likely possibility is that α-MSH is transported primarily in precursor form. This suggestion would be consistent with the observation that arcuate perikarya normally show only faint immunocytochemical fluorescence. Furthermore, the arcuate nucleus perikarya also contain corticotropin, β-endorphin, β-MSH, and β-lipotropin. Because these peptides are probably derived from a common precursor containing α-MSH in brain [as occurs in pituitary (29,31, 43,44)], all these related peptides may show diurnal variations. The rhythm of α-MSH and perhaps these peptides may play a role in modulating arousal processes of the CNS.

The pineal gland α-MSH rhythm is similar to the rhythm in brain regarding

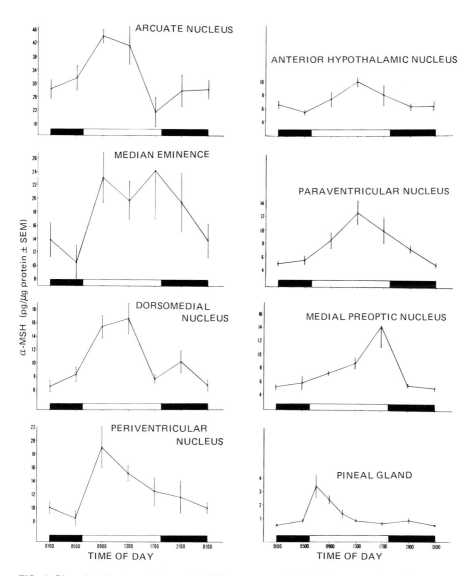

FIG. 6. Diurnal rhythmic variation of α-MSH immunoreactivity in discrete regions of rat brain and pineal gland. Male rats were housed in a colony room with a 12:2 light-to-dark schedule.

the times of peak and nadir. The likely sources of pineal α-MSH are the pituitary, the arcuate nucleus (reaching the pineal by cerebroventricular flow), or the pineal itself. Interestingly, lesion of the arcuate nucleus, which markedly depletes brain α-MSH, fails to affect concentrations of pineal α-MSH (35) (Table 3). Furthermore, there is still a rhythm of α-MSH in the pineal after hypophysectomy (35). These data suggest that the pineal may synthesize α-MSH, but this possibility must be further investigated.

The pineal α-MSH rhythm may be related to the pineal rhythm of melatonin. The peak pineal concentration of these two hormones are approximately 180 degrees out-of-phase as melatonin concentrations increase after the lights are turned off. Furthermore, chronic light has similar effects on the pineal melatonin (42) and α-MSH rhythm. In rats housed in chronic light for 7 days, the α-MSH rhythm was significantly suppressed. In contrast, animals maintained in chronic dark for 7 days maintained an α-MSH rhythm, but the time of the peak was shifted and increased in amplitude (35). A major difference between the regulating mechanisms of the pineal α-MSH and melatonin rhythms can be deduced from the differential effects of superior cervical ganglionectomy (35). The α-MSH rhythm in ganglionectomized rats is unchanged, whereas sympathectomy completely abolishes the circadian variations of melatonin and serotonin-N-acetyltransferase, a melatonin biosynthetic enzyme (42).

The role of the pineal α-MSH rhythm is yet to be determined. One possibility is that the rhythm of α-MSH modulates the pineal indoleamine rhythm. In the dark, sympathetic norepinephrine is released at a high rate and stimulates, via cyclic AMP formation, the biosynthetic processes that lead to the formation of melatonin (1,2). The early morning peak of α-MSH occurs at exactly the same time the presence of light is inhibiting sympathetic norepinephrine release, cyclic AMP formation, and melatonin biosynthesis. The reciprocal relationship between the increasing α-MSH concentrations and the decreasing melatonin concentrations at this time may reflect an antagonistic relationship between the hormones. This suggestion is supported by the findings that α-MSH inhibits both noradrenergic depolarization of pineal cells and noradrenergic stimulation of cyclic AMP formation (48). In this manner, α-MSH could inhibit noradrenergic stimulation of the pineal cells and help "turn off" melatonin biosynthesis. The physiological significance of this effect requires further investigation, however, as α-MSH has no effect on noradrenergic stimulation of N-acetyl transferase activity (O'Donohue, Klein, Weller, and Jacobowitz, *unpublished observations*).

SUMMARY AND PERSPECTIVES

An extensive neuronal system containing α-MSH and deacetylated α-MSH emanates from perikarya of the arcuate nucleus to innervate diverse regions of the brain. These neurons release α-MSH, deacetylated α-MSH, and related compounds in a calcium-dependent manner *in vitro* and probably *in vivo,* as these compounds are also detected in human and rat CSF. The brain α-MSH neuronal system is anatomically distinct and, probably chemically independent from the pituitary, since the hypothalamus and pituitary contain different immunoreactive compounds. Certain chemical similarities between biosynthesis of α-MSH in brain and pituitary, however, appear evident. In the pituitary, α-MSH is believed to be derived from a precursor that contains not only α-MSH, but also β-MSH, ACTH, β-liprotropin, endorphin, and enkephalin (29,31,43,44). In the pituitary, as well as in brain, a parallel anatomical distribution of α-MSH, β-endorphin, ACTH, and β-lipotropin has been noted (7,21,34,59,60,63). Furthermore, Bloch et al. (6) have recently localized the MSH, ACTH, and opiate peptides in the same neuronal perikarya of the arcuate nucleus. The role of these neurons containing multiple neuroactive compounds remains conjectural at this time.

Behavioral studies suggest that α-MSH and closely related structural peptides play a role in CNS mediation of attention and arousal processes (10,22,62). It is interesting to speculate that diurnal variations of α-MSH-like compounds may play a role in these processes. Another behavioral effect of α-MSH administration is the induction of grooming and a stretch-yawn syndrome (15). Structure activity studies have shown that the *N*-terminally acetylated serine of α-MSH is important for elicitation of these behaviors (17). As α-MSH and ACTH-like peptides are contained in the same neurons with endorphin peptides, it may be significant that deacetylated α-MSH and ACTH peptides also have affinity for the opiate receptor and antagonize morphine analgesia (16,52,61). In contrast with effects on grooming and the stretch-yawn syndrome, the *N*-acetylation of serine to form α-MSH markedly decreases affinity for the opiate receptor (52). These data suggest the possibility that both acetylated and deacetylated α-MSH may play neurotransmitter or neuromodulatory roles. The presence of both peptides in rat and human brain and CSF support such a hypothesis. Similarly, β-endorphin has recently been shown to exist in deacetylated and acetylated forms in brain and the acetylated form is completely inactive in opiate receptor binding or in providing analgesia (50). The intraneuronal interrelationships of acetylated and deacetylated forms of α-MSH and their relationship to other MSH, ACTH, and opioid peptides could provide the basis of a sensitive interneuronal modulatory system. Further evidence will be required to support or refute such a hypothesis.

ACKNOWLEDGMENTS

We would like to thank Ms. Judy G. Blumenthal and Ms. Doreen E. White for their expert editorial and secretarial aid. T. L. O'Donohue was supported by National Institute of General Medical Studies grant No. 5-702-GM05001.

REFERENCES

1. Axelrod, J. (1974): The pineal gland: A neurochemical transducer. *Science,* 184:1341–1348.
2. Baker, B. J. (1973): The separation of different forms of melanocyte-stimulating hormone from the rat neurointermediate lobe by polyacrylamide gel electrophoresis, with a note on rat neurophysins. *J. Endocrinol.,* 57:393–404.
3. Barnea, A., Neaves, W. B., Cho, G., and Porter, J. C. (1978): A subcellular pool of hypoosmotically resistant particles containing thyrotropin releasing hormone, α-melanocyte stimulating hormone, and luteinizing hormone releasing hormone in the rat hypothalamus. *J. Neurochem.,* 30:937–948.
4. Barnea, A., Oliver, C., and Porter, J. C. (1977): Subcellular localization of α-melanocyte stimulating hormone in the rat hypothalamus. *J. Neurochem.,* 29:619–624.
5. Barondes, S. H. (1974): Synaptic macromolecules: Identification and metabolism. *Annu. Rev. Biochem.,* 43:147–168.
6. Bloch, B., Bugnon, C., Fellman, D., and Unys, D. (1978): Immunocytochemical evidence that the same neurons in the human infundibular nucleus are stained with anti-endorphins and antisera of other related peptides. *Neuroscience Lett.,* 10:147–152.
7. Bloom, F., Battenberg, E., Rossier, J., Ling, N., and Guilleman, R. (1978): Neurons containing β-endorphin in rat brain exist separately from those containing enkephalin: Immunocytochemical studies. *Proc. Natl. Acad. Sci. USA,* 75:1591–1595.
8. Coons, A. H. (1958): Fluorescent antibody methods. In: *General Cytochemical Methods,* edited by J. F. Danielli, pp. 399–422. Academic Press, New York.
9. Désy, L., and Pelletier, G. (1978): Immunohistochemical localization of alphamelanocyte stimulating hormone (α-MSH) in the human hypothalamus. *Brain Res.,* 154:377–381.
10. de Wied, D. (1971): Pituitary control of avoidance behavior. In: *The Hypothalamus,* edited by L. Martini, M. Motta, and F. Fraschini, pp. 1–8. Academic Press, New York.
11. Dube, D., Lissitzky, J. C., Leclerc, R., and Pelletier, G. (1978): Localization of α-melanocyte stimulating hormone in rat brain and pituitary. *Endocrinology,* 102:1283–1291.
12. Dunn, J. D., Kastin, A. J., and Carrillo, A. J. (1976): Circadian variation in plasma melanocyte stimulating hormone activity in the rat. *Int. J. Chronobiol.,* 4:163–169.
13. Eskay, R. L., Brownstein, M. J., and Long, R. T. (1979): Reduction of α-MSH levels in the adult rat brain following monosodium glutamate treatment of neonatal animals. *Science,* 205:827–829.
14. Eskay, R. L., Giraud, P., Oliver, C., and Brownstein, M. J. (1979): Distribution of α-melanocyte stimulating hormone in the rat brain: Evidence that α-MSH-containing cells in the arcuate region send projections to extra-hypothalamic areas. *Brain Res.,* 178:55–67.
15. Ferrari, W., Gessa, G. L., and Uorgiu, L. (1963): Behavioral effects induced by intracisternally injected ACTH and MSH. *Ann. N.Y. Acad. Sci.,* 104:330–345.
16. Gispen, W. H., Buitelaar, J., Wiegart, V. N., Terenius, L., and de Wied, D. (1976): Interaction between ACTH fragments, brain opiate receptors and morphine-induced analgesia. *Eur. J. Pharmacol.,* 39:393–397.
17. Gispen, W. H., Wiegart, V. N., Averae, H. N., and de Wied, D. (1975): The induction of excessive grooming in the rat by intraventricular application of peptides derived from ACTH: Structure activity studies. *Life Sci.,* 17:645–652.
18. Guillemin, R., Schally, A. V., Lipscomb, H. S., Andersen, R. N., and Long, J. M. (1962): On the presence in hog hypothalamus of β-corticotrophin-releasing factor and α- and β-melanocyte-stimulating hormones, adrenocorticotropin, lysine vasopressin, and oxytocin. *Endocrinology,* 70:471–477.
19. Harris, J. I., and Lerner, A. B. (1957): Amino-acid sequence of the α-melanocyte-stimulating hormone. *Nature,* 179:1346–1347.
20. Holmquist, G. E., O'Donohue, T. L., Thoa, N. B., Moody, T. W., and Jacobowitz, D. M. (1980): Release of α-melanotropin (α-MSH) from hypothalamic slices *in vitro. Neuroscience Abstr. (in press).*
21. Jacobowitz, D. M., and O'Donohue, T. L. (1978): α-Melanocyte stimulating hormone: Immunocytochemical identification and mapping in neurons of the rat brain. *Proc. Natl. Acad. Sci. USA,* 75:6300–6304.
22. Kastin, A. J., Plotnikoff, N. P., Schally, A. V., and Sandman, C. A. (1976): Endocrine and

CNS effects of hypothalamic peptides and MSH. In: *Reviews of Neuroscience, Vol. 2,* edited by S. Ehrenpreis and I. J. Kopin, pp. 111–148. Raven Press, New York.

23. Kastin, A. J., and Schally, A. V. (1967): Autoregulation of release of melanocyte stimulating hormone from the rat pituitary. *Nature,* 213:1238–1240.

24. Kastin, A. J., Viosca, S., Nair, R. M. G., Schally, A. V., and Miller, M. C. (1973): Interactions between pineal, hypothalamus and pituitary involving melatonin, MSH release-inhibiting factor and MSH. *Endocrinology,* 91:1323–1328.

25. Lewis, D., Lee, F. C., and Astwood, E. B. (1937): Some observations on intermedin. *Bull. Johns Hopkins Hosp.,* 61:198–209.

26. Li, C. H., Danho, W. O., Chung, D., and Rao, A. J. (1975): Isolation, characterization, and amino acid sequence of melanotropins from camel pituitary glands. *Biochemistry,* 14:947–952.

27. Loh, Y. P., and Gainer, H. (1977): Heterogeneity of melanotropic peptides in the pars intermedia and brain. *Brain Res.,* 130:169–175.

28. Lowry, O., Rosebrough, M., Farr, A., and Randall, R. (1951): Protein measurement with the Folin phenol reagent. *J. Biol. Chem.,* 193:265–275.

29. Mains, R. E., Eipper, B. A., and Ling, N. (1977): Common precursor to corticotropins and endorphins. *Proc. Natl. Acad. Sci. USA,* 74:3014–3018.

30. Miller, L. H., Kastin, A. J., and Sandman, C. A. (1977): Psychobiological actions of MSH in man. *Front. Horm. Res.,* 4:153–161.

31. Nakanishi, S., Inoue, A., Kita, T., Nakamura, M., Chang, A. C. Y., Cohen, S. N., and Numa, S. (1979): Nucleotide sequence of cloned cDNA for bovine corticotropin-β-lipotropin precursor. *Nature,* 278:423–427.

32. O'Donohue, T. L., Holmquist, G. E., and Jacobowitz, D. M. (1980): Effects of hypophysectomy on α-melanocyte stimulating hormone in discrete regions of the rat brain. *Neuroscience Lett.,* 14:271–274.

33. O'Donohue, T. L., Massari, V. J., Tizabi, Y., and Jacobowitz, D. M. (1979): Identification and distribution of α-melanotropin in the cat brain. *Brain Res. Bull.,* 4:829–832.

34. O'Donohue, T. L., Miller, R. L., and Jacobowitz, D. M. (1979): Identification, characterization, and stereotaxic mapping of intraneuronal α-melanocyte stimulating hormone-like immunoreactive peptides in discrete regions of the rat brain. *Brain Res.,* 186:145–155.

35. O'Donohue, T. L., Miller, R. L., Pendleton, R. C., and Jacobowitz, D. M. (1980): Demonstration of an endogenous circadian rhythm of α-melanocyte stimulating hormone in the rat pineal gland. *Brain Res. (in press).*

36. O'Donohue, T. L., Miller, R. L., Pendleton, R. C., and Jacobowitz, D. M. (1980): A diurnal rhythm of immunoreactive α-melanocyte stimulating hormone is discrete regions of the rat brain. *Neuroendocrinology,* 29:281–287.

37. Oliver, C., and Porter, J. C. (1978): Distribution and characterization of α-melanocyte-stimulating hormone in the rat brain. *Endocrinology,* 102:697–705.

38. Palkovits, M. (1975): Isolated removal of hypothalamic nuclei for neuroendocrinological and neurochemical studies. In: *Anatomical Neuroendocrinology,* edited by W. E. Stumpf and L. D. Grant, pp. 72–80. Karger, Basel.

39. Parker, C. R., and Porter, J. C. (1979): Regional and subcellular localization of α-MSH-like immunoreactive substances in adult human brain. *Fed. Proc.,* 38:1130 (Abstr. 4769).

40. Pelletier, G., and Dube, D. (1977): Electron microscopic immunohistochemical localization of α-MSH in the rat brain. *Am. J. Anat.,* 150:201–205.

41. Preslock, J. P., and Brinkley, H. J. (1979): Melanophore and adrenocortical stimulating activities of substances from the pars intermedia, pars distalis, hypothalamus and cerebral cortex of the frog, *Rana pipiens. Life Sci.,* 9:1369–1380.

42. Quay, W. B. (1974): *Pineal Chemistry in Cellular and Physiological Mechanisms.* Charles C Thomas, Springfield, Illinois.

43. Roberts, J. L., and Herbert, E. (1977): Characterization of a common precursor to corticotropin and β-lipotropin: Cell-free synthesis of the precursor and identification of corticotropin peptides in the molecule. *Proc. Natl. Acad. Sci. USA,* 74:4826–4830.

44. Roberts, J. L., and Herbert, E. (1977): Characterization of a common precursor to corticotropin and β-lipotropin: Identification of β-lipotropin peptides and their arrangement relative to corticotropin in the precursor synthesized in a cell-free system. *Proc. Natl. Acad. Sci. USA,* 74:5300–5304.

45. Rudman, D., Del Rio, A. E., Hollins, B., and Houser, D. H. (1971): Observations on lipolytic and melanotropic activities of the pineal gland. *J. Biol. Chem.*, 246:324–330.

46. Rudman, D., Del Rio, A. E., Hollins, B. M., Houser, D. H., Keeling, M. E., Sutin, J., Scott, J. W., Sears, R. A., and Rosenberg, M. Z. (1973): Melanotropic-lipolytic peptides in various regions of bovine, simian and human brains and in simian and human cerebrospinal fluid. *Endocrinology*, 92:372–379.

47. Rudman, D., Scott, J. W., Del Rio, A. E., Houser, D. H., and Shenn, S. (1974): Melanotropic activity in regions of rodent brain. *Am. J. Physiol.*, 226:682–686.

48. Sakai, K. K., Schneider, D., Felt, B., and Marks, B. H. (1976): The effect of α-MSH on β-adrenergic receptor mechanisms in the rat pineal. *Life Sci.*, 19:1145–1150.

49. Scott, A. P., Lowry, P. J., Ratcliffe, J. G., Rees, L. H., and Landon, J. (1974): Corticotrophin-like peptides in the rat pituitary. *J. Endocrinol.*, 61:355–367.

50. Smyth, D. G., and Zakarian, S. (1979): Isolation and characterization of endogenous [α]-N-acyl derivatives of the C and C' fragments of lipotropin. In: *Endorphins in Mental Health Research*, edited by E. Usdin, W. E. Bunney, and N. S. Kline, pp. 84–92. MacMillan Press, London.

51. Swaab, D. F., and Fisser, B. (1977): Immunocytochemical localization of α-melanocyte stimulating hormone (α-MSH)-like compounds in the rat nervous system. *Neuroscience Lett.*, 7:313–317.

52. Terenius, L., Gispen, W. H., and DeWeid, D. (1975): ACTH-like peptides and opiate receptors in the rat brain: Structure-activity studies. *Eur. J. Pharmacol.*, 33:395–399.

53. Tilders, F. J. H., and Smelik, P. G. (1975): A diurnal rhythm in melanocyte-stimulating hormone content of the rat pituitary gland and its independence from the pineal gland. *Neuroendocrinology*, 17:296–308.

54. Turner, C. D., and Bagnara, J. T. (1971): *General Endocrinology*, Saunders, Philadelphia.

55. Usategui, R., Oliver, C., Vaudry, H., Lombardi, G., Rozenberg, I., and Mourre, A. M. (1976): Immunoreactive α-MSH and ACTH levels in rat plasma and pituitary. *Endocrinology*, 98:189–196.

56. Vaudry, H., Oliver, C., Jegou, S., Leboulenger, F., Tonon, M. C., Delarve, C., Morin, J. P., and Vaillant, R. (1978): Immunoreactive melanocyte-stimulating hormone (α-MSH) in the brain of the frog (*Rana esculenta* L.). *Gen. Comp. Endocrinol.*, 34:391–401.

57. Vaudry, H., Tonon, M. C., Delarve, R., Vaillaint, R., and Kraicer, J. (1978): Biological and radioimmunological evidence for melanocyte stimulating hormones (MSH) of extrapituitary origin in the rat brain. *Neuroendocrinology*, 27:9–24.

58. Warberg, J., Oliver, C., Eskay, R. L., Parker, C. R., Barnea, A., and Porter, J. C. (1977): Release of α-MSH from a synaptosome-enriched fraction prepared from rat hypothalamic tissue. *Front. Horm. Res.*, 4:167–169.

59. Watson, S. J., Barchas, J. D., and Li, C. H. (1977): β-Lipotropin: Localization of cells and axons in rat brain by immunocytochemistry. *Proc. Natl. Acad. Sci. USA*, 74:5155–5158.

60. Watson, S. J., Richard, C. W., and Barchas, J. D. (1978): Adrenocorticotropin in rat brain: Immunocytochemical localization in cells and axons. *Science*, 200:1180–1182.

61. Wiegart, V. M., Gispen, W. H., Terenius, L., and de Wied, D. (1977): ACTH-like peptides and morphine: Interaction at the level of the CNS. *Psychoneuroendocrinology*, 2:63–69.

62. Wimersma Greidanus, T. B. van (1977): Effects of MSH and related peptides on avoidance behavior in rats. *Front. Horm. Res.*, 4:129–139.

63. Zimmerman, E. A., Liotta, A., and Krieger, D. T. (1978): β-Lipotropin in brain: Localization in hypothalamic neurons by immunoperoxidase technique. *Cell Tissue Res.*, 186:393–398.

64. Zondek, B., and Krohn, H. (1932): Hormon des Zwischenloppens der Hypophyse (Intermedin). II. Intermedin im Organismus (Hypophyse, Gehirn). *Klin. Wochenschr.*, 11:849–853.

Polypeptide Hormones, edited by
R. F. Beers, Jr. and E. G. Bassett.
Raven Press, New York © 1980.

21. Hypothalamic Peptides Affect Behavior after Systemic Injection

Abba J. Kastin, James E. Zadina, David H. Coy,
Andrew V. Schally, and Curt A. Sandman

*Veterans Administration Medical Center and Tulane University School of Medicine,
New Orleans, Louisiana 70146*

INTRODUCTION

In the last few years, our concept of multiple independent actions of brain peptides has received additional attention due to work with the opiate peptides (45). Originally described in 1971 as a dissociation of the endocrine from the "extra-endocrine" effects of the hypothalamic peptides (75), the concept was extended in 1976 to include the separation of behavioral from analgesic effects of the enkephalins (56). Earlier work (52) on the distinction between the pigmentary and "extra-pigmentary" effects of melanocyte-stimulating hormone (MSH) also contributed to the formation of this concept; however, in retrospect this concept may have its origins in the series of neuroendocrine studies we began reporting in 1964 concerning the dissociation between the release of MSH and that of ACTH from the pituitary gland even though both peptides share a behaviorally active core of amino acids.

OBSERVATIONS AND DISCUSSION

Dissociation of MSH from ACTH Release

Our concept that the hypothalamus inhibits the release of MSH in mammals despite its known stimulatory control of the release of ACTH and most of the other pituitary hormones was not initially accepted (52). As late as 1968 (63) prominent endocrinologists still considered MSH release, like ACTH release, to be mainly stimulated by the hypothalamus in the rat, although inhibitory control of MSH release by the hypothalamus in the frog was acknowledged. Reports by a group of influential investigators that MSH and ACTH were released in parallel (1,61,71) also might have made it seem unlikely that an inhibitory process would regulate the release of one substance while an excitatory process governed the other. However, much of this evidence was based on radioimmunoassay (RIA) of human β-MSH (β_h-MSH). Conflicting studies using

223

RIA of β_h-MSH showed dissociated release of MSH and ACTH (17,31,62) and we now know that β_h-MSH is an artifact of extraction rather than a naturally occurring substance in man. Thus, even though the nature of the physiological inhibitor of MSH was uncertain (50) there was little compelling evidence against the concept that control of MSH release is dissociated from ACTH release and is inhibitory in nature.

On the other hand, a series of studies conducted in our laboratory over a 10-year period showed that hypothalamic control of MSH release did not necessarily coincide with that of ACTH release. These studies concentrated on conditions in which changes in pigmentary responses associated with MSH activity could not be accounted for by changes in the concentrations of ACTH, a larger peptide which possessed intrinsic, MSH-like biological activity. They included removal of the pituitary from direct hypothalamic control by transplantation of the pituitary (48), destruction of the hypothalamus (49), injection of hypothalamic extracts (51), pinealectomy (47), stress induced by ether (37,54) adrenalectomy (30), injection of morphine (19,54), septal lesions (8), variations associated with circadian rhythms (18), and related conditions in the human (38,42).

All of our studies on the dissociation of MSH and ACTH release used bioassays. The results have now been confirmed by other investigators, some of whom have also used the bioassay (20,24,34,94). This technique has the advantage of measuring total MSH activity and obviates any disagreement concerning various forms of the hormone. Some have used immunohistochemical techniques to arrive at the same conclusion (60). Most of the other investigators, however, have used RIA to confirm our findings (95–97,99). One of these recent studies involved incubated rat pituitary tissue that showed a progressive decline in the ratio of ACTH to MSH released over time (95). An even more marked dissociation of ACTH and MSH release was found in human fetal pituitary tissue cultured for longer periods (91).

Melanocyte-Stimulating Hormone

Although both de Wied's group and our own arrived at the same conclusion that MSH exerts direct effects on the brain, the conceptual approaches were entirely different. de Wied was interested in finding the amino acid sequence of ACTH responsible for its effects on the central nervous system (CNS) and then apparently assumed that ACTH and MSH contained redundant information. We were influenced to a large extent by the dissociated release of MSH and ACTH described in the previous section and believed from the beginning that MSH itself would have distinctive CNS effects. Recently we (Sandman, Beckwith, and Kastin) have observed that different learning tasks may be uniquely influenced by specific sequences of the MSH/ACTH fragments. For certain phases of learning, such as the initial learning of a visual discrimination task, the 4–10 fragment seems to exert the most prominent influence followed by molecules of increasing molecular weight. For the reversal learning phase of the task, the α- and β-MSH molecules (1–13 and 1–18 amino acids) were found to exert the most influence, whereas the smallest (4–10) and largest (1–24) sequences have the least effects. Thus, the structure-activity relationships observed in this reversal phase were different from those observed during the early learning phase. These preliminary findings support our previous belief that, although the ACTH and MSH peptides may produce similar effects, each of these compounds also contains nonredundant information and influences discrete arrays of behavior. This principle should also apply to clinical studies with these peptides and their analogs.

Initially we used appetitive tasks involving hunger-motivated rats (88) rather than avoidance of shock, the method favored by the Utrecht group. Although early findings showed that MSH delayed extinction, the few times we used the conditioned avoidance response favored by de Wied, we found facilitated extinction in rats (6) and no effect in man (64). When we (89) used shock as a reinforcer during more complex learning tasks, we showed that MSH enhanced information processing by its effects on attention rather than memory. Subsequently, de Wied and colleagues confirmed our studies with appetitive paradigms (26).

Neither group of investigators had seen any reliable effect on acquisition in their early studies, although a tendency in that direction had been noted (83,88). We reasoned that the effect of MSH might be more evident in more difficult tasks, a hypothesis substantiated by the observation that hungry rats receiving MSH ran a 12-choice maze faster and with fewer errors than the controls (93). In an aversive task, we were also able to demonstrate facilitated learning by varying the level of shock (92). Although the effects of MSH in adult animals seemed to be transient, long-term effects have been observed by us after injection of newborns with MSH (4,6). The possible organizing influence of MSH and other peptides on the developing brain has been suggested by the enhanced spectrum of learning and social behaviors we have observed.

Electroencephalographic (EEG) changes after MSH were found by us several years ago in rats (84) and frogs (15). These were expected because of our earlier study in humans (43). A variety of electrocortical changes of the human brain after administration of MSH or its fragments has been found. In 1971, we demonstrated that in the somatosensory cortex, averaged evoked responses to threshold electrical stimulation of the median nerve were increased by MSH and that the increases were greatest when the subject was attentive to the task (44). Power spectral analysis showed the EEG of normal men to be significantly changed by MSH 4–10 as was the persistence of α-blocking (66). In another study, visual evoked potentials recorded from the occipital region showed changes in latency and magnitude of the negative component which normally peaks at about 200 msec and the presence of an additional negative element at about 350 msec (65).

Human subjects receiving MSH or its active core evidenced improved attention as measured by additional tasks such as the Benton Visual Retention test (44,

65,66,86,87), a visual discrimination task involving concept formation (86,87), the heart rate response during an orienting procedure (85), perceptual integration of patterned information (85), and a continuous performance task (65). Mentally retarded (87) as well as normal subjects were tested in these studies, all but one being double-blind in design. In addition to their improvement in the processing of information, the subjects were significantly less anxious (66,86).

MSH-Release Inhibiting Factor

Manipulations that selectively alter the release of MSH or of ACTH were involved in the dissociation discussed in the first section of this chapter. In addition to its well known effects on the skin, the separate actions of MSH on the CNS, described in the previous section, characterize a second type of dissociation. The extra-endocrine effects of a hypothalamic peptide on the brain rather than on the pituitary represent a third type of dissociation. This dissociation was first illustrated by the tripeptide Pro-Leu-Gly-NH$_2$ (MIF-I), a compound that, under some circumstances, may be representative of the inhibitor(s) responsible for the dissociation between MSH and ACTH release discussed earlier. The role of biogenic amines in MSH release has lately been reviewed elsewhere (53). Recently, some ironic evidence has appeared that, although MIF-I can selectively influence the release of either MSH or ACTH, it may be ACTH that can be inhibited (104,105). Nevertheless, evidence continues to accumulate that MIF-I does inhibit MSH release. Some of this work involves bioassay of MSH and other work involves RIA. Using bioassay, Vivas and Celis (101) showed that MIF-I inhibited the release of MSH into medium that contained incubated pituitaries of rats obtained at different stages of their estrous cycles. Using RIA, van Wimersma Greidanus et al. (99) recently reported that MIF-I inhibited the release of α-MSH induced by β-endorphin.

The tripeptide Pro-Leu-Gly-NH$_2$ has been called MIF-I for the past several years due to the uncertainty as to whether it is the physiological inhibitor of MSH release and to distinguish it from other proposed MIFs. Apart from its limited endocrine effects, we thought that it would also have direct effects on the CNS. This was demonstrated in the DOPA-potentiation test in which both intact and hypophysectomized animals responded to MIF-I (75). Later we (79) reported that the pineal, adrenals, ovaries, testes, thyroid, parathyroids, thymus, kidney, and spleen are also unnecessary for the actions of MIF-I. The activity of MIF-I in the DOPA-potentiation test has been confirmed by other investigators (32,33,103).

Two other systems that are sometimes also considered animal models of Parkinson's disease and mental depression are the oxotremorine and deserpidine reversal tests. MIF-I was active in reversing the tremors induced by oxotremorine (76), a finding confirmed in Sweden (7,10). Oral administration of MIF-I reversed the sedation induced by the *Rauwolfia* derivative deserpidine in both mice and monkeys (77). MIF-I has also been found to affect attention and learning (5,

83,93). In a number of other systems, including assessment of peripheral dopa-minergic receptors in the cardiovascular system, MIF-I has been found inactive (74).

The somewhat conflicting studies concerning the mechanism of action of MIF-I have been summarized elsewhere (46). Recently, we have again tried without success to detect a change in striatal dopamine synthesis after MIF-I (53). Moreover, the failure of MIF-I to potentiate the action of apomorphine in several studies did not fit with other evidence for activity at a postsynaptic site, but it now appears that the use of a smaller dose of apomorphine (14) or animals with sensitized dopamine receptors (59) results in potentiation.

Regardless of the mechanism of action, the initial report in 1972 of the benefi-cial effect of MIF-I in Parkinson's disease (36) has been confirmed in studies performed in several countries (2,3,11,23,27,28,90). Two intriguing findings emerge from these investigations. First, the most dramatic effects of MIF-I in parkinsonism occurred in those patients already ingesting DOPA (2,28,90), as might be expected from the animal work mentioned above. Second, mood was improved in some parkinsonian patients after MIF-I administration, a finding first indicated by our double-blind studies in mental depression (21,22) in which it was found that small doses of MIF-I were more effective than larger doses, as has been seen in some animal studies (75,77).

Brain Opiates

Several of the experimental models in which MIF-I was shown to be active have been used to test the opiate peptides. One of these, the 12-choice Warden maze, was used by us to introduce the fourth example of dissociation discussed in this review, namely that between the behavioral and analgesic effects of the brain opiates.

The peripheral administration of 80 μg/kg Met-enkephalin, a dose essentially devoid of any analgesic activity even if given centrally, resulted in hungry rats negotiating the complex maze quicker and with fewer errors than control rats injected with the diluent (56). The dissociation was further confirmed by similar results obtained with two analogs, one of which was much more potent, and the other much less potent, than the parent Met-enkephalin when tested for opiate activity (13,107). Yet injection of either analog appeared to cause the same degree of improved acquisition of the maze as did Met-enkephalin. The same dose of morphine was ineffective (56).

Another model in which enkephalin and MIF-I were found to have similar effects was the DOPA-potentiation test. These two peptides were the most active among hundreds of compounds tested in this system for potential antidepressant effects and antiparkinsonian agents. As in most of the behavioral tasks we have used, testing does not begin until 15 to 60 min after systemic injection of the peptide. This time is longer than the half-time disappearance of the brain peptides tested (40).

A third animal system that has been described as a model of mental depression involves the placement of rats in a cylinder containing water from which escape is impossible (80). One hour after injection of either enkephalin or the tricyclic antidepressant amitriptyline, rats show less "passive immobility" than was found after injection of the diluent or morphine (55). As in the maze study, an analog of enkephalin with little analgesic activity was active, whereas some superactive analogs showed no reversal of the "helpless" behavior. We have also found behavioral changes after injections of enkephalins in goldfish (68), monkeys (69,70), and chicks (72). Despite the initial opposition to the idea that peripherally administered enkephalins could exert any effects (40), other investigators (12,16,29,83,106) have now reported support for this concept, which has been applied clinically in schizophrenic patients (58,100). Because of the results in the three animal systems described earlier in this section, trials of enkephalins in mental depression could be worthwhile.

Thyrotropin-Releasing Hormone

Although to a lesser extent than MIF-I or enkephalin, thyrotropin-releasing hormone (TRH) was also active in the DOPA-potentiation test, but it did not reverse the tremors caused by oxotremorine or the immobility in the swimming task described in the previous section. Researchers from Chapel Hill recently extended their series of studies with TRH to show that rats could be trained in a two-lever operant task to discriminate between saline and TRH regardless of whether the TRH was administered systemically or centrally (35).

Clinically, most studies of TRH in the treatment of mental depression have been much less encouraging than the inital ones (46). Nevertheless, the finding of a blunted TSH response to TRH in some depressed patients has been repeatedly confirmed and considered by some to distinguish subgroups of depression (25,57,102).

Somatostatin

Although the possibility of hypothalamic peptides acting on neurotransmission had been obvious for some time (75), it was first put forth in a study of somatostatin in the DOPA-potentiation test (78). Other studies have shown that its actions are generally opposite to those of TRH on the sedation and hypothermia induced by pentobarbital as well as seizures induced by strychnine (9,81). Its other effects, particularly after central administration, have been reviewed recently (39).

Luteinizing Hormone-Releasing Hormone

The ability of luteinizing hormone-releasing hormone (LH-RH) to increase mating behavior in female rats without releasing gonadotropins from the pituitary has attracted much attention (67,73). It appears to be more difficult to apply the results of these animal studies to the clinical situation, but the possibility still exists. This information has been discussed lately (41).

Other Hypothalamic Peptides

This chapter has discussed peptides found in the hypothalamus, regardless of whether they are usually associated with the pituitary (e.g., MSH) or brain (e.g., enkephalin), and others will undoubtedly be found. Vasopressin fits in this category, and the fine work of DeWied and his collaborators, discussed extensively elsewhere, should be mentioned. Like the other peptides reviewed here, vasopressin is active when given peripherally (98).

It is not known whether the hypothalamic peptides administered systemically exert their effects initially in the periphery, cross the blood-brain barrier, affect enzymes in the endothelial cells lining the barrier, or enter the brain intact. Now that our concept that hypothalamic peptides administered peripherally can exert extra-endocrine effects on the brain is becoming more generally accepted, more attention can be given to the mechanisms involved.

SUMMARY

Although the hypothalamic hormones were isolated on the basis of their endocrine effects on the pituitary gland, their extra-endocrine effects on the CNS are now well known. Other peptides such as MSH and the brain opiates, also found in the hypothalamus but not usually classified as hypothalamic hormones, similarly exert behavioral effects on the CNS. Dissociations can be found between the release of MSH and that of ACTH from the pituitary, between the pigmentary and extra-pigmentary effects of MSH, between the endocrine and extra-endocrine effects of the hypothalamic hormones, and between the analgesic and behavioral effects of the opiate peptides. These peptides are potentially useful in optimizing normal as well as in treating abnormal functioning of the brain.

ACKNOWLEDGMENTS

Supported in part by the Medical Research Service of the Veterans Administration, Mrs. Lois Stevens, the Wacker Foundation, Mrs. Louise Dunagan Kramer, and grant NS 07664 from the National Institutes of Health.

REFERENCES

1. Abe, K., Nicholson, W. E., Liddle, G. W., Orth, D. N., and Island, D. P. (1969): Normal and abnormal regulation of β-MSH in man. *J. Clin. Invest.*, 48:1580–1585.
2. Barbeau, A. (1975): Potentiation of levodopa effect by intravenous L-prolyl-L-leucyl-glycine amide in man. *Lancet*, 2:683–684.

3. Barbeau, A., and Kastin, A. J. (1976): Polypeptide therapy in Parkinson's disease. In: *Advances in Parkinsonism,* edited by W. Birkmayer and O. Hornykeiwicz, pp. 483–487. Roche, Basel.

4. Beckwith, B. E., O'Quinn, R. K., Petro, M. S., Kastin, A. J., and Sandman, C. A. (1977): The effects of neonatal injections of α-MSH on the open field behavior of juvenile and adult rats. *Physiol. Psychol.,* 5:295–299.

5. Beckwith, B. E., Sandman, C. A., Hothersall, D., and Kastin, A. J. (1976): The influence of 3 short-chain peptides (α-MSH, MSH/ACTH 4–10, MIF-I) on dimensional attention. *Pharmacol. Biochem. Behav., (Suppl.* 1)5:11–16.

6. Beckwith, B. E., Sandman, C. A., Hothersall, D., and Kastin, A. J. (1977): Influence of neonatal injections of α-MSH on learning, memory and attention in rats. *Physiol. Behav.,* 18:63–71.

7. Bjorkman, S., and Sievertsson, H. (1977): On the optimal dosage of Pro-Leu-Gly-NH₂ (MIF) in neuropharmacological tests and clinical use. *Naunyn Schmiedebergs Arch. Pharmacol.,* 298:79–81.

8. Brown, G. M., Uhlir, I. V., Seggie, J., Schally, A. V., and Kastin, A. J. (1974): Effect of septal lesions on plasma levels of MSH, corticosterone, GH, and prolactin before and after exposure to novel environment: Role of MSH in septal syndrome. *Endocrinology,* 94:583–587.

9. Brown, M., and Vale, W. (1975): Central nervous system effects of hypothalamic peptides. *Endocrinology,* 96:1333–1336.

10. Castensson, S., Sievertsson, H., Lindeke, B., and Sum, C. Y. (1974): Studies on the inhibition of oxotremorine induced tremors by a melanocyte-stimulating hormone release-inhibiting factor, thyrotropin releasing hormone and related peptides. *FEBS Lett.,* 44:101–105.

11. Chase, T. N., Woods, A. C., Lipton, M. A., and Morris, C. E. (1974): Hypothalamic releasimg factors and Parkinson's disease. *Arch. Neurol.,* 31:55–56.

12. Chipkin, R. E., Stewart, J. M., Morris, D. H., and Crowley, T. J. (1978): Generalization of [D-Ala²] enkephalin but not of substance P to morphine cue. *Pharmacol. Biochem. Behav.,* 9:129–132.

13. Coy, D. H., Kastin, A. J., Schally, A. V., Morin, O., Caron, N. G., Labrie, F., Walker, J. M., Fertel, R., Berntson, G. G., and Sandman, C. A. (1976): Synthesis and opioid activities of stereoisomers and other D-amino acid analogs of methionine-enkephalin. *Biochem. Biophys. Res. Commun.,* 73:632–638.

14. Davis, K. L., Kastin, A. J., Beilstein, B. A., and Vento, A. L. (1980): α-MSH and MIF-I in animal models of tardive dyskinesia. *Brain Res. Bull. (in press).*

15. Denman, P. M., Miller, L. H., Sandman, C. A., Schally, A. V., and Kastin, A. J. (1972): Electrophysiological correlates of melanocyte-stimulating hormone activity in the frog. *J. Comp. Physiol. Psychol.,* 80:59–65.

16. de Wied, D., Kovacs, G. L., Bohus, B., Van Ree, J. M., and Greven, H. M. (1978): Neuroleptic activity of the neuropeptide β-LPH, (Des-Tyr¹)-γ-endorphin DT-γ-E. *Eur. J. Pharmacol.,* 49:427–436.

17. Donald, R. S., and Toth, A. (1973): A comparison of the β-melanocyte-stimulating hormone and corticotropin response to hypoglycemia. *J. Clin. Endocrinol. Metab.,* 36:925–930.

18. Dunn, J. D., Kastin, A. J., and Carrillo, A. J. (1976): Circadian variation in plasma melanocyte stimulating hormone activity in the rat. *Int. J. Chronobiol.,* 4:163–169.

19. Dunn, J. D., Kastin, A. J., Carrillo, A. J., and Schally, A. V. (1972): Additional evidence for dissociation of melanocyte-stimulating hormone and corticotropin release. *J. Endocrinol.,* 55:463–464.

20. Egge, P. R., Peaslee, M. H., and Einhellig, F. A. (1978): Tannic acid-induced dissociation of pituitary melanocyte-stimulating hormone and adrenocorticotropic hormone levels. *Gen. Pharmacol.,* 9:33–35.

21. Ehrensing, R. H., and Kastin, A. J. (1974): Melanocyte-stimulating hormone release inhibiting hormone as an antidepressant. *Arch. Gen. Psychiatry,* 30:63–65.

22. Ehrensing, R. H., and Kastin, A. J. (1978): Dose-related biphasic effect of prolyl-leucyl-glycinamide (MIF-I) in depression. *Am. J. Psychiatry,* 135:562–566.

23. Fischer, P., Schneider, E., Jacobi, P., and Maxion, H. (1975): Effect of melanocyte-stimulating hormone release inhibiting hormone (MIF) in Parkinson's syndrome. *Eur. Neurol.,* 12:360–368.

24. Francis, M. G., and Barnawell, E. B. (1978): The influence of the nervous system upon adrenal gland weight and assayable pituitary MSH. *Neuroendocrinology,* 27:228–238.

25. Furlong, F. W., Brown, G. M., and Beeching, M. F. (1976): Thyrotropin-releasing hormone: Differential antidepressant and endocrinological effects. *Am. J. Psychiatry,* 133:1187–1190.

26. Garrud, P., Gray, J. A., and DeWied, D. (1974): Pituitary adrenal hormones and extinction of rewarded behavior in the rat. *Physiol. Behav.,* 12:109–119.

27. Gerstenbrand, V. J., Binder, H., Kozma, C., Pusch, S., and Reisner, T. (1975): Infusiontherapie mit MIF (Melanocyte Inhibiting Factor) beim Parkinson-Syndrom. *Wien. Klin. Wochenschr.,* 87:822–823.

28. Gerstenbrand, V. J., Poewe, W., Archner, F., and Kozma, C. (1979): Clinical utilization of MIF-I. In: *Central Nervous System Effects of Hypothalamic Hormones and Other Peptides,* edited by R. Collu, A. Barbeau, J. R. Ducharme, and J. G. Rochefort, pp. 415–426. Raven Press, New York.

29. Gorelick, D., Catlin, D., George, R., and Li, C. H. (1978): Beta endorphin is behaviorally active in rats after chronic intravenous administration. *Pharmacol. Biochem. Behav.,* 9:385–386.

30. Gosbee, J. L., Kraicer, J., Kastin, A. J., and Schally, A. V. (1979): A functional relationship between pars intermedia and ACTH secretion in the rat. *Endocrinology,* 86:560–567.

31. Hirata, Y., Sakamoto, N., Matsukura, S., and Imura, H. (1975): Plasma levels of β-MSH and ACTH during acute stresses and metyrapone administration in man. *J. Clin. Endocrinol. Metab.,* 41:1092–1097.

32. Huidobro-Toro, J. P., Scottie de Carolis, A., and Longo, V. G. (1974): Action of two hypothalamic factors (TRH, MIF) and angiotensin II on the behavioral effects of L-DOPA and 5-hydroxytryptophan in mice. *Pharmacol. Biochem. Behav.,* 2:105–109.

33. Huidobro-Toro, J. P., Scottie de Carolis, A., and Longo, V. G. (1975): Intensification of central catecholaminergic and serotonergic processes by the hypothalamic factors MIF and TRF and by angiotensin II. *Pharmacol. Biochem. Behav.,* 3:235–242.

34. Iturriza, F. C., Celotti, F., Estivariz, F. E., and Martini, L. (1976): Lack of detectable secretion of ACTH from pituitary homografts of pars intermedia. *Neuroendocrinology,* 22:175–182.

35. Jones, C. N., Grant, L. D., and Prange, A. J., Jr. (1978): Stimulus properties of thyrotropin-releasing hormone. *Psychopharmacology,* 59:217–224.

36. Kastin, A. J., and Barbeau, A. (1972): Preliminary clinical studies with L-prolyl-L-leucyl-glycine amide in Parkinson's disease. *Can. Med. Assoc. J.,* 107:1079–1081.

37. Kastin, A. J., Barrett, L., Viosca, S., Arimura, A., and Schally, A. V. (1976): MSH activity in rat pituitaries after stress. *Neuroendocrinology,* 2:200–208.

38. Kastin, A. J., Beach, G. D., Hawley, W. D., Kendally, J. W., Jr., Edwards, M. S., and Schally, A. V. (1973): Dissociation of MSH and ACTH release in man. *J. Clin. Endocrinol. Metab.,* 36:770–772.

39. Kastin, A. J., Coy, D. H., Jacquet, Y., Schally, A. V., and Plotnikoff, N. P. (1978): CNS effects of somatostatin. *Metabolism (Suppl. 1),* 5:1247–1252.

40. Kastin, A. J., Coy, D. H., Schally, A. V., Miller, L. H. (1978): Peripheral administration of hypothalamic peptides results in CNS changes. *Pharmacol. Res. Commun.,* 10:293–312.

41. Kastin, A. J., Ehrensing, R. H., Coy, D. H., Schally, A. V., and Kostrzewa, R. M. (1979): Behavioral effects of brain peptides, including LH-RH. In: *Proceedings of the Symposium on Clinical Psycho-Neuroendocrinology in Reproduction,* edited by L. Zichella. Elsevier, Amsterdam.

42. Kastin, A. J., Hawley, W. D., Miller, M. C., Schally, A. V., and Lancaster, C. (1974): Plasma MSH and cortisol levels in 567 patients with special reference to brain trauma. *Endocrinol. Exper. (Bratisl.),* 8:97–105.

43. Kastin, A. J., Kullander, S., Borglin, N. E., Dyster-Aas, K., Dahlberg, B., Ingvar, D., Krakau, C. E. T., Miller, M. C., Bowers, C. Y., and Schally, A. V. (1968): Extrapigmentary effects of melanocyte-stimulating hormone in amenorrheic women. *Lancet,* 1:1007–1010.

44. Kastin, A. J., Miller, L. H., Gonzalez-Barcena, D., Hawley, W. D., Dyster-Aas, K., Schally, A. V., Velasco-Parra, M. L., and Velasco, M. (1971): Psychophysiologic correlates of MSH activity in man. *Physiol. Behav.,* 7:893–896.

45. Kastin, A. J., Olson, R. D., Schally, A. V., and Coy, D. H. (1979): CNS effects of peripherally administered brain peptides. *Life Sci.,* 25:401–414.

46. Kastin, A. J., Plotnikoff, N. P., Schally, A. V., and Sandman, C. A. (1976): Endocrine and CNS effects of hypothalamic peptides and MSH. In: *Reviews of Neuroscience, Vol. 2,* edited by S. Ehrenpries and I. J. Kopin, pp. 111–148. Raven Press, New York.

47. Kastin, A. J., Redding, T. W., and Schally, A. V. (1967): MSH activity in rat pituitaries after pinealectomy. *Proc. Soc. Exp. Biol. Med.,* 124:1275–1277.

48. Kastin, A. J., and Ross, G. T. (1964): Melanocyte stimulating hormone (MSH) and ACTH activities of pituitary transplants in the rat. *Endocrinology,* 75:187–191.

49. Kastin, A. J., and Ross, G. T. (1965): Melanocyte-stimulating hormone (MSH) and ACTH activities in pituitaries of frogs with hypothalamic lesions. *Endocrinology,* 77:45–48.

50. Kastin, A. J., Sandman, C. A., Miller, L. H., and Schally, A. V. (1976): Some questions related to melanocyte-stimulating hormone. *Mayo Clin. Proc.,* 51:632–636.

51. Kastin, A. J., and Schally, A. V. (1966): MSH activity in pituitaries of rats treated with hypothalamic extracts. *Gen. Comp. Endocrinol.,* 7:452–456.

52. Kastin, A. J., and Schally, A. V. (1971): Control of MSH release in mammals. In: Proceedings VII Pan American Congress of Endocrinology, *Excerpta Medica Int. Congr. Ser.,* 238:311–317.

53. Kastin, A. J., Schally, A. V., and Kostrzewa, R. M. (1980): Possible adrenergic mediation of MSH release and of the CNS effects of MSH and MIF-I. *Fed. Proc. (in press).*

54. Kastin, A. J., Schally, A. V., Viosca, S., and Miller, M. C. (1969): MSH activity in plasma and pituitaries of rats after various treatments. *Endocrinology,* 84:20–27.

55. Kastin, A. J., Scollan, E., Ehrensing, R. H., Schally, A. V., and Coy, D. H. (1978): Enkephalins and other peptides reduce passiveness. *Pharmacol. Biochem. Behav.,* 9:515–519.

56. Kastin, A. J., Scollan, E. L., King, M. G., Schally, A. V., and Coy, D. H. (1976): Enkephalin and a potent analog facilitate maze performance after intraperitoneal administration in rats. *Pharmacol. Biochem. Behav.,* 5:691–695.

57. Kirkegaard, C., Bjorum, N., Cohn, D., Faber, J., Lauridsen, U. B., and Nerup, J. (1977): Studies on the influence of biogenic amines and psycho-active drugs on the prognostic value of the TRH stimulation test in endogenous depression. *Psychoneuroendocrinology,* 2:131–136.

58. Kline, N. S., Li, C. H., Lehmann, H. E., Lajtha, A., Laskie, E., and Cooper, T. (1977): β-Endorphin induced changes in schizophrenic and depressed patients. *Arch. Gen. Psychiatry,* 34:1111–1113.

59. Kostrzewa, R. M., Kastin, A. J., and Sobrian, S. K. (1978): Potentiation of apomorphine action in rats by L-prolyl-L-leucyl-glycine-amide. *Pharmacol. Biochem. Behav.,* 9:375–378.

60. Kruseman, A. C. N., and Schroder-van der Elst, J. P. (1976): The immunolocalization of ACTH and α-MSH in human and rat pituitaries. *Virchows Arch.* [*Cell Pathol.*], 22:263–272.

61. Liddle, G. W. (1973): Regulation of secretion. In: *Peptide Hormones,* edited by S. A. Berson and R. S. Yalow, pp. 421–422. Elsevier, New York.

62. Lombardi, G., Oliver, C., Lupoli, G., and Minozzi, M. (1977): Corticotrophic and melano-trophic functions in congenital adrenal hyperplasia. *Acta Endocrinol. (Kbh.),* 85:118–125.

63. McCann, S. M., Dhariwal, A. P. S., and Porter, J. C. (1968): Regulation of the adenohypophysis. *Annu. Rev. Physiol.,* 30:589–640.

64. Miller, L. H., Fischer, S. C., Groves, G. A., Rudrauff, M. E., and Kastin, A. J. (1977): MSH/ACTH 4–10 influences on the CAR in human subjects: A negative finding. *Pharmacol. Biochem. Behav.,* 7:417–419.

65. Miller, L. H., Harris, L., Van Riezen, H., and Kastin, A. J. (1976): A neuroheptapeptide influence on attention and memory in man. *Pharmacol. Biochem. Behav. (Suppl. 1),* 5:17–21.

66. Miller, L. H., Kastin, A. J., Sandman, C. A., Fink, M., and Van Veen, W. J. (1974): Polypeptide influence on attention, memory and anxiety in man. *Pharmacol. Biochem. Behav.,* 2:663–668.

67. Moss, R. L., and McCann, S. M. (1973): Induction of mating behavior in rats by luteinizing hormone-releasing factor. *Science,* 181:177–179.

68. Olson, R. D., Kastin, A. J., Michell, G. F., Olson, G. A., Coy, D. H., and Montalbano, D. M. (1978): Effects of endorphin and enkephalin analogs on fear habituation in goldfish. *Pharmacol. Biochem. Behav.,* 9:111–114.

69. Olson, G. A., Olson, R. D., Kastin, A. J., Castellanos, F. X., Kneale, M. J., Coy, D. H., and Wolf, R. H. (1978): Behavioral effects of D-Ala²-β-endorphin in squirrel monkeys. *Pharmacol. Biochem. Behav.,* 9:687–691.

70. Olson, G. A., Olson, R. D., Kastin, A. J., Green, M. T., Roig-Smith, R., Hill, C. W., and

Coy, D. H. (1979): Effects of enkephalin analog on complex learning in the rhesus monkey. *Pharmacol. Biochem. Behav.,* 11:341–345.

71. Orth, D. N., Nicholson, W. E., Mitchell, W. M., Island, D. P., Shapiro, M., and Byyny, R. L. (1973): ACTH and MSH production by a single cloned mouse pituitary tumor cell line. *Endocrinology,* 92:385–393.

72. Panksepp, J., Vilberg, T., Bean, N. J., Coy, D. H., and Kastin, A. J. (1978): Reduction of distress vocalization in chicks by opiate-like peptides. *Brain Res. Bull.,* 3:663–667.

73. Pfaff, D. W. (1973): Luteinizing hormone-releasing factor potentiates lordosis behavior in hypophysectomized ovariectomized female rats. *Science,* 182:1148–1149.

74. Plotnikoff, N. P., and Kastin, A. J. (1974): Pharmacological studies with a tripeptide prolyl-leucyl-glycineamide. *Arch. Int. Pharmacodyn. Ther.,* 211:211–224.

75. Plotnikoff, N. P., Kastin, A. J., Anderson, M. S., and Schally, A. V. (1971): DOPA potentiation by a hypothalamic factor, MSH release-inhibiting hormone (MIF). *Life Sci.,* 10:1279–1283.

76. Plotnikoff, N. P., Kastin, A. J., Anderson, M. S., and Schally, A. V. (1972): Oxotremorine antagonism by a hypothalamic hormone, melanocyte-stimulating hormone release-inhibiting factor (MIF). *Proc. Soc. Exp. Biol. Med.,* 140:811–814.

77. Plotnikoff, N. P., Kastin, A. J., Anderson, M. S., and Schally, A. V. (1973): Deserpidine antagonism by a tripeptide, L-prolyl-L-leucylglycinamide. *Neuroendocrinology,* 11:67–71.

78. Plotnikoff, N. P., Kastin, A. J., and Schally, A. V. (1974): Growth hormone release inhibiting hormone: Neuropharmacological studies. *Pharmacol. Biochem. Behav.,* 2:693–696.

79. Plotnikoff, N. P., Minard, F. N., and Kastin, A. J. (1974): DOPA potentiation in ablated animals and brain levels of biogenic amines in intact animals after prolyl-leucylglycinamide. *Neuroendocrinology,* 14:271–279.

80. Porsolt, R. D., Le Pichon, M., and Jalfre, M. (1977): Depression: A new animal model sensitive to antidepressant treatments. *Nature,* 266:730–732.

81. Prange, A. J., Jr., Breese, G. R., Jahnke, G. D., Martin, B. R., Cooper, B. R., Cott, J. M., Wilson, I. C., Alltop, L. B., Lipton, M. A., Bissette, G., Nemeroff, C. B., and Loosen, P. T. (1975): Modification of pentobarbital effects by natural and synthetic polypeptides: Dissociation of brain and pituitary effects. *Life Sci.,* 16:1907–1914.

82. Rigter, H., Greven, H., and Van Riezen, H. (1977): Failure of naloxone to prevent reduction of amnesia by enkephalins. *Neuropharmacology,* 16:545–547.

83. Sandman, C. A., Alexander, W. D., and Kastin, A. J. (1973): Neuroendocrine influences on visual discrimination and reversal learning in the albino and hooded rat. *Physiol. Behav.,* 11:613–617.

84. Sandman, C. A., Denman, P. M., Miller, L. H., Knott, J. R., Schally, A. V., and Kastin, A. J. (1971): Electroencephalographic measures of melanocyte-stimulating hormone activity. *J. Comp. Physiol. Psychol.,* 76:103–109.

85. Sandman, C. A., George, J., McCanne, T. R., Nolan, J. D., Kaswan, J., and Kastin, A. J. (1977): MSH/ACTH 4–10 influences behavioral and physiological measures of attention. *J. Clin. Endocrinol. Metab.,* 44:884–891.

86. Sandman, C. A., George, J., Nolan, J., Van Riezen, H., and Kastin, A. J. (1975): Enhancement of attention in man with ACTH/MSH 4–10. *Physiol. Behav.,* 15:427–431.

87. Sandman, C. A., George, J., Walker, B., Nolan, J. D., and Kastin, A. J. (1976): The neuropeptide MSH/ACTH 4–10 enhances attention in the mentally retarded. *Pharmacol. Biochem. Behav. (Suppl. 1),* 5:23–28.

88. Sandman, C. A., Kastin, A. J., and Schally, A. V. (1969): Melanocyte-stimulating hormone and learned appetitive behavior. *Experientia,* 25:1001–1002.

89. Sandman, C. A., Miller, L. H., Kastin, A. J., and Schally, A. V. (1972): Neuroendocrine influence on attention and memory. *J. Comp. Physiol. Psychol.,* 80:54–58.

90. Schneider, V. E., Fischer, P. A., Jacobi, P., and Reh, W. (1978): Der Einfluss von MIF (Melanozyteninhibierender Faktor) auf Psychomotorik und Stimmungsverhalten von Parkinsonkranken. *Arzneim. Forsch.,* 28:1296–1297.

91. Siler-Khodr, T. M., Morgenstern, L. L., and Greenwood, F. C. (1974): Hormone synthesis and release from human fetal adenohypophyses *in vitro. J. Clin. Endocrinol. Metab.,* 39:891–904.

92. Stratton, L. O., and Kastin, A. J. (1974): Avoidance learning at two levels of motivation in rats receiving MSH. *Horm. Behav.,* 5:149–155.

93. Stratton, L. O., and Kastin, A. J. (1975): Increased acquisition of a complex appetitive task after MSH and MIF. *Pharmacol. Biochem. Behav.,* 3:901–904.
94. Thody, A. J., and Hinks, W. M. (1973): The secretion of melanocyte-stimulating hormone after adrenalectomy and dexamethasone treatment in the rat. *J. Endocrinol.,* 59:657–658.
95. Tilders, F. J. H. (1979): Relationship between the release of corticotropin and melanocyte-stimulating hormone from the pars intermedia of the rat pituitary gland. *J. Endocrinol.,* 80:8P.
96. Usategui, R., Gillioz, P., and Oliver, C. (1977): Effect of cold exposure on α-MSH and ACTH release in the rat. *Horm. Metab. Res.,* 9:519.
97. Usategui, R., Oliver, C., Vaudry, H., Lombardi, G., Rozenberg, I., and Mourre, A. M. (1976): Immunoreactive α-MSH and ACTH levels in rat plasma and pituitary. *Endocrinology,* 98:189–196.
98. van Wimersma Greidanus, T. B., and de Wied, D. (1976): Dorsal hippocampus: A site of action of neuropeptides on avoidance behavior? *Pharmacol. Biochem. Behav. (Suppl. 1),* 5:29–33.
99. van Wimersma Greidanus, T. B., Thody, T. J., Verspaget, H., de Rotte, G. A., Goedemans, H. J. H., Croiset, G., and Van Ree, J. M. (1979): Effects of morphine and β-endorphin on basal and elevated plasma levels of α-MSH and vasopressin. *Life Sci.,* 24:579–586.
100. Verhoeven, W. M. A., Van Praag, H. M., Van Ree, J. M., and DeWied, D. (1979): Improvement of schizophrenic patients treated with [Des-Tyr¹]-γ-endorphin (DTγE). *Arch. Gen. Psychiatry,* 36:294–298.
101. Vivas, A., and Celis, M. E. (1977): Differences in the release of melanocyte-stimulating hormone *in vitro* by rat pituitary glands collected at various times during the oestrous cycle. *J. Endocrinol.,* 78:1–6.
102. Vogel, H. P., Benkert, O., Illig, R., Muller-Oerlinghausen, B., and Poppenberg, A. (1977): Psychoendocrinological and therapeutic effects of TRH in depression. *Acta Psychiatr. Scand.,* 56:223–232.
103. Voith, K. (1977): Synthetic MIF analogues. Part II: DOPA potentiation and fluphenazine antagonism. *Arzneim. Forsch.,* 27:2290–2293.
104. Voigt, K. H., Fehm, H. L., Lang, R. E., Beinert, K. E., and Pfeiffer, E. F. (1977): Suppression of ACTH secretion by synthetic MSH-release inhibiting factor Pro-Leu-Gly-NH₂ in Addison's disease. *Horm. Metab. Res.,* 9:150–152.
105. Voigt, K. H., Fehm, H. L., Lang, R. E., and Walter, R. (1976): The effect of somatostatin and of prolyl-leucyl-glycinamide (MIF) on ACTH release in dispersed pituitary cells. *Life Sci.,* 21:739–746.
106. von Graffenried, B., Del Pozo, E., Roubicek, J., Krebs, E., Poldinger, W., Burmeister, P., and Kerp, L. (1978): Effects of the synthetic enkephalin analogue FK-33-844 in man. *Nature,* 272:729–730.
107. Walker, J. M., Berntson, G. G., Sandman, C. A., Coy, D. H., Schally, A. V., and Kastin, A. J. (1977): An analogue of enkephalin having a prolonged opiate-like effect *in vivo. Science,* 196:85–87.

Polypeptide Hormones, edited by
R. F. Beers, Jr. and E. G. Bassett.
Raven Press, New York © 1980.

22. Mechanisms of Action of Hypothalamic Hormones in the Anterior Pituitary

F. Labrie, P. Borgeat, N. Barden, M. Godbout, M. Beaulieu, L. Ferland, and M. Lavoie

MRC Group in Molecular Endocrinology, Le Centre Hospitalier de l'Université Laval, Quebec G1V 4G2, Canada

INTRODUCTION

The rate of secretion of the six main anterior pituitary hormones is controlled by neurohormones released from the hypothalamus and transported to their adenohypophyseal site of action by a short portal blood system. The secretion of luteinizing hormone (LH), follicle-stimulating hormone (FSH), and adrenocorticotropin (ACTH) is thought to be exclusively under positive control, whereas that of growth hormone (GH), thyrotropin (TSH), and prolactin results from the balance of action of inhibitory and stimulatory neurohormones. The overall influence of the hypothalamus on GH and TSH secretion is stimulatory, whereas it is inhibitory on prolactin secretion.

It is only recently that the concept of neurohormonal control of adenohypophyseal secretion could be translated into biochemical and chemical terms. The discovery of hypothalamic hormones and the relative ease of synthesis of three hypothalamic peptides [TRH, (TSH-releasing hormone), LH-RH (LH-releasing hormone), and somatostatin], (5,32,39,45,53,58) and their analogs has opened new possibilities for studies of their mechanism of action and has led to a rapid increase of our knowledge of the physiology of the hypothalamo-pituitary complex. The availability of synthetic hypothalamic peptides and their analogs has permitted a detailed analysis of not only the specific effects of these neuropeptides on pituitary hormone secretion, but also of the important modulatory role exerted by peripheral hormones (gonadal, adrenocortical, and thyroid hormones) at the pituitary level.

Although peripheral hormones had been known for many years to play a major role in the control of adenohypophyseal activity in man and experimental animals, *in vivo* approaches could not clearly dissociate between hypothalamic and pituitary sites of action. This area of research has been much facilitated by the development of the pituitary cell culture system (45,69). In fact, adenohypophyseal cells in primary culture have been extremely useful, not only for assessment of the biological activity of analogs of TRH, LH-RH, and somatostatin but also for precise analysis of the interactions between hypothalamic and peripheral hormones at the adenohypophyseal level (18,20–22). These studies performed in adenohypophyseal cells in primary culture have clearly demonstrated that the effect of peripheral hormones at the pituitary level can sometimes overcome the hypothalamic influence and that proper assessment of the control of anterior pituitary function must take into account the simultaneous influence of hypothalamic and peripheral hormones.

This chapter attempts to summarize the evidence obtained so far on the effect of three synthetic hypothalamic hormones, namely TRH, LH-RH, and somatostatin, as well as one catecholamine, dopamine, on cyclic AMP accumulation in the anterior pituitary gland. Since the characteristics of binding of TRH and properties of cyclic AMP-dependent adenohypophyseal protein kinase and some of its substrates have been described in a recent review (39), these aspects will not be included in the present chapter.

OBSERVATIONS AND DISCUSSION

Stimulatory Effect of LH-RH on Pituitary Cyclic AMP Accumulation

Indirect evidence for a role of cyclic AMP in the action of LH-RH on LH and FSH secretion first derived from the observations that theophylline and cyclic AMP derivatives (45,60) have a stimulatory effect on LH release and that theophylline potentiates the effect of a crude preparation of FSH-releasing hormone on FSH release (31). Definitive proof that the adenylyl cyclase system is a mediator of the action of LH-RH had to be obtained, however, by measurement of adenohypophyseal adenylyl cyclase activity or cyclic AMP concentration under the influence of the pure neurohormone.

It is now well known that addition of LH-RH leads to stimulation of cyclic AMP accumulation in rat anterior pituitary gland *in vitro* (5,7,32,45,53,55,59), the concentration of LH-RH required for half-maximal stimulation of cyclic AMP accumulation being 0.1 to 1 nM. Moreover, when LH-RH analogs having a spectrum of biological activity ranging from 0.001% and 500% to 1,000% the activity of LH-RH itself were used, a close parallelism was found between stimulation of cyclic AMP accumulation and both LH and FSH release was found under all experimental conditions (7). That LH-RH exerts its action by activating adenylyl cyclase and not by inhibiting cyclic nucleotide phosphodiesterase is indicated by the observation that a similar effect of the neurohormone is observed in the presence or absence of theophylline (5).

The possibility of developing a contraceptive method based on inhibitory LH-RH analogs has led to the synthesis of many such substances, some of which are potent inhibitors of LH-RH action both *in vivo* (23) and *in vitro* (46). The availability of such LH-RH antagonists offered the possibility of investigating the correlation between their inhibitory effect on LH-RH-induced cyclic AMP accumulation and LH and FSH release.

As an example, Fig. 1 shows the inhibitory effect of increasing concentrations of [D-Phe^2,D-Leu^6]-LH-RH on cyclic AMP accumulation and LH and FSH release in rat anterior pituitary gland *in vitro*. The close correlation observed between inhibition of LH-RH-induced cyclic AMP accumulation and LH and FSH release adds strong support to the concept of an obligatory role of the adenylyl cyclase system as mediator of LH-RH action in the anterior pituitary gland.

As additional direct evidence for a stimulatory effect of LH-RH on pituitary adenylyl cyclase activity, the neurohormone has been found to stimulate cyclic AMP formation in rat anterior pituitary homogenate (14) and membrane fractions (53). A stimulatory effect of LH-RH on adenylate cyclase activity has also been reported in homogenate from the ventral lobe of the pituitary of the dogfish (15).

Since gonadotrophs represent about 5% of the total cell population in the anterior pituitary gland, it is not surprising that addition of LH-RH leads to only a 100 to 300% stimulation (over control) of anterior pituitary cyclic AMP concentration (5,7,45,57,58). In order to induce a significant increase of total cyclic AMP accumulation, LH-RH must then stimulate specific cyclic AMP formation at least 20- to 60-fold in gonadotrophs.

We have recently found (22) that estrogens increase the sensitivity of the LH responsiveness to LH-RH by a direct action at the pituitary level whereas androgens have the opposite effect. Such a gonadal hormone-induced change

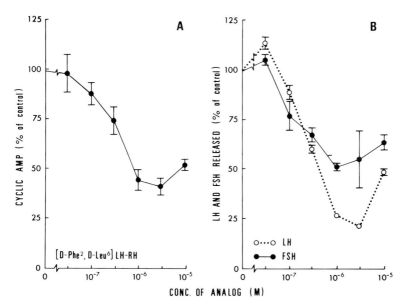

FIG. 1. Effect of increasing concentrations of [D-Phe^2, D-Leu^6]-LH-RH on 3 nM LH-RH-induced cyclic AMP accumulation **(A)** and LH and FSH **(B)** release in male rat hemipituitaries *in vitro*.

of pituitary responsiveness to LH-RH may explain why pituitaries obtained from male rats show a consistent increase of pituitary cyclic AMP levels under the influence of LH-RH, whereas no significant effect could be observed when female rat pituitaries were used (59; P. Borgeat, M. Beaulieu, and F. Labrie, *unpublished observations*). The higher sensitivity of the gonadotropin response to LH-RH in female animals is expected to require lower changes of cyclic AMP levels to induce LH and FSH release, whereas higher changes of intracellular cyclic AMP concentration are likely to be needed in male pituitaries. Such a possibility is supported by the finding that the cyclic AMP response to LH-RH observed in pituitaries obtained from intact male rats is lost after castration and is restored after androgen administration in castrated animals (59).

Suggestions against an obligatory role of cyclic AMP as mediator of LH-RH action are based on the expected observation that nonspecific agents leading to changes of total pituitary cyclic AMP accumulation (such as theophylline, prostaglandins or inhibitors of their synthesis, and cholera toxin) do not lead to parallel changes of LH release and cyclic AMP concentration (11,58,67). Since it is now clear that prostaglandins are not involved in LH-RH action at the level of the anterior pituitary gland (19,21,41,54) and, as mentioned earlier, gonadotrophs represent only 5% of the total cell population in the anterior pituitary gland, it is most likely that the changes of cyclic AMP levels observed with the above-mentioned compounds take place in cell types other than gonadotrophs. In fact, somatotrophs represent approximately 50% of the total adenohypophyseal cell population in male rat pituitaries and are highly sensitive to all the substances tested in the above-mentioned studies (1,21,43,44). All these negative attempts to correlate changes of cyclic AMP levels with alterations of LH release can be explained by the lack of specificity of the substances used that the heterogeneity of the pituitary cell population was not taken into account. In fact, the preferential effects of prostaglandins and cholera toxin in cell types other than gonadotrophs could explain all the reported changes of cyclic AMP levels that were not accompanied by specific effects on LH secretion (11,40,57,58,67).

Stimulatory Effect of TRH on Pituitary Cyclic AMP Accumulation

Although the changes of cyclic AMP levels were of relatively small magnitude, a significant increase (30% over control) was measured after 15 min of incubation with TRH, while a maximal effect at 50% over control was found after 2 hr of incubation (39,44). As found previously with LH-RH for LH and FSH release, the changes of cyclic AMP levels induced by TRH were accompanied by parallel changes of TSH release. Since the experiments were performed in the presence of 5 mM theophylline, it is likely that the observed changes of cyclic AMP concentrations are secondary to parallel modifications of adenylyl cyclase activity rather than to inhibition of cyclic nucleotide phosphodiesterase.

Inhibitory Effect of Somatostatin on Pituitary Cyclic AMP Accumulation

Since we had found that a purified fraction of GH-RH (GH-releasing hormone) led to a marked stimulation of pituitary cyclic AMP accumulation and GH release (9), it was of interest to study the effect of somatostatin on pituitary cyclic AMP accumulation. It was then found that somatostatin led to a rapid inhibition of cyclic AMP accumulation in anterior pituitary gland *in vitro* (8,32), this inhibitory effect being accompanied by a marked inhibition of both GH and TSH release.

Since GH- and TSH-secreting cells account for 50 to 70% of the total adenohypophyseal cell population in adult male rats, the 50% inhibition of cyclic AMP accumulation observed in total pituitary tissue suggests an almost complete inhibition of cyclic AMP accumulation in the GH- and TSH-secreting cells. The inhibitory effect of somatostatin is observed under both basal and prostaglandin E_2- or theophylline-induced conditions, thus suggesting an inhibitory action of somatostatin on adenylyl cyclase activity.

The correlation observed between inhibition of cyclic AMP levels and GH release was further demonstrated by an experiment performed in pituitary cells in primary culture (Fig. 2). It can be seen that the approximately 10-fold increase of cyclic AMP levels induced by 10^{-5} M PGE_2 is 60% inhibited by somatostatin

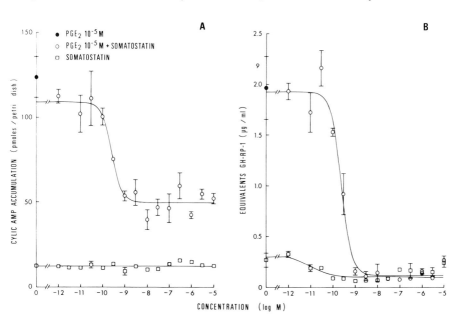

FIG. 2. Effect of increasing concentrations of somatostatin alone (□) or in the presence of 10^{-5} M PGE_2 (○) on cyclic AMP accumulation **(A)** and GH release **(B)** in rat anterior pituitary cells in primary culture. Cells were incubated for 30 min in the presence of the indicated substances as described (45) and cyclic AMP measured by RIA.

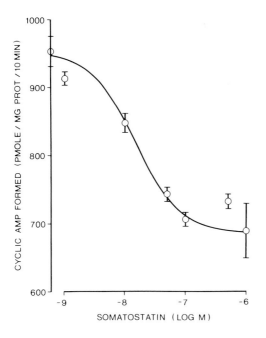

FIG. 3. Inhibition by somatostatin of anterior pituitary PGE₁-stimulated adenylyl cyclase activity. Rat anterior pituitary homogenate was incubated with 1 mM [³²Pα]-ATP, 10^{-4} M PGE₁, and different concentrations of somatostatin for 10 min at 30°C. Cyclic AMP formed was isolated by chromatography on successive columns of Dowex and alumina. Results are the means ± SE of triplicate determinations.

at an ED_{50} value of 0.3 nM. Under the same experimental conditions, GH release was 90 to 95% inhibited at maximal concentrations of somatostatin. The inhibitory effect of somatostatin on cyclic AMP levels and GH release was measured at the same ED_{50} value (0.3 nM). The absence of a significant effect of somatostatin on basal cyclic AMP levels in cells in culture in the presence of an approximately 50% inhibitory effect on basal GH release can probably be explained by the presence of fibroblasts in the culture.

As illustrated in Fig. 3, a similar inhibitory effect of somatostatin on PGE₁-induced adenylyl cyclase activity was observed in rat anterior pituitary gland homogenate, an half-maximal inhibition ($p < 0.01$) being observed at 15 nM somatostatin. Besides its intrinsic interest, this system could be advantageous as a model for studies of the mechanisms of action of substances having opposite effects on cyclic AMP accumulation, GH-RH or PGE₁ leading to stimulation and somatostatin to inhibition of enzymatic activity, respectively.

Inhibitory Effect of Dopamine on Pituitary Cyclic AMP Accumulation

Strong evidence obtained in the rat indicates that dopamine (DA) secreted by the tuberoinfundibular system is the main factor involved in the control of prolactin secretion (37,52,66,68). According to these data, DA released from nerve endings in the median eminence is transported to the pituitary prolactin-secreting cells by the hypothalamo-adenohypophyseal portal blood system. In support of such a physiological role of DA at the pituitary level on prolactin secretion, DA has recently been measured in portal blood (4) and a typical dopaminergic receptor has been characterized in anterior pituitary gland (10,37).

Indirect evidence for a role of cyclic AMP in the control of prolactin secretion originated from the observations that cyclic AMP derivatives or theophylline, an inhibitor of cyclic nucleotide phosphodiesterase, stimulated prolactin release (29,50,56,62,70). These data, obtained with theophylline and cyclic AMP derivatives, already suggested that the cyclic nucleotide has a stimulatory role in the control of prolactin secretion.

More direct evidence for a role of cyclic AMP in the action of dopamine on prolactin secretion had to be obtained, however, by measurement of adenohypophyseal adenylyl cyclase activity or cyclic AMP concentration under the influence of the catecholamine. As illustrated in Fig. 4, addition of 100 nM dopamine to male rat hemipituitaries led to a rapid inhibition of cyclic AMP accumulation, a maximal effect (30% inhibition) being already obtained 5 min after addition of the catecholamine.

In order to investigate further the effect of DA on adenohypophyseal adenylyl cyclase, cyclic AMP measurements were performed after treatments known to inhibit DA release at the hypothalamic level, thus resulting in a marked elevation of prolactin secretion. As illustrated in Fig. 5, 30 min after administration of a DA antagonist, haloperidol (10 mg/kg, s.c.), pituitary cyclic AMP levels were increased sixfold in both saline and estrogen-treated ovariectomized rats. A similar effect was observed after treatment with reserpine, an inhibitor of catecholamine uptake, in estrogen-treated animals. This effect of reserpine is

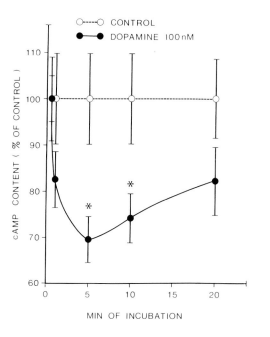

FIG. 4. Effect of dopamine (100 nM) on cyclic AMP accumulation in male rat anterior pituitaries. The experiment was performed as described (5).

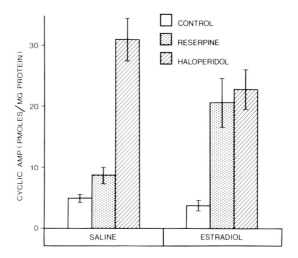

FIG. 5. Stimulation by reserpine and haloperidol of rat anterior pituitary cyclic AMP content *in vivo*. Ovariectomized rats treated with saline or 17β-estradiol (1 μg, twice a day for 7 days) were injected with saline, reserpine (5 mg/kg, s.c.) or haloperidol (10 μg/kg, s.c.) 30 min before sacrifice by concentrated microwave irradiation of the head. Cyclic AMP was extracted from anterior pituitary tissue by homogenization in 1 *N* HCl and measured by RIA. Results, expressed per milligram of anterior pituitary protein are the mean ± SE of six replicates. Haloperidol caused a significant stimulation of cyclic AMP content in both vehicle and estradiol injected animals ($p < 0.01$) whereas reserpine led to a significant stimulation only in estradiol-treated rats ($p < 0.01$).

in agreement with the data of Guidotti et al. (24), who have observed a stimulation of pituitary cyclic AMP levels 30 min after the administration of reserpine, the levels of the cyclic nucleotide being still elevated 5 hr after administration of the drug (25). That the stimulatory effect of reserpine treatment is related to diminished catecholamine availability at the hypothalamo-pituitary level was suggested by the reversal of the reserpine effect by the administration of pargylline, a monoamine oxidase inhibitor.

That the inhibitory effect of DA agonists on prolactin (PRL) release is mediated by inhibition of adenylyl cyclase is also suggested by the observation that $N^6,O^{2'}$-dibutyryl cyclic AMP can reverse the inhibitory effects of DA, apomorphine, or 2α-bromoergocryptine on PRL release (29).

Further support for a direct inhibitory effect of DA on adenylyl cyclase activity in mammotrophs has also been obtained in prolactin-secreting adenomas. At 10 μM DA, De Camilli et al. (13) have found a 13 to 39% inhibition of adenylyl cyclase activity in homogenates obtained from human prolactin-secreting pituitary adenomas. The inhibitory effect of DA was exerted at IC_{50} values of 3×10^{-7} to 10^{-5} M in individual cases, whereas norepinephrine [in agreement with its potency to inhibit prolactin secretion (37)] was approximately one-tenth as potent.

The existence of two classes of DA receptors has been suggested on the basis of their coupling to DA-sensitive adenylyl cyclase (34). The DA receptors stimulating adenylyl cyclase were called D-1 whereas those uncoupled to the enzyme were designated D-2. As mentioned earlier, there is, however, good evidence that the pituitary DA receptor is linked to adenylyl cyclase although coupling to the enzyme in this tissue leads to inhibition instead of stimulation of adenylyl cyclase.

The fairly good similarity of the specificity of binding to the DA receptor in striatum and anterior pituitary gland and the opposite effects of DA agonists on adenylyl cyclase in the two tissues [stimulation in striatum (35) and inhibition in anterior pituitary gland (41)] indicate the importance of different coupling mechanisms in the two tissues. This represents the first example where the same neurotransmitter interacting with receptors having similar binding characteristics leads to opposite effects in two different tissues.

The data presented so far clearly show that two stimulatory hypothalamic hormones, TRH and LH-RH, lead to parallel stimulation of cyclic AMP accumulation and specific hormone release, whereas one inhibitory peptide (somatostatin) and one catecholamine (dopamine) lead to parallel inhibition of cyclic AMP accumulation and hormone release (Fig. 6). Such findings strongly suggest that changes of adenylyl cyclase activity are involved in the mechanism of action of these three peptides and dopamine in the anterior pituitary gland.

Prostaglandins and Adenohypophyseal Cyclic AMP

Prostaglandins (PGs) are well known to stimulate cyclic AMP accumulation in anterior pituitary tissue (6,45,51,53,61,71,72).

As evidenced by the effect of increasing concentrations from 10^{-7} to 10^{-4} M, the various PGs exhibit markedly different potencies to induce cyclic AMP accumulation in rat adenohypophysis after 2 hr of incubation. As shown in Fig. 7, the order of potency is: $PGE_1 \simeq E_2 > A_1 \simeq A_2 > F_{1\alpha} \simeq F_{2\alpha}$. In control groups, cyclic AMP levels varied from 5 to 10 pmoles per adenohypophysis.

At 1×10^{-7} M, the stimulatory effect of PGE_2 was already significant at 2 min and became maximal at 30 min (6). This maximal effect was followed by a progressive decrease to basal levels at 2 hr. On addition of higher concentrations of PGE_2, cyclic AMP levels remained higher than controls at least up to 3 hr (6). When studied at short-time intervals (15 and 30 min), PGA_1 stimulated cyclic AMP accumulation only at high concentrations (10^{-4} M) and $PGF_{1\alpha}$ had only a minimal effect (6). PGs of the E type are thus the most potent activators of cyclic AMP accumulation in anterior pituitary tissue. PGE_1 and PGE_2 are in fact more potent than PGA_1 and PGA_2, and slight stimulation by $PGF_{1\alpha}$ can be observed only at high concentrations (10^{-4} M).

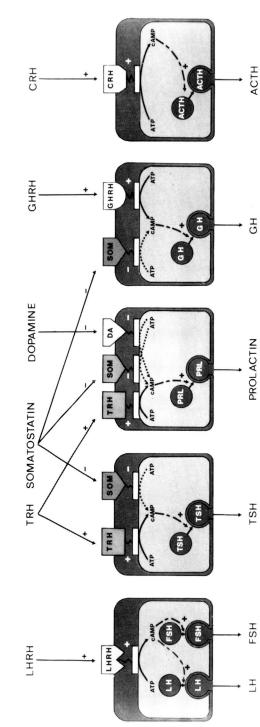

FIG. 6. Schematic representation of the role of the adenylyl cyclase system in the action of hypothalamic hormones in the anterior pituitary gland. Direct evidence has been obtained for a stimulatory effect of two hypothalamic hormones, LH-RH and TRH, on adenohypophyseal cyclic AMP accumulation and parallel changes of specific hormone release whereas opposite effects have been found with somatostatin and dopamine. A stimulatory effect of purified GH-RH has also been found on cyclic AMP accumulation while the stimulation of ACTH release induced by cyclic AMP derivatives suggests a similar role of the cyclic nucleotide in the action of CRH (ACTH-releasing hormone) in corticotrophs.

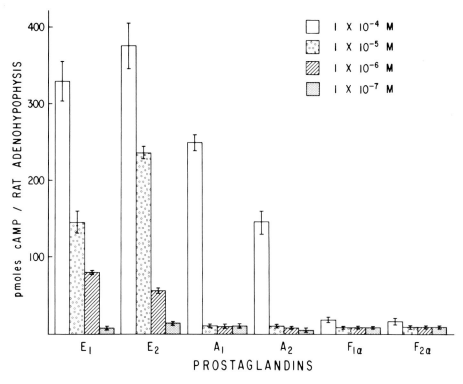

FIG. 7. Effect of increasing concentrations of prostaglandins E_1, E_2, A_1, A_2, $F_{1\alpha}$, and $F_{2\alpha}$ on cyclic AMP accumulation in rat anterior pituitary gland *in vitro*. The experiment was performed as described (6). Cyclic AMP was measured after 2 hr of exposure to the indicated concentrations of prostaglandins (43).

Prostaglandins and Adenohypophyseal Hormone Release

Data obtained from many *in vitro* studies using ox pituitary slices (12,65) and rat hemipituitaries (3,6,26–28,33,51,61) leave no doubt about the stimulatory effect of PGs of the E series on GH release. The order of potency of various PGs in stimulating GH release from rat anterior pituitary cells in culture closely parallels the potency previously observed on cyclic AMP accumulation. In fact, half-maximal stimulation of GH release by PGE_1 and PGE_2 is observed at 5×10^{-7} M, at 8 to 10×10^{-6} M for PGA_1 and PGA_2, and approximately 3×10^{-4} M for $PGF_{1\alpha}$ and $PGF_{2\alpha}$ (21). This potent *in vitro* stimulatory effect of PGE_1 and PGE_2 on GH release was confirmed *in vivo* (43). In fact, both PGE_1 and PGE_2 injected into the right superior vena cava in conscious rats led to rapid and markedly elevated plasma GH levels, the effect of PGE_2 being approximately twice that of PGE_1. At doses up to 250 μg, PGA_1 and PGA_2 had no effect on plasma GH levels. These data obtained in unanesthetized animals agree with the stimulatory effect of PGE_1 on plasma GH levels found in rats anesthetized with pentobarbital (28) or urethane (33).

Since the reports concerning the *in vitro* effects of PGs on LH release were conflicting (6,53,61,63,71), it was felt of interest to study in more detail the effect of PGs on basal and LH-RH-induced LH release *in vitro,* using adenohypophyseal cells in culture.

In anterior pituitary cells in primary culture, the presence of 10^{-6} M PGE_1 had no influence on the dose-response curve of LH release to increasing concentrations of LH-RH. In both groups, a 45-fold stimulation of LH release was found at 1×10^{-8} M LH-RH, a half-maximal response being measured at 3×10^{-10} M. Moreover, 10^{-6} M PGE_2 did not alter the time-course of basal or LH-RH-induced LH release in cells in culture up to 10 hr of incubation (19).

Since it seemed clear from the above-mentioned studies that PGEs do not stimulate LH release and do not change the LH responsiveness to LH-RH or the time-course of basal and stimulated LH release in cultured cells, it became of great interest to study the site of action of PGs injected *in vivo.* The availability of a specific LH-RH antiserum offered the ideal means of assessing the role of LH-RH in the previously observed PG-induced LH release and to discriminate between a hypothalamic or pituitary site of action of PGEs on LH release. Under appropriate conditions, the presence of excess circulating LH-RH antiserum should neutralize any PG-induced LH-RH secretion. Not only was the basal plasma LH concentration reduced by approximately 75% 1 hr after injection of the antiserum, but also the treatment almost completely obliterated the plasma LH rise observed after injection of PGE_1 or PGE_2 (19).

The above-mentioned data show that PGs have two effects on hormone release by anterior pituitary cells in culture: a direct stimulatory effect on GH and TSH release and a potentiation of the stimulatory effect of TRH on TSH release. The effect of PGs appears to be specific for somatotrophs and thyrotrophs, no effect being detected on LH, FSH, or prolactin release.

Adenohypophyseal Cyclic AMP-Dependent Protein Kinase and Its Protein Substrates

The finding of a cyclic AMP-dependent protein kinase that catalyzes the phosphorylation of phosphorylase kinase (16) and glycogen synthetase (64) with respective stimulation and inhibition of enzymic activity, led to the explanation of how cyclic AMP acts on glycogen metabolism at the chemical level. Convincing evidence supports the hypothesis that, in many systems, cyclic AMP-dependent protein kinase mediates the intracellular effects of the cyclic nucleotide. In fact, besides the well-known effect of cyclic AMP-dependent phosphorylation of phosphorylase kinase and glycogen synthetase, there is evidence that cyclic AMP stimulates the phosphorylation of other physiologically important protein substrates.

Properties of adenohypophyseal protein kinase including interaction of the catalytic and receptor subunits with various nucleotides and GTP, have been described in detail (38,42,47,48). Moreover, cyclic AMP-dependent phosphorylation of proteins from the ribosomes (2), secretory granules (42), plasma membranes (49), and nuclei (30) have been described. This information has been described in recent reviews (39,44).

Proposed Mode of Action of Hypothalamic Hormones in the Anterior Pituitary Gland

The proposed mode of action is based on the following considerations: (a) the characteristics of TRH binding (17,36); (b) the close association between changes of pituitary cyclic AMP levels and specific hormone release under the influence of LH-RH, TRH, and somatostatin (5,7,8,39,41,44); (c) the properties of adenohypophyseal adenylyl cyclase (49), cyclic AMP-dependent protein kinase (38,48); and (d) phosphorylation of adenohypophyseal substrates (2,30,39,49). The mode of action schematically illustrated in Fig. 6 is thus proposed for the three hypothalamic peptides (LH-RH, TRH, and somatostatin) and one catecholamine (dopamine) studied so far. There is extremely convincing physiological and pharmacological evidence for the presence of hypothalamic GH-RH and CRH and indirect observations also suggest that cyclic AMP is involved in their action on GH and ACTH secretion, respectively.

CONCLUSIONS

The observation of a close parallelism between changes of cyclic AMP accumulation and specific hormone release under the influence of two stimulatory hypothalamic hormones (TRH and LH-RH), one inhibitory peptide (somatostatin), and dopamine strongly suggests that the adenylyl cyclase system is involved in the mechanism of action of these three peptides and dopamine in the anterior pituitary gland. Such a mechanism is supported by data obtained on the characteristics of the TRH receptor and properties of adenohypophyseal cyclic AMP-dependent protein kinase and its substrates. Concerning the role of prostaglandins, their action at the pituitary level appears to be limited to the control of GH and TSH secretion.

REFERENCES

1. Barden, N., Bergeron, L., and Betteridge, A. (1976): Effects of prostaglandin synthetase inhibitors and prostaglandin precursors on anterior pituitary cyclic AMP and hormone secretion. In: *Prostaglandin and Thromboxane Research,* edited by B. Samuelsson and R. Paoletti, pp. 341–344. Raven Press, New York.
2. Barden, N., and Labrie, F. (1973): Cyclic adenosine $3',5'$-monophosphate-dependent phosphorylation of ribosomal proteins from bovine anterior pituitary gland. *Biochemistry,* 12:3096–3102.
3. Bélanger, A., Labrie, F., Borgeat, P., Savary, M., Côté, J., Drouin, J., Schally, A. V., Coy, D. H., Coy, E. J., Immer, H., Sestanj, K., Nelson, V., and Götz, M. (1974): Inhibition of

growth hormone and thyrotropin release by growth hormone-release-inhibiting hormone. *Mol. Cell. Endocrinol.,* 1:329–339.

4. Ben-Jonathan, N., Oliver, C., Weiner, H. J., Mical, R. S., and Porter, J. C. (1977): Dopamine in hypophysial portal plasma of the rat during the estrous cycle and throughout pregnancy. *Endocrinology,* 100:452–458.

5. Borgeat, P., Chavancy, G., Dupont, A., Labrie, F., Arimura, A., and Schally, A. V. (1972): Stimulation of adenosine $3',5'$-cyclic monophosphate accumulation in anterior pituitary gland *in vitro* by synthetic luteinizing hormone-releasing hormone. *Proc. Natl. Acad. Sci. USA,* 69:2677–2681.

6. Borgeat, P., Garneau, P., and Labrie, F. (1975): Characteristics of action of prostaglandins on cyclic AMP accumulation in rat anterior pituitary gland. *Can. J. Biochem.,* 53:455–460.

7. Borgeat, P., Labrie, F., Côté, J., Ruel, F., Schally, A. V., Coy, D. H., Coy, E. J., and Yanaihara, N. (1974): Parallel stimulation of cyclic AMP accumulation and LH and FSH release by analogs of LHRH *in vitro. Mol. Cell. Endocrinol.,* 1:7–20.

8. Borgeat, P., Labrie, F., Drouin, J., Bélanger, A., Immer, I., Sestanj, K., Nelson, V., Götz, M., Schally, A. V., Coy, D. H., and Coy, E. J. (1974): Inhibition of adenosine $3',5'$-monophosphate accumulation in anterior pituitary gland *in vitro* by growth hormone release-inhibiting hormone. *Biochem. Biophys. Res. Commun.,* 56:1052–1059.

9. Borgeat, P., Labrie, F., Poirier, G., Chavancy, G., and Schally, A. V. (1973): Stimulation of adenosine $3',5'$-cyclic monophosphate accumulation in anterior pituitary gland by purified growth hormone-releasing hormone. *Trans. Assoc. Am. Physicians,* 86:284–299.

10. Caron, M. G., Beaulieu, M., Raymond, V., Gagné, B., Drouin, J., Lefkowitz, R. J., and Labrie, F. (1978): Dopaminergic receptors in the anterior pituitary gland. Correlation of [^{3}H]dihydroergocryptine binding with the dopaminergic control of prolactin release. *J. Biol. Chem.,* 253:2244–2253.

11. Conn, P. M., Morrell, D. V., Dufau, M. L., and Catt, K. J. (1979): Gonadotropin-releasing hormone action in cultured pituicytes: Independence of luteinizing hormone release and adenosine $3',5'$-monophosphate production. *Endocrinology,* 104:448–453.

12. Cooper, R. H., McPherson, M., and Schofield, J. G. (1972): The effect of prostaglandins on ox pituitary content of adenosine $3':5'$-cyclic monophosphate and the release of growth hormone. *Biochem. J.,* 127:143–154.

13. De Camilli, P., Macconi, D., and Spada, A. (1979): Dopamine inhibits adenylate cyclase in human prolactin-secreting pituitary adenomas. *Nature,* 278:252–254.

14. Deery, D. J., and Howell, S. L. (1973): Rat anterior pituitary adenylyl cyclase activity: GTP requirement of prostaglandin E_1 and E_2 and synthetic luteinizing hormone-releasing hormone activation. *Biochim. Biophys. Acta,* 329:17–22.

15. Deery, D. J., and Jones, A. C. (1975): Effects of hypothalamic extracts, neurotransmitters and synthetic hypothalamic releasing hormones on adenylyl cyclase activity in the lobes of the pituitary of the dogfish (*Scyliorhinus canicula* L.). *J. Endocrinol.,* 64:49–57.

16. DeLange, R. J., Kemp, R. G., Riley, W. D., Cooper, R. A., and Krebs, E. G. (1968): Activation of skeletal muscle phosphorylase kinase by adenosine triphosphate and adenosine $3',5'$-monophosphate. *J. Biol. Chem.,* 243:2200–2208.

17. De Léan, A., Ferland, L., Drouin, J., Kelly, P. A., and Labrie, F. (1977): Modulation of pituitary thyrotropin releasing hormone receptor levels by estrogens and thyroid hormones. *Endocrinology,* 100:1496–1504.

18. Drouin, J., De Léan, A., Rainville, D., Lachance, R., and Labrie, F. (1976): Characteristics of the interactions between thyrotropin-releasing hormone and somatostatin for the thyrotropin and prolactin release. *Endocrinology,* 98:514–521.

19. Drouin, J., Ferland, L., Bernard, J., and Labrie, F. (1976): Site of the *in vivo* stimulatory effect of prostaglandins on LH release. *Prostaglandins,* 11:367–375.

20. Drouin, J., and Labrie, F. (1976): Selective effect of androgens on LH and FSH release in anterior pituitary cells in culture. *Endocrinology,* 98:1528–1534.

21. Drouin, J., and Labrie, F. (1976): Specificity of the stimulatory effect of prostaglandins on hormone release in anterior pituitary cells in culture. *Prostaglandins,* 11:355–365.

22. Drouin, J., Lagacé, L., and Labrie, F. (1976): Estradiol-induced increase of the LH responsiveness to LH releasing hormone (LHRH) in anterior pituitary cells in culture. *Endocrinology,* 99:1477–1481.

23. Ferland, L., Labrie, F., Coy, D. H., Coy, E. J., and Schally, A. V. (1975): Inhibitory activity of four analogs of luteinizing hormone-releasing hormone *in vivo. Fertil. Steril.,* 26:889–893.

24. Guidotti, A., Naik, S. R., and Kurosawa, A. (1977): Possible role of gamma aminobutyric acid (GABA) in the regulation of cAMP system in rat anterior pituitary. *Psychoneuroendocrinology,* 2:227–235.
25. Guidotti, A., Zivkovic, B., and Costa, E. (1974): Possible involvement of cyclic nucleotides in the stimulation of pituitary function elicited by reserpine. In: *Psychoneuroendocrinology,* edited by H. Hatotani, pp. 259–266. Karger, Basel.
26. Hertelendy, F. (1971): Studies on growth hormone secretion. II. Stimulation by prostaglandins *in vitro. Acta Endocrinol. (Kbh.),* 68:355–362.
27. Hertelendy, F., Peake, G. T., and Todd, H. (1971): Studies on growth hormone secretion. III. Inhibition of prostaglandin, theophylline and cyclic AMP stimulated growth hormone release by valinomycin *in vitro. Biochem. Biophys. Res. Commun.,* 44:253–260.
28. Hertelendy, F., Todd, H., Ehrhart, K., and Blute, R. (1972): Studies on growth hormone secretion. IV. *In vivo* effects of prostaglandin E₁. *Prostaglandins,* 2:79–91.
29. Hill, M. K., MacLeod, R. M., and Orcutt, P. (1976): Dibutyryl cyclic AMP, adenosine and guanosine blockade of the dopamine, ergocryptine and apomorphine inhibition of prolactin release *in vitro. Endocrinology,* 99:1612–1617.
30. Jolicoeur, P., and Labrie, F. (1974): Phosphorylation of nuclear proteins from bovine anterior pituitary gland induced by adenosine 3′:5′-monophosphate. *Eur. J. Biochem.,* 48:1–9.
31. Jutisz, M., and Paloma de la Llosa, M. (1970): Requirement of Ca⁺⁺ and Mg⁺⁺ ions for the *in vitro* release of follicle-stimulating hormone from rat pituitary glands and its subsequent biosynthesis. *Endocrinology,* 86:761–768.
32. Kaneko, T., Saito, S., Oka, H., Oda, T., and Yanaihara, N. (1973): Effects of synthetic LH-RH and its analogs on rat anterior pituitary cyclic AMP and LH and FSH release. *Metabolism,* 22:77–80.
33. Kato, Y., Dupre, J., and Beck, J. C. (1973): Plasma growth hormone in the anesthetized rat: Effects of dibutyryl cyclic AMP, prostaglandin E₁, adrenergic agents, vasopressin, chlorpromazine, amphetamine and L-DOPA. *Endocrinology,* 93:135–146.
34. Kebabian, J. W., and Calne, D. B. (1979): Multiple receptors for dopamine. *Nature,* 277:93–96.
35. Kebabian, J. W., Petzold, G. L., and Greengard, P. (1972): Dopamine-sensitive adenylate cyclase in caudate nucleus of rat brain, and its similarity to the "dopamine receptor." *Proc. Natl. Acad. Sci. USA,* 69:2145–2149.
36. Labrie, F., Barden, N., Poirier, G., and De Léan, A. (1972): Binding of thyrotropin-releasing hormone to plasma membranes of bovine anterior pituitary gland. *Proc. Natl. Acad. Sci. USA,* 69:283–287.
37. Labrie, F., Beaulieu, M., Caron, M. G., and Raymond, V. (1978): The adenohypophyseal dopamine receptor: Specificity and modulation of its activity by estradiol. In: *Progress in Prolactin Physiology and Pathology,* edited by C. Robyn and M. Harter, pp. 121–136. Elsevier/North-Holland, Amsterdam.
38. Labrie, F., Béraud, G., Gauthier, M., and Lemay, A. (1971): Actinomycin-insensitive stimulation of protein synthesis in rat anterior pituitary *in vitro* by dibutyryl adenosine 3′,5′-monophosphate. *J. Biol. Chem.,* 246:1902–1908.
39. Labrie, F., Borgeat, P., Lemay, A., Lemaire, S., Barden, N., Drouin, J., Lemaire, I., Jolicoeur, P., and Bélanger, A. (1975): Role of cyclic AMP in the action of hypothalamic regulatory hormones. In: *Advances in Cyclic Nucleotide Research, Vol. 5,* edited by G. I. Drummond, P. Greengard, and G. A. Robison, pp. 787–801. Raven Press, New York.
40. Labrie, F., De Léan, A., Drouin, J., Barden, N., Ferland, L., Borgeat, P., Beaulieu, M., and Morin, O. (1976): New aspects of the mechanism of action of hypothalamic regulatory hormones. In: *Hypothalamus and Endocrine Functions,* edited by F. Labrie, J. Meites, and G. Pelletier, pp. 147–159. Plenum Press, New York.
41. Labrie, F., Di Paolo, T., Raymond, V., Ferland, L., and Beaulieu, M. (1980): The pituitary dopamine receptor. In: *Ergot Compounds and Brain Function,* edited by M. Goldstein, D. B. Calne, A. Lieberman, and M. O. Thorner, pp. 217–227. Raven Press, New York.
42. Labrie, F., Lemaire, S., Poirier, G., Pelletier, G., and Boucher, R. (1971): Adenohypophyseal secretory granules. I. Their phosphorylation and association with protein kinase. *J. Biol. Chem.,* 246:7311–7317.
43. Labrie, F., Pelletier, G., Borgeat, P., Drouin, J., Ferland, L., and Bélanger, A. (1976): Mode of action of hypothalamic regulatory hormones. In: *Frontiers in Neuroendocrinology, Vol. 4,* edited by W. F. Ganong and L. Martini, pp. 63–94. Raven Press, New York.

44. Labrie, F., Pelletier, G., Borgeat, P., Drouin, J., Savary, M., Côté, J., and Ferland, L. (1975): Aspects of the mechanism of action of hypothalamic hormone (LH-RH). In: *Gonadotropins and Gonadal Functions, Vol. 1,* edited by J. A. Thomas and R. L. Singhal, pp. 77–127. University Park Press, Baltimore.

45. Labrie, F., Pelletier, G., Lemay, A., Borgeat, P., Barden, N., Dupont, A., Savary, M., Côté, J., and Boucher, R. (1973): Control of protein synthesis in anterior pituitary gland. *Acta Endocrinol. [Suppl.] (Kbh.),* 180:301–340.

46. Labrie, F., Savary, M., Coy, D. H., Coy, E. J., and Schally, A. V. (1976): Inhibition of luteinzing hormone release by analogs of luteinizing hormone-releasing hormone (LH-RH) *in vitro. Endocrinology,* 98:289–294.

47. Lemaire, S., Labrie, F., and Gauthier, M. (1974): Adenosine 3',5'-monophosphate-dependent protein kinase from bovine anterior pituitary gland. III. Structural specificity of the ATP site of the catalytic subunit. *Can. J. Biochem.,* 52:137–141.

48. Lemaire, S., Pelletier, G., and Labrie, F. (1971): Adenosine 3',5'-monophosphate-dependent protein kinase from bovine anterior pituitary gland. II. Subcellular distribution. *J. Biol. Chem.,* 246:7303–7310.

49. Lemay, A., Deschenes, M., Lemaire, S., Poirier, G., Poulin, L., and Labrie, F. (1974): Phosphorylation of adenohypophyseal plasma membranes and properties of associated protein kinase. *J. Biol. Chem.,* 249:323–328.

50. Lemay, A., and Labrie, F. (1972): Calcium dependent stimulation of prolactin release in rat anterior pituitary *in vitro* by N^6-monobutyryl adenosine 3',5'-monophosphate. *FEBS Lett.,* 20:7–10.

51. MacLeod, R. M., and Lehmeyer, J. F. (1970): Release of pituitary growth hormone by prostaglandins and dibutyryl adenosine cyclic 3':5'-monophosphate in the absence of protein synthesis. *Proc. Natl. Acad. Sci. USA,* 67:1172–1179.

52. MacLeod, R. M., and Lehmeyer, J. E. (1974): Restoration of prolactin synthesis and release by the administration of monoaminergic blocking agents to pituitary tumor-bearing rats. *Cancer Res.,* 34:345–350.

53. Makino, T. (1973): Study of the intracellular mechanism of LH release in the anterior pituitary. *Am. J. Obstet. Gynecol.,* 115:606–614.

54. McCann, S. R., Ojeda, P. G., Harms, J. E., Wheaton, D. K., Sundberg, K., and Fawcett, G. P. (1976): Role of prostaglandins (PGs) in the control of adenophpophyseal hormone secretion. In: *Hypothalamus and Endocrine Functions,* edited by F. Labrie, J. Meites and G. Pelletier, pp. 21–36. Plenum Press, New York.

55. McCullagh, D. R. (1932): Dual endocrine activity of the testis. *Science,* 76:19–20.

56. Nagasawa, H., and Yanai, R. (1972): Promotion of pituitary prolactin release in rats by dibutyryl adenosine 3',5'-monophosphate. *J. Endocrinol.,* 55:215–216.

57. Naor, F., Koch, Y., Bauminger, S., and Zor, U. (1975): Action of luteinizing hormone-releasing hormone and synthesis of prostaglandin in the pituitary gland. *Prostaglandins,* 9:211–219.

58. Naor, Z., Koch, Y., Chobsieng, P., and Zor, U. (1975): Pituitary cyclic AMP production and mechanism of luteinizing hormone release. *FEBS Lett.,* 58:318–321.

59. Naor, Z., Zor, U., Meidan, R., and Koch, Y. (1978): Sex difference in pituitary cyclic AMP response to gonadotropin-releasing hormone. *J. Physiol.,* 235:E37–E41.

60. Ratner, A. (1970): Stimulation of luteinizing hormone release *in vitro* by dibutyryl-cyclic AMP and theophylline. *Life Sci.,* 9:1221–1226.

61. Ratner, A., Wilson, M. C., Srivastava, L., and Peake, G. T. (1974): Stimulatory effects of prostaglandin E_1 on rat anterior pituitary cyclic AMP and luteinizing hormone release. *Prostaglandins,* 5:165–171.

62. Samli, M. H., and Lai, M.-F. (1973): Protein synthesis in the rat anterior pituitary. III. The fate of total protein, prolactin and growth hormone labeled in an *in vitro* incubation. *Endocrinology,* 93:767–776.

63. Sato, T., Hirono, M., Jyujo, T., Ieseka, T., Taya, K., and Igarashi, M. (1975): Direct action of prostaglandins on rat pituitary. *Endocrinology,* 96:45–49.

64. Schlender, K. K., Wei, S. H., and Villar-Palassi, C. (1969): UDP-glucose:glycogen α-4-glucosyltransferase I kinase activity of purified muscle protein kinase: Cyclic nucleotide specificity. *Biochim. Biophys. Acta,* 191:272–278.

65. Schofield, J. G. (1970): Prostaglandin E_1 and the release of growth hormone *in vitro. Nature,* 228:179–180.

66. Shaar, C. J., and Clemens, J. A. (1974): The role of catecholamines in the release of anterior pituitary prolactin *in vitro. Endocrinology,* 95:1202–1212.
67. Sundberg, D. K., Fawcett, C. P., and McCann, S. M. (1976): The involvement of cyclic 3′,5′-cyclic AMP in the release of hormones from the anterior pituitary *in vitro. Proc. Soc. Exp. Biol. Med.,* 151:149–154.
68. Takahara, J., Arimura, A., and Schally, A. V. (1974): Suppression of prolactin release by a purified porcine PIF preparation and catecholamines infused into a rat hypophysial portal vessel. *Endocrinology,* 95:462–465.
69. Vale, W., Grant, G., Amoss, M., Blackwell, R., and Guillemin, R. (1972): Culture of enzymatically dispersed pituitary cells: Functional validation of a method. *Endocrinology,* 91:562–572.
70. Wakabayashi, K., Date, Y., and Tamaoki, B. (1973): On the mechanism of action of luteinizing hormone-releasing hormone factor and prolactin release inhibiting factor. *Endocrinology,* 92:698–704.
71. Zor, U., Kaneko, T., Schneider, H. P. G., McCann, S. M., and Field, J. B. (1970): Further studies of stimulation of anterior pituitary cyclic adenosine 3′,5′-monophosphate formation by hypothalamic extract and prostaglandins. *J. Biol. Chem.,* 245:2883–2888.
72. Zor, U., Kaneko, T., Schneider, H. P. G., McCann, S. M., Lowe, I. P., Bloom, S., Borland, B., and Field, J. B. (1969): Stimulation of anterior pituitary adenyl cyclase activity and adenosine 3′:5′-cyclic phosphate by hypothalamic extract and prostaglandin E_1. *Proc. Natl. Acad. Sci. USA,* 63:918–925.

Polypeptide Hormones, edited by
R. F. Beers, Jr. and E. G. Bassett.
Raven Press, New York © 1980.

23. Clinical Applications of Hypothalamic Regulatory Peptides

Michael O. Thorner

*Department of Internal Medicine, University of Virginia School of Medicine,
Charlottesville, Virginia 22908*

INTRODUCTION

The hypothesis proposed by Harris and colleagues 39 years ago that the control of pituitary secretion was mediated by the synthesis and release into the hypothalamo-hypophyseal portal capillaries of hypothalamic regulatory factors (39,46,102) was finally proven with the isolation, characterization, and synthesis of three hypothalamic regulatory hormones. This was achieved by the perseverance and ingenuity of the groups of Guillemin and Schally. In this chapter, I shall review some results of studies in both laboratory animals and man that have been performed using these hormones.

The overall relationship of the hypothalamus to the pituitary and target organs is summarized in Fig. 1. Besser (6) has emphasized two important characteristics of this relationship that he has termed the "hypothalamic pituitary amplifier":

(a) The *integrative nature* of the neuroendocrine connection such that neurological input from higher centers enables circadian rhythms to be maintained, reflex hormonal responses to take place, and appropriate hormonal responses to stress; and

(b) *"Cascade amplification"* such that minute quantities of hypothalamic hormones cause release of larger quantities of pituitary hormones that, in turn, lead to release of even larger quantities of target gland hormone secretion. The latter system has the advantage of permitting modulation at any level; thus, the target gland secretion may feedback in a negative (or positive) manner at the next higher one, two, or three levels, e.g., thyroid hormone at the pituitary, hypothalamus, and higher centers to ultimately inhibit thyrotropin-releasing hormone (TRH) and thyrotropin (TSH) secretion. Furthermore, the pituitary hormones may themselves feedback at the hypothalamus or higher centers to produce "short-loop feedback" systems.

After the isolation and synthesis of these hypothalamic hormones, specific antibodies were raised to enable the development of radioimmunoassays (RIAs) and for immunohistochemical studies to measure levels of, and map the distribution respectively, of these peptides. Such studies have shown these peptides,

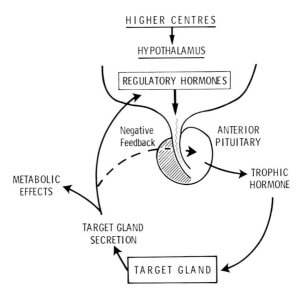

FIG. 1. Diagrammatic representation of the relationships between hypothalamic regulatory hormones and target organs. (From ref. 42.)

initially believed to be specific to the hypothalamus, to be more widely distributed throughout the body and thus may be better considered in a more general sense as *peptide neurotransmitters* rather than simply hypothalamic regulatory hormones. Although the question of opioid peptides is timely, these will be omitted since the 11th Miles Symposium was devoted, at least in part, to that subject. Furthermore, the nature of the opioid peptides in the hypothalamus is still unclear as is their physiological function.

The three peptides that I shall address are thyrotropin-releasing hormone, gonadotropin-releasing hormone (GnRH), and growth hormone release-inhibiting hormone (somatostatin), giving particular emphasis to their role in the control of anterior pituitary hormone secretion.

THYROTROPIN-RELEASING HORMONE

Thyrotropin-releasing hormone was the first hypothalamic regulatory hormone to be isolated, characterized, and synthesized (15,41,79,98). TRH is a tripeptide containing glutamic acid, histidine, and proline in the form of L-pyroglutamyl-L-histidyl-L-prolinamide. The synthetic hormone is biologically effective *in vivo* in man and laboratory animals and is indistinguishable from that found in porcine, ovine, and human hypothalami (96).

To maintain the euthyroid state, TRH is secreted by the hypothalamus to stimulate the synthesis and release of thyrotropin from the pituitary that, in turn, stimulates thyroxine synthesis by the thyroid gland. Thyroxine is the predominant secretory product from the thyroid although triiodothyronine (T_3), the major metabolically active thyroid hormone, is also secreted by the thyroid; however, a major portion of T_3 is derived from peripheral monodeiodination of thyroxine. In the euthyroid state the pituitary is exquisitely sensitive to exogenous TRH. However, very small changes in circulating thyroid hormone levels may lead to marked changes in the thyrotrope sensitivity. Thus, changes of T_3 levels within the normal range, by administration of thyroid hormone (104) or iodide (92) to raise and lower thyroid hormone levels, respectively, profoundly alter pituitary thyrotrope responsiveness to TRH. Burger and Patel (13) have concluded from such data that T_3 may be the physiological modulator of the TSH response to TRH and that small changes in thyroid hormone levels, even within the normal range, may lead to marked changes in the response of the thyrotrope to TRH.

The clinical application of TRH is, from a practical point of view, the greatest of any of the hypothalamic regulatory hormones. From the discussion above, it is clear that minor degrees of thyroid dysfunction will be associated with major changes in thyrotrope sensitivity. Thyrotoxicosis is almost never due to hypothalamic-pituitary disease, but either to an adenoma of the thyroid or, more commonly, to Graves' disease, where the thyroid is stimulated by human thyroid-stimulating immunoglobulins. In Fig. 2, the patterns of circulating TSH responses to TRH administration (200 μg intravenously) are shown. Blood samples were drawn before and at 20 and 60 min after TRH injection in a group of normal subjects, patients with thyrotoxicosis, and those with primary hypothyroidism. The peak level of serum TSH was seen at 20 min and fell by 60 min. The presence of elevated peripheral thyroid hormone levels (as in thyrotoxicosis) results in increased negative feedback and extinction of the thyrotrope's ability to respond to TRH. Low levels of thyroid hormone, (as in primary hypothyroidism) are associated with reduced negative feedback, elevated basal TSH levels, and exaggerated TSH responses (84). In patients with equivocal hyperthyroidism, particularly before the days of serum T_3 RIAs, T_3 suppression tests were performed. This test has been replaced by the TRH test that shows suppressed TSH levels after TRH in patients whose radioactive iodine uptake does not suppress with exogenous T_3 (13). However, in patients with hypothyroidism, it is essential to measure the peripheral TSH levels to distinguish between primary and secondary (due to hypothalamic/pituitary disease) hypothyroidism. Clearly, a markedly elevated serum TSH level (greater than 20 μU/ml) obviates the need for a TRH test. However, it should be stressed that mildly elevated TSH levels may occur in secondary hypothyroidism. The delayed TSH response to TRH (peak level observed at 60 rather than 20 min) in patients with hypothalamic disease was initially thought to be pathognomonic of hypothalamic dysfunction (45). However, it is now clear that normal, delayed, impaired, or even exaggerated response may occur in patients with any form of hypothalamic/pituitary disease (29,85), and a delayed response may also be seen in some patients with primary hypothyroidism.

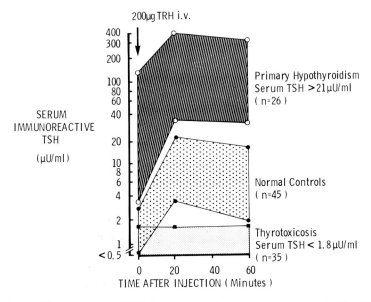

FIG. 2. Serum TSH response to TRH in normal controls, and in patients with thyrotoxicosis and primary hypothyroidism (values at **right** refer to levels 20 min after TRH). (From ref. 42.)

Therapeutic applications of TRH are limited, particularly since thyroid hormone is inexpensive and simple to administer orally. However, in view of the distribution of TRH outside the hypothalamus (50), several groups have investigated its other biological properties. Some initial reports suggested it to be effective in treating depression (53,89) and also to have a role in the treatment of Parkinsonism (70), but neither has been confirmed (18,44,78). One group has used TRH to enhance TSH secretion to augment radioactive iodine uptake in the treatment of thyroid carcinoma (26) but this has not been widely applied.

TRH is also a highly potent stimulator of prolactin release both *in vitro* (105) and *in vivo* (11,19,52,83). In some patients with primary hypothyroidism, prolactin levels are elevated; however, with thyroid hormone replacement therapy, TSH levels suppress more readily and prolactin levels may take several months to return to the normal range.

The physiological role of TRH in control of prolactin release is yet to be established, since prolactin levels may rise independently of TSH, e.g., during suckling (35) and sleep. Immunization of sheep agonist TRH led to marked alterations in TSH secretions and thyroid status, but only minor alterations in prolactin secretion (A. S. McNeilly, *personal communication*), suggesting that it may indeed have a physiological role. It has been proposed that the prolactin response to TRH may be a useful index for the presence or absence of a pituitary tumor (19); however, in our and others' experience neither the absence of the response to TRH nor its presence confirms or excludes the diagnosis of tumor in these patients (47,51,61,108).

HYPOTHALAMIC REGULATORY PEPTIDES

GONADOTROPIN-RELEASING HORMONE

The second hypothalamic regulatory hormone to be isolated (95) characterized (69,80), and synthesized (68) was GnRH, the decapeptide pyroGlu-His-Trp-Ser-Tyr-Gly-Leu-Arg-Pro-Gly-NH$_2$. It was subsequently isolated and characterized in sheep hypothalamus, where the structure was identical to porcine GnRH (14). Although initially based on biological assays, it was believed that there were two distinct and separate releasing hormones for luteinizing hormone (LH) and follicle-stimulating hormone (FSH), it now seems clear that the decapeptide gonadotropin releasing hormone is responsible for the release of both LH and FSH (97). This especially makes sense since LH and FSH are probably secreted by the same cells in the pituitary and may occur even within the same secretory granules (72). In all *in vitro* systems, the decapeptide releases both LH and FSH and the proportions in which they are released is dependent on the characteristics of the system. Furthermore, *in vivo* the GnRH is effective in releasing gonadotropins in a variety of species ranging from avian to primate (94).

GnRH is responsible for the synthesis and release of LH and FSH by the pituitary to stimulate the gonad. Its importance is exemplified by the observations reviewed by Schally and Arimura (94). Rabbits immunized to GnRH who developed antibodies demonstrated testicular atrophy and azospermia associated with *reduction* of the pituitary content of LH. Passive immunization of rats with GnRH antibodies prevents the post-castration rise of LH and FSH and prevents the development of "castration cells" in the pituitary. Furthermore, in a variety of female rodents, depending on the timing of the passive transfer of antibodies, either follicular development or the proestrus rise of gonadotropins can be prevented.

Using bioassays and RIAs for GnRH, several groups have reported changes in peripheral circulating levels in women at different stages of the menstrual cycle (3,67). However, Mortimer and colleagues were unable to show consistent changes (76). Several reports of immunoreactive GnRH levels in the hypothalamo-hypophyseal portal blood have been published and there appears to be no agreement as to whether even in portal blood there are changes at different phases of the menstrual estrus cycle or after gonadectomy (Table 1).

The gonadotropin response in the human to exogenous GnRH depends on the developmental status of the patient, the presence or absence of gonads, and the hormonal environment. In the prepubertal child, GnRH leads to a greater FSH than LH release (31,54). However, as puberty progresses, the LH response increases and becomes greater than that of FSH (32). In the adult, LH (and to a lesser extent FSH) is secreted in an asynchronous pulsatile fashion; in boys the nocturnal rise in LH seen in puberty disappears with maturity.

In women the basal gonadotropin levels vary depending on the state of the menstrual cycle. Using very small doses of GnRH, Yen and colleagues have been able to define changes in pituitary sensitivity and pools at different stages of the menstrual cycle, which probably reflect the results of feedback effects. These changes are reviewed in depth by Yen (111).

TABLE 1. GnRH levels in portal blood[a]

Species	Sex	Stage of cycle	Time (hr)	Portal blood GnRH (pg/ml)	Reference
Rat	F	Estrus	1400		25
		Diestrus	to	50–55	
		Oöphorectomized	1700		
		Proestrus	1400–1700	< 12	
	M	Intact	1100	30–35	25
			to		
		Castrate	1400	50–65	
Rat	F	Diestrus	1800	54 ± 11	28
		Proestrus	0900	92 ± 18	
			1300	73 ± 28	
			1400–1600	46 ± 5	
			1800	107 ± 29	
		Estrus	1800	43 ± 10	
Monkey	F	Follicular		20–75	16
		Mid-cycle		800	
Monkey	F	Follicular		66 ± 6.6	17
		Oöphorectomized	(1 month)	51 ± 5.3	
Monkey	F	Follicular		23 ± 5	81
		Preovulatory		104 ± 34	
		Oöphorectomized	(0.5 or 3 months)	19/32	
			(18 months)	100/226	

[a] Cannulation of portal vessels and anesthesia may affect GnRH levels.

Very early studies with administration of purified porcine GnRH resulted in a rise in gonadotropins in men and women (55,56). Subsequently, when the synthetic decapeptide became available, many groups developed tests for LH and FSH reserve. Mortimer and colleagues studied 155 patients and found that only 9 of 137 hypogonadal patients with hypothalamic/pituitary disease lacked gonadotropin responses to GnRH. Some of the most exciting data on the mode of action and physiological secretion of the gonadotropins has been collected in clinical studies and in some elegant studies performed by Knobil and colleagues in monkeys. In many patients with hypothalamic/pituitary disease, the gonadal dysfunction is due to hyperprolactinemia rather than frank gonadotropin deficiency (2,33,107). They also found that patients with primary gonadal disease had exaggerated gonadotropin responses to GnRH. Tests utilizing the single intravenous bolus dose of GnRH (100 μg) are unable to distinguish between a hypothalamic and/or a pituitary site of gonadotropin deficiency; however, therapy for 1 week or longer with GnRH followed by a repeat test appears to distinguish those patients with intact gonadotropes from those with presumed pituitary destruction (74,75,103).

Isolated Gonadotropin Deficiency

Isolated gonadotropin deficiency is one of nature's most interesting experiments. The use of GnRH therapy in this condition has yielded insight into the pathophysiology of isolated gonadotropin deficiency. Furthermore, the lessons learned from attempting to treat this condition with GnRH have highlighted the complexity and sophistication of the hypothalamic-pituitary-gonadal axis. Patients with isolated gonadotropin deficiency have normal hypothalamic/pituitary function with the exception of gonadotropin secretion. Their development is normal except that at puberty gonadal development does not proceed nor do secondary sexual characteristics appear. Many of these patients have anosmia (Kalman's syndrome). Mortimer, McNeilly, and Besser (74,75) treated a group of six patients having an isolated gonadotropin deficiency with GnRH, 500 μg subcutaneously every 8 hr, for many months. Potency was restored in between 2 and 17 days even before there was a rise in androgen levels suggesting that, as in the rat, GnRH may have behavioral effects. Two of these patients were treated from 12 to 18 months. Before treatment low or undetectable LH and FSH levels were present with low androgen levels. During therapy the patients' LH and FSH response patterns changed as seen in a normal child going through puberty—a prepubertal response (FSH > LH) was seen followed by achievement of an adult pattern wherein LH > FSH. The testes increased in size and pubertal development progressed. Interestingly, the FSH response fell before spermatozoa were seen on semen analysis. One woman with isolated gonadotropin deficiency was also treated with the same regimen for 1 and then for 4 months. Cyclical increases in 24 hr total urinary estrogens, but no ovulation or menstruation, resulted. However, Rabin and colleagues, using a different regimen of 1 mg twice daily have had very disappointing results. The explanation for the discrepancy may be partially explained in the studies reported by Crowley and colleagues (21), who treated four men with isolated gonadotropin deficiency with a long-acting analog of GnRH (D-Trp⁶-Pro⁹-NEt-LRF) in a dose of 50 μg every 2 days. They developed changes of puberty similar to those described by Mortimer and colleagues. However, normal testosterone levels and full puberty were not achieved. They, therefore, increased the frequency of administration to 50 μg daily. Instead of increasing the response, they observed a decline in gonadotropin levels and reversal of the increase in testicular size previously noted. When the frequency of administration was kept constant, but the dose decreased to 10 μg daily, development proceded once more. However, the optimal gonadotropin responses were seen not with the superactive analog, but with a pulsatile regimen previously employed by Knobil and colleages in monkeys, using synthetic GnRH. Administration of a 6-min pulse each 2 hr for 7 days of the natural synthetic GnRH (50 ng/kg) produced far higher levels of FSH than ever seen during analog therapy. Thus, it is clear that isolated gonadotropin deficiency is, in many cases, not due to an abnormality at the pituitary level, but is more likely due to an abnormality in GnRH synthesis and/or release. Furthermore, patients with structural or functional derangement of hypothalamic function, e.g., with craniopharyngiomas or anorexia nervosa show similar responses to GnRH therapy (74,75,82). However, the ovulatory response in women has been poor except in those patients who have only very mild dysfunction and are clomiphene responsive (101,113,114). In general, GnRH therapy requires supplementation with HCG to produce normal luteal function (82).

At present therapy with GnRH is not optimal, either with the natural hormone or with long-acting analogs. The reasons for these rather disappointing results may be explained by the very sophisticated and elegant studies of Knobil and colleagues. Their experimental model was the adult female rhesus monkey. These monkeys were submitted to radiofrequency lesions of the arcuate nucleus that effectively prevented synthesis and secretion of GnRH and thus lowered plasma gonadotropins and abolished the positive feedback of estrogen. These monkeys had previously undergone oophorectomy and were then infused for 14 days with GnRH (6 μg/hr) either as a continuous infusion or in one 6-min pulse/ hr (4). The LH and FSH levels rose during the first 24 hr in the monkeys exposed to the continuous infusions, but then fell progressively. In contrast, the monkeys exposed to the pulses showed increasing LH and FSH secretion and maintained high levels for as long as they were exposed to GnRH. In these experiments, both experimental groups were exposed to the same total dose of GnRH. Thus, the mode of exposure is critical to the pattern of response. Furthermore, in another group of female monkeys, whose ovaries were not removed, but who also had arcuate nucleus lesions and were exposed to a 6-min pulse/hr regimen of GnRH for 3 months, regular menstrual cycles of 29–33 days in four of the seven animals developed; furthermore, these monkeys had normal luteal phases as documented by a rise in serum progesterone (58). It is, therefore, clear that if GnRH is administered in an appropriate, albeit intermittent regimen, on a minute-to-minute basis but constant in terms of the cycle, normal ovulatory function may be restored, at least in the rhesus monkey. GnRH acts as a permissive but essential component of the control of the female reproductive cycle. However, the ovary dictates its own gonadotropin requirements by feedback at the pituitary level (58).

The implications of these studies are that for successful clinical therapy, GnRH will have to be given in a pulsatile fashion; thus, perhaps long-acting analogs will not hold promise for the treatment of hypogonadotropic hypogonadism. Perhaps a superactive, short-acting analog would be optimal to enable it to be given intranasally and only in small quantities for cost containment.

As mentioned above, there is an increase in potency within a few days in the boys treated with GnRH for hypogonadism, at a time well before any substantial change in gonadal steroid levels occurred. In the rat sexual behavior was induced in oophorectomized, hypophysectomized rats, suggesting a direct effect of GnRH on this behavior (77,87). However, in a double-blind study in patients with psychogenic impotence, no salutory effects were observed (23).

Children with delayed puberty or boys with undescended testes have posed both diagnostic and therapeutic problems for pediatric endocrinologists. In the past, initiation of puberty or descent of the testes has been achieved with the use of injections of human chorionic gonadotropins. More recently, a more physiological approach of the use of GnRH has achieved excellent results (34, 49,91).

Antigonadal Effects

The understanding of the structure-activity relationships and metabolism of GnRH has enabled several groups to develop analogs of GnRH that are superactive or have blocking activity. These have been reviewed by Schally and Arimura (94) and Guillemin (40). However, as indicated above, the regimen by which GnRH is administered is extremely important and it is clear that superactive agonists are capable of having antigonadal effects both in laboratory animals and in man (57,60,112). Not only do they lead to "down regulation" of the pituitary GnRH receptors to reduce gonadotropin release (93), but there is some evidence, albeit conflicting, that GnRH agonists may also have direct effects at the gonadal level to block the action of the gonadotropins (48,57,59, 60,93). Male rats treated with high doses of GnRH or several GnRH analogs developed testicular atrophy and gonadotropin deficiency together with a rise in prolactin concentrations (59). Female rats treated in the initial days of pregnancy or at mid-gestation with a superactive GnRH analog led to the interruption of pregnancy with resorption of the fetuses (9). Furthermore, normal women treated throughout the cycle with a superactive GnRH analog became amenorrheic (S. J. Nillius, *personal communication*) and injection of two doses of a single analog, one for each of two days at mid-cycle, led to shortening of the luteal phase in normal women (112). Similar effects have been described with five injections of GnRH (250 μg) 4-hourly in the luteal phase of the cycle (62). Thus, perhaps there is no need for antigonadotropic analogs—the superactive analogs may be equally or even more effective, particularly if, as it now appears, they may act at the gonadal level as well. These peptides may lead to new approaches to the problem of contraception, particularly if they are effective after ovulation and fertilization have occurred, i.e., to inhibit or interrupt implantation.

GROWTH HORMONE RELEASE-INHIBITING HORMONE (SOMATOSTATIN)

Somatostatin was the third hypothalamic regulatory hormone to be isolated (12,99), characterized, and synthesized (20,90). Its widespread distribution outside the hypothalamus, in the brain (with the exception of the cerebellum), the gut (88), stomach, and pancreas (D cells) (64,88) emphasizes that it should be considered as a peptide neurotransmitter rather than a hormone, although it subserves a hormonal function in the inhibition of growth hormone (GH) release. It is a tetradecapeptide with a cyclic structure:

H-Ala-Gly-Cys-Lys-Asn-Phe-Trp-Lys-Thr-Phe-Thr-Ser-Cys-OH

The isolation and characterization of somatostatin depended on its growth hormone release-inhibiting effects. However, it is now recognized that somatostatin is capable of inhibiting secretion of many, but not all, hormones. The effects of somatostatin in man are summarized in Table 2 and references for these effects may be found in the excellent review by Gomez-Pan and Hall (38).

The discussion of the clinical applications of somatostatin will be limited to its uses in acromegaly, diabetes, and in certain tumors. However, review of its widespread effects (see Table 2) indicates that it is not a practical therapeutic agent in its present form. The studies performed in man indicate that it is effective in decreasing GH secretion when infused at a rate of 1.3 μg/min or greater (43). Unfortunately, it is very short acting and the effects wear off within 5 min (43) after the termination of an infusion. Intravenous, intramuscular, or subcutaneous injections of 500 μg somatostatin produced suppression of GH that persisted for less than 2 hr. This effect could be prolonged for 4 to

TABLE 2. *Effects of somatostatin on hormone secretion in man[a]*

	Normal subject		Pathological hypersecretion
	Basal	Stimulated	
Anterior pituitary hormones			
Growth hormone	↓[b]	↓	↓
Thyrotropin	↓	↓	↓
Luteinizing hormone	→[c]	→	
Follicle stimulating hormone	→	→	
Prolactin	→	→	→↓
Corticotropin	→	→	↓
Pancreas			
Insulin	↓	↓	↓
Glucagon	↓	↓	↓
Gut			
Pepsin	↓		
Gastrin	↓	↓	↓
Cholecystokinin	↓		
Secretin	↓		
Vasoactive intestinal peptide			↓
Enteroglucagon	↓		
Motilin	↓		
Pancreatic polypeptide	↓		
Gastric inhibiting peptide			
Hydrochloric acid (stomach)	↓	↓	↓
Other systems			
Renin	↓		
Salivary amylase	↓		
Thyroxine triodothyronine	→		
Steroid secretion by adrenal or gonads (12)	→		

[a] References for these effects may be found in the excellent review, ref. 38.
[b] ↓ Secretion inhibited.
[c] → No change in secretion.

5 hr by giving somatostatin as a protamine zinc suspension (7). In normal man, both spontaneous and stimulated GH secretion, e.g., by exercise, hypoglycemia, arginine, levodopa) may be inhibited by somatostatin (reviewed in ref. 38).

In acromegalic patients, somatostatin infusions suppress GH levels for as long as the infusion continues. However, within 30 min of discontinuing the infusion, GH levels rise. We have performed 28-hr infusions of somatostatin in a number of acromegalic patients. During these infusions, GH levels fell and remained suppressed, even during meals and sleep, and there was a fall in urinary GH (8). There were also changes in insulin and glucagon secretion associated with changes in blood sugar (7,8,43). The monomeric, biologically most active form of GH was preferentially suppressed by somatostatin (5).

In normal subjects, insulin and glucagon levels are also suppressed by somatostatin infusions, with a resulting fall in blood sugar concentration (24). This effect can be prevented by infusing physiological doses of glucagon (1). It appears, therefore, that glucagon is physiologically important in maintaining normal fasting blood sugar levels. However, when Mortimer and colleagues infused somatostatin into a patient with an insulinoma, not only did the insulin levels fall, but also the glucagon levels decreased and the patient became even more profoundly hypoglycemic (73).

Somatostatin infusion has been used experimentally to suppress gastrin levels in patients with the Zollinger-Ellison syndrome (10), vasoactive intestinal peptide in Verner-Morrison syndrome (63), and to suppress insulin (22) and glucagon (73) in β and α cell tumors of pancreas as well as pancreatic polypeptide in a tumor secreting that hormone. However, the availablility of safe and effective histamine-2 blocking drugs has obviated the need for its use in the Zollinger-Ellison syndrome. Although somatostatin may be useful in the short-term to prepare a patient for surgery for removal of one of these gastrointestinal or pancreatic tumors, it is of no use in long-term therapy due to its short half-life, widespread effects, and the need to administer it parenterally.

Unger and Orci have suggested that the hyperglycemia in diabetes mellitus is due not only to insulin deficiency, but also to glucagon excess (109). This is supported by studies of glucagon levels in diabetic patients. Thus, as might be expected, insulin therapy, together with suppression of glucagon by somatostatin in patients with diabetes, leads to a fall in blood sugar levels, improvement in glucose tolerance, and diabetic control (36); insulin requirements fall by approximately 50% (71). Furthermore, ketoacidosis may be prevented by somatostatin infusions (37), but once established it cannot be reversed by somatostatin alone (65). At the present time, somatostatin in its natural form has little therapeutic role apart from the rare patient with a gastrointestinal or pancreatic tumor needing preparation for surgery. However, somatostatin has served as an extremely useful research tool for suppression of a variety of hormones to investigate their physiological role, e.g., glucagon. Two further observations are worthy of note:

(a) The many effects and widespread distribution of somatostatin make it clear that the reported effects of somatostatin infusions, during which circulating levels of somatostatin in the peripheral blood are at least 10- to 100-fold higher than those normally observed, may well be pharmacologic effects (110). However, if somatostatin is considered part of the paracrine system, [as proposed by Feyrter (27) with local release and only a short distance for diffusion] then its physiological role in so many different hormonal systems may more easily be understood. Somatostatin neurons appear to be clearly part of the amine precursor uptake and decarboxylation (APUD) system proposed by Pearse (86); confirmatory evidence is the observation that somatostatin has been found in a thymic "carcinoid" tumor that secreted ACTH and GnRH.

(b) It is conceivable that somatostatin receptors on the various endocrine cells may differ. It may, therefore, be possible to develop analogs specific for inhibition of a single hormone, e.g., GH or glucagon. Although such analogs have been described, the author is skeptical that they will show sufficient specificity to be of therapeutic value.

MODEL OF AN ANALOG OF A HYPOTHALAMIC REGULATORY HORMONE: BROMOCRIPTINE AND PROLACTIN SECRETION

It is generally accepted that one and probably the most important factor controlling prolactin secretion is the catecholamine, dopamine (66,100). Prolactin is unique among the anterior pituitary hormones in that it is under tonic hypothalamic inhibition. Dopamine is secreted by the tuberoinfundibular neurons into the portal capillaries to be transported to and finally to act directly on the pituitary to inhibit prolactin release. Schelesnyak noted that certain ergot alkaloids inhibit prolactin release and Flückiger took this observation and developed a drug, bromocriptine, that was potent in its prolactin lowering effect, but devoid of the toxic cardiovascular and oxytocic effect of its parent compound, ergokryptine (30). Only later was it discovered to act by stimulating dopamine receptors and recently thereafter did firm data become available to suggest dopamine to be the physiologically relevant prolactin inhibiting factor. The most common hypothalamic pituitary disease is, in fact, hyperprolactinemia, which may be associated with gonadal dysfunction.

Bromocriptine is effective in lowering pathologically elevated prolactin levels after a single oral dose. During chronic treatment it sustains suppression of prolactin into the normal range and allows recovery of gonadal function.

Dopamine, like somatostatin and the other hypothalamic regulatory hormones, is widely distributed throughout the body (106). Bromocriptine, a functional orally effective analog of dopamine, mimics the effect of the hypothalamic dopamine and lowers prolactin levels to normal, resulting in a restoration of normal pituitary and gonadal functions. However, dopamine is not a peptide. Furthermore, its effects are not "down regulated," at least at the clinical level. The story of the successful use of bromocriptine gives us a perspective into what might be achieved when physiologically active analogs (physical or functional) of the hypothalamic regulatory hormones become available. The data derived from the studies of GnRH suggest that perhaps the receptor mechanism on the gonadotrope may not be as easy to manipulate as the dopamine receptor on the lactotrope; furthermore, the extra-pituitary antigonadotropic effects of GnRH at the gonadal level pose further problems. However, the first synthetic hypothalamic regulatory hormone has been available for physiological and clinical studies for only the past 8 years, and the progress made in their use is remarkable. Neuroendocrinology as a science is here to stay and to progress. It will eventually achieve its rightful place as one, if not the most important functional system of organization of higher organisms in clinical medicine— not only in endocrinology but also in neurology, psychiatry, gastroenterology, cardiology, and gynecology, to mention just a few disciplines.

REFERENCES

1. Alford, F. P., Bloom, S. R., Nabarro, J. D. N., Hall, R., Besser, G. M., Coy, D. H., Kastin, A. J., and Schally, A. V. (1974): Glucagon control of fasting glucose in man. *Lancet,* 2:974–976.
2. Antunes, J. L., Housepian, E. H., Frantz, D. A., Holub, D. A., Hui, R. M., Carmel, P. W., and Quest, D. O. (1977): Prolactin-secreting pituitary tumors. *Ann. Neurol.,* 2:148–153.
3. Arimura, A., Kastin, A. J., and Schally, A. V. (1974): Immunoreactive LH-releasing hormone in plasma: Midcycle elevation in women. *J. Clin. Endocrinol. Metab.,* 38:510–513.
4. Belchetz, P. E., Nakai, Y., Keogh, E. J., Plant, T. M., and Knobil, E. (1978): Pituitary responses to pulsatile and continuous luteinizing hormone releasing hormone (LH-RH) stimulation. *Fed. Proc.,* 37:225(Abstr. 69).
5. Benker, G., Mortimer, C. H., Chait, A., Lowry, P. J., Besser, G. M., Coy, D. H., Kastin, A. J., and Schally, A. V. (1975): Heterogeneity of human growth hormone in plasma and urine: Influence of growth hormone-release inhibiting hormone. *Acta Endocrinol. [Suppl.], (Kbh.),* S193:72.
6. Besser, G. M. (1974): Hypothalamus as an endocrine organ. *Br. Med. J.,* 3:560–564.
7. Besser, G. M., Mortimer, C. H., Carr, D., Schally, A. V., Coy, D. H., Evered, D. C., Kastin, A. J., Tunbridge, W. M. G., Thorner, M. O., and Hall, R. (1974): Growth hormone-release inhibiting hormone in acromegaly. *Br. Med. J.,* 1:352–355.
8. Besser, G. M., Mortimer, C. H., McNeilly, A. S., Thorner, M. O., Batistoni, G. A., Bloom, S. R., Kastrup, K. W., Hansen, K. F., Hall., R., Coy, D. H., Kastin, A. J., and Schally, A. V. (1974): Long-term infusions of growth hormone-release inhibiting hormone in acromegaly: Effects on pituitary and pancreatic hormones. *Br. Med. J.,* 4:622–627.
9. Bex, F. H., and Corbin, A. (1979): LHRH or LHRH agonist-induced termination of pregnancy in hypophysectomised (HPYX) rats: Extrapituitary site of action. *Program, 61st Annual Meeting of the Endocrine Society,* Abstr. 436.
10. Bloom, S. R., Mortimer, C. H., Thorner, M. O., Besser, G. M., Hall, R., Gomez-Pan, A., Roy, V. M., Russell, R. C. G., Coy, D. H., Kastin, A. J., and Schally, A. V. (1974): Inhibition of gastrin and gastric acid secretion by growth hormone-release inhibiting hormone. *Lancet,* 2:1106–1109.
11. Bowers, C. Y., Friesen, H. G., Hwang, P., Guyda, J. J., and Folkers, K. (1971): Prolactin and thyrotropin release in man by synthetic pyroglutamyl-histidyl-prolinamide. *Biochem. Biophys. Res. Commun.,* 45:1033–1041.
12. Brazeau, P., Vale, W., Burgus, R., Ling, N., Butcher, M., Rivier, J., and Guillemin, R. (1973): Hypothalamic polypeptide that inhibits the secretion of immunoreactive pituitary growth hormone. *Science,* 179:77–79.
13. Burger, H. G., and Patel, Y. C. (1977): Thyrotropin releasing hormone—TSH. *Clin. Endocrinol. Metab.,* 6:83–100.

14. Burgus, R., Butcher, M., Amoss, M., Ling, N., Monahan, M., Rivier, J., Fellows, R., Blackwell, R., Vale, W., and Guillemin, R. (1972): Primary structure of the ovine hypothalamic luteinizing hormone-releasing factor (LRF). *Proc. Natl. Acad. Sci. USA*, 69:278–282.

15. Burgus, R., Dunn, T. F., Desiderio, D., and Guillemin, R. (1969): Structure moleculaire du facteur hypothalamique hypophysiotrope TRF d'origine ovine: Mise en evidence par spectrometrie de masse de la sequence PCA-His-Pro-NH$_2$. *C.R. Acad. Sci. [D] (Paris)*, 269:1870–1873.

16. Carmel, P. C., Araki, S., and Ferin, M. (1975): Prolonged stalk portal blood collection in rhesus monkey: Pulsatile release of gonadotropin-releasing hormone. *Program, 57th Annual Meeting of the Endocrine Society*, Abstr. 107.

17. Carmel, P. C., Araki, S. and Ferin, M. (1976): Prolonged stalk portal blood collection in rhesus monkeys: Evidence for pulsatile release of gonadotropin-releasing hormone (GnRH). *Endocrinology*, 99:243–248.

18. Coppen, A., Montgomery, S., Peet, M., Bailey, J., Marks, V., and Woods, P. (1974): Thyrotropin-releasing hormone in the treatment of depression. *Lancet*, 2:433–435.

19. Cowden, E., Ratliffe, J. G., Thompson, J. A. MacPherson, D. D., and Teasedale, G. M. (1979): Tests of prolactin secretion in diagnosis of prolactinomas. *Lancet*, 1:1155–1158.

20. Coy, D. H., Coy, E. J., Arimura, A., and Schally, A. V. (1973): Solid phase synthesis of growth hormone release inhibiting factor. *Biochem. Biophys. Res. Commun.*, 54:1267–1273.

21. Crowley, W., Vale, W., Beitins, I., Rivier, J., Rivier, C., and McArthur, J. (1979): Chronic administration of a long acting LRF agonist D-Trp^6-Pro^9-NEt-LRF) in hypogonadotropic hypogonadism: The critical nature of dosage and frequency in enhancement, extinction, and restoration of gonadotropin responsiveness, *Program, 61st Annual Meeting of the Endocrine Society*, Abstr. 16.

22. Curnow, R. T., Carey, R. M., Taylor, A., Johanson, A., and Murad, F. (1975): Somatostatin inhibition of insulin and gastrin in pancreatic islet cell carcinoma. *N. Engl. J. Med.*, 292:1385–1386.

23. Davies, T. F., Mountjoy, C. Q., Gomez-Pan, A., Watson, M. J., Hanker, J. P., Besser, G. M., and Hall, R. (1976): A double-blind crossover trial of gonadotropin releasing hormone (LHRH) in sexually impotent men. *Clin. Endocrinol. (Oxf.)*, 5:601–608.

24. DeVane, G. W., Siler, T. M., and Yen, S. S. C. (1974): Acute suppression of insulin and glucose levels by synthetic somatostatin in normal human subjects. *J. Clin. Endocrinol. Metab.*, 38:913–915.

25. Eskay, R. L., Mical, R. S., and Porter, J. C. (1977): Relationship between luteinizing hormone releasing hormone concentration in hypophyseal portal blood and luteinizing hormone release in intact, castrated, and electrochemically stimulated rats. *Endocrinology*, 100:263–270.

26. Fairclough, P. D., Cryer, R. J., McAllister, J., Hawkins, L., Jones, A. E., McKendrick, M., Hall, R., and Besser, G. M. (1973): Serum TSH responses to intravenously and orally administered TRH after thyroidectomy for carcinoma of the thyroid. *Clin. Endocrinol. (Oxf.)*, 2:351–359.

27. Feyrter, F. (1953): *Über die Peripheren Endokrinen (Parakrinen) Drusen des Menschen.* Maudrich, Vienna.

28. Fink, G., and Jamieson, M. G. (1976): Immunoreactive lutenizing hormone releasing factor in rat pituitary stalk blood: Effects of electrical stimulation of the medial preoptic area. *J. Endocrinol.*, 68:71–87.

29. Fleischer, N., Lorente, M., Kirkland, J., Kirkland, R., Clayton, G., and Calderon, M. (1972): Synthetic thyrotropin releasing factor as a test of pituitary thyrotropin response. *J. Clin. Endocrinol. Metab.*, 34:617–624.

30. Flückiger, E., and Wagner, H. (1968): 2-Br-α-Ergokryptin: Beeinflussung von Fertilität und Laktation bei der Ratte. *Experientia*, 24:1130–1131.

31. Franchimont, P., Becker, H., Ernould, C., Trys, C., Demoulin, A., Bourguignon, J. P., Legros, J. J., and Valcke, J. C. (1973): Action de l'hormone hypothalamique liberant l'hormone luteninisante (LH-RH) sur les gonadotrophines chez le sujet normal. *Ann. Endocrinol. (Paris)*, 34:477–490.

32. Franchimont, P., and Roulier, R. (1977): Gonadotropin secretion in male subjects. In: *Clinical Neuroendocrinology*, edited by L. Martini and G. M. Besser, pp. 197–212. Academic Press, New York.

33. Franks, S., Nabarro, J. D. N., and Jacobs, H. S. (1977): Prevalance and presentation of hyperprolactinemia in patients with "functionless" pituitary tumours. *Lancet*, 1:778–780.

34. Garnier, P. E., Chaussain, J.-L., Binet, E., Schlumberger, A., and Job, J.-C. (1974): Effect

of synthetic luteinizing hormone release hormone (LH-RH) on the release of gonadotrophins in children and adolescents. VI. Relations to age, sex, and puberty. *Acta Endocrinol. (Khb.),* 77:422–434.

35. Gautvick, K. M., Tashjian, A. H., Jr., Kourides, I. A., Weintraub, B. D., Graeber, C. T., Maloof, F., Suzuki, K. and Zuckerman, J. E. (1974): Thyrotropin-releasing hormone is not the sole physiologic mediator of prolactin release during suckling. *N. Engl. J. Med.,* 290:1162–1165.

36. Gerich, J. E., Lorenzi, M., Schneider, V., Kwan, C. W., Karam, J. H., Guillemin, R., and Forsham, P. H. (1974): Effects of somatostatin on plasma glucose and glucagon levels in human diabetes mellitus: Pathophysiologic and therapeutic implications. *N. Engl. J. Med.,* 291:544–547.

37. Gerich, J. E., Lorenzi, M., Bier, D. M., Schneider, V., Tsalikian, E., Karam, J. H., and Forsham, P. H. (1974): Prevention of human diabetic ketoacidosis by somatostatin. Evidence for an essential role of glucagon. *N. Engl. J. Med.,* 292:985–989.

38. Gomez-Pan, A., and Hall, R. (1977): Somatostatin (growth hormone-release inhibiting hormone). *Clin. Endocrinol. Metabol.,* 6:181–200.

39. Green, J. D., and Harris, G. W. (1947): The neurovascular link between the neurohypophysis and adenohypophysis. *J. Endocrinol.,* 5:136–146.

40. Guillemin, R. (1978): Peptides in the brain: The new endocrinology of the neuron. *Science,* 202:390–402.

41. Guillemin, R., Yamazaki, E., Jutisz, M., and Sakiz, E. (1962): Presence dans un extract des tissus hypothalamiques d'une substance stimulant la secretion de l'hormone hypophysaire thyreotrope (TSH). Premier purification par filtration sur gel sephadex. *C.R. Acad. Sci. [D] (Paris),* 255:1018–1020.

42. Hall, R., Anderson, J., Smart, G. A., and Besser, G. M. (1974): *Fundamentals of Clinical Endocrinology, 2nd ed.,* Pitman Medical, London.

43. Hall, R., Besser, G. M., Schally, A. V., Coy, D. H., Evered, D. C., Goldie, D. J., Kastin, A. J., McNeilly, A. S., Mortimer, C. H., Phenekos, C., Tunbridge, W. M. G., and Weightman, D. R. (1973): Actions of growth-hormone-release inhibiting hormone in healthy men and in acromegaly. *Lancet,* 2:581–584.

44. Hall, R., Hunter, P. R., Price, J. S., and Mountjoy, C. O. (1975): Thyrotrophin releasing hormone in depression. *Lancet,* 1:162.

45. Hall, R., Ormston, B. J., Besser, G. M., Cryer, R. J., and McKendrick, M. (1972): The thyrotrophin-releasing hormone test in diseases of the pituitary and hypothalamus. *Lancet,* 1:759–763.

46. Harris, G. W. (1955): *Neural Control of the Pituitary Gland,* Edward Arnold, London.

47. Healy, D. C., Pepperell, R. J., Stockdale, J. Bremner, W. J., and Burger, H. G. (1977): Pituitary autonomy in hyperprolactinemic secondary amenorrhea: Results of hypothalamic-pituitary testing. *J. Clin. Endocrinol. Metab.,* 44:809–819.

48. Hsueh, A. J. W. (1979): Extrapituitary action of gonadotropin releasing hormone (GnRH): Direct inhibition of ovarian and testicular responses. *Program, 61st Annual Meeting of the Endocrine Society,* Abstr. 198.

49. Illig, R., Kollmann, F., Borkenstein, M., Kuber, W., Exner, G. U., Kellerer, K., Lunglmayer, L., and Prader, A. (1977): Treatment of crypto-orchidism by intranasal synthetic luteinising-hormone-releasing-hormone. *Lancet,* 2:518–520.

50. Jackson, I. M., and Reichlin, S. (1974): Thyrotropin releasing hormone (TRH): Distribution in the brain, blood, and urine of the rat. *Life Sci.,* 14:2259–2266.

51. Jacobs, H. S., Franks, S., Murray, M. A. F., Hull, M. G. R., Steele, S. J., and Nabarro, J. D. N. (1976): Clinical and endocrine features of hyperprolactinaemic amenorrhoea. *Clin. Endocrinol. (Oxf.),* 5:439–454.

52. Jacobs, L. S., Snyder, P. J., Wilber, J. F., Utiger, R. D., and Daughaday, W. H. (1971): Increased serum prolactin after administration of synthetic thyrotropin releasing hormone (TRH) in man. *J. Clin. Endocrinol. Metab.,* 33:996–998.

53. Kastin, A. J., Ehrensing, R. H., Schalch, D. S., and Anderson, M. A. (1972): Improvement in mental depression with decreased thyrotropin release after administration of thyrotropin releasing hormone. *Lancet,* 2:740–742.

54. Kastin, A. J., Gual, C., and Schally, A. V. (1972): Clinical experience with hypothalamic releasing hormones. Part 2. Luteinizing hormone-releasing hormone and other hypophysiotropic releasing hormones. *Recent Prog. Horm. Res.,* 28:201–227.

55. Kastin, A. J., Schally, A. V., Gual, C., Midgley, A. R., Jr., Bowers, C. Y., and Diaz-Infante, A., Jr. (1969): Stimulation of hormone release in men and women by LH releasing hormone purified from porcine hypothalami. *J. Clin. Endocrinol. Metab.,* 29:1046–1050.

56. Kastin, A. J., Schally, A. V., Gual, C., Midgley, A. R., Jr., Bowers, C. Y., and Gomez-Perez, E. (1970): Administration of LH-releasing hormone to selected subjects. *Am. J. Obstet. Gynecol.,* 108:177–182.

57. Kledzik, G. S., Cusan, L., Auclair, C., Kelly, P. A., and Labrie, F. (1978): Inhibition of ovarian luteinizing hormone (LH) and follicle stimulating hormone receptor levels by treatment with an LH-releasing hormone agonist during the estrus cycle in the rat. *Fertil. Steril.,* 30:348–353.

58. Knobil, E., Plant, T. M., Wildt, L., and Belchetz, P. (1979): The induction of ovulatory menstrual cycles in rhesus monkeys with hypothalamic lesions by an unvarying pulsatile GnRH replacement regimen. *Program, 61st Annual Meeting of the Endocrine Society,* Abstr. 18.

59. Labrie, F., Auclair, C., Cusan, L., Kelly, P. A., Pelletier, G., and Ferland, L. (1978): Inhibitory effect of LHRH and its agonists in testicular gonadotropin receptors and spermatogenesis in the rat. *Int. J. Androl. (Suppl. 2),* :303–318.

60. Labrie, F., Auclair, C., Lemay, A., Kledzik, G. S., Cusan, L., Kelly, P. A., Ferland, L., Sequin, D., Belanger, A., Azadian-Boulanger, G., and Raynaud, J.-P. (1979): Inhibition of ovarian receptor levels and function by treatment with LHRH or its agonists in the rat and possible luteolytic effects of LHRH in normal women. In: *Clinical Neuroendocrinology,* edited by G. Tolis, F. Labrie, J. B. Martin, and F. Naftolin, pp. 115–128. Raven Press, New York.

61. Lamberts, S. W. J., Birkenhager, J. C., and Kwa, H. G. (1976): Basal and TRH-stimulated prolactin in patients with pituitary tumors. *Clin. Endocrinol.,* 5:709–711.

62. Lemay, A., Labrie, F., Ferland, L., and Raynaud, J.-P. (1979): Possible luteolytic effects of luteinizing hormone-releasing hormone in normal women. *Fertil. Steril.,* 31:29–34.

63. Lennon, J. R., Sircus, W., Bloom, S. R., Mitchel, S. J., Polak, J. M., Besser, G. M., Hall, R., Coy, D. H., Kastin, A. J., and Schally, A. V. (1975): Investigation and treatment of a recurrent vipoma. *Gut,* 16:821–822.

64. Luft, R., Efendic, S., Hokfelt, T., Johansson, O., and Arimura, A. (1974): Immunohistochemical evidence for localization of somatostatin-like immunoreactivity in a cell population of the pancreatic islets. *Med. Biol.,* 52:428–430.

65. Lundbaek, K., Christensen, S. E., Prange-Hansen, A., Iversen, J., Orskov, H., Seyer-Hansen, K., Alberti, G. M. M., and Whitefoot, R., (1976): Failure of somatostatin to correct manifest diabetic ketoacidosis. *Lancet,* 1:215–218.

66. MacLeod, R. M. (1976): Regulation of prolactin secretion. In: *Frontiers in Neuroendocrinology,* edited by L. Martini and W. F. Ganong, pp. 169–194, Raven Press, New York.

67. Malacara, J. M., Seyler, L. E., Jr., and Reichlin, S. (1972): Luteinizing hormone releasing factor activity in peripheral blood from women during the midcycle luteinizing hormone ovulatory surge. *J. Clin. Endocrinol. Metab.,* 34:271–278.

68. Matsuo, H., Arimura, A., Nair, R. M. G., and Schally, A. V. (1971): Synthesis of the porcine LH- and FSH-releasing hormone by the solid-phase method. *Biochem. Biophys. Res. Commun.,* 45:822–827.

69. Matsuo, H., Nair, R. M. G., Arimura, A., and Schally, A. V. (1971): Structure of the porcine LH- and FSH-releasing hormone. I. The proposed amino acid sequence. *Biochem. Biophys. Res. Commun.,* 43:1334–1339.

70. McCaul, J. A., Cassel, K. J., and Stern, G. M. (1974): Intravenous thyrotropin-releasing hormone in Parkinson's disease. *Lancet,* 1:735.

71. Meissner, C., Thum, C., Beischer, W., Winkler, G., Schroder, K. E. and Pfeiffer, E. F. (1975): Antidiabetic action of somatostatin assessed by artificial pancreas. *Diabetes,* 24:988–996.

72. Moriarty, G. (1973): Adenohypophysis: Ultrastructural cytochemistry. A review. *J. Histochem. Cytochem.,* 21:855–894.

73. Mortimer, C. H., Carr, D., Lind, T., Bloom, S. R., Mallinson, C. N., Schally, A. V., Tunbridge, W. M. G., Yeomans, L., Coy, D. H., Kastin, A. J., Besser, G. M., and Hall, R. (1974): Effects of growth hormone-release inhibiting hormone on circulating glucagon, insulin, and growth hormone in normal, diabetic, acromegalic and hypopituitary patients. *Lancet,* 1:697–701.

74. Mortimer, C. H., McNeilly, A. S., Fisher, R. A., Murray, M. A. F., and Besser, G. M. (1974): Gonadotrophin-releasing hormone therapy in hypogonadal males with hypothalamic or pituitary dysfunction. *Br. Med. J.,* 4:619–621.

75. Mortimer, C. H., McNeilly, A. S. and Besser, G. M. (1976): Gonadotrophin releasing hormone therapy. *Ann. Biol. Anim. Biochim. Biophys.,* 16:235–243.
76. Mortimer, C. H., McNeilly, A. S., Rees, L. H., Lowry, P. J., Gilmore, D., and Dobbie, H. G. (1976): Radioimmunoassay and chromatographic similarity of circulating endogenous gonadotrophin releasing hormone and hypothalamic extracts in man. *J. Clin. Endocrinol. Metab.,* 43:882–888.
77. Moss, R. L., and McCann, S. M. (1973): Induction of mating behavior in rats by luteinizing hormone-releasing factor. *Science,* 181:177–179.
78. Mountjoy, C. Q., Price, I. S., Weller, M., Hunter, P., Hall, R., and Dewar, J. H. (1974): A double-blind crossover sequential trial of oral thyrotropin-releasing hormone in depression. *Lancet,* 1:958–960.
79. Nair, R. M. G., Barrett, J. F., Bowers, C. Y., and Schally, A. V. (1970): Structure of porcine thyrotropin releasing hormone. *Biochemistry,* 9:1103–1106.
80. Nair, R. M. G., and Schally, A. V. (1972): Structure of a hypothalamic peptide possessing gonadotropin-releasing activity. *Int. J. Pept. Protein Res.,* 4:421–430.
81. Neill, J. D., Patton, J. M., Dailey, R. A., Tsou, R. C., and Tindall, G. T. (1977): Luteinizing hormone releasing hormone (LHRH) in pituitary stalk blood of rhesus monkeys: Relationship to level of LH release. *Endocrinology,* 101:430–434.
82. Nillius, S. J., and Wide, L. (1975): Gonadotrophin-releasing hormone treatment for induction of follicular maturation and ovulation in amenorrhoeic women with anorexia nervosa. *Br. Med. J.,* 3:405–408.
83. Noel, G. K., Diamond, R. C., Wartofsky, L., Earll, J. M., and Frantz, A. G. (1974): Studies of prolactin and TSH secretion by continuous infusion of small amounts of thyrotropin-releasing hormone (TRH). *J. Clin. Endocrinol. Metab.,* 39:6–17.
84. Ormston, B. J., Garry, R., Cryer, R. J., Besser, G. M., and Hall, R. (1971): Thyrotropin-releasing hormone as a thyroid function test. *Lancet,* 2:10–16.
85. Patel, Y. C., and Burger, H. G. (1973): Serum thyrotropin (TSH) in pituitary and/or hypo-thalamic hypothyroidism: Normal or elevated basal levels and paradoxical response to thyrotropin releasing hormone. *J. Clin. Endocrinol. Metab.,* 37:190–196.
86. Pearse, A. G. E., and Takor, T. T. (1976): Neuroendocrine embryology and the APUD concept. *Clin. Endocrinol. (Oxf.),* 5:229S–244S.
87. Pfaff, D. W. (1973): Luteinizing hormone-releasing factor potentiates lordosis behaviour in hypophysectomised, ovariectomised female rats. *Science,* 182:1148–1149.
88. Polak, J. M., Pearse, A. G. E., Grimelius, L., Bloom, S. R., and Arimura, A. (1975): Growth-hormone releasing inhibiting hormone (GH-RIH) in gastro-intestinal and pancreatic D cells. *Lancet,* 1:1220–1222.
89. Prange, A. J., Jr., Wilson, I. C., Lara, P. P., Alltop, L. B., and Breese, G. R. (1972): Effects of thyrotropin-releasing hormone in depression. *Lancet,* 2:990–1002.
90. Rivier, J., Brazeau, P., Vale, W., Ling, N., Burgus, R., Gilon, C., Yardley, J., and Guillemin, R. (1973): Synthese totale par phase solide d'un tetradecapeptide ayant les proprietes chimiques et biologiques de la somatostatine. *C.R. Acad. Sci. [D] (Paris),* 276:2737–2740.
91. Roth, J. C., Kelch, R. P., Kaplan, S. L., and Grumbach, M. M. (1972): FSH and LH response to luteinizing hormone-releasing factor in prepubertal children, adult males and patient with hypogonadotropic and hypergonadotropic hypogonadism. *J. Clin. Endocrinol. Metab.,* 35:926–930.
92. Saberi, M., and Utiger, R. D. (1975): Augmentation of thyrotropin responses to thyrotropin releasing hormone following small decreases in serum thyroid hormone concentration. *J. Clin. Endocrinol. Metab.,* 40:435–441.
93. Sandow, J., von Rechenberg, W., Krauss, B., and Jerzabek, G. (1978): Direct pituitary inhibition by an LH-RH analog. *Program, 60th Annual Meeting of the Endocrine Society,* Abstr. 185.
94. Schally, A. V., and Arimura, A. (1977): Physiology and nature of hypothalamic regulatory hormones. In: *Clinical Neuroendocrinology,* edited by L. Martini and G. M. Besser, pp. 1–42, Academic Press, New York.
95. Schally, A. V., Arimura, A., Baba, Y., Nair, R. M. G., Matsuo, H., Redding, T. W., Debeljuk, L., and White, W. F. (1971): Isolation and properties of the FSH and LH releasing hormone. *Biochem. Biophys. Res. Commun.,* 43:393–399.
96. Schally, A. V., Arimura, A., Bowers, C. Y., Wakabayaski, I., Kastin, A. J., Redding, T. W., Mittler, J. C., Nair, R. M. G., Pizzolato, P., and Segal, A. J. (1970): Purification of hypothalamic releasing hormones of human origin. *J. Clin. Endocrinol.,* 31:291–300.

97. Schally, A. V., Arimura, A., Kastin, A. J., Matsuo, H., Baba, Y., Redding, T. W., Nair, R. M. G., Debeljuk, L., and White, W. F. (1971): Gonadotropin-releasing hormone: One polypeptide regulates secretion of luteinizing and follicle-stimulating hormones. *Science,* 173:1036–1037.

98. Schally, A. V., Bowers, C. Y., Redding, T. W., and Barrett, J. F. (1966): Isolation of thyrotropin releasing factor (TRF) from porcine hypothalamus. *Biochem. Biophys. Res. Commun.,* 25:165–169.

99. Schally, A. V., Dupont, A., Arimura, A., Redding, T. W. and Linthicum, G. L. (1975): Isolation of porcine GH-release inhibiting hormone: The existence of three forms of GH-RIH. *Fed. Proc.,* 34:584 (Abstr. 2065).

100. Schally, A. V., Dupont, A., Arimura, A., Takahara, J., Redding, T. W., Clemens, J., and Shaar, C. (1976): Purification of a catecholamine-rich fraction with prolactin release-inhibiting factor (PIF) activity from porcine hypothalami. *Acta Endocrinol. (Kbh.),* 82:1–14.

101. Schally, A. V., Kastin, A. J., and Arimura, A. (1975): The hypothalamus and reproduction. *Am. J. Obstet. Gynecol.,* 122:857–862.

102. Scharrer, E., and Scharrer, B. (1954): Hormones produced by neurosecretory cells. *Recent Prog. Horm. Res.,* 10:183–240.

103. Snyder, P. J., Rudenstein, R. S., Gardner, D. F., and Rothman, J. G. (1979): Repetitive infusion of gonadotropin-releasing hormone distinguishes hypothalamic from pituitary hypogonadism. *J. Clin. Endocrinol. Metab.,* 48:864–868.

104. Snyder, P. J., and Utiger, R. D. (1972): Inhibition of thyrotropin response to thyrotropin releasing hormone by small quantities of thyroid hormones. *J. Clin. Invest.,* 51:2077–2084.

105. Tashjian, A. H., Barowsky, N. J., and Jensen, D. J. (1971): Thyrotropin releasing hormone: Direct evidence for stimulation of prolactin production by pituitary cells in culture. *Biochem. Biophys. Res. Commun.,* 43:516–523.

106. Thorner, M. O. (1975): Dopamine is an important neurotransmitter in the autonomic nervous system. *Lancet,* 1:662–664.

107. Thorner, M. O. (1977): Prolactin: Clinical physiology and the significance and management of hyperprolactinemia. In: *Clinical Neuroendocrinology,* edited by L. Martini and G. M. Besser, pp. 319–361, Academic Press, New York.

108. Tolis, G., Somma, M., Campenhout, J. V., and Friesen, H. (1974): Prolactin secretion in sixty-five patients with galactorrhea. *Am. J. Obstet. Gynecol.,* 118:91–101.

109. Unger, R. H., and Orci, L. (1975): The essential role of glucagon in the pathogenesis of the endogenous hyperglycemia in diabetes mellitus. *Lancet,* 2:14–16.

110. Wass, J. A. H., Penman, E., Medbak, S., Webb, J. P. W., Dawson, A. M., Besser, G. M., and Rees, L. H. (1979): Circulating and C.S.F. immunoreactive somatostatin levels in normal and acromegalic subjects basally and during glucose loading. *Program, 61st Annual Meeting of the Endocrine Society,* Abstr. 282.

111. Yen, S. S. C. (1977): Neuroendocrine aspects of the regulation of cyclic gonadotropin release in women. In: *Clinical Neuroendocrinology,* edited by L. Martini and G. M. Besser, pp. 175–196, Academic Press, New York.

112. Yen, S. S. C., and Casper, R. F. (1979): Induction of luteolysis in the human by a superactive LRF agonist: Implication for fertility control. *Program, 61st Annual Meeting of the Endocrine Society,* Abstr. 435.

113. Zanartu, J., Dabancens, A., Kastin, A. J., and Schally, A. V. (1974): Effect of synthetic hypothalamic gonadotropin-releasing hormone (FSH/LH-RH) in anovulatory sterility. *Fertil. Steril.,* 25:160–169.

114. Zarate, A., Canales, E. S., Soria, J., Gonzalez, A., Schally, A. V., and Kastin, A. V. (1974): Further observations on the therapy of anovulatory infertility with synthetic luteinizing hormone-releasing hormone. *Fertil. Steril.,* 25:3–10.

Polypeptide Hormones, edited by
R. F. Beers, Jr. and E. G. Bassett.
Raven Press, New York © 1980.

24. Discussion

Moderator: A. V. Schally

J. Ramachandran: Dr. Kastin, with regard to the behavioral effects you described as due to MSH, I wonder whether they can truly be called MSH effects. If only the heptapeptide MSH 4–10, and not the α-MSH, was used in these studies, it might just as well be an ACTH effect.

Also, is there any evidence that MSH 4–10 is generated in any way from these precursors?

A. J. Kastin: We know of no substantial evidence for *natural* generation of the 4–10 sequence from MSH, although we have examined this issue [Marks et al. (1972): *Brain Res. Bull.,* 1:591–593]. The first two clinical studies with the MSH substance were performed with the complete, intact α-MSH.

The primary reason why the subsequent studies were done with the 4–10 sequence was a matter of simple feasibility: A pharmaceutical company had manufactured this sequence and assumed the legal responsibility for the tests.

At the time of these clinical trials, the evidence seemed to indicate that there was no difference between the effects of the 4–10 sequence and the α-MSH.

Indeed, the de Wied studies, which had initially looked for the effects of ACTH on the brain and found them to be due to the 4–10 sequence shared with MSH, showed this similarity.

However, Sandman, Beckwill, and I now have evidence that suggests that indeed this information is not necessarily redundant and that different sequences of the same molecule can have slightly different effects in different behavioral tests.

J. Ramachandran: Wouldn't it be better to attribute this effect specifically to MSH 4–10 and not classify it as an effect of α-MSH?

A. J. Kastin: Not necessarily. To be accurate, one should designate the particular compound used in each study. The conclusion should be that the results of that study are only applicable to the compounds that were tested.

J. Ramachandran: Dr. Labrie, in the February issue of *Endocrinology,* Conn, Morrell, Dufan, and Catt reported that, using dispersed primary cultures of rat pituitary cells, there was absolutely no evidence of increase of cyclic AMP production by synthetic gonadotropin-releasing hormones. In addition, the agents that inhibit phosphodiestrase, such as MIX and theophylline, had no effect on the release of LH.

Would you care to comment on these results?

F. Labrie: These studies were based on the effects of prostaglandins and cholera toxin on cyclic AMP. Cholera toxin and prostaglandins, as I mentioned earlier, have nothing to do with LH release.

When prostaglandins and cholera toxin are added to pituitary cells in culture, they stimulate formation of cyclic AMP in cell types other than LH-secreting cells.

We must realize that LH-secreting cells represent only 5% of the total pituitary cell population. Prostaglandins are acting preferentially in GH-secreting cells, the stimulatory effect of prostaglandins on cyclic AMP accumulation being parallel to changes of GH secretion. It is a mistake to attempt to correlate total changes of cyclic AMP with a specific hormone release, especially when using a substance known to be specific for GH-secreting cells and having no action on LH secretion. Then, it is not too surprising to find that prostaglandin-induced increases of cyclic AMP accumulation are not accompanied by changes of LH release.

J. Ramachandran: No, I was talking about the gonadotropin-releasing hormone.

They reported that there is no increase in either intracellular or extracellular cyclic AMP, nor is there any change in the occupancy on the cyclic AMP binding site.

F. Labrie: I was coming to that, too.

Since LH secreting cells are only 5% of the total population, a 100% increase of total cyclic AMP indicates that the level of cyclic AMP in LH-secreting cells must have increased 20-fold. Thus, there is the very important problem of background which has to be taken into account. In intact rat hemipituitaries, a 2- to 3-fold increase of total cyclic AMP is observed on addition of LH-RH, which means that the levels of cyclic AMP have increased 40- to 60-fold in this cell type. However, when using pituitary cells in culture, the proportion of LH-secreting cells is markedly reduced, due to the rapid growth of fibroblasts, which account for a large proportion of the cells containing cyclic AMP in the Petri dish.

E. Gross: Dr. Kastin, the fact is that the peptides have a relatively short half-life; nevertheless the biological effect lasts about 4 hr. Can you address yourself further to this question? Have you published any studies on this topic?

A. J. Kastin: Any interpretation I could offer would be pure speculation.

My main purpose in emphasizing that point during my presentation was to stimulate ideas and research that would explain these observations.

E. Gross: Dr. Labrie, you mentioned phosphorylation. Can you tell us what proteins are being phosphorylated and what is the significance of such phosphorylation?

F. Labrie: This is a difficult problem that I have not discussed. This has been done with purified plasma membranes; we found that 11 of 36 proteins were phosphorylated, this phosphorylation being cyclic AMP-dependent. However, we do not know the role of these phosphorylated membranes in the biology of the pituitary cell.

A. J. Kastin: Dr. Gross' question has stimulated me enough to finally indulge in some of the speculation he encouraged.

There are many possibilities to explain how a peptide with a brief existence in the circulation exerts its long-lasting effects in the brain. The first possibility is that indeed the peptide doesn't penetrate into the brain directly but exerts its primary effect in the periphery. That effect would be exerted immediately. It then could generate some other compound that would require some time to get into the brain tissue.

Another related possibility is that the peptide doesn't enter the brain directly, but changes the permeability of the blood brain barrier to other substances. Again, this would take some time and perhaps could account for some of the delay, but not necessarily the persistence of effects.

An additional possibility, of course, is an effect on the pituitary, even though we have shown in some cases that the pituitary isn't necessary for the CNS actions; this could then act through the retrograde flow in the portal vessels.

Or, since hypophysectomy does not necessarily affect the levels of MSH and other peptides in the brain, the administered peptide could perhaps just stimulate the endogenous production of peptides or other compounds in the brain.

Certainly even more appealing is the possibility that the entire molecule enters the brain, but it is quite possible that a degradation product or fragment enters directly.

With any of these possibilities, the peptide could exert an immediate effect, for example, on cyclic AMP, as Dr. Labrie has just mentioned, or directly in the cell and therefore its continued presence would not be necessary.

T. L. O'Donohue: One comment, Dr. Schally.

We do have some data on the effect of hypophysectomy on α-MSH in the brain and the manipulation does affect α-MSH concentrations. Although we have observed no change in the number of α-MSH-positive neurons by immunocytochemical techniques, radioimmunoassay has uncovered some interesting long-term effects of hypophysectomy.

After 2, 3, and 4 weeks of hypophysectomy there is a gradual decline of α-MSH in α-MSH nerve terminal regions but, interestingly, there is no change in concentrations in the arcuate nucleus, a region containing α-MSH perikarya sites.

We are not quite sure how to interpret this data at present.

C. P. Fawcett: Dr. Schally, you alluded to the production of GI disturbances after the administration of TRH to patients. Some work by Dr. Bruce and myself has shown that, *in vitro,* TRH can stimulate directly several smooth muscle tissues. This TRH increases the amplitude, but not the frequency of, say, antral contractions. We think that this may be acting via a histaminergic type pathway.

I admire your tenacity in continuing to search for the true CRF. Does your peptide with CRF-like activity release ACTH in any system other than your monolayer cultures?

A. V. Schally: Your comments were well taken.

As to the CRF, there is ample evidence from the work of many investigators that such a hormone exists and is different from ACTH and vasopressin. However, the work on CRF is very difficult. Tremendous interference is caused by ACTH-like peptides, catecholamines, and vasopressin.

Catecholamines cause about 40% stimulation of ACTH release. I have been studying CRF since my undergraduate days because I felt completely sure that it exists. For our bioassays, we use not only monolayer cell cultures but also pituitary quarters and *in vivo* systems.

The simplest and cheapest system is, of course, monolayer cell culture assay. Using it, we can examine dozens and dozens of fractions. We isolated these CRF-like peptides and characterized them principally on the basis of *in vitro* stimulation of ACTH release from monomeric cultures of pituitary cells. Our recent papers describe the results obtained during *in vivo* experiments.

C. P. Fawcett: Dr. Labrie, as your know, several investigators including myself have detected early changes in cyclic nucleotides, particularly cyclic GMP, in association with TRH and LH-LRH activities. What would you think of the possibility that cyclic GMP may also have a role in the stimulating pituitary hormone release?

F. Labrie: Due to the shortage of time I did not discuss this subject. With the cyclic AMP system, when you add the exogenous cyclic AMP derivative, you can mimic the effect of the endogenous hormone, thus making more convincing the argument in favor of cyclic AMP as the mediator of the action of the neurohormone.

It is also clear that changes of hormone release induced by LH-RH are associated with changes of cyclic GMP levels. However, when cyclic GMP derivatives are added extracellularly, they do not lead to any change of hormone release. One would be tempted to associate these changes of cyclic GMP levels to changes of rates of hormone secretion, although the exact role of this cyclic nucleotide in these mechanisms remains to be elucidated. The role of cyclic GMP could, in fact, be very important but the present data do not permit association of it with specific cell function.

A. J. Kastin: Drs. Christensen, Spirtes, Kostrzewa, and I have also looked at possible mediation of the nucleotides on the extra-endocrine effects in the brain. There is some indication that cyclic AMP may modify the actions of α-MSH in the region of the occipital cortex and that cyclic GMP may modify the actions of MIF-I in the region of the thalamus.

P. H. Seeburg: Dr. Labrie, do you have an idea about what the T_3 or T_4 do in pituitary secreting cells?

F. Labrie: We studied the effect of T_3 and T_4 on TSH and prolactin secretion and found that it is inhibitory. We have not, however, looked at the possible effect of these hormones on LH and FSH secretion.

N. Khazam: Dr. Schally, you stated or speculated, as I recall, that GABA has a direct effect on pituitary prolactin. Was the experiment done *in vitro* or *in vivo* conditions?

A. V. Schally: I didn't speculate. We reported, in an elaborate paper, trials in which both pituitary halves and cell cultures were used. We also used an *in vivo* system based on haloperidol and other pharmacological agents such as perphenazine, sulpiride, and reserpine. In any case, *in vitro* GABA clearly and significantly inhibited the *in vitro* and *in vivo* release of prolactin.

Subsequent experiments, in which the *in vivo* release of prolactin was stimulated by TRH and the agents mentioned above, demonstrated that GABA was able to significantly decrease prolactin secretion. These results were confirmed recently in MacLeod's laboratory, and also by Libertun in Argentina using lactating rats that had higher levels of prolactin. Further, E. E. Müller published on agonists and antagonists of GABA; he also reached the conclusion that GABA may play a role in physiological control of prolactin secretion. We never said GABA is the true prolactin-release inhibiting factor (PIF), but stated that, under a variety of conditions, it inhibits the release of prolactin [Schally, A. V. et al. (1977): *Endocrinology,* 100:681–691].

We have noticed that following administration of large doses of GABA (200 mg i.v. or 10 g orally), one observes a fall in prolactin levels. The problem encountered in clinical work with GABA is that it has severe side effects, including a drop in diastolic blood pressure, cramps, nausea, and so forth.

N. Khazam: A question to Dr. Thorner regarding bromocriptine, the dopamine agonist. Would L-DOPA do the same thing or have selective effect here? Can you contrast this effect with the L-DOPA effect in reducing prolactin and increasing gonadotropin release?

M. O. Thorner: I think the effects of bromocriptine are very clear and that it directly affects the pituitary to inhibit prolactin release. It works through dopamine receptors. It is different from L-DOPA in that it does not need to be converted to dopamine and it has a much longer duration of action. I don't really wish to get into the controversy about the effects of dopamine on gonadotropin secretion. I think at the present time that is a growing thing in endocrinology.

E. M. Bogdanove: Dr. Labrie, would you like to speculate about the curious lack of down-regulation, or development of desensitization, or unresponsiveness observed with the inhibitory factors?

The stimulator factors, particularly LH-RH, do seem to down-regulate. If you give them continuously, the gland ceases to respond; however, you can keep suppressing the gland with either dopamine or SRIF. Do you think anyone has any idea as to why this may be?

F. Labrie: I can try to answer this question. We must admit that we do not know all that much about the inhibitory peptides or have not administered them for periods of time as long as those during which we gave LH-RH and TRH, for example. It did, in fact, take some time before we realized that LH-RH treatment leads to desensitization.

We can take the example of dopamine where, at least in the brain, prolonged treatment with domaminergic agonists leads to inhibition of the response, an effect that is similar to that observed with stimulatory peptides. This responsiveness to dopaminergic agonists can be observed on acetylcholine release in the striatum.

A. V. Schally: With reference to the question of down-regulation, caused by paradoxical effects of superactive LH-RH analogs, I would like to emphasize that inhibitory analogs can attach themselves to the receptors and block the access of endogenous LH-RH and thereby prevent normal processes of ovulation.

In the case of superactive and long-acting analogs, we are also dealing with a possible direct effect on the gonads. One of these explanations could thus be down-regulation of receptors, but this is not the complete story.

So I don't think you can speak about down-regulation with regard to inhibitory LH-RH analogs.

L. Recant: I was very struck by Dr. Coy's remarks concerning the lack of correlation between the effects of somatostatin analogs during *in vitro*—such as pancreatic perfusion—and the whole animal. I would like to know if he has any data regarding the effects of these analogs on the gastrointestinal hormones that could explain the lack of correlation between the *in vitro* and *in vivo* data.

D. H. Coy: It has really never been proven that the distinctions in somatostatin receptors actually exist. I think all the effects that have been observed could indeed be explained by effects on other hormones, on transport processes, or things like that.

Still a very confusing situation exists, particularly with the C-14 analogs. In some systems, for instance, using a perfused pancreas, we simply observe dissociated activity, but in normal animals the situation is nowhere near as clear.

It is just going to take awhile longer before we figure out what is going on. Does that answer your question?

L. Recant: No.

A. V. Schally: Well, really it shouldn't be unexpected that some analogs of somatostatin should exert selective effects on different tissues. The effect of somatostatin analogs on release of GH doesn't have to correspond to their effect on inhibition of pepsin or hydrochloric acid secretion. So the receptors in different tissues must be studied.

Most important is what each analog does in humans. But of course we can't test every analog in humans. We can only test the more promising ones that have been proven safe.

D. H. Coy: If you compare effects on GH release and, say, gastric acid release with most of the assays in use, you will go to different animal species for measuring acid and GH, so you have another variable. It is a major problem with somatostatin that you have to look at so many assays, and to unify them is very difficult at this stage.

A. J. Kastin: I think your speculation makes very good sense. I believe the body is very efficient and I advocate teleological reasoning even though it might be considered unscientific by many.

As we heard this morning from Brownstein, O'Donohue, and others, these peptides are being found all over the body. In this regard, we should recall that the term, hormone, was coined for a gastrointestinal substance. So if these hormones are being found all over the body, if they are exerting many different effects, and if the brain and blood levels don't necessarily correlate, then the body would be faced during evolution with two choices: Either it evolves an enormous number of different peptides for the many different types of cells and functions or it takes some common precursor(s) that provides the required peptides as needed. This can be mediated by permeability into brain tissue for CNS effects or by some other mechanism.

I thought the principle we showed with the opiate peptides, that is, the association of narcotic and behavioral effects depending on the route of administration, may serve as an illustration of an efficient use of the same peptides. As Dr. O'Donohue indicated today, it is probable that α-MSH does not exist in human blood, although it does in rats, but it seems to occur in the human brain, where its presumed functions would be selectively exerted.

This concept of multiple independent actions of the peptides, on perhaps a more general basis, would indeed substantiate your suggestion.

T. L. O'Donohue: Dr. Kastin, in keeping with your thoughts on teleological consistency or conservatism, do you feel that the extraendocrine and endocrine effects of neuropeptides and neurohormones are related?

A. J. Kastin: The answer to that is difficult.

Essentially, the answer is yes but proof is a step away. I am reminded of the situation when, 10 years ago, Dr. Schally and our group as well as others were busy at meetings like this defending the very existence of the hypothalamic hormones; they were compared with the Loch Ness Monster and the Abominable Snowman—elusive and never to be found. At the time we were debating whether these hormones even existed, some people would ask us questions about what controls them or how they act. These were questions we wanted to know the answers for but it was just premature. Similarly, your excellent question may be ahead of the time.

When we introduced, in 1971, the concept of the extra-endocrine effects of the hypothalamic peptides, somewhat similar skepticism greeted us. Most of our work was therefore directed to determining the nature of these extra-endocrine effects. In fact, I would imagine there are still some people who remain skeptical of it. It is only recently that we have been able to look at the mechanism of actions on the brain.

I think your question deals with the next step. Will we find that the efficient human body uses the same compounds for independent actions as I think it does?

But overriding it should be some kind of integrative mechanism where independent actions might indeed coincide.

J. E. Villarreal: Just a comment. What is an extraendocrine action? For example, ACTH inhibits acetylcholine release in the stimulated myenteric plexus of the guinea pig ileum. But there are many such nonendocrine actions of hormones. In other words, to measure the nonendocrine effect of a hormone, do we have to measure the change in the secretion of another hormone?

F. Labrie: Although the effect of an hormone can be modulation of the secretion of another hormone, it is more frequent to find that the end effect is modulation of intracellular events with no secondary message being sent into circulation. The response of the tissue can be, for example, growth (estrogens in the uterus).

A. V. Schally: I wish to thank the panelists and discussants for participating in this interesting discussion period.

Polypeptide Hormones, edited by
R. F. Beers, Jr. and E. G. Bassett.
Raven Press, New York © 1980.

25. Introduction to Section D: Pituitary Hormones

Choh Hao Li

*Hormone Research Laboratory, University of California,
San Francisco, California 94143*

The pituitary gland consists of three lobes. The anterior and intermediate lobes, together, are generally known as the adenohypophysis, and the posterior lobe is synonomous with the neurohypophysis. The adenohypophysis is perhaps the most far-reaching in its control of the body's functioning, since its hormones are either metabolic, regulating the chemistry of the body, or gonadotropic, being concerned with sexual activity.

As noted in Fig. 1, the neurohypophysis secretes two hormones (oxytocin and vasopressin) and the adenohypophysis 11 hormones (thyrotropin, lutropin, follitropin, prolactin, somatotropin, α-melanotropin, β-melanotropin, β-lipotropin, γ-lipotropin, β-endorphin, and corticotropin). The isolation, structure, and synthesis of pituitary hormone began in early 1950 with the work of Vincent duVigneaud and colleagues on oxytocin and vasopressin. About the same time, similar investigations were carried out on corticotropin (ACTH) by four groups of investigators. All of the eleven adenohypophysial hormones have now been isolated in pure form and their amino acid sequences are known. Eight of them have been partially or totally synthesized. It is impossible to discuss recent developments of these 13 hormones within the limitations of this section. Instead, we have chosen to present some basic and clinical data on ACTH, oxytocin, β-endorphin, and human somatotropin.

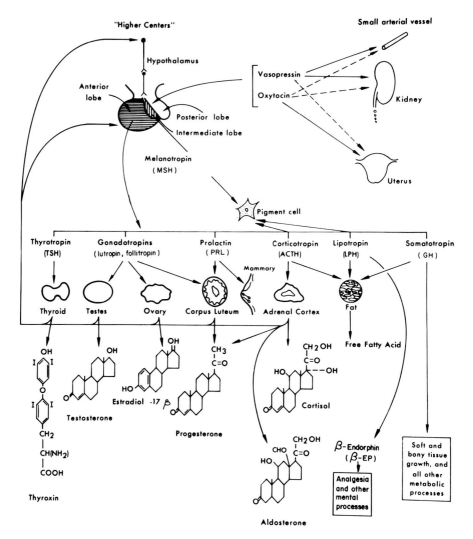

FIG. 1. Diagrammatic summary of biological properties of pituitary hormones.

Polypeptide Hormones, edited by
R. F. Beers, Jr. and E. G. Bassett.
Raven Press, New York © 1980.

26. Chemical Messengers of the Anterior Pituitary with Special Reference to Human Somatotropin and β-Endorphin

Choh Hao Li

*Hormone Research Laboratory, University of California,
San Francisco, California 94143*

INTRODUCTION

From the studies on primary structures of anterior pituitary hormones, it is possible to divide them into three groups (13) having certain structural features in common (Table 1). Because of these common structures, they exhibit overlapping biological activities. A high degree of structural resemblance has been found to exist among the glycoprotein hormones thyrotropin, lutropin, and follitropin. Somatotropin and prolactin comprise the second group, exhibiting considerable structural homology as well as common biological properties. Corticotropin, the melanotropins, the lipotropins, and β-endorphin fall into the third group of structurally and biologically related molecules.

The three glycoprotein hormones (lutropin, follitropin, and thyrotropin) consist of α and β subunits. In solutions of acidic pH and denaturants, the native hormones dissociate into α and β subunits that can be isolated by countercurrent distribution or chromatographic procedures (36–38,40). The amino acid sequences of the α subunits in FSH, LH, and TSH are nearly identical, whereas the primary structures of the β subunit of these three hormones are different. Apparently, the β subunit is hormonally specific. When the β subunit of TSH recombines with FSH-α, it generates thyrotropic activity. Similarly, when TSH-α recombines with FSH-β, it generates follitropic activity. The complete amino acid sequences of human FSH (41) and TSH (39) have recently been determined.

Since 1937, highly purified prolactin preparations have been obtained from cattle, sheep, rat, human [for a review, see (17)] and fish (8) pituitary glands. The primary structure of prolactin from sheep pituitary gland was finally shown, in 1969, to consist of 199 amino acids with linear sequence (15,27).

Growth hormone (somatotropin) was first isolated in highly purified form from bovine pituitary glands (28). Although the effects of bovine somatotropin were readily evident in the rat and mouse, it seemed to be ineffective in humans. Evidence was gathered by a number of investigators that pointed to an important

TABLE 1. *The eleven hormones of the adenohypophysis*

Group	Hormone	Number of amino acids		Principal function
Simple peptides	Corticotropin (ACTH)		39	Stimulates the adrenal cortex to produce cortical hormones
	Melanotropins			Darkening of skin
	α-MSH	Human	13	(pigmentation)
	β-MSH	Bovine	18	
		Human	22	
	Lipotropins			Fat mobilizing activity; β-LPH
	β-LPH		91	is the prohormone for en-
	γ-LPH		58	dorphins
	β-Endorphin		31	Opiate-like activities
Simple proteins	Somatotropin (growth hormone, GH)		191	General body growth
	Prolactin (lactogenic hormone)		199	Development and lactation of the mammary gland
Glycoproteins	Lutropin (LH, ICSH)	Ovine	215	Affects reproduction
		Human	204	
	Follitropin (FSH)	Ovine	196	Affects reproduction
		Human	210	
	Thyrotropin (TSH)	Bovine	209	Stimulates thyroid gland to produce thyroid hormones
		Human	211	

connection between the biological effectiveness of the hormone and the species from which it was derived. This was borne out in 1956, when highly purified preparations of growth hormone were successfully isolated from both human and monkey pituitaries (11,32). Chemical studies on these preparations have clearly demonstrated a difference between the human growth hormone (HGH) and the bovine hormone; for example, HGH is a monomer in neutral solutions, whereas bovine hormone is a dimer. The amino acid sequence of HGH has been determined (25,26).

Corticotropin (ACTH) has been isolated in highly purified form from sheep, pig, cattle, human, fish, whale, and ostrich. Although all ACTHs have similar biological properties, they differ slightly in amino acid composition and in chemical structure (24). They are single-chain polypeptides composed of 39 amino acids with serine and phenylalanine as NH_2-terminal and COOH-terminal residues, respectively. Human ACTH has been synthesized by both solution (42) and solid-phase (46) methods.

Two melanotropins are present in pituitary extracts (10), namely, α-MSH and β-MSH. α-Melanotropin consists of 13 amino acid residues and its sequence is identical to the first 13 residues of ACTH, except that the amino group of serine in position 1 is acetylated and the carboxyl group of valine in position 13 is present as an amide. Synthesis of α-MSH was achieved by both solution (9) and solid-phase (2) methods.

β-Melanotropins from various species consist of 18 amino acids, whereas the human hormone consists of 22 amino acids. Human β-MSH has been synthesized by both solution (45) and solid-phase (44) methods.

Lipotropins (LPHs) were discovered only 15 years ago. During the course of improving the yield of ACTH from sheep pituitary extracts, a new component was isolated and characterized to be different chemically from all known pituitary hormones (1,12). It was first assayed for lipolytic activity in rabbit fat pad and shown to be a potent lipotropic agent. There are two lipotropins: β-LPH

```
                              5                 10
Human:    H- Glu- Leu- Thr- Gly- Gln- Arg- Leu- Arg- Gln- Gly-
Ovine:    H- Glu- Leu- Thr- Gly- Glu- Arg- Leu- Glu - Gln- Ala-
Porcine:  H- Glu- Leu- Ala - Gly- Ala- Pro- Pro- Glu - Pro- Ala-


                             15                 20
          Asp- Gly - Pro- Asn- Ala- Gly - Ala- Asn- Asp- Gly-
          Arg- Gly - Pro- Glu - Ala- Gln - Ala- Glu - Ser - Ala-
          Arg- Asp- Pro- Glu - Ala- Pro- Ala- Glu - Gly - Ala-


                             25                 30
          Glu- Gly- Pro- Asn- Ala- Leu- Glu- His- Ser- Leu-
          Ala- Ala- Arg- Ala - Glu- Leu- Glu- Tyr- Gly- Leu-
          Ala- Ala- Arg- Ala - Glu- Leu- Glu- His- Gly- Leu-


                             35                 40
          Leu- Ala- Asp- Leu- Val- Ala- Ala- Glu- Lys- Lys-
          Val - Ala- Glu - Ala - Glu- Ala- Ala- Glu- Lys- Lys-
          Val - Ala- Glu - Ala - Gln- Ala- Ala- Glu- Lys- Lys-


                             45                 50
          Asp- Glu- Gly- Pro- Tyr- Arg- Met- Glu- His- Phe-
          Asp- Ser- Gly- Pro- Tyr- Lys- Met- Glu- His- Phe-
          Asp- Glu- Gly- Pro- Tyr- Lys- Met- Glu- His- Phe-


                             55                 60
          Arg- Trp- Gly- Ser- Pro- Pro- Lys- Asp- Lys- Arg-
          Arg- Trp- Gly- Ser- Pro- Pro- Lys- Asp- Lys- Arg-
          Arg- Trp- Gly- Ser- Pro- Pro- Lys- Asp- Lys- Arg-


                             65                 70
          Tyr- Gly- Gly- Phe- Met- Thr- Ser- Glu- Lys- Ser-
          Tyr- Gly- Gly- Phe- Met- Thr- Ser- Glu- Lys- Ser-
          Tyr- Gly- Gly- Phe- Met- Thr- Ser- Glu- Lys- Ser-


                             75                 80
          Gln- Thr- Pro- Leu- Val- Thr- Leu- Phe- Lys- Asn-
          Gln- Thr- Pro- Leu- Val- Thr- Leu- Phe- Lys- Asn-
          Gln- Thr- Pro- Leu- Val- Thr- Leu- Phe- Lys- Asn-


                             85                 91
          Ala- Ile- Ile  - Lys- Asn- Ala- Tyr- Lys- Lys- Gly- Glu- OH
          Ala- Ile- Ile  - Lys- Asn- Ala- His - Lys- Lys- Gly- Gln- OH
          Ala- Ile- Val - Lys- Asn- Ala- His - Lys- Lys- Gly- Gln- OH
```

FIG. 1. Amino acid sequence of various β-lipotropins.

(18) and γ-LPH (6). β-Lipotropin consists of 91 amino acids with the sequence as shown in Fig. 1 (18,22). γ-Lipotropin has a structure corresponding to the 58 NH$_2$-terminal residues of β-LPH. Total synthesis of sheep β-LPH was recently accomplished by the solid-phase method (47).

In the search for β-lipotropin from camel pituitary glands, a new peptide with 31 amino acids was discovered. Its sequence (23) was identical to the COOH-terminal 31 residues of β-LPH (Fig. 1). It possesses significant opiate activity *in vitro* (7,23) and *in vivo* (35). This untriakontapeptide was designated β-endorphin (β-EP) (23). Both camel (31) and human (34) β-EPs have been synthesized by the solid-phase method.

RESULTS AND DISCUSSION

Semisynthetic Human Somatotropin and Analogs

Human somatotropin is a globular protein with a molecular weight of 22,000, an isoelectric point at pH 4.9, and an α-helical content of 55%. Its primary structure is known (Fig. 2) and contains 191 amino acid residues with the tryptophan residue at position 86. There are two disulfide bridges that are easily reduced and reoxidized to the native state. In addition, the hormone molecule can be reduced and alkylated by iodoacetamide. The resulting tetra-*S*-carbamido-methylated (RCAM) derivative retains all biological activities including those in human subjects. The secondary and tertiary structures of the RCAM derivatives are indistinguishable from the native molecule (14).

It has recently been found that hydrolysis of HGH with human plasmin does not cause any changes of the biological properties of the hormone. It was shown subsequently that the predominant action of plasmin on HGH is the cleavage of the Arg-Thr and Lys-Gln bonds at positions 134–135 and 140–141, respectively. Thus, the main point of a limited plasmin digestion of the hormone is composed of the NH$_2$-terminal portion (residues 1–134) and the COOH-terminal portion (residues 141–191) of HGH. They are connected to each other by a disulfide linkage at sequence positions 53 and 165. The removal of the hexapeptide (residues 135–140) from the structure of HGH does not alter the conformation of the molecule as evidenced by the circular dichroism (CD) spectra. Moreover, the biological potency of the plasmin-modified HGH (PL-HGH) remains the same as the native hormone (29).

When PL-HGH is submitted to reduction and alkylation, two peptide fragments are easily separated by exclusion chromatography on Sephadex G-50 in 10% acetic acid: [Cys(Cam)^{53}-HGH-(1–134)] and [Cys(Cam)^{165,182,189}-HGH-(141–191)]. Bioassay data showed both fragments to be biologically active. The biological activity of NH$_2$-terminal 1–134 fragment is about 14% of that for native HGH by both the rat tibia and pigeon crop-sac tests. The COOH-terminal fragment (residue 141–191) also exhibits activity in both tests, although it is less active in comparison with the NH$_2$-terminal fragment (14,29).

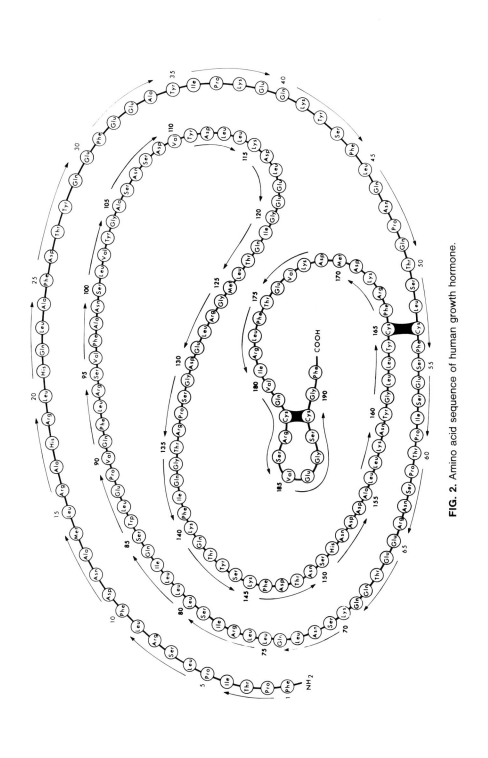

FIG. 2. Amino acid sequence of human growth hormone.

It is possible to regenerate full biological activity by noncovalent interaction of these two fragments in 0.1 M Tris-HCl buffer of pH 8.4 containing 5% *n*-butanol (16,19,30). As shown in Fig. 3, the immunoreactivity of recombined solutions increases to a maximal value within 24 hr, indicating that the complementation reaction is a rapid process. Purification of the recombined solution was achieved by exclusion chromatography on Sephadex G-100 in 0.01 M NH₄HCO₃ at pH 8.2. Figure 4 shows the elution pattern of the reaction mixture and the material appears in peak III at a Ve/Vo ratio of 2.08, which is the same for HGH under identical experimental conditions. The recovered protein (yield, 40%) from peak III was assayed for biological activities (Table 2). The circular dichroism spectra of the recombinant is not significantly different from

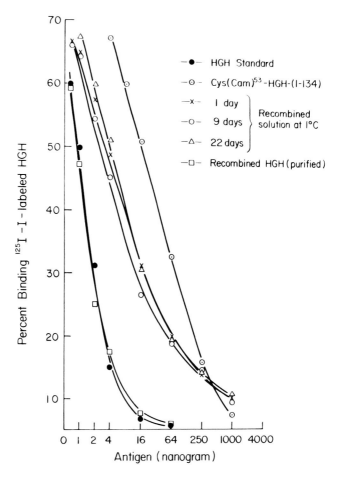

FIG. 3. Immunoreactivity of recombined solutions at various intervals and purified recombinant human growth hormone (HGH) by radioimmunoassay. Final dilution of guinea pig antiserum to HGH was 1:100,000.

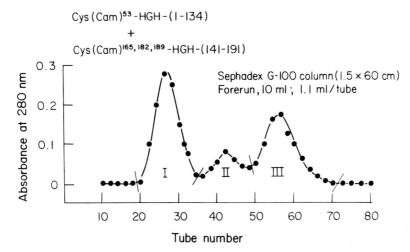

FIG. 4. Exclusion chromatography of the reaction mixture on a Sephadex G-100 column (1.5 × 60 cm) in 0.01 M NH_4CO_3 at pH 8.4.

that of the natural hormone, indicating that the three-dimensional structure has also been restored (19).

The recombinant hormone obtained by noncovalent interaction of the natural NH_2-terminal 1–134 fragment with a synthetic COOH-terminal fragment of 52 amino acids [Cys-(Cam)[165,182,189]-HGH-(140–191)] (3) is also found to exhibit full biological activity (Table 3) of the native hormone as evidenced by the tibia test (20). Radioimmunoassay (RIA) data indicate that the semisynthetic recombinant hormone possesses essentially full immunoreactivity as compared with the native one.

Two synthetic analogs of COOH-terminal fragments of HGH, [Nle[170],

TABLE 2. *Prolactin and growth-promoting activities of the recombinant obtained by noncovalent interaction of the two fragments of HGH*

Preparation	Pigeon crop-sac assay		Rat tibia assay	
	Total dose (nmoles)	Response[a]	Total dose (nmoles)	Response[b]
HGH	0.093	18.5 ± 0.7	0.47[c]	216.8 ± 2.6
	0.279	25.0 ± 2.1	1.40	261.3 ± 2.2
Recombinant	0.093	19.2 ± 0.8	0.47[d]	223.8 ± 10.8
	0.279	24.6 ± 0.8	1.40	257.8 ± 10.4
Saline	0	10.7 ± 0.2	0	155.3 ± 4.7

[a] Dry mucosal weight in mg; mean ± SE; four birds in each group.
[b] Tibia width in microns; mean ± SE; four animals in each group.
[c] Relative potency to PL-HGH, 102% with 95% confidence limit of 59–176 and $\lambda = 0.22$.
[d] Relative potency to PL-HGH, 108% with 95% confidence limit of 70–158 and $\lambda = 0.15$.

TABLE 3. *Growth-promoting activity of the semisynthetic hormone by rat tibia assay*

Preparation	Total dose (μg)	Response[a]
HGH	20	226 ± 0.8
	60	273 ± 5.8
Semisynthetic HGH[b]	20	233 ± 3.3
	60	267 ± 2.8
Saline	0	162 ± 1.9

[a] Tibia width in microns; mean $\pm$ SE; six animals in each group.
[b] Relative potency to HGH, 101% with 95% confidence limit of 82–124 and $\lambda = 0.11$.

Ala[165,182,189]-HGH-(140–191) and [Nle[170],Ala[165,182,189]]-HGH-(145–191) have been described (4). As shown in Table 4, complementation of these two synthetic analogs with the natural NH$_2$-terminal fragment (consisting of 134 amino acid residues) gave recombinants with full growth-promoting activity (21). Immunoreactivity of semisynthetic HGH analogs was nearly identical to the natural hormone as evidenced by the RIA data (21).

Aspects of Structure-Activity Relationship of β-Endorphin

Among various fragments of β-LPH-(61–91) (Fig. 1) having opioid activity, only β-endorphin (β-EP) exhibits potent analgesic activity by intravenous injection (43). In addition, it is the most active peptide when administered directly into the brain (35). Amino acid sequences of various β-EP are shown in Fig. 5.

TABLE 4. *Growth-promoting activity of recombinant hormones by rat tibia assay*

Preparation	Total dose (μg)	Response[a]
HGH	20	245.0 ± 9.5
	60	290.2 ± 2.9
Recombinant I[b,c]	20	249.2 ± 9.2
	60	286.0 ± 2.1
Recombinant II[d,e]	20	248.5 ± 7.7
	60	297.2 ± 10.0
Saline	0	167.0 ± 1.3

[a] Tibia width in microns; mean $\pm$ SE; four animals in each group.
[b] Recombinant I: [Cys(Cam)[53]]-HGH-(1–134) + [Nle[170],ALa[165,182,189]]-HGH-(140–191).
[c] Relative potency to HGH, 100%, with 95% confidence limits of 65–154 and $\lambda = 0.16$.
[d] Recombinant II: [Cys(Cam)[53]]-HGH-(1–134) + [Nle[170],Ala[165,182,189]]-HGH-(145–191).
[e] Relative potency to HGH, 113%, with 95% confidence limits of 74–180 and $\lambda = 0.16$.

HUMAN:

$$\overset{5}{\text{H–Tyr–Gly–Gly–Phe–Met}}\text{–Thr–Ser–Glu–Lys–Ser–}\overset{10}{}$$

$$\overset{15}{\text{Gln–Thr–Pro–Leu–Val}}\text{–Thr–Leu–Phe–Lys–Asn–}\overset{20}{}$$

$$\overset{25}{\text{Ala–Ile–Ile–Lys–Asn}}\text{–Ala–Tyr–Lys–Lys–Gly–Glu–OH}\overset{31}{}$$

| PORCINE: | VAL | HIS | GLN-OH |
| CAMEL, OVINE, BOVINE: | ILE | HIS | GLN-OH |

FIG. 5. Amino acid sequences of various β-endorphins.

Synthetic Analogs with Various Amino Acid Residues in Positions 1,2,4, and 5

Tables 5 and 6 summarized the *in vivo* and *in vitro* opiate activities of synthetic analogs with various amino acid residues (48,49) in positions 1,2,4, and 5. It may be noted that substitutions of Tyr[1] with D-isomer residue in position 2 with Sar, Ala, D-Leu, and D-Lys, position 4 with D-Phe, and position 5 with D-Met, Pro, Leu, and D-Leu decrease the activity. Substitution of Gly[2] with D-Ala retains full analgesic activity. The synthetic analog containing a Lue-enkephalin segment has only 17% the analgesic activity of the parent molecule and replacement of Leu with D-isomer lowers the activity to only 0.2%. Apparently, residue 5 in the β-EP structure is more important for its analgesic activity.

Synthetic Analogs with Various Chain Lengths

The syntheses of β_h-EP-(1–15), -(1–21), -(1–26), -(1–28), -(1–29), and -(1–30) have been accomplished (33,50) by an improved procedure of the solid-phase method. Table 7 summarizes various biological activities of synthetic

TABLE 5. *Opiate activity of synthetic β_c-endorphin with D-amino acids in positions 1, 2, 4, and 5*

Synthetic peptides	Relative potency	
	Guinea pig ileum assay	i.c.v. in mice
β_c-EP	100	100
[D-Tyr[1]]-β_c-EP	<1	0.5
[D-Ala[2]]-β_c-EP	43	100
[D-Phe[4]]-β_c-EP	4	<0.3
[D-Met[5]]-β_c-EP	4	1

TABLE 6. *Opiate activity of synthetic β-endorphin with substitutions in positions 2 and 5*

| | Relative potency | |
Synthetic peptides	Guinea pig ileum assay	i.c.v. in mice
β_h-EP	100	100
[Sar^2]-β_c-EP	13	0.3
[Ala^2]-β_c-EP	6	12
[D-Leu^2]-β_c-EP	12	48
[D-Lys^2]-β_c-EP	8	15
[Pro^5]-β_h-EP	<0.01	0.6
[Leu^5]-β_h-EP	18	17
[D-Leu^5]-β_h-EP	<0.01	0.2
[D-Ala^2,D-Leu^5]-β_h-EP	3	8

β_h-EP analogs with different chain lengths. In the guinea pig ileum assay, the extension of β-EP-(1–5) at its COOH-terminus to give β-EP-(1–15) leads to loss in potency. Further extension to give β-EP-(1–21) restores activity exceeding that of the NH$_2$-terminal pentapeptide. No significant increment of activity is observed by further addition of five more residues to form β-EP-(1–26). The most dramatic gain in activity occurs as the chain is lengthened by addition of the next three residues. Thus, β-EP-(1–29) displays the full activity of β_h-EP in the guinea pig ileum assay.

The immunoreactivities of analogs of various chain lengths as measured by the β_h-EP RIA system (5) are also summarized in Table 7. β-EP-(1–15) and -(1–21) are practically inactive. On the other hand, β_h-EP-(1–28) and -(1–29) are equally potent as the intact molecule on a weight basis, whereas β_h-EP-(1–26) is partially active.

The analgesic activity of synthetic peptides was assessed in mice by the tail-flick method after the test substances were injected directly into the brain. As shown in Table 7, the removal of one amino acid at a time starting with the COOH-terminus of β_h-EP reduced the potency of analgesic activity of β_h-EP

TABLE 7. *Relative potency of synthetic analogs with various chain lengths*

Synthetic peptide	Guinea pig ileum assay	Analgesic activity in mice	Immunoreactivity by RIA
β_h-Endorphin(β_h-EP)	100	100	100
β_h-EP-(1–30)	—	72	100
β_h-EP-(1–29)	104	20	95
β_h-EP-(1–28)	89	6	90
β_h-EP-(1–26)	48	8	65
β_h-EP-(1–21)	46	0.3	<2
β_h-EP-(1–15)	17	<0.1	<1
β_h-EP-(1–5)	25	nil	0

in a stepwise fashion. Thus, removal of COOH-terminal Glu reduced analgesic activity by 28%, removal of -Gly-Glu reduced it by 80%, and removal of -Lys-Gly-Glu by 94%. These data indicate that all 31 amino acid residues are required for full analgesic activity.

SUMMARY

The chemistry of anterior pituitary hormones is briefly reviewed. Recent studies on the complementation of two plasmin fragments of HGH are presented with the data of semisynthetic molecules with full biological activities. Aspects of structure-activity relationship of β-endorphin are discussed. It is noted that complete primary structure is required for full analgesic activity of β-endorphin. In addition, residues 1 and 5 in the β-endorphin structure are essential for its analgesic activity.

ACKNOWLEDGMENT

I thank my collaborators whose names are cited in the references for their contributions to these investigations. Experimental work was supported in part by NIH grants GM-2907, AM-18677, and NIMH grant MH-30245.

REFERENCES

1. Birk, Y., and Li, C. H. (1964): Isolation and properties of a new, biologically active peptide from sheep pituitary glands. *J. Biol. Chem.,* 239:1048–1052.
2. Blake, J. T., and Li, C. H. (1971): The solid-phase synthesis of alpha-melanotropin. *Int. J. Pept. Protein Res.,* 3:185–189.
3. Blake, J. T., and Li, C. H. (1975): The synthesis and biological activity of [165,182,189-*S*-carbamidomethylcysteine]-human growth hormone-(140–191). *Int. J. Pept. Protein Res.,* 7:495–501.
4. Blake, J. T., and Li, C. H. (1978): Human somatotropin. 55. Synthesis and growth-promoting activity of peptide analogs of the carboxyl terminal plasmin fragment. *Int. J. Pept. Protein Res.,* 11:315–322.
5. Chang, W. C., Yeung, H. W., and Li, C. H. (1979): Human β-endorphin: Immunoreactivity of synthetic analogs with various chain lengths. *Int. J. Pept. Protein Res.,* 13:278–281.
6. Chrétien, M., and Li, C. H. (1967): Isolation, purification, and characterization of γ-lipotropic hormone from sheep pituitary glands. *Can. J. Biochem.,* 45:1163–1174.
7. Cox, M. B., Goldstein, A., and Li, C. H. (1976): Opioid activity of a peptide, β-lipotropin-(61–91), derived from β-lipotropin. *Proc. Natl. Acad. Sci. USA,* 73:1821–1823.
8. Farmer, S. W., Papkoff, H., Bewley, T. A., Hayashida, T., Nishioka, R. S., Bern, J. A., and Li, C. H. (1977): Isolation and properties of teleost prolactin. *Gen. Comp. Endocrinol.,* 31:60–71.
9. Guttman, S., and Boissonnas, R. A. (1959): Synthése de l'α-mélanotropin (α-MSH) de porc. *Helv. Chim. Acta,* 42:1257–1264.
10. Lerner, A. B., and Lee, T. H. (1962): The melanocyte-stimulating hormone. *Vitam. Horm.,* 20:337–346.
11. Li, C. H. (1957): Properties and structural investigations on growth hormones isolated from bovine, monkey and human pituitary glands. *Fed. Proc.,* 16:775–783.
12. Li, C. H. (1964): Lipotropin, a new active peptide from pituitary glands. *Nature,* 201:924.
13. Li, C. H. (1972): Hormones of the adenohypophysis. *Proc. Am. Phil. Soc.,* 116:365–382.

14. Li, C. H. (1975): The chemistry of human pituitary growth hormone, 1967–1973. In: *Hormonal Proteins and Peptides, Vol. 3,* edited by C. H. Li, pp. 1–40. Academic Press, New York.
15. Li, C. H. (1976): Studies on pituitary lactogenic hormone. The primary structure of the porcine hormone. *Int. J. Pept. Protein. Res.,* 8:205–224.
16. Li, C. H. (1978): Noncovalent interaction of the NH₂-terminal fragment of human somatotropin with the COOH-terminal fragment of human choriomammotropin to generate growth-promoting activity. *Proc. Natl. Acad. Sci. USA,* 75:1700–1702.
17. Li, C. H. (1979): The chemistry of prolactin. In: *Hormonal Proteins and Peptide, Vol. 8,* edited by C. H. Li, pp. 1–36. Academic Press, New York.
18. Li, C. H., Barnafi, L., Chrétien, M., and Chung, D. (1966): Isolation and structure of β-LPH from sheep pituitary glands. In: *Proceedings VIth Pan American Congress of Endocrinology,* edited by C. Gual, pp. 349–364. Excerpta Medica, New York.
19. Li, C. H., and Bewley, T. A. (1976): Human pituitary growth hormone: Restoration of full biological activity by non-covalent interaction of two fragments of the hormones. *Proc. Natl. Acad. Sci. USA,* 73:1476–1479.
20. Li, C. H., Bewley, T. A., Blake, J., and Hayashida, T. (1977): Human somatotropin: Restoration of full biological activity by noncovalent interaction of a natural and a synthetic fragment of the hormone. *Proc. Natl. Acad. Sci. USA,* 74:1016–1019.
21. Li, C. H., Blake, J., and Hayashida, T. (1978): Human somatotropin: Semisynthesis of the hormone by noncovalent interaction of the NH₂-terminal fragment with synthetic analogs of the COOH-terminal fragment. *Biochem. Biophys. Res. Commun.,* 82:217–222.
22. Li, C. H., and Chung, D. (1976): Primary structure of human β-lipotropin. *Nature,* 260:623–624.
23. Li, C. H., and Chung, D. (1976): Isolation and structure of an untriakontapeptide with opiate activity from camel pituitary glands. *Proc. Natl. Acad. Sci. USA,* 73:1145–1148.
24. Li, C. H., Chung, D., Oelofsen, W., and Naudé, R. J. (1978): Adrenocorticotropin 53. The amino acid sequence of the hormone from the ostrich pituitary glands. *Biochem. Biophys. Res. Commun.,* 81:900–906.
25. Li, C. H., and Dixon, J. S. (1971): Human pituitary hormone. XXXII. The primary structure of the hormone. Revision. *Arch. Biochem. Biophys.,* 146:233–236.
26. Li, C. H., Dixon, J. S., and Liu, W. K. (1969): Human pituitary growth hormone. XIX. The primary structure of the hormone. *Arch. Biochem. Biophys.,* 133:70–91.
27. Li, C. H., Dixon, J. S., Lo, T. B., Pankov, Y. A., and Schmidt, K. D. (1969): Amino acid sequence of ovine lactogenic hormone. *Nature,* 223:695–696.
28. Li, C. H., and Evans, H. M. (1944): The isolation of pituitary growth hormone. *Science,* 99:183–184.
29. Li, C. H., and Gráf, L. (1974): Human pituitary growth hormone: Isolation and properties of two biologically active fragments from plasmin digests. *Proc. Natl. Acad. Sci. USA,* 71:1197–1201.
30. Li, C. H., Hayashida, T., Doneen, B. A., and Rao, A. J. (1976): Human somatotropin: Biological characterization of the recombinant molecule. *Proc. Natl. Acad. Sci. USA,* 73:3463–3465.
31. Li, C. H., Lemaire, S., Yamashiro, D., and Doneen, B. A. (1976): The synthesis and opiate activity of β-endorphin. *Biochem. Biophys. Res. Commun.,* 71:19–25.
32. Li, C. H., and Papkoff, H. (1956): Preparation and properties of growth hormone from human and monkey pituitary glands. *Science,* 124:1293–1294.
33. Li, C. H., Tseng, L. F., and Yamashiro, D. (1978): β-Endorphin: Complete primary structure is required for full analgesic activity. *Biochem. Biophys. Res. Commun.,* 85:795–800.
34. Li, C. H., Yamashiro, D., Tseng, L. F., and Loh, H. H. (1977): Synthesis and analgesic activity of human β-endorphin. *J. Med. Chem.,* 20:325–328.
35. Loh, H. H., Tseng, L. F., Wei, E., and Li, C. H. (1976): β-Endorphin is a potent analgesic agent. *Proc. Natl. Acad. Sci. USA,* 73:2895–2898.
36. Papkoff, H., Ryan, R. J., and Ward, D. N. (1977): The gonadotropic hormones. In: *Frontiers in Reproduction and Fertility Control,* edited by R. O. Greep and M. A. Koblinsky, pp. 1–10. MIT Press, Cambridge, Massachusetts.
37. Pierce, J. G. (1971): The subunits of pituitary thyrotropin: Their relationship to other glycoprotein hormones. *Endocrinology,* 89:1331–1344.
38. Pierce, J. G., Liao, T.-H., and Carlsen, R. B. (1973): The chemistry of pituitary thyrotropin. In: *Hormonal Proteins and Peptides, Vol. 1,* edited by C. H. Li, pp. 17–57. Academic Press, New York.

39. Sairam, M. R., and Li, C. H. (1977): Human pituitary thyrotropin. The primary structure of the α and β subunits. *Can. J. Biochem.,* 55:755–760.
40. Sairam, M. R., and Li, C. H. (1978): Chemistry of human pituitary thyrotropin. In: *Hormonal Proteins and Peptides, Vol. 6,* edited by C. H. Li, pp. 1–56. Academic Press, New York.
41. Shome B., and Parlow, A. F. (1974): Human follicle stimulating hormone: First proposal for the amino acid sequence of the hormone-specific β subunit (hFSHβ). *J. Clin. Endocrinol. Metab.,* 39:203–205.
42. Sieber, P., Rittel, W., and Riniker, B. (1972): Die Synthese von menschlichem adrenocorticotropem Hormon (α$_h$-ACTH) mit revidierter Aminosäuresequenz. *Helv. Chim. Acta,* 55:1243–1248.
43. Tseng, L. F., Loh, H. H., and Li, C. H. (1976): β-Endorphin as a potent analgesic by intravenous injection. *Nature,* 263:239–240.
44. Wang, K. T., Blake, J., and Li, C. H. (1973): The solid-phase synthesis of human and monkey beta-melanotropins. *Int. J. Pept. Protein Res.,* 5:33–36.
45. Yajima, H., Okada, Y., Kimomura, Y., Mizokami, N., and Kawatami, H. (1969): Studies on peptides. XXIII. Total synthesis of monkey β-melanocyte-stimulating hormone. *Chem. Pharm. Bull. (Tokyo),* 17:1237–1245.
46. Yamashiro, D., and Li, C. H. (1973): Adrenocorticotropins 44. Total synthesis of human hormone by the solid-phase method. *J. Am. Chem. Soc.,* 95:1310–1315.
47. Yamashiro, D., and Li, C. H. (1978): Total synthesis of ovine β-lipotropin by the solid-phase method. *J. Am. Chem. Soc.,* 100:5174–5179.
48. Yamashiro, D., Li, C. H., Tseng, L. F., and Loh, H. H. (1978): β-Endorphin: Synthesis and analgesic activity of several analogs modified in positions 2 and 5. *Int. J. Pept. Protein Res.,* 11:251–257.
49. Yamashiro, D., Tseng, L. F., Doneen, B. A., Loh, H. H., and Li, C. H. (1977): β-Endorphin: Synthesis and morphine-like activity of analogs with D-amino acid residues in positions 1, 2, 4, and 5. *Int. J. Pept. Protein Res.,* 10:159–166.
50. Yeung, H. W., Yamashiro, D., Chang, W. C., and Li, C. H. (1978): Synthesis and opiate activity of human β-endorphin analogs with various chain lengths. *Int. J. Pept. Protein Res.,* 12:42–46.

Polypeptide Hormones, edited by
R. F. Beers, Jr. and E. G. Bassett.
Raven Press, New York © 1980.

27. Studies of Adrenocorticotropin Receptors

J. Ramachandran, *C. Y. Lee, György Keri,
and Maria Kenez-Keri

Hormone Research Laboratory, University of California, San Francisco, California 94143

INTRODUCTION

Although the involvement of cyclic AMP in the actions of adrenocorticotropin (ACTH) was proposed more than 20 years ago (5), there is still considerable debate as to the nature of the second messenger mediating the steroidogenic action of the hormone. Doubts about the role of cyclic AMP in ACTH-induced steroidogenesis first surfaced in 1972 when it was observed that physiological concentrations of the hormone could stimulate corticosterone synthesis in isolated rat adrenocortical cells without causing detectable changes in the intracellular concentration of cyclic AMP (1,13,14,18). Studies from our laboratory (16) showed that the o-nitrophenylsulfenyl derivative of ACTH (NPS-ACTH) was able to stimulate steroidogenesis to the same extent as ACTH (albeit at higher concentrations) but caused only a marginal increase in cyclic AMP. Studies with several other analogs of ACTH also emphasized the discrepancy between the peptide concentrations required for eliciting steroid synthesis and cyclic AMP production (24). These results have been explained in two ways.

Proponents of the cyclic AMP theory of hormone action invoke the spare receptor concept (26) to account for the apparent dissociation between steroidogenesis and cyclic AMP formation (1,13). According to this, the adrenocortical cells contain receptors much in excess of that necessary for maximal stimulation of the physiological response. The spare receptor concept implies that only a very small fraction of the total cyclic AMP, which can be generated by interaction of the hormone with all the receptors, is required for mediating the steroidogenic response.

The alternative explanation of the discrepancy between the steroidogenic and cyclic AMP responses is that the two responses are mediated by two different receptors. In this scheme, steroidogenesis is stimulated by the interaction of ACTH with the high-affinity sites and the large increase in cyclic AMP is caused by the action of the hormone on lower affinity sites. In the two receptor

---

* Permanent address: Department of Biochemistry, Chinese University of Hong Kong, Shatin, N.T., Hong Kong.

formulation, the second messenger could be cyclic AMP or some other factor. If cyclic AMP mediated steroidogenesis, it would have to be generated in a special compartment of the adrenocortical cell in response to the interaction of the hormone with the high-affinity sites. Recently, both cyclic GMP (4,20) and Ca^{2+} (19,21,25,28) have been proposed as second messengers involved in the stimulation of steroidogenesis by ACTH. Irrespective of what the second messenger is, it would be of great value to know if there are one or two classes of receptors for ACTH on adrenocortical cells.

The presence of two types of receptors for ACTH in extracts of a mouse adrenal tumor was inferred from early binding studies with ^{125}I-ACTH (9). Lefkowitz et al. (9) reported that the adrenal tumor cell contained 60 high-affinity sites of $k_d = 1.1 \times 10^{-12}$ M and 360,000 low-affinity sites of $K_d = 3.3 \times 10^{-8}$ M. Studies of the binding of ^{125}I-ACTH preparations to isolated rat adrenocortical cells have also suggested the presence of high- and low-affinity receptors. McIlhinney and Schulster (14) found sites with $K_d = 2.5 \times 10^{-10}$ M (3,000 sites/cell) and $K_d = 1 \times 10^{-8}$ M (30,000 sites/cell). Yanagibashi et al. (28) estimated that there are 7,350 high-affinity sites per cell ($K_d = 2.6 \times 10^{-10}$ M) and 57,400 low-affinity sites/cell ($K_d = 7.1 \times 10^{-9}$ M). However, in view of the low biological activities of ^{125}I-ACTH preparations and the strong tendency of ACTH to bind to inert materials and nonreceptor components of target cells (2), it is important to confirm these observations by other methods. We are attempting to answer this question by three experimental approaches, namely, (a) direct binding studies with specifically tritiated ACTH of full biological activity, (b) analysis of the inhibition of ACTH-induced steroidogenesis and cyclic AMP formation by corticotropin inhibiting peptide (CIP), a naturally occurring inhibitor, and (c) study of the desensitization of the steroidogenic and cyclic AMP responses after stimulation with ACTH. The results of these studies are discussed below.

RESULTS AND DISCUSSION

Binding Studies with Tritiated ACTH

[3,5-^{3}H]-Tyr$^{2,23}\alpha_h$-ACTH (^{3}H-ACTH) was prepared by catalytic dehalogenation of 3,5-diiodoTyr$^{2,23}\alpha_h$-ACTH (10) with pure tritium in the presence of palladium as previously described (23). ^{3}H-ACTH was purified by gel filtration on Sephadex G-25 and ion-exchange chromatography on carboxymethylcellulose. This preparation of ^{3}H-ACTH was found to be homogeneous by paper electrophoresis at pH 3.7 and 6.7 and comigrated with synthetic human ACTH. Electrophoresis of a tryptic digest of ^{3}H-ACTH at pH 6.7 showed that the radioactivity was equally distributed in the peptides corresponding to α_h^{1-8}-ACTH and α_h^{22-39}-ACTH. The ultraviolet absorption spectrum of ^{3}H-ACTH was identical to that of synthetic human ACTH, indicating that the iodine atoms on the tyrosine residues were quantitatively removed. The amino acid composition of an acid hydrolysate of ³H-ACTH agreed well with that of human ACTH. The ability of ³H-ACTH to stimulate glycerol release in isolated rat adipocytes or corticosterone synthesis in isolated rat adrenocortical cells was indistinguishable from that of synthetic human ACTH. The potency of ³H-ACTH was identical to that of synthetic human ACTH in both assays. The specific radioactivity of this preparation of ³H-ACTH was found to be 90 Ci/mmole (200 dpm/fmole) or approximately 80% of the theoretically attainable radioactivity.

The binding of ³H-ACTH to isolated rat adrenocortical cells was studied by incubating the radioactive hormone with 0.5 to 1.0×10^6 cells in phosphate-buffered saline (PBS) containing 0.5% bovine serum albumin and 0.01% lima bean trypsin inhibitor in polypropylene microfuge tubes. Free and bound hormone were separated by centrifugation, aspiration of the supernatant, and washing once with ice-cold incubation buffer. The tip of the microfuge tube containing the cell pellet was cut, digested in 0.5 ml NCS solubilizer for 16 hr at 37°C, mixed with scintillant, and counted.

It was found that about 5% of the added ³H-ACTH was bound optimally to the adrenocortical cells and nearly 50% of this was displaced by a large excess of unlabeled ACTH (Table 1). However, under these conditions, various other hormones including insulin, prolactin, and luteinizing hormone (LH) also displaced significant amounts of radioactivity. Basic peptides such as cardiotoxin and polylysine were almost as effective as ACTH in displacing the bound radioactivity. These results suggested that there was considerable nonreceptor binding of ³H-ACTH even though the concentration of ³H-ACTH was only 3 nM. In view of the efficacy of polylysine in displacing ³H-ACTH from apparent nonreceptor sites on adrenocortical cells, we employed this basic polypeptide to mask these sites. As shown in the right hand column of Table 1, 70% of the total bound radioactivity could be displaced by nonradioactive ACTH when the binding studies were performed in the presence of 0.01% polylysine. This binding was quite specific since insulin, prolactin, LH, and cardiotoxin did not displace the bound hormone. NPS-ACTH, which stimulates steroidogenesis and inhibits ACTH-induced cyclic AMP production, competed effectively with ³H-ACTH. Polylysine preparations of 15,000 and 85,000 M.W. did not stimulate corticosterone synthesis or cyclic AMP production at any concentration tested (0.01–100 μg/ml) and had no effect on the ability of ACTH to stimulate steroid synthesis and cyclic AMP formation.

In the presence of 0.01% polylysine the binding of ³H-ACTH was found to be rapid and saturable. The specific binding of ³H-ACTH as a function of concentration is shown in Fig. 1. Significant specific binding of ³H-ACTH could not be detected at concentrations below 1 nM. In the near physiological range of concentrations (1–10 nM), the binding studies reveal the presence of one class of receptors with a K_d of 2 to 4 nM. At saturation, about 7 fmoles of ³H-ACTH were bound per 10⁶ cells. This amounts to approximately 4,000 sites per cell. The results of an experiment in which binding, corticosterone synthesis,

TABLE 1. *Specificity of binding of ³H-ACTH to adrenocortical cells*[a]

	Displacement (%)	
Peptide	Polylysine absent	Polylysine (0.01%)
ACTH	47.3	71.6
NPS-ACTH	31.0	39.4
Insulin	22.9	0
LH	26.7	0
Prolactin	23.8	0
Cardiotoxin	40.2	0

[a] Isolated rat adrenocortical cells were incubated overnight at 4°C with 3 nM ³H-ACTH in the presence and absence of the peptides (30 µg/ml, except unlabeled ACTH which was present at 100 µg/ml). Binding was measured as described in the text.

and cyclic AMP accumulation were measured with the same batch of cells is shown in Fig. 2. Maximal steroidogenesis was produced by concentrations of ACTH at which no binding of ³H-ACTH or cyclic AMP accumulation could be detected. The binding of ³H-ACTH appears to correlate better with cyclic

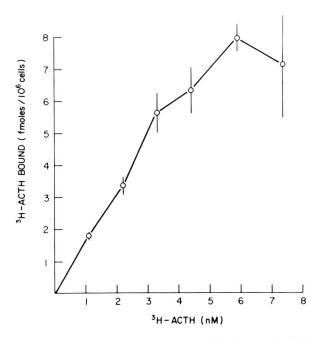

FIG. 1. Binding of ³H-ACTH to adrenocortical cells as a function of ³H-ACTH concentration. Adrenocortical cells were incubated with ³H-ACTH in PBS-0.5% BSA-0.01% LTI-0.01% polylysine for 16 hr. Radioactivity not displaced by a large excess of unlabeled ACTH (10^{-5} M) has been subtracted to obtain the amount of ³H-ACTH bound specifically. *Vertical bars* extend to the limits of the SE for triplicate incubations at each point.

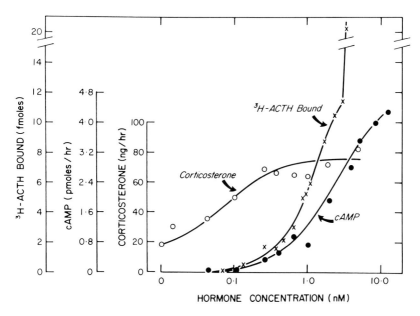

FIG. 2. Correlation of corticosterone production, cyclic AMP formation, and ³H-ACTH binding to adrenocortical cells. Specific binding was measured as described for Fig. 1. Corticosterone and cyclic AMP were measured by radioimmunoassay with the same batch of cells.

AMP production. The concentration of ACTH required for half-maximal stimulation of cyclic AMP formation in the presence of polylysine was also found to be 2 to 4 nM.

These studies indicate that the adrenocortical cells contain a large number of nonfunctional sites in addition to a limited number of high-affinity sites that appear to be related to cyclic AMP production. Higher affinity sites capable of interacting with ACTH at steroidogenic concentrations could not be detected with ³H-ACTH even though the ³H-ACTH had high specific radioactivity (90 Ci/mmole) and full biological activity. This does not rule out the presence of higher affinity sites and, therefore, these binding studies are not sufficient to decide whether the spare receptor concept or the two-receptor thesis is applicable in the case of adrenocortical cells. These results also emphasize the enormous technical difficulties in the direct identification of ACTH receptors.

Studies with Corticotropin-inhibiting Peptide (α_h^{7-38}-ACTH)

The presence of a basic peptide in the sheep pituitary with an amino acid composition corresponding to that of residues 7–38 of ovine ACTH was first reported by Pickering et al. (22). A similar peptide has subsequently been isolated from human pituitary glands, characterized, and synthesized by Li et al. (12). We have found that this peptide, designated corticotropin-inhibiting peptide (CIP), has no intrinsic steroidogenic or cyclic AMP generating activity but is able to block these actions of ACTH in a competitive manner (8). We have analyzed the inhibition of ACTH-induced steroidogenesis and cyclic AMP formation by CIP and compared the results with the inhibition expected on the basis of the spare receptor concept.

The effects of ACTH and CIP (α_h^{7-38}-ACTH) on steroidogenesis and cyclic AMP production in isolated rat adrenocortical cells are shown in Fig. 3. CIP failed to stimulate corticosterone synthesis or cyclic AMP formation at all concentrations tested. However, the analog was able to inhibit ACTH-induced stimulation of corticosterone and cyclic AMP synthesis. The inhibition is competitive in nature, as shown by the fact that although 0.455 μM α_h^{7-38}-ACTH caused a shift in the concentration of ACTH required for half-maximal stimulation of steroidogenesis from 0.05 to 0.85 nM and that for cyclic AMP production from 2.9 to 24 nM, in neither response was the maximal stimulation achievable affected by the analog.

The apparent inhibitory constants of CIP for inhibition of ACTH-induced steroidogenesis and cyclic AMP production were estimated by analyzing the CIP concentration-inhibition relationship at various concentrations of ACTH.

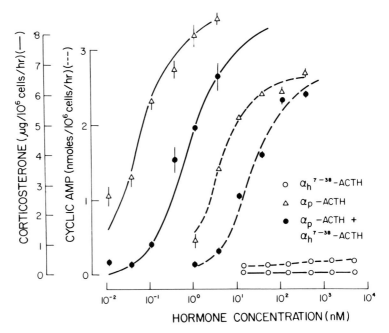

FIG. 3. Effects of ACTH and α_h^{7-38}-ACTH on corticosterone and cyclic AMP production. Isolated adrenocortical cells were incubated with varying concentrations of ACTH (Δ) or α_h^{7-38}-ACTH ($\bigcirc$) or ACTH + 0.455 μM α_h^{7-38}-ACTH ($\bullet$). Corticosterone and cyclic AMP were determined by radioligand binding assay. *Vertical bars* extend to the limits of the SE for triplicate incubations at each point.

Typical inhibition curves for submaximal and maximal stimulation of the two responses are shown in Fig. 4. In each experiment, the concentration of hormone required for half-maximal stimulation of each response (H_{50}) in the absence of the inhibitor was separately determined with the same batch of cells as that employed for the inhibition studies. The values of the apparent inhibitory constants for the responses measured at different ACTH concentrations, together with those of H_{50} and I_{50} are listed in Table 2. It is clear that the apparent K_i for the inhibition of cyclic AMP production is significantly higher than that for the inhibition of steroidogenesis. The average values from five experiments are 301 ± 62 nM and 21.6 ± 6.8 nM, respectively. The difference is highly significant ($p < 0.01$).

The results in Table 2 suggest that if there is one class of receptors mediating both responses (spare receptor model), half-maximal stimulation of steroidogenesis can be achieved by activating less than 0.3% of the receptors, assuming a linear relationship between binding and cyclic AMP production. This model predicts that much higher concentrations of CIP would be needed for inhibiting

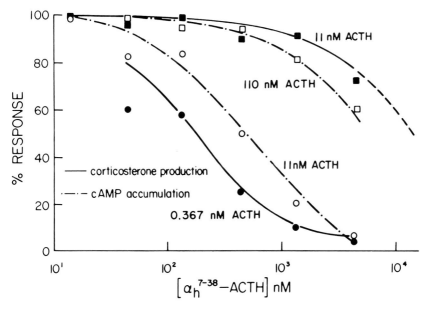

FIG. 4. Inhibition of ACTH-induced corticosterone and cyclic AMP production by α_h^{7-38}-ACTH. One hundred percent response was that observed for each concentration of ACTH in the absence of α_h^{7-38}-ACTH. *Points* represent experimental values. *Curves* trace the computer-generated points derived from weighted, nonlinear least squares fit to the equation

$$\text{percent response} = \frac{100}{1 + \dfrac{H_{50}I}{(H_{50} + H)\,K_i}}$$

I, concentration of α_h^{7-38}-ACTH; H, concentration of ACTH; H_{50}, concentration of ACTH required for half-maximal response in the absence of inhibitor; K_i, inhibitory constant.

TABLE 2. Pharmacologic parameters for the effect of ACTH and CIP on corticosterone and cyclic AMP production in isolated rat adrenal cells[a]

ACTH (nM)	Steroidogenesis			Cyclic AMP production		
	H_{50}^s	I_{50}^s	K_i^s	H_{50}^c	I_{50}^c	K_i^c
0.367	0.0167	178 ± 45	7.9	—	—	—
0.734	0.0160	1,404 ± 152	30.0	—	—	—
1.84	0.0160	4,681 ± 340	40.4	—	—	—
3.67	0.0167	1,041 ± 427	4.5	9.90	510 ± 130	334
7.34	—	—	—	2.95	467 ± 98	134
11.0	0.019	14,754 ± 4,840	25.0	7.00	504 ± 60	239
18.4	—	—	—	2.95	2,088 ± 204	289
110.0	—	—	—	7.00	6,209 ± 600	509
Average	0.0169 ± 0.001		21.6 ± 6.8	5.96 ± 1.34		301 ± 62

[a] Values are nanomolar concentrations ± SE of hormone or analog required to achieve the desired effect indicated by the parameter. H_{50}^s, concentration of ACTH required for half-maximal stimulation of steroidogenesis in the absence of inhibitor, determined on the same batch of cells as that used for the inhibition studies; I_{50}^c, concentration of CIP required for inhibiting ACTH-induced steroidogenesis by 50%; K_i^s, inhibitory constant for the steroidogenic response calculated from $K_i = I_{50}/1 + H/H_{50}$. The superscript c refers to the same parameters for cyclic AMP production.

TABLE 3. *Comparison of I_{50}^s measured experimentally with that predicted by the spare receptor model[a]*

		I_{50}^s	
ACTH	I_{50}^c	Measured	Predicted
3.67	510	1,041	82,139
11.0	504	14,754	113,670

[a] Values are nanomolar concentrations. The predicted values were obtained from

$$I_{50}^s = \frac{I_{50}^c \left(1 + \dfrac{H}{H_{50}^s}\right)}{1 + \dfrac{H}{H_{50}^c}}$$

which can be derived for the spare receptor model. (From C. Y. Lee et al., *Arch. Biochem. Biophys., in press.*)

steroidogenesis compared with cyclic AMP formation. Knowing the values of H_{50} for steroidogenesis and cyclic AMP formation and the I_{50} for the cyclic AMP response, it is possible to predict the I_{50} for the steroidogenic response for any given concentration of ACTH. In Table 2, the I_{50} values for CIP inhibition of steroidogenesis and cyclic AMP production were both determined for ACTH concentrations of 3.67 and 11 nM. The measured I_{50} values for CIP inhibition of steroidogenesis are compared with the I_{50} values calculated for the one-receptor model in Table 3. It is apparent that the observed values are much smaller than the values predicted.

Inhibition studies with CIP thus appear to favor the two-receptor hypothesis. The differences in the inhibitory constants for steroidogenesis and cyclic AMP formation may, therefore, be due to differences in the affinities of the hormone as well as the inhibitor for the two sites. These results also indicate that the first six residues of ACTH (missing in CIP) are more important for binding to the steroidogenic site than for interaction with the lower affinity site involved in cyclic AMP formation since the K_i for steroidogenesis is more than 1,000-fold larger than the H_{50} for steroidogenesis, but the K_i for cyclic AMP formation is only 50 times the H_{50} for cyclic AMP production.

Desensitization of Steroid and Cyclic AMP Responses in Adrenocortical Cells

The existence of hormone-induced refractoriness or desensitization has been reported in several tissues (3,6,7,11,17). In most systems, the desensitization of adenylate cyclase to hormonal stimulation has been correlated with a loss of receptors. It has been recently reported that treatment of mouse adrenal tumor cells (Y_1) with ACTH induced cell refractoriness to further hormonal stimulation (15). We have started studies of desensitization of steroid and cyclic AMP responses in normal rat adrenocortical cells in the hope of utilizing this

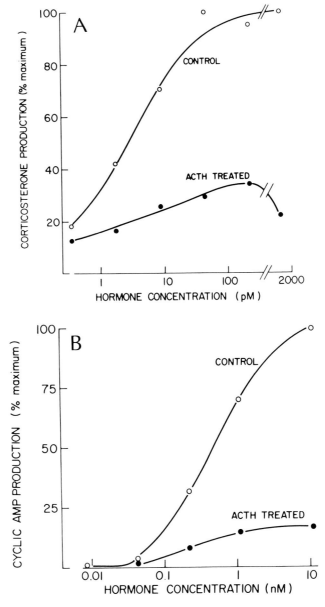

FIG. 5. Effects of ACTH pretreatment on responsiveness of adrenocortical cells. Rat adrenocortical cells maintained in culture for 4 days were incubated with or without 10 nM ACTH for 6 hr. Cells were washed (twice), incubated 1 hr without hormone, washed again (twice), and reincubated in the presence of varying concentrations of ACTH for 2 hr. Corticosterone **(A)** and cyclic AMP **(B)** in the medium were analyzed by radioimmunoassay.

TABLE 4. Effects of pretreatment with ACTH and NPS-ACTH on subsequent responses to ACTH[a]

	Corticosterone production			Cyclic AMP formation		
		Pretreatment			Pretreatment	
ACTH (nM)	Control	ACTH	NPS-ACTH	Control	ACTH	NPS-ACTH
0	6.4	8.6	21.2	0.9	1.0	0.6
0.02	71.5	58.7	57.1	1.1	0.9	0.5
0.20	100.0	68.4	83.3	13.8	19.4	16.0
2.20	92.0	60.7	78.6	72.0	73.9	73.3
22.0	113.0	63.5	83.4	100.0	115.0	101.0

[a] Rat adrenocortical cells were maintained in culture for 3 days and then incubated with no hormone (control), ACTH (0.2 nM) or NPS-ACTH (20 nM) for 6 hr. Cells were washed twice, incubated 1 hr without hormone, washed again (twice), and then incubated in the presence of different concentrations of ACTH for 2 hr. Corticosterone and cyclic AMP in the medium were measured by radioimmunoassay. All values are expressed as a percent of the maximal stimulation produced in the control cells.

phenomenon to elucidate whether there are one or two types of ACTH receptors present in these cells.

Treatment of rat adrenocortical cells with 10 nM ACTH for 6 hr resulted in nearly 85% loss of the cyclic AMP response to further stimulation with ACTH (Fig. 5). If desensitization is solely due to receptor loss, the steroidogenic response should not be impaired (according to spare receptor model), since there would still be an excess of receptors to mediate this response. However, it was observed that steroidogenesis was also desensitized nearly 70% after the 6-hr treatment with 10 nM ACTH (Fig. 5). When adrenocortical cells were pretreated with a concentration of ACTH (0.2 nM) sufficient to produce maximal steroidogenesis but not for maximal cyclic AMP formation, the steroidogenic response was attenuated 30% but the cyclic AMP response was unaffected (Table 4). Similarly, when cells were pretreated with NPS-ACTH (an analog that stimulates steroid production but not cyclic AMP formation), only the steroidogenic response to subsequent ACTH stimulation was decreased (Table 4). These results can be construed as evidence for two distinct receptors mediating the steroidogenic and cyclic AMP responses. However, desensitization is recognized to be a complex process and it is not clear that it involves only loss of receptors. Defects in the steroidogenic pathway have been noted in the desensitization of gonadotropin action on Leydig cells (27) as well as in the action of ACTH on mouse adrenal tumor cells (15). Further studies are necessary to elucidate the mechanism of desensitization in the adrenocortical cells.

CONCLUSIONS

Although ACTH was among the first polypeptide hormones to be utilized in direct binding studies, the identification, quantitation, and characterization of specific receptors for the hormone have been hampered by technical difficulties. Binding studies with specifically tritiated ACTH of high specific radioactivity and full biological activity have shown that normal rat adrenocortical cells contain a limited number of sites with a K_d of 2 to 4 nM that appear to be related to the generation of cyclic AMP. Higher affinity sites that may be involved in stimulating steroidogenesis through the mediation of cyclic AMP or other factors could not be detected. Analysis of the inhibition of ACTH-induced steroidogenesis and cyclic AMP formation by CIP (α_h^{7-38}-ACTH) indicated that there are two distinct receptors for ACTH in the adrenocortical cell. Preliminary studies of the desensitization of the steroidogenic and cyclic AMP responses of adrenocortical cells also favor the two-receptor model.

ACKNOWLEDGMENTS

We wish to thank Professor C. H. Li for his interest and Dr. Vojtech Licko for help in analyzing the results of the inhibition studies. This work was supported by grant CA-16417 from the National Institutes of Health.

REFERENCES

1. Beall, J. R., and Sayers, G. (1972): Isolated adrenal cells: Steroidogenesis and cyclic AMP accumulation in response to ACTH. *Arch. Biochem. Biophys.*, 148:70–76.
2. Cuatrecasas, P., and Hollenberg, M. D. (1976): Membrane receptors and hormone action. *Adv. Protein Chem.*, 30:251–451.
3. Gavin, J. R., Roth, J., Neville, D. M., De Meyts, P., and Buell, D. N. (1974): Insulin-dependent regulation of insulin receptor concentrations: A direct demonstration in cell culture. *Proc. Natl. Acad. Sci. USA*, 71:84–88.
4. Harrington, C. A., Fenimore, D. C., and Farmer, R. W. (1978): Regulation of adrenocortical steroidogenesis by cyclic 3',5'-guanosine monophosphate in isolated rat adrenal cells. *Biochem. Biophys. Res. Commun.*, 85:55–61.
5. Haynes, R. C., and Berthet, L. (1957): Studies on the mechanism of action of adrenocorticotropic hormone. *J. Biol. Chem.*, 225:115–124.
6. Hinkle, P. M., and Tashijian, A. H., Jr. (1975): Thyrotropin-releasing hormone regulates the number of its own receptors in the GH_3 strain of pituitary cells in culture. *Biochemistry*, 14:3845–3851.
7. Kebabian, J. W., Zatz, M., Romero, J. A., and Axelrod, J. (1975): Rapid changes in rat pineal β-adrenergic receptor: Alterations in 1-[^{3}H]-alprenolol binding and adenylate cyclase. *Proc. Natl. Acad. Sci. USA*, 72:3735–3739.
8. Lee, C.-Y., Ramachandran, J., and Li, C. H. (1978): Inhibition of corticotropin-induced steroidogenesis by α^{7-38}-ACTH. In: *Program, 60th Annual Meeting of the Endocrine Society*, Abstr. 307.
9. Lefkowitz, R. J., Roth, J., and Pastan, I. (1971): ACTH-receptor interaction in the adrenal: A model for the initial step in the action of hormones that stimulate adenyl cyclase. *Ann. N.Y. Acad. Sci.*, 185:195–209.
10. Lemaire, S., Yamashiro, D., Behrens, C., and Li, C. H. (1977): Adrenocorticotropin 51. Synthesis and properties of analogues of the human hormone with tyrosine residues replaced by 3,5-diiodotyrosine. *J. Am. Chem. Soc.*, 99:1577–1580.
11. Lesniak, M. A., and Roth, J. (1976): Regulation of receptor concentration by homologous hormone: Effect of human growth hormone on its receptor in IM-9 lymphocytes. *J. Biol. Chem.*, 251:3720–3729.
12. Li, C. H., Yamashiro, D., Chung, D., and Lee, C.-Y. (1978): Isolation, characterization and synthesis of a corticotropin-inhibiting peptide from human pituitary glands. *Proc. Natl. Acad. Sci. USA*, 75:4306–4309.
13. Mackie, C., Richardson, M. C., and Schulster, D. (1972): Kinetics and dose-response characteristics of adenosine 3',5'-monophosphate production by isolated rat adrenal cells stimulated with adrenocorticotrophic hormone. *FEBS Lett.*, 23:345–348.
14. McIlhinney, R. A. J., and Schulster, D. (1975): Studies on the binding of ^{125}I-labelled corticotropin to isolated rat adrenocortical cells. *J. Endocrinol.*, 64:175–184.
15. Morera, A.-M., Cathiard, A.-M., and Saez, J. M. (1978): ACTH-induced refractoriness in cultured adrenal cell line Y_1. *Biochem. Biophys. Res. Commun.*, 83:1553–1560.
16. Moyle, W. R., Kong, Y-C., and Ramachandran, J. (1973): Steroidogenesis and cyclic adenosine 3',5'-monophosphate accumulation in rat adrenal cells: Divergent effects of adrenocorticotropin and its *o*-nitrophenyl sulfenyl derivative. *J. Biol. Chem.*, 348:2409–2417.
17. Mukherjee, C., Caron, M. J., and Lefkowitz, R. J. (1975): Catecholamine-induced subsensitivity of adenylate cyclase with loss of β-adenergic receptor binding sites. *Proc. Natl. Acad. Sci. USA*, 72:1945–1949.
18. Nakamura, M., Ide, M., Okabayashi, J., and Tanaka, A. (1972): Relation between steroidogenesis and 3',5'-cyclic AMP production in isolated adrenal cells. *Endocrinol. Jpn.*, 19:443–448.
19. Neher, R., and Milani, A. (1978): Calcium-induced steroidogenesis in isolated rat adrenal cells. In: *Hormones and Cell Regulation, Vol. 2*, edited by J. Dumont and J. Nunez, pp. 71–73. North-Holland, Amsterdam.
20. Perchellet, J.-P., Shanker, G., and Sharma, R. K. (1978): Regulatory role of guanosine 3',5'-monophosphate in adrenocorticotropin hormone-induced steroidogenesis. *Science*, 199:311–312.
21. Perchellet, J.-P., and Sharma, R. K. (1979): Mediatory role of calcium and guanosine 3',5'-monophosphate in adrenocorticotropin-induced steroidogenesis by adrenal cells. *Science*, 203:1259–1261.

22. Pickering, B. T., Andersen, R. N., Lohman, P., Birk, Y., and Li, C. H. (1963): Adrenocorticotropin 27. On the presence of pig-type adrenocorticotropin in sheep pituitaries and a simple method for the isolation of α_s-adrenocorticotropin. *Biochim. Biophys. Acta,* 74:763–773.
23. Ramachandran, J., and Behrens, C. (1977): Preparation and characterization of specifically tritiated ACTH. *Biochim. Biophys. Acta,* 496:321–328.
24. Ramachandran, J., and Moyle, W. R. (1977): Correlation of ACTH-induced steroidogenesis with cyclic AMP synthesis. In: *Proceedings 5th International Congress of Endocrinology,* edited by V. H. T. James, pp. 520–525. Excerpta Medica, New York.
25. Rubin, R. P., and Laychock, S. G. (1978): Prostaglandins and calcium-membrane interactions in secretory glands. *Ann. N.Y. Acad. Sci.,* 307:377–390.
26. Stephenson, R. P. (1956): A modification of receptor theory. *Br. J. Pharmacol. Chemother.,* 11:379–393.
27. Tsuruhara, T., Dufau, M. L., Cigorraga, S., and Cah, K. J. (1977): Hormonal regulation of testicular luteinizing hormone receptors. *J. Biol. Chem.,* 252:9002–9006.
28. Yanagibashi, K., Kamiya, N., Ling, G., and Matsuba, M. (1978): Studies on adrenocorticotropic hormone receptor using isolated rat adrenocortical cells. *Endocrinol. Jpn.,* 25:545–551.

Polypeptide Hormones, edited by
R. F. Beers, Jr. and E. G. Bassett.
Raven Press, New York © 1980.

28. Clinical Studies with Human Somatotropin

Salvatore Raiti

*National Pituitary Agency, University of Maryland School of Medicine,
Baltimore, Maryland 21201*

INTRODUCTION

Growth hormone (GH) was discovered in the 1920s, and methods for its bioassay were well established in the 1930s and 1940s. However, the GH of animals was ineffective in humans. It was therefore widely believed by clinicians that humans did not need or have a specific hormone for growth. In 1956, the species-specificity for growth hormone was first recognized (9,16,23); that is, GH from higher animals and man will work in lower animals, but the hormone of lower animals will not work in higher animals or in humans. Human growth hormone (HGH) extracted from human pituitary glands was first administered to humans in 1958 (24). In the United States, the discovery of HGH led to a scramble among parents of hypopituitary children and interested endocrinologists to collect as many human pituitaries as possible. In 1963, the National Institute of Arthritis, Metabolism and Digestive Diseases with the full cooperation of the College of American Pathologists formed a single collection program called the National Pituitary Agency (NPA). Since 1967, the NPA has been housed, under contract, at the University of Maryland School of Medicine. Its function (25) is to collect all human pituitary glands within the United States, organize the extraction of HGH and all other anterior pituitary hormones, and distribute these within the country for hypopituitary children and for other clinical, metabolic, and laboratory studies.

Currently, about 60,000 human pituitaries (40,000 frozen and 20,000 stored in acetone) are collected each year. From these glands, about 650,000 International Units (IU) of highly monomeric HGH are produced (activity of 2 IU/ mg). Frozen pituitaries yield 12 IU and acetone glands yield 8 IU of HGH. The total production and distribution cost of this HGH is about 75¢/IU. This HGH is distributed to about 1,600 hypopituitary patients per year in the United States.

Technical advances in the mid 1960s led to the more definitive diagnosis of hypopituitarism. In the earlier years, the metabolic response to HGH (nitrogen retention and calcium excretion) over a 4- to 6-week period was used as the clinical guide to HGH responsiveness. The widespread availability of the radioimmunoassay (RIA) for HGH (first reported in 1962 and 1963) supplanted the tedious, laborious, and expensive metabolic studies. Initially, the immunochemical HGH response to hypoglycemia induced by insulin infusion was used alone. Several years later it was discovered, empirically, that arginine infusion will stimulate HGH release in normal, but not hypopituitary, children. In 1967, Raiti et al. (26) reported that both stimuli must be used to diagnose hypopituitarism because some normal children respond to one stimulus and not to the other.

PATHOLOGIES AND THERAPIES

Hyposomatotropism

The criteria for diagnosis of growth hormone deficiency, as recommended by the National Pituitary Agency, are as follows.

(a) The subject is of short stature, with its height at least two standard deviations below the mean. These children have normal body proportions, as distinct from the abnormal proportions found with the dyschondroplasias. They tend to be obese as well as short, although obesity is often absent in the children who also have symptomatic hypoglycemia.

(b) Current rate of growth is 4.0 to 4.5 cm/year or less, in children over 2 years of age.

(c) Skeletal and dental ages are delayed by 2 or more years in children over 2 years of age. The poor rate of growth and delayed skeletal age can be considered as the clinical equivalent of a bioassay showing low or absent HGH.

(d) Screening tests for HGH may be used and, if no HGH is found, these must be followed by definitive tests. Screening tests currently used include exercise, propanolol (19), sleep studies, and somatomedin-C measurement by RIA (8).

(e) The patient, in a definitive test, must show failure of adequate HGH response (a rise below 10 ng/ml of HGH) to at least two of the following: insulin hypoglycemia, arginine infusion, L-DOPA, and intramuscular glucagon.

Clinical Types of Hyposomatotropism

Organic and idiopathic

The most common cause of compression or destruction of the pituitary is craniopharyngioma. These patients not only are short, but also may have neurological and visual symptoms, headaches, and vomiting. Diabetes insipidus occurs only in organic hypopituitarism. Skull radiographs and visual field evaluations are mandatory.

Patients with idiopathic hypopituitarism have GH deficiency alone, or a combination of this and one or several other anterior pituitary hormones.

Abnormally circulating GH

Patients with abnormally circulating GH have immunologically intact HGH as measured by RIA, but the hormone is biologically inactive (15). These patients have all the clinical features of hypopituitarism including skeletal and dental age delay, but display a normal radioimmunological HGH response to stimuli. They respond to administration of HGH therapeutically.

Peripheral resistance

In peripheral resistance, there is inability to produce somatomedin, which is thought to be the true intermediate between HGH and tissues. These patients have the clinical features of hypopituitarism, but have low somatomedin levels that fail to increase after HGH is administered. Pygmies fall into this category (27).

Psychosocial dwarfism

In 1966, Powell et al. (21,22) described reversible hypopituitarism in children who were emotionally and mentally battered although they were not harmed physically. Bizarre behavior included polydipsia, polyphagia, polyuria, stealing of food, eating from garbage cans, and shyness. They did not have renal or gastrointestinal dysfunction. Testing at time of diagnosis showed deficiency of HGH with or without other anterior pituitary hormone deficiencies. However, when they were moved from their adverse environment, anterior pituitary function returned to normal within weeks or a few months.

Treatment of Hyposomatotropism

Either of two dose schedules are commonly used in the United States to treat hyposomatotropism. The initial, empirically selected dose of 2 IU of HGH given intramuscularly three times a week (6 IU/week) has proved to be effective for most patients except for obese adolescents, who require more. On such doses, patients grew at 9.3 ± 2.3 cm during the first year of therapy (1). This compared very favorably with growths of 10.7 cm/year using 4 to 7 times this dose (24 to 40 IU/week) (29) and 11.9 ± 2.5 cm/year using 5 times that dose (30 IU/week) (1). Patients with multiple anterior pituitary hormone deficiencies or with organic hypopituitarism responded less well, with growths of 5.4 to 7.3 cm in the first year (1). Glucocorticoid replacement, even in smaller doses of 20 mg/m²/day, interfered and resulted in a lower than expected growth rate (1). In the second and subsequent years of therapy, these patients have grown at 6 and 4 to 5 cm/year, respectively. Some patients have been treated continuously for as long as 10 years. The adult height expectation for these hyposomatotropic patients has been increased from 100 cm (40 inches) to 160 to 170 cm (63 to 67 inches).

The alternative dose schedule is to use 0.06 IU of HGH per kilogram body weight three times a week (7). The expected growth response in the first year is about 7.3 cm. This is an effective and practical dose (in terms of limited HGH supply), but not necessarily the most effective dose.

Failure of growth response to HGH therapy can be due to wrong diagnosis, high cortisone replacement dose, irregular administration of HGH by parents or the adolescent child, and formation of fibrous areas with poor absorption of HGH (if continually administered in one area). Gradual onset of thyrotropin-stimulating hormone (TSH) deficiency—with consequent decrease in serum thyroxine—can and will result in decreased growth. Antibody production was once an important cause of failure to grow 6 to 9 months or more after HGH therapy was initiated (20). While many patients develop HGH antibodies, the incidence of growth failure due to high titer antibodies is now so low as to account for only one to two patients per year (0.1% of patients on therapy). This sudden decline in incidence of these antibodies in the United States since 1977 is due to the widespread use of HGH exclusively in the highly monomeric form.

Once the skeletal age (bone age) reaches 14 years, little or no further growth-stimulating effect can be expected from HGH. The resultant growth is due primarily to sex hormone action on epiphyseal maturation and fusion.

Puberty and Hyposomatotropism

While HGH therapy alone stimulates growth, the addition of androgens to affected males will potentiate and increase the growth-stimulating effect. The androgens, however, do cause rapid maturation and fusion of epiphyses and should rarely be added unless the patient is approaching an acceptable adult height in excess of 158 to 160 cm.

Other Forms of Short Stature

Primordial Dwarfism

HGH in physiological doses does not stimulate growth acceleration in patients who have normal GH production. Indeed, there is the theoretical risk of antibody production and resultant inhibition of the patient's own GH.

Constitutional Delay

Patients with constitutional delay have normal HGH response to stimuli, although usually they must be primed prior to testing with androgens or estrogens for up to 7 days. Characteristically, these adolescent patients have normal weight for height and grow at a steady rate of 4.0 to 4.5 cm/year after the age of 6 years. HGH therapy may produce a growth spurt that continues after HGH is stopped, probably due to stimulation of increased gonadal androgen production.

Low Birthweight Dwarfs

HGH has not produced a sustained long-term growth acceleration in low birthweight dwarfs, although the short-term studies might suggest otherwise. By using larger doses of 5 IU daily, a few patients have grown better than might otherwise be expected, although many have not. There is no way of differentiating these two groups.

Turner's Syndrome (Gonadal Dysgenesis)

HGH has not produced any sustained increase in growth of Turner's syndrome patients when administered over a 2 to 3-year period.

Dwarfism Resulting from Renal Dialysis or Transplants

Such patients may grow poorly and this condition cannot be improved by HGH therapy.

Dwarfism Due to Bone/Cartilage Disorders

Bone/cartilage disorders include achondroplasia, dyschondroplasia, vitamin D-resistant rickets, metaphyseal dysplasia, and osteogenesis imperfecta. HGH therapy has been ineffective in stimulating an increased rate of growth or altering the bone or cartilage disorder.

Hypoglycemia, Carbohydrate Metabolism, and HGH

Although asymptomatic hypoglycemia is found in as many as 30% of documented hypopituitary patients, symptoms of hypoglycemia are found in only about one-half of them (thus, 17% of hypopituitary patients) (11). Hypoglycemia occurs as frequently in organic as in idiopathic hypopituitarism and is most commonly found in the first 4 years of life. Even after 6 years of age, 25% of patients tested (oral glucose tolerance test) show a hypoglycemic tendency. The hypoglycemic patients tend to have low body weight for their height and are lean and young, as distinct from the non-hypoglycemic group who tend to be obese for height and older.

With HGH deficiency, there is increased insulin sensitivity with a tendency to hypoglycemia, low insulin responses to such stimuli as arginine infusion, defective free fatty acid mobilization, and deficient protein synthesis. HGH replacement produces an insulinotropic effect with increased insulin synthesis and release, increased release of free fatty acids, increased uptake of amino acids, and increased protein synthesis.

HGH replacement is one of the most effective forms of therapy for the hypoglycemia of hypopituitarism. Although hydrocortisone or ACTH therapy can control such hypoglycemia, these hormones also inhibit even more the poor statural growth of such patients. HGH, on the other hand, not only controls and eliminates the hypoglycemia but also produces catch-up growth. Children under 4 years of age respond well to HGH doses of 1 to 2 IU three times weekly. In the occasional patient, this does not suffice and the HGH must be given in doses of 0.5 to 1.0 IU daily.

HGH and Stress Ulcer

Massive, recurrent, and continuous upper gastrointestinal bleeding may occur from the multiple superficial erosions of the body of the stomach or the antrum in such disorders as extensive burns (Curling's ulcer), central nervous system lesions (Cushing's ulcer), and cancer (extensive malignancies) (31). Animals subjected to stress show reduced gastric proliferation, reduced DNA synthesis, and loss of RNA from the gastric mucosa. Hypophysectomy shows gastric mucosal atrophy and administration of bovine GH reduces the degree of gastric erosions.

There is a high mortality from the massive and uncontrolled hemorrhage of stress ulcer. A study was carried out in eight patients with endoscopically documented stress ulcers with uncontrolled massive bleeding. HGH was given intramuscularly in doses of 10 IU daily for 6 days in conjunction with other therapy for hemorrhage. The survival of six such patients was striking. This preliminary study suggests that HGH is not only helpful in survival of such patients, but may also be useful in the management of other ulcerative diseases of the gastrointestinal tract and other organs.

Effects of HGH on Muscular Dystrophy

Myotonic and Limb-girdle Types

Male patients with premyopathic myotonic muscular dystrophy were found to be hyperresponsive to HGH by 18 years of age even in the premyotonic state (10). They showed up to a 10-fold increase in retention of nitrogen, phosphorus, potassium, sodium, and chloride. Such hyperresponsive changes were not found in females before menopause, probably due to the counteracting estrogenic effect in the menstruating woman. HGH showed an anabolic and hyperresponsive effect and increased protoplasm in patients with frank myotonic dystrophy. A similar hyperresponsiveness was found in the limb-girdle type of dystrophy.

Long-term (6 months) HGH therapy did not produce any advantage (28). Muscle strength was reduced although performance time increased, and there were increases in levels of such enzymes as CPK, SGOT, and LDH.

Duchenne Type

HGH therapy in patients with Duchenne type muscular dystrophy produced a catabolic effect with negative element balance, nitrogen, and weight loss (loss of protoplasm and of extracellular fluid) (28).

Osteoporosis and HGH Therapy

Senile osteoporosis occurs in up to 25% of postmenopausal women and is responsible for a high incidence of hip fractures in the geriatric age group. HGH has an anabolic effect and stimulates calcium absorption and bone formation. HGH therapy alone in large doses has not been of benefit to these patients (3). No anabolic effect (no increase in total body levels of sodium, potassium, chloride, calcium, and phosphorus) was noted. The urinary excretion of calcium and hydroxyproline increased, whereas the mineral content of bone decreased. Bone biopsies showed some increased bone formation and resorption surfaces, but these changes were not statistically significant. HGH did not increase the skeletal mass. Several acromegalic side effects including hyperglycemia, hypertension, arthralgia, and carpal tunnel syndrome were noted.

The same high doses of HGH were then combined with calcium supplements and with salmon calcitonin (to inhibit bone resorption); this combined therapy produced an increased skeletal mass (4).

Males with severe osteoporosis have also been studied with HGH therapy for up to 15 months (14). There was no marked improvement either clinically or in the ^{47}Ca kinetic data. However, there were undisputed and encouraging histomorphometric changes in the bone biopsies, including increased periosteal new bone formation as well as intracortical bone resorption and increased activity of osteoblasts on the endosteal surfaces.

Use of HGH in Fractures

Fresh Fractures

HGH was given in doses of 16 IU every second day for 5 weeks, in association with orthopedic treatment for management of fresh fractures of the lower leg (18). No difference was found in the rate or degree of healing between the control group of 8 patients and the study group of 12 patients who received HGH. No harmful effects were observed from the HGH administration.

Non-Healing Fractures

This study included 20 patients with delayed or non-union of long bone fractures (15 were of the tibial shaft) (13). HGH was given in doses of 16 IU every second day for 5 weeks, in association with orthopedic management. Bony union occurred in all 20 patients and was complete within 3 months in 85% or 17 patients. No excessive callus formation was observed.

Hemopoietic Effects of HGH Therapy

Untreated hypopituitary patients have a reduced plasma cell volume (by about 15%) and a reduced red cell mass, compared with normal or with children with idiopathic short stature (17). These parameters are corrected by HGH administration. HGH, therefore, stimulates erythropoiesis in hypopituitary patients. In panhypopituitary or hypophysectomized patients, HGH probably acts synergistically with thyroxine in stimulating erythropoiesis.

The anemia of prepubertal hypopituitary dwarfs was found to be associated with reduced levels of erythropoietin-stimulating factor in the urine (12). In this one study, HGH therapy not only expanded the plasma volume and increased erythropoiesis (as manifested by the increased red cell mass), but also increased bone marrow lymphocytosis and improved the iron kinetics.

Dermal Effects of HGH Therapy

Patients with senile osteoporosis have abnormally thin skin (2). Administration of HGH for 1 year produced changes approaching normality. There was consistent proliferation of blood vessels and increased numbers of mast cells and fibrocytes. Collagen bundles and elastic tissue fibers became hyperplastic and more horizontally oriented. The fine vertical elastic fibrils of the papillary dermis were restored to their normal configuration. There was no evidence of stimulation of hair, sebum, or melanin as is found in acromegaly. Therefore, the scope of HGH action on the skin appears to be limited to the mesenchymal tissues.

HGH Effects on Healing of Burns

In a study of three patients, HGH showed little or no effect on the speed of the regenerative and healing process of burns (6).

Cholesterol Changes with HGH Therapy

HGH lowers plasma cholesterol and increases plasma triglycerides. It might have a role in management of hypercholesterolemia (5).

HGH and Nutrition

Obese patients characteristically show a blunted HGH response to stimuli and this is reversed with weight reduction (30). Forced feeding of prisoners has produced a progressive decrease in the HGH response to stimuli with increasing weight gain; there is also a blunting of the HGH increases expected during deep sleep.

Increased plasma GH responses are found in subjects with anorexia nervosa and with kwashiorkor (30). In the latter, there is reversal of this effect after protein repletion. Low plasma GH concentrations are found in patients afflicted with marasmus.

SUMMARY AND SPECULATIONS

HGH has proved to be effective physiological replacement therapy for hyposomatotropism. Further studies are needed to evaluate the effects of pharmacological doses (5–10 times physiological) on patients with primordial and genetic dwarfism and low birthweight or intrauterine dwarfs. The side effects of such large doses of HGH are not yet well documented. HGH in combination with other hormones is useful for senile osteoporosis in females. HGH is effective for management of the critically dangerous hemorrhage of peptic ulcer and in the treatment of fractures exhibiting non-union or delayed healing. It is one of the most useful forms of therapy for the hypoglycemia of hyposomatotropism. HGH may have an effect on management of cholesterol disorders. Its effect on nutrition and obesity is not well studied. HGH has a definite hemopoietic effect. It is useful in management of acute liver failure and regeneration of hepatic cells.

HGH does not appear to be useful in the management of burns (although more studies are needed), fresh fractures, muscular dystrophies, growth problems after renal transplants, the chondrodystrophies, and Turner's syndrome.

Because of its anabolic action, HGH might play a useful role in the management of poor nutritional states due, for example, to gastrointestinal disorders in infancy and adulthood. It may play a role in increasing muscle mass and mobility in the senile and, more particularly, in premature senility. It would be tempting to speculate that HGH might play a role in the regeneration of damaged myocardium after infarcts and that it would have a direct role in the management of primary muscular atrophy. Obese patients show poor HGH response to stimuli and they have excessive deposits of fat. It would be tempting to speculate that HGH could play a role in the management of this disorder because of its anabolic effects in directing intermediary metabolites into the amino acid-protein building pathway rather than into the unneeded and unwanted deposits of lipids.

Finally, malignancies represent growth of abnormal cells and tissues. It would be tempting to speculate that either HGH itself or one of its fragments might correct this abnormal cell growth either by competing or interfering with some vital step in the abnormal cell growth pathway. The recent successful production of GH by bacteria may lead us one step closer to such understanding and achievements.

Studies such as those outlined will await the more ready availability of HGH. They will also require courage and conviction of clinical scientists to test such newer ideas and of society to acquiesce to such studies even though there may appear little logic in them. For it is often in challenging the accepted and established ideas of scientists and society that great advances are made.

REFERENCES

1. Aceto, T., Jr., Frasier, S. D., Hayles, A. B., Meyer-Bahlburg, H. F. L., Parker, M. L., Munschauer, R., and Di Chiro, G. (1972): Collaborative study of the effects of human growth hormone in growth hormone deficiency. I. First year of thérapy. *J. Clin. Endocrinol. Metab.,* 35:483–496.
2. Aloia, J. F., and Grover, R. W. (1976): Dermal changes in osteoporosis following prolonged treatment with human growth hormone. *J. Cutan. Pathol.,* 3:222–223.
3. Aloia, J. F., Zanzi, I., Ellis, K., Jowsey, J., Roginsky, M., Wallach, S., and Cohn, S. H. (1976): Effects of growth hormone in osteoporosis. *J. Clin. Endocrinol. Metab.,* 43:992–999.
4. Aloia, J. F., Zanzi, I., Vaswani, A., Ellis, K., and Cohn, S. H. (1977): Combination therapy for osteoporosis. *Metabolism,* 26:787–792.
5. Byers, S. O., and Friedman, M. (1973): Reduction of hypercholesterolemia by growth hormone. In: *Advances in Human Growth Hormone Research* (DHEW-NIH 74–612), edited by S. Raiti, pp. 843–852. Government Printing Office, Washington, D.C.
6. Crawford, J. D., Bode, H. H., and Botstein, P. M. (1973): Human growth hormone and nonhypopituitary disorders. In: *Advances in Human Growth Hormone Research* (DHEW-NIH 74–612), edited by S. Raiti, pp. 757–764. Government Printing Office, Washington, D.C.
7. Frasier, S. D., Aceto, T., Jr., Hayles, A. B., and Mikity, V. G. (1977): Collaborative study of the effects of human growth hormone in growth hormone deficiency. IV. Treatment with low doses of human growth hormone based on body weight. *J. Clin. Endocrinol. Metab.,* 44:22–31.
8. Furlanetto, R. W., Underwood, L. E., Van Wyk, J. J., and D'Ercole, A. J. (1977): Estimation of somatomedin-C levels in normals and patients with pituitary disease by radioimmunoassay. *J. Clin. Invest.,* 60:648–657.
9. Gemzell, C. A., and Heijkenskojold, F. (1956): Growth hormone content in human pituitaries. *Endocrinology,* 59:681.
10. Heymsfield, S. B., Bethel, R. A., and Rudman, D. (1977): Hyperresponsiveness of patients with clinical and premyopathic myotonic dystrophy. *J. Clin. Endocrinol. Metab.,* 45:147–158.
11. Hopwood, N. J., Forsman, P. J., Kenny, F. M., and Drash, A. (1973): The relationship between hypopituitarism and hypoglycemia. In: *Advances in Human Growth Hormone Research* (DHEW-NIH 74–612), edited by S. Raiti, pp. 819–842. Government Printing Office, Washington, D.C.
12. Jepson, J. H., and McGarry, E. E. (1972): Hemopoiesis in pituitary dwarfs treated with human growth hormone and testosterone. *Blood,* 39:238–248.
13. Koskinen, E. V. S., Nieminen, R. A., Lindholm, R. V., Puranen, J., and Attila, U. (1977): Human growth hormone in bone regeneration of non-healing fractures. *Calcif. Tissue Res.,* 22:521–523.
14. Kruse, H. P., and Kuhlencordt, F. (1975): On an attempt to treat primary and secondary osteoporosis. *Horm. Metab. Res.,* 7:488–491.
15. Laron, Z., Pertzelan, A., and Mannheimer, S. (1966): Genetic pituitary dwarfism with high serum concentration of human growth hormone—a new inborn error of metabolism? *Isr. J. Med. Sci.,* 2:152.
16. Li, C. H., and Papkoff, H. (1956): Preparation and properties of growth hormone from human and monkey pituitary glands. *Science,* 124:1293–1294.
17. Linderkamp, O., Butenandt, O., Mader, T., Knorr, D., and Riegel, K. P. (1977): The effect of growth hormone deficiency and of growth hormone substitution on blood volume and red cell parameters. *Pediatr. Res.,* 11:885–889.
18. Lindholm, R. V., Koskinen, E. V. S., Puranen, J., Nieminen, R. A., Kairaluoma, M., and Attila, U. (1977): Human growth hormone in the treatment of fresh fractures. *Horm. Metab. Res.,* 9:245–246.
19. Maclaren, N. K., Taylor, G. E., and Raiti, S. (1975): Propranolol augmented, exercise induced human growth hormone release. *Pediatrics,* 56:804–807.
20. Parker, M. L., Mariz, I. K., and Daughaday, W. H. (1964): Resistance to human growth hormone in pituitary dwarfism: Clinical and immunological studies. *J. Clin. Endocrinol. Metab.,* 24:997.
21. Powell, G. F., Brasel, J. A. and Blizzard, R. M. (1967): Emotional deprivation and growth retardation simulating idiopathic hypopituitarism. I. Clinical evaluation of the syndrome. *N. Engl. J. Med.,* 276:1271–1278.

22. Powell, G. F., Brasel, J. A., Raiti, S., and Blizzard, R. M. (1967): Emotional deprivation and growth retardation simulating idiopathic hypopituitarism: II. Endocrinologic evaluation of the syndrome. *N. Engl. J. Med.,* 276:1279–1283.

23. Raben, M. S. (1957): Preparation of growth hormone from pituitaries of man and monkey. *Science,* 125:883.

24. Raben, M. S. (1978): Treatment of pituitary dwarf with human growth hormone. *J. Clin. Endocrinol. Metab.,* 18:901.

25. Raiti, S. (1973): The National Pituitary Agency. In: *Advances in Human Growth Hormone Research* (DHEW-NIH 74–612), edited by S. Raiti, pp. 11–24. Government Printing Office, Washington, D.C.

26. Raiti, S., Davis, W. T., and Blizzard, R. M. (1967): A comparison of the effects of insulin hypoglycemia and arginine infusion on release of human growth hormone. *Lancet,* 2:1182–1183.

27. Rimoin, D. L., Merimee, T. J., Rabinowitz, D., McKusick, V. A., and Cavalli-Sforza, L. L. (1969): Growth hormone in African pygmies. *Lancet,* 2:523.

28. Rudman, D., Chyatte, S. B., Patterson, J. H., Gibbas, D. L., Richardson, T. J., Awrich, A. E., Anthony, A. E., and Bixler II, T. J. (1973): Quantitative studies on the responsiveness of human subjects to human growth hormone: Effects of endogenous growth hormone deficiency and the muscular dystrophies. In: *Advances in Human Growth Hormone Research* (DHEW-NIH 74–612), edited by S. Raiti, pp. 877–898. Government Printing Office, Washington, D.C.

29. Tanner, J. M., Whitehouse, R. H., Hughes, P. C. R., and Vince, F. P. (1971): Effect of human growth hormone treatment for 1 to 7 years on growth of 100 children with growth hormone deficiency, low birthweight, inherited short stature, smallness, Turner's syndrome and other complaints. *Arch. Dis. Child.,* 46:745–782.

30. Vanderlaan, W. P. (1973): Growth hormone and nutrition. In: *Advances in Human Growth Hormone Research* (DHEW-NIH 74–612), edited by S. Raiti, pp. 853–861. Government Printing Office, Washington, D.C.

31. Winawer, S. J., Sherlock, P., Lipkin, M., Sonenberg, M., and Vanamee, P. (1973). Cancer and stress ulcer hemorrhage: Effect of growth hormone. In: *Advances in Human Growth Hormone Research* (DHEW-NIH 74–612), edited by S. Raiti, pp. 862–876. Government Printing Office, Washington, D.C.

Polypeptide Hormones, edited by
R. F. Beers, Jr. and E. G. Bassett.
Raven Press, New York © 1980.

29. Central Nervous System Effects of Posterior Pituitary Hormones, Fragments, and Their Derivatives on Drug Tolerance/Dependence and Behavior

Roderich Walter, *Louis B. Flexner, Ronald F. Ritzmann, **Hemendra N. Bhargava, and Paula L. Hoffman

*Departments of Physiology and Biophysics and **Pharmacognosy and Pharmacology, University of Illinois Medical Center, Chicago, Illinois 60612; and *Department of Anatomy, University of Pennsylvania School of Medicine, Philadelphia, Pennsylvania 19174*

INTRODUCTION

Arginine vasopressin and oxytocin, (Cys-Tyr-$\frac{\text{Ile}}{\text{Phe}}$-Gln-Asn-Cys-Pro-$\frac{\text{Leu}}{\text{Arg}}$-Gly-NH$_2$),[1] the hormones of the mammalian posterior pituitary, elicit both endocrine (e.g., ref. 22) and extra-endocrine (e.g., 10,30,42,44) responses in animals and humans. These latter activities include centrally mediated influences on learning and memory, which have been interpreted as modifications of consolidation or retrieval of information (11,12,42,44,48,54). In addition, the neurohypophyseal hormones [and not other central nervous system (CNS)-active peptides, such as substance P, somatostatin, angiotensin III, and neurotensin (A. J. Dunn, R. L. Delanoy, and R. Walter, *unpublished observations*)] induce specific behavioral patterns in mice and rats (10,25; Table 1).

While the hormones per se cause well-characterized responses, oxytocin has also been shown to serve as a precursor for a peptide, Pro-Leu-Gly-NH$_2$ (PLG), with divergent biological activities. This COOH-terminal tripeptide of oxytocin, which can be released enzymatically from the hormone by a membrane-bound hypothalamic enzyme (7,47,53), was originally proposed to be the natural factor that inhibits melanocyte-stimulating hormone (MSH) release from the pituitary (6). PLG was isolated from bovine hypothalamic tissue and was shown to inhibit MSH release, both *in vitro* and *in vivo* (6,31). As yet, the role of PLG as the MSH-release-inhibiting hormone is not universally accepted, and its efficacy

---

[1] Abbreviations: Z, benzlyoxycarbonyl protecting group; AVP, arginine vasopressin, [Arg^8] vasopressin; LVP, lysine vasopressin, [Lys^8] vasopressin; DGLVP, [desglycinamide^9, Lys^8] vasopressin; DGAVP, [desglycinamide^9, Arg^8] vasopressin; cLG, cyclo(Leu-Gly); cAG, cyclo(Arg-Gly); PLG, prolyl-leucyl-glycinamide; PLysG, prolyl-lysyl-glycinamide; PAG, prolyl-arginyl-glycinamide.

TABLE 1. Comparison of potencies of various neurohypophyseal hormones and analogs among various behavioral assays in mice and rats

	Mouse behavior (i.c.v. peptide)[a]		Rat barrel rotation (i.c.v. peptide)[b]		Mouse amnesia (s.c. peptide)[c]		Rat extinction (s.c. peptide)[d]
	ED_{25} (ng)	Efficacy	ED_{50} (ng)	Efficacy	Savings (%)	Efficacy	Approx. potency (%)
AVP	54	**	200	**	76	**	100
LVP	60	**	10	**	76	**	63
AVT	10	***	200	**		0	7
OXT	180	**	11,000	*		0	13
[Thi³]LVP	28	**					13
[Abu⁴]AVP	80	**					1
[Abu⁴]LVP	250	**					2
[Δ³-Pro⁷]AVP	16	**					
[Hly⁸]LVP	13	***					
[Leu⁴]LVP	7,000	*			68	**	13
DDAVP	11,000	*			79	**	3
[Ala²]AVP	>10,000	0			10	0	4
[Ala⁵]LVP	>>10,000	0					2
AVP-acid	>>10,000	0			2	0	
DG-LVP	>50,000	0	>>5,000	0	61	**	67

Abbreviations: Δ³-Pro, 3,4-dehydroproline; Thi, thienylalanine; Abu, aminobutyric acid; Hly, homolysine; DDAVP, [β-mercaptopropionic acid, D-Arg⁸] vasopressin; AVP acid, [Gly⁹, Arg⁸] vasopressin; DGLVP, [desglycinamide⁹, Arg⁸] vasopressin.

[a] Male CD-1 mice were injected intracerebroventricularly (i.c.v.) with various doses of the indicated peptides. The behavior of each animal was monitored every 30 sec for 30 min after injection. Behaviors recorded were quiet (Q), moving (M), grooming (G), foraging (F), scratching (Sc), squeaking (Sq), and ingesting (I). The sum of F + Sc + Sq (Σ) was used as the index that most reflected the characteristic response to neurohypophyseal hormones. Data are presented as dose of peptide eliciting an average Σ score of 15 out of 60 possible responses. (From ref. 10.)

[b] Values represent the dose of peptide, given i.c.v., which was effective in producing barrel rotation in 50% of the rats. (From ref. 25.)

[c] Swiss-Webster mice were treated subcutaneously with 100 μg of peptide immediately after training in a Y-maze. Puromycin (90 μg in 12 μl H₂O) was given intracerebrally 24 hr later. Puromycin alone caused amnesia in retention tests given 1 week after training. Savings represents the ability of the various peptides to attenuate the amnesia (see text). High percentage savings indicates attenuation of amnesia. (From ref. 48.)

[d] Rats were trained in a conditioned avoidance response (pole-jumping). Immediately after the last acquisition session, they were injected subcutaneously with peptide, and 24, 48, and 72 hr later, extinction sessions were carried out (see text). Approximate potency is the minimal dose of peptide which was effective in inhibiting extinction. Data are expressed as percent minimal effective dose of AVP (~ 0.1 μg). (From ref. 54.)

in humans has not been demonstrable (20). However, this peptide has attracted a great deal of attention for its actions in the CNS. In animals, PLG potentiated the behavioral effects of small amounts of DOPA and reversed the tremor induced by oxotremorine and the sedation caused by deserpidine (21). These responses to PLG occurred in the absence of the pituitary and other endocrine glands (21), indicating a direct action in the CNS. Because of these exciting results, PLG was tested clinically in Parkinsonian patients and, at least in some cases (2,16), was found to ameliorate the symptoms of rigidity and tremor as well as to potentiate the response to DOPA. A "side effect" noted in the patients was improved mood. These studies indicated for the first time that a low-molecular weight, COOH-terminal peptide fragment (such as PLG)—in contrast with an analog of a hormone (e.g., [Ala^2]oxytocin)—could directly affect CNS function.

RESULTS AND DISCUSSION

Central Nervous System Effects Shared by Neurohypophyseal Hormones and Their COOH-Terminal Fragments

Another first was the discovery that fragments of neurohypophyseal hormones, in addition to the hormones themselves, could affect the same CNS functions. One activity that was shared by the hormones and by peptides comprising the COOH-terminal sequence of the hormones was the ability to attenuate the amnesia caused by puromycin in mice (48). Animals were trained in a Y-maze to a criterion of nine out of ten correct responses, with foot-shock given for failure to move from the stem of the "Y" or errors of left-right discrimination. Retention tests, using the same procedure, were carried out 1 week after training, when the animal had recovered from the effects of puromycin. It had been shown that intracerebral injections of puromycin, given 24 hr after training, resulted in complete loss of memory in retention tests and, in an initial study, it was found that subcutaneous treatment of animals with an analog of lysine vasopressin, des-9-glycinamide lysine vasopressin (DGLVP), immediately after training, could prevent this amnesia (27). DGLVP was chosen because it does not produce the endocrinological effects of lysine vasopressin (LVP) and, therefore, peripheral responses would not be a complicating factor in interpreting CNS effects.

In a more extensive study, neurohypophyseal hormones and analogs, as well as peptide fragments and derivatives, were administered subcutaneously at a single dose immediately after training, and certain structural requirements were shown to exist for the demonstration of CNS effects (48). Although oxytocin did not appear active, the COOH-terminal tripeptide of oxytocin, PLG, and peptides related structurally to PLG, such as N-carbobenzoxy-PLG (Z-PLG), Leu-Gly-NH$_2$, D-Leu-Gly-NH$_2$, and the cyclic derivative of Leu-Gly-NH$_2$, [cyclo(Leu-Gly)], all attenuated the amnesia, as did Pro-Lys-Gly-NH$_2$, the COOH-terminal peptide of lysine vasopressin. In order to more accurately compare the potency of the hormones and fragments, dose-response studies were carried out (13) (Fig. 1). By this method, oxytocin was found to be active at high doses and, on a molar basis, PLG and Z-PLG were more potent than oxytocin. Cyclo(Leu-Gly) was about equipotent with oxytocin. It was of interest to find that, in this system, Z-PLG was about equally as effective as the potent antidiuretic hormone, arginine vasopressin (AVP). We recently conducted further dose-response studies using COOH-terminal peptides related to the vasopressins (Fig. 1). As previously found, Pro-Lys-Gly-NH$_2$ (PLysG) had activity comparable to that of LVP, whereas Z-Pro-Lys-Gly-NH$_2$ (Z-PLysG) was again more active than LVP. Furthermore, Z-Pro-Lys-Gly-NH$_2$, as well as Z-PLG and Pro-Arg-Gly-NH$_2$ (PAG), were all more active in attenuating amnesia than AVP. Cyclo(Arg-Gly) (cAG) was equipotent with AVP as cyclo(Leu-Gly) (cLG) had been with oxytocin (13).

The influence of vasopressin on various memory-related processes is long term (12), in spite of the short half-life of the hormone (28). It is not clear, therefore, whether intact hormone must be present in the animal to induce a response. It may be speculated that either the hormone can trigger an event that results in longer term changes, or that a long-acting metabolite may be formed from the hormone. Although attenuation of puromycin-induced amnesia was initially determined by giving the peptide immediately after training (13, 48), it was shown that both arginine and lysine vasopressin, as well as cyclo (Leu-Gly), at doses giving similar responses, were effective when given up to 24 hr before training (14). Z-PLG was active even if given 5 days before training (14). Therefore, in this system, as in others (11,12), the effects of the hormones were relatively long-lived. In addition, it appeared that the COOH-terminal peptides had long-term activities.

In order to evaluate the amount of peptide present in brain at a given time after injection, the diketopiperazine cyclo(Leu-Gly) was synthesized as a labeled compound. This peptide was found to enter readily the cerebrospinal fluid (CSF) after intravenous injection into the cat (Fig. 2) and to be resistant to enzymatic degradation by brain, liver, and kidney extracts *in vitro* (19) for up to 22 hr, and by mouse brain *in vivo* for up to 96 hr (34). Vasopressin, in contrast and in line with previous findings (28), was rapidly degraded (19). Cyclo(Leu-Gly) was, therefore, useful as a model compound for determining peptide distribution in brain after subcutaneous injection, since radioactivity alone could be measured without complications arising from interference by metabolites. Cyclo(Leu-Gly) was not found to accumulate in any particular brain area after subcutaneous injection (34). Peptide disappearance from plasma and brain was biphasic, and relatively long half-lives were calculated, both for the rapid (0.8 hr for plasma and 1.0 hr for brain) and slow (83 hr for plasma and 42 hr for brain) components of the disappearance curves (34; Fig. 3). There was no selective retention of cyclo(Leu-Gly) by the cytosolic or synaptosomal fractions.

The amount of cyclo(Leu-Gly) present in the cytosolic fraction of brain at 24 hr after injection was 25 pmoles/g; the amount in the synaptosomal fraction

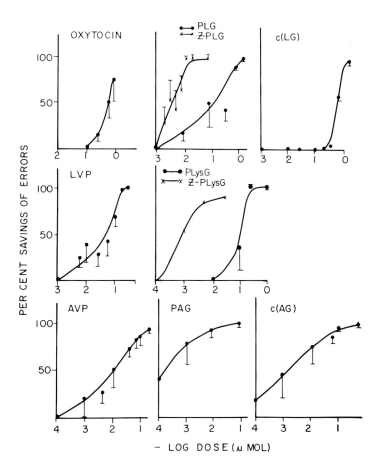

FIG. 1. Degree of attenuation of puromycin-induced amnesia as a function of the dose of neurohypophyseal peptide administered. Peptides were injected subcutaneously, immediately after training in a Y-maze, and puromycin was given by intracerebral injection 24 hr later (48). Animals were tested for retention at 1 week after training. The number of errors to criterion (9 correct responses in 10 consecutive runs) in training minus the number of errors in the retention test, divided by the number in training and multiplied by 100 represents "percent savings of errors." Perfect memory is indicated by 100% savings; total amnesia by 0% (puromycin alone). Negative savings were scored as zero. Values represent the median ±SE for 4 to 8 mice; where no standard errors are indicated, only three mice per dose were tested. Abbreviations: PLG, Pro-Leu-Gly-NH₂; PLysG, Pro-Lys-Gly-NH₂; PAG, Pro-Arg-Gly-NH₂; cLG, cyclo(Leu-Gly); cAG, cyclo(Arg-Gly); AVP, arginine vasopressin; LVP, lysine vasopressin.

was 4.5 pmoles/g. Since 24 hr was the longest time over which cyclo(Leu-Gly) was shown to be active (14), it may be theorized that such a small amount of peptide injected into brain immediately after training would attenuate puromycin-induced amnesia.

It was found that the amount of cyclo(Leu-Gly) present in the synaptosomal fraction at a given time after injection correlated positively with the ability of

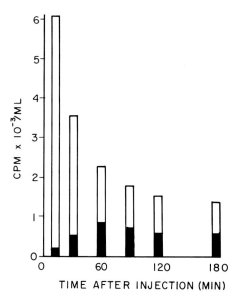

FIG. 2. Uptake of cyclo(Leu-Gly) into cat brain. Uniformly labeled ^{14}C-Gly was incorporated into the peptide, giving a specific activity of 106 Ci/mole. A single injection of 2.8 μCi/3ml saline was given via a cannula in the femoral vein of the cat over a period of 1 min. Cerebrospinal fluid (CSF) samples were obtained through a cannula introduced into the cisterna magna, and blood samples through a cannula in the femoral artery, at the indicated times after injection. Radioactivity in plasma *(open column)* and CSF *(solid column)* was determined by scintillation counting; all radioactivity was shown to represent intact cyclo(Leu-Gly). (From ref. 19.)

the peptide to protect against puromycin-induced amnesia (34; Fig. 4). There was no significant correlation for any other subcellular fraction studied (see Fig. 4 for cytosol data). Such results could indicate that the peptide interacts with receptors on synaptic membranes in order to exert its effects, although much more direct evidence is needed to support such a theory.

The results obtained with COOH-terminal fragments of the neurohypophyseal hormones and derivatives of the fragments in this system are in line with the possibility that, at least for certain CNS activities, neurohypophyseal hormones may act as precursors for producing even more active compounds, with a longer half-life than that of the hormones. For example, *in vivo*, cyclo(Leu-Gly) could be formed in several steps from oxytocin, the first involving the enzymatic release of PLG (6,47), followed by the release of Pro from this tripeptide (32,49). Although the resulting Leu-Gly-NH$_2$ is subject to rapid degradation by aminopeptidases, (e.g., 49), a minor amount of this dipeptide could spontaneously cyclize to yield cyclo(Leu-Gly).

In our previous studies of the enzymatic inactivation of arginine vasopressin by kidney of many species, we found that after release of the dipeptide Arg-Gly-NH$_2$ by the post-proline cleaving enzyme (39,53), the resultant linear dipeptide did, in fact, spontaneously cyclize (39). Our recent findings, showing that cyclo(Arg-Gly) is as active as AVP in attenuating puromycin-induced amnesia, and preliminary studies indicating a high degree of resistance of cyclo(Arg-Gly) to enzymatic degradation in brain, lend further support to the idea that arginine vasopressin, which was more active than oxytocin in attenuating amnesia (48), may exert its central effects (in particular, certain long-term actions) in part via formation of an active metabolite.

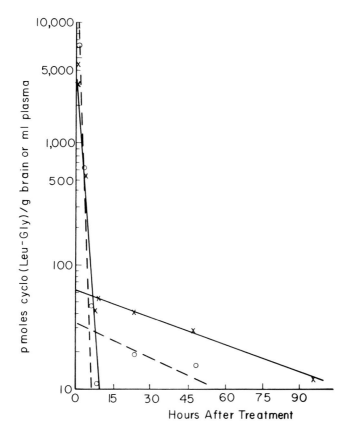

FIG. 3. Disappearance of cyclo(Leu-^{14}C(U)Gly) from cerebral cortex (X—X) and plasma ○—○) of mouse after subcutaneous injection. Male ICR mice were injected with 1 μmole of cyclo-(Leu-^{14}C(U)Gly), at a specific activity of 1μCi/μmole for the 10-, 30-, and 60-min time points; 3 μCi/μmole for 4-, 7-, and 10-hr time points; and 5 μCi/μmole for the 24-, 48-, and 96-hr time points. At the indicated times, animals were killed and brains were dissected. Blood was collected by cardiac puncture. Blood and brain tissue were treated with 6% trichloroacetic acid, precipitated protein was removed, and aliquots were subjected to liquid scintillation counting. Since all radioactivity represented intact peptide, dpm/g tissue was converted to pmole/g tissue, based on peptide specific activity. All values were corrected for contamination by blood. Peptide concentrations in cortex were indistinguishable from those found in other brain regions (i.e., brainstem, hippocampus plus entorhinal cortex, diencephalon, and corpus striatum) except at 10 min after injection. Extrapolated values of the slow exponential phase of disappearance were subtracted from the observed values of the rapid phase. Not shown in the figure: plasma at 0.17, 0.5, and 96 hr (20,124; 13,124; and 4.1 pmoles/ml, respectively). Values are medians (three to four determinations per time point). Half-lives were estimated from the regression lines. (From ref. 34.)

The finding that cyclo(Leu-Gly) was resistant to inactivation for up to 96 hr, but was behaviorally active for only 24 hr, probably reflects its excretion and resulting low brain levels after 24 hr. Z-PLG, on the other hand, was active for up to 5 days (14), and preliminary results suggest that Z-Pro-Lys-Gly-NH$_2$ is also active for this length of time. These peptides are most likely

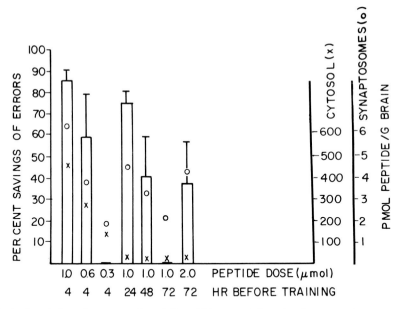

FIG. 4. Correlation of amount of cyclo(Leu-Gly) present in cytosol or synaptosomes after subcutaneous injection with degree of protection against puromycin-induced amnesia. ICR mice were injected with various doses of cyclo(Leu-^{14}C(U)Gly) and the amount of peptide present in cytosol (x) or synaptosomes (○) at the indicated times was determined as described in the legend to Fig. 3. The degree of protection against puromycin-induced amnesia was evaluated as described in the legend to Fig. 1; peptide was injected at the time indicated and puromycin at 24 hr after training. *Bars* represent mean ±SE percent savings of errors. Animals receiving water in place of puromycin showed 88.0 ± 5.5% savings ($N = 5$), those receiving puromycin had 0.0 ± 0.0% savings ($N = 5$). There were four to five animals in each group. The correlation coefficient for the relationship between peptide concentration in the synaptosomal fraction and degree of protection against amnesia was highly significant ($r = 0.921$, df $= 5$, $p < 0.005$), whereas those for cytosol as well as for the other fractions studied (data not shown) were not significant. (From ref. 34.)

active per se and, moreover, may be resistant to enzymatic degradation, whereas PLG itself appears to be inactivated by a peptidase activity (32,49). In addition, the physicochemical properties of the Z-tripeptide derivatives may allow them to accumulate in brain to a greater degree than the cyclic derivatives. If it is postulated that the neurohypophyseal hormones exert certain of their CNS effects via production of long-acting metabolites, the effect of the *N*-protected analogs may represent a synthetic improvement over the natural compounds, as has been attempted for the enkephalins (17) and endorphins (56).

Although our results are in line with the hypothesis that centrally active fragments released from the neurohypophyseal hormones can modulate memory processes, it is not likely that the smaller peptides are totally responsible for all hormone-induced CNS effects. The structure-activity relationships of neurohypophyseal hormone analogs, with respect to attenuation of puromycin-induced amnesia, indicated that the characteristics that distinguish vasopressin from oxytocin, i.e., the presence of the aromatic residues in positions 2 and 3 of the ring structure of the hormones, in combination with a basic residue in position 8, were important features for activity (48). Such findings are not consistent with the idea that the hormones serve solely as precursors for smaller peptides with CNS activity. Even more strikingly, structure-activity studies have shown that the COOH-terminal peptides are dramatically less active or inactive, when compared with the hormones, as inhibitors of extinction of an active avoidance response (54). The COOH-terminal peptides were also inactive in inducing spontaneous behaviors in mice (A. J. Dunn, R. L. Delanoy, and R. Walter, *unpublished observations*), a system in which LVP and a series of neurohypophyseal hormone analogs were found to be very effective (*see below;* 10).

For many behavioral activities, only the neurohypophyseal hormones (and analogs thereof) have been tested (5,10,25,37); therefore, the activity of peptides related to the COOH-terminal structure has not been evaluated. However, in every case where a structure-activity study has been carried out, certain distinct hormonal structural features have been found to be required (10,25,48,54; Table 1). One such study was performed by evaluating the ability of various neurohypophyseal hormones and analogs to inhibit the extinction of an active avoidance response. Rats were trained to jump onto a pole on presentation of a conditioned stimulus, in order to avoid foot-shock (54). Animals reaching a criterion of seven positive responses·after three acquisition trials were injected subcutaneously with placebo or peptide and then three extinction sessions were run. It was found that the amino acid residues in positions 2, 3, and 5 of the ring structure of the hormones made critical contributions to their ability to inhibit extinction. Modifications in the COOH-terminal peptide portion, i.e., positions 8 and 9, had much less effect on this behavioral activity.

Another system that has been evaluated is the response of mice to intraventricular hormone injection, in which spontaneous behaviors, such as foraging, scratching, and squeaking, were determined (10). Vasopressins increase these activities and it was found that the presence of tyrosine in position 2 and asparagine in position 5 of the hormones was most crucial, whereas the requirements for amino acid residues in positions 3, 4, 7, and 8 were less restrictive and showed greater tolerance to chemical changes. The requirements for these particular behavioral effects agreed well with those found for the peripheral effects of vasopressin (3,52). For attenuation of amnesia and inhibition of extinction, the structural requirements also agree to a certain extent with those for the endocrinological effects of vasopressin. Such findings are in line with the presence of CNS receptors that recognize the neurohypophyseal hormones and that are different from receptors for various smaller peptides. Thus, it seems likely that for certain CNS actions, the initial event triggered by hormone–receptor interaction must have consequences that persist, even after the hormone itself has been metabolized or excreted, regardless of the formation of longer lasting metabolites.

Central Nervous System Effects Not Shared by Neurohypophyseal Hormones and Their COOH-Terminal Fragments

As more studies on the central effects of neurohypophyseal hormones accumulate, it appears that the hormones and fragments may differentially affect various memory-related processes. Nevertheless, the hypothesis that processes such as memory consolidation represent CNS adaptations, which may share underlying mechanisms with other CNS adaptive phenomena (29,40), has led to a number of further studies. In particular, tolerance to drugs may be viewed as such an adaptive function. It has been reported that arginine vasopressin is capable of maintaining tolerance to the hypothermic and sedative effects of ethanol, once this tolerance has been established (18). Such an action might be viewed as being similar to the inhibition of extinction of an avoidance response, once that response has been established. Our preliminary studies have shown that [desglycinamide[9]]lysine vasopressin (DGLVP) can also maintain ethanol tolerance, and further structure-activity studies are in progress.

The situation with respect to morphine tolerance and dependence is somewhat more complicated. Tolerance to and physical dependence on morphine, as opposed to ethanol (41), may be viewed as two aspects of a single phenomenon (55). Although initial reports indicated that oxytocin, DGLVP (24), and [desglycinamide[9]]arginine vasopressin (DGAVP) (43), as well as PLG (43), could facilitate the development of morphine tolerance/dependence (measured by analgesia and changes in body weight and temperature, respectively), more recent findings do not support these results (38). In fact, it has been found that PLG and a number of peptides related to the COOH-terminal structure of the neurohypophyseal hormones are able to *block* the development in mice of tolerance to the analgesic effects of morphine, as well as certain signs of physical dependence (4,50,51). Various strains of mice were made tolerant to and dependent on morphine by subcutaneous implantation of morphine pellets for 3 days (50). Control animals received placebo pellets. Tolerance to the analgesic effects of morphine was determined by measuring the jump threshold to an increasing electric current and tolerance to the hypothermic effects by measuring body temperature, after intraventricular morphine injection. Physical dependence was quantitated either after abrupt or naloxone-precipitated withdrawal by monitoring changes in body weight, body temperature, and stereotyped jumping behavior. When animals were injected subcutaneously with PLG, Z-PLG, cyclo(Leu-Gly), or various structurally related peptides, such as Z-Pro-D-Leu (4,50,51), once daily during morphine exposure, it was found that tolerance to the analgesic effects and (for Z-Pro-D-Leu) the hypothermic effect of morphine did not develop. Similarly, animals receiving peptide treatment and morphine did not differ from control animals (those receiving peptide or vehicle plus placebo pellet) in terms of change in body weight or change in body temperature after abrupt or precipitated withdrawal.

Later studies showed that these same results could be obtained with only a single injection of peptide prior to morphine exposure (4). Peptide treatment given only on the last day of morphine exposure did not affect the expression of tolerance or of signs of physical dependence once these had developed (4,50,51) and no differences were observed between peptide- and vehicle-treated, morphine-implanted mice on the first day of morphine exposure, indicating that the peptides did not affect the acute response to morphine. Furthermore, no alterations in morphine metabolism were noted in peptide-treated animals, so that the effects of the peptides were related to functional, rather than metabolic changes.

These results indicated, in general, that the various peptides did not act by interfering with the primary morphine-receptor interaction, but rather by modifying or preventing some step subsequent to this interaction. Dose-response studies, using subcutaneous injection, showed an all-or-none effect of the peptides on body temperature after naloxone-precipitated withdrawal, with cyclo(Leu-Gly) being most potent, followed by PLG. Z-PLG, Z-Pro-Leu and Z-Pro-D-Leu required higher doses for activity (Table 2; 51).

One significant finding in these studies was that not all of the responses by

TABLE 2. *Dose-response relationship of effects of PLG and derivatives on naloxone-precipitated withdrawal in mice*[a]

Treatment	Dose (μg)	N	Δt (°C)	p
Pro-Leu-Gly-NH$_2$	50	8	$+0.25 \pm 0.24$	0.001
	5	4	$+0.08 \pm 0.28$	0.001
	0.5	5	$+0.18 \pm 0.39$	0.001
	0.05	4	-1.50 ± 0.14	NS
	0.005	4	-1.05 ± 0.17	NS
Z-Pro-Leu-Gly-NH$_2$	50	9	$+0.08 \pm 0.93$	0.01
	5	4	$+0.33 \pm 0.26$	0.01
	0.5	6	-1.17 ± 0.17	NS
Z-Pro-D-Leu	50	11	-0.09 ± 0.58	0.001
	5	4	-0.05 ± 0.37	0.01
	0.5	6	-1.47 ± 0.12	NS
Cyclo(Leu-Gly)	50	15	-0.19 ± 0.58	0.001
	5	5	$+0.47 \pm 0.32$	0.001
	0.5	10	$+0.30 \pm 0.29$	0.001
	0.05	10	$+0.27 \pm 0.70$	0.01
Vehicle	0	33	-1.18 ± 0.43	—

[a] Male Swiss-Webster mice were injected subcutaneously with the indicated dose of peptide (in 0.1 ml) or with 0.1 ml water 2 hr prior to subcutaneous implantation of morphine pellets containing 75 mg of morphine free base (51). The injections of vehicle or peptide were repeated 24 and 48 hr after the first injection. Pellets were removed 24 hr after the last peptide injection and the morphine antagonist, naloxone (0.1 mg/kg), was injected i.p. 1 hr later. Mice were monitored for changes in body temperature using a probe (inserted 2.5 cm into the rectum) and telethermometer (Model 43TA, Yellow Springs Instrument Company). The first measurement was made just prior to naloxone injection and then after 15, 30, and 60 min. Results are expressed as the difference between zero time and the 30-min readings (Δt); values are mean $\pm$ SD. Mean values for peptide-treated animals were compared with the mean for the vehicle-treated animals by the Student's *t*-test. $p > 0.05$ was considered to be nonsignificant (NS).

which tolerance to and physical dependence on morphine were measured were equally affected by peptide treatment. Although hypothermia and body weight loss after withdrawal were prevented, peptide treatment did not alter the occurrence of stereotyped jumping behavior (4). Similarly, tolerance to the analgesic and hypothermic effects of morphine were blocked by peptide treatment, but tolerance to the effects of morphine on contraction of the guinea pig ileum *in vitro* was not prevented by prior exposure of the tissue to cyclo(Leu-Gly) *in vitro* (36). These results emphasize the importance of evaluating several measures of tolerance and/or physical dependence when manipulations thought to modulate these phenomena are being studied (1). A particular treatment may modify biochemical processes that are common only to certain tests being used and not to the generalized mechanism whereby tolerance or dependence develop.

On the other hand, the results provided by the present work have indicated certain neurochemical processes that may be altered by COOH-terminal neurohypophyseal peptide fragments and derivatives, since different symptoms can be influenced by different neuronal pathways. It has been proposed, on the basis of pharmacological and behavioral studies using dopaminergic agonists, that chronic treatment with morphine gives rise to increased sensitivity of CNS dopaminergic receptors (26). This effect was suggested not to be due to blocking of dopamine (DA) receptors by morphine itself, but to a decrease in dopaminergic transmission caused by the opiate during chronic administration (26). It is most important to note that dopaminergic mechanisms are not involved in all withdrawal symptoms (1), and that expression of the signs that are related to DA function may be due to an increase or a decrease in dopaminergic activity, depending on the symptom measured. Withdrawal hypothermia is one symptom that appears to have a dopaminergic component (1). Because treatment with neurohypophyseal peptides prevented the development of morphine dependence as measured by withdrawal hypothermia, the effect of peptide treatment on the hypothermic response to DA agonists after chronic morphine treatment was assessed (35). Mice were treated with cyclo(Leu-Gly) (0.2 μmole per animal) or vehicle prior to being implanted with morphine or placebo pellets. After 3 days, pellets were removed and 24 hr later, the hypothermic response of the animals to the DA agonist piribedil was determined. Morphine-treated, vehicle-injected animals were more sensitive than placebo-treated controls in terms of drop in body temperature. However, cyclo(Leu-Gly)-injected, morphine-treated animals did not have a significantly different response, as compared with controls (Table 3; 35). Similar results were found when the effects of apomorphine on locomotor activity were determined (35). Peptide treatment alone did not affect the response to DA agonists in animals that were already dependent on morphine. Thus, these results suggested that peptide treatment could block the development of certain aspects of morphine dependence by preventing a change in response to DA that occurs during chronic morphine treatment.

Since changes in DA receptor sensitivity in morphine-treated animals have been attributed to decreased dopaminergic activity, exposure to peptide treatment

TABLE 3. *Hypothermic response of morphine-treated mice to piribedil*[a]

Group	Δt (30 min)
Vehicle/Morphine (N = 14)	−2.2 ± 0.4[b]
Cyclo(Leu-Gly)/Morphine (N = 14)	−1.1 ± 0.4
Vehicle/Placebo (N = 6)	−1.2 ± 0.4
Cyclo(Leu-Gly)/Placebo (N = 6)	−1.0 ± 0.2

[a] Male Swiss-Webster mice were injected subcutaneously with cyclo(Leu-Gly) (0.2 μmole) or water. Two hr later, animals were implanted with morphine (75 mg morphine, free base) or placebo pellets. Pellets were removed 72 hr later and 24 hr after pellet removal, the hypothermic response to i.p. injection of the DA agonist piribedil (20 mg/kg) was determined. Body temperature was measured at zero time and 30 min after injection of piribedil. At zero time (prior to piribedil injection) there were no significant differences in body temperature among the groups. Values represent mean ± SD of change in body temperature at 30 min. (From ref. 35.)

[b] Different from all other groups, $p < 0.05$.

may directly or indirectly increase DA transmission. Earlier findings that PLG, which also blocks the development of morphine dependence *(see above)*, potentiated DOPA action in animals (33) and humans (2) led to a number of studies of the effects of this peptide on dopaminergic systems in brain. No consistent effects were found on DA turnover in caudate nucleus, striatum, or whole brain (2,15,23,45), or in uptake of DA by synaptosomes *in vitro* (2), indicating that, in these cases, PLG did not interact with presynaptic DA receptors (2). It has been postulated that PLG may act at postsynaptic DA receptors, but no direct evidence has been found for such an action. PLG has been demonstrated to antagonize morphine-induced catalepsy in rats and the most significant effects occurred after chronic treatment with high doses (8). PLG was also found to reverse neuroleptic-induced catalepsy (46) after prolonged treatment. These results suggest that PLG may act both on nigrostriatal and mesolimbic dopaminergic pathways, since the latter have been shown to be involved in the cataleptogenic effects of morphine. Whether such interaction occurs via DA receptors themselves or via specific receptors for PLG remains to be elucidated. One intriguing possibility is that PLG and related peptides may interact with the recently identified striatopallidal enkephalinergic pathway (9).

CONCLUSIONS

It appears that neurohypophyseal hormones are effective per se in modifying memory-related processes and may also serve as precursors for long-acting, smaller peptides that share certain activities of the hormones and also have diverse, unique CNS effects. The results indicate that various CNS adaptive processes must be mediated by distinct receptors and/or pathways, since the neurohypophyseal peptides that facilitate certain aspects of memory consolidation (i.e., attenuate amnesia) have been found, in contrast, to block the development of morphine tolerance/dependence. In addition, dose-response studies indicate that the relative potency of particular peptides varies, depending on the response being measured (10,25,48,54). As more actions of the hormones and related peptides are discovered, specific receptors for each action may be elucidated. Alternatively, it may be evident that peptide-receptor interactions in particular brain areas lead to divergent results, depending on influences on other neuronal systems that respond in complex ways to pharmacological and physiological intervention.

ACKNOWLEDGMENTS

This work was supported in part by USPHS grant AM-18399, National Science Foundation grants GB-42753 and BNS-76-11779, and by the Illinois Department of Mental Health and Developmental Disabilities (904).

REFERENCES

1. Ary, M., Cox, B., and Lomax, D. (1977): Dopaminergic mechanisms in precipitated withdrawal in morphine-dependent rats. *J. Pharmacol. Exp. Ther.*, 200:271–276.
2. Barbeau, A. (1979): Role of peptides in the pathogenesis and treatment of Parkinson's disease. In: *Central Nervous System Effects of Hypothalamic Hormones and Other Peptides*, edited by R. Collu, A. Barbeau, J. R. Ducharme, and J.-G. Rochefort, pp. 403–414. Raven Press, New York.
3. Berde, B., and Boissonnas, R. A. (1968): Basic pharmacological properties of synthetic analogues and homologues of the neurohypophysial hormones. In: *Neurohypophysial Hormones and Similar Polypeptides (Handbook of Experimental Pharmacology, Vol. 23)*, edited by B. Berde, pp. 802–870. Springer-Verlag, Berlin.
4. Bhargava, H. N., Walter, R., and Ritzmann, R. F. (1980): Development of narcotic tolerance and physical dependence: Effects of Pro-Leu-Gly-NH$_2$ and cyclo(Leu-Gly). *Pharmacol. Biochem. Behav.*, 12:73–77.
5. Bookin, H. B., and Pfeifer, W. D. (1977): Effect of lysine vasopressin on pentylenetetrazole-induced retrograde amnesia in rats. *Pharmacol. Biochem. Behav.*, 7:51–54.
6. Celis, M. E., Taleisnik, S., and Walter, R. (1971): Regulation of formation and proposed structure of the factor inhibiting the release of melanocyte-stimulating hormone. *Proc. Natl. Acad. Sci. USA*, 68:1428–1433.
7. Celis, M. E., and Taleisnik, S. (1971): Formation of a melanocyte-stimulating hormone-release inhibiting factor by hypothalamic extracts from rats. *Int. J. Neurosci.*, 1:223–230.
8. Chiu, S., and Mishra, R. K. (1979): Antagonism of morphine-induced catalepsy by L-prolyl-L-leucyl-glycinamide. *Eur. J. Pharmacol.*, 53:119–125.
9. Cuello, A. D., and Paxinos, G. (1978): Evidence for a long Leu-enkephalin striato-pallidal pathway in rat brain. *Nature*, 271:178–180.
10. Delanoy, R. L., Dunn, A. J., and Walter, R. (1979): Neurohypophyseal hormones and behavior: Effects of intracerebroventricularly injected hormone analogs in mice. *Life Sci.*, 24:651–658.
11. de Wied, D. (1973): Long-term effect of vasopressin on the maintenance of a conditioned avoidance response in rats. *Nature*, 232:137–143.
12. de Wied, D., Bohus, B., Urban, I., van Wimersma Griedanus, Tj. B., and Gispen, W. H. (1975): Pituitary peptides and memory. In: *Peptides: Chemistry, Structure, Biology*, edited by R. Walter and J. Meienhofer, pp. 635–643, Ann Arbor Science Publications, Ann Arbor, Michigan.

13. Flexner, J. B., Flexner, L. B., Hoffman, P. L., and Walter, R. (1977): Dose-response relationships in attenuation of puromycin-induced amnesia by neurohypophyseal peptides. *Brain Res.,* 134:139–144.

14. Flexner, J. B., Flexner, L. B., Walter, R., and Hoffman, P. L. (1978): ADH and related peptides: Effect of pre- or post-training treatment on puromycin amnesia. *Pharm. Biochem. Behav.,* 8:93–95.

15. Friedman, E., Friedman, J., and Gershon, S. (1973): Dopamine synthesis: Stimulation by a hypothalamic factor. *Science,* 182:831–832.

16. Gerstenbrand, F., Kozma, C., Poewe, W., and Aichner, F. (1979): Clinical utilization of MIF-I. In: *Central Nervous System Effects of Hypothalamic Hormones and Other Peptides,* edited by R. Collu, A. Barbeau, J.-G. Rochefort, and J. R. Ducharme, pp. 415–426. Raven Press, New York.

17. Hambrook, J. M., Morgan, B. A., Rance, M. J., and Smith, C. F. C. (1976): Mode of deactivation of the enkephalins by rat and human plasma and rat brain homogenates. *Nature,* 262:782–783.

18. Hoffman, P. L., Ritzmann, R. F., Walter, R., and Tabakoff, B. (1978): Arginine vasopressin maintains ethanol tolerance. *Nature,* 276:614–616.

19. Hoffman, P. L., Walter, R., and Bulat, M. (1977): An enzymatically stable peptide with activity in the central nervous system; its penetration through the blood-CSF barrier. *Brain Res.,* 122:87–94.

20. Kastin, A. J., Barbeau, A., Plotnikoff, N. P., Schally, A. V., and Ehrensing, R. H. (1979): MIF-I: Actions in man. In: *Clinical Neuroendocrinology,* edited by L. Martini and G. M. Besser, pp. 393–400. Academic Press, New York.

21. Kastin, A. J., Plotnikoff, N. P., Sandman, C. A., Spirtes, M. A., Kostrzewa, R. M., Paul, S. M., Stratton, L. O., Miller, L. H., Labrie, F., Schally, A. V., and Goldman, H. (1975): The effects of MSH and MIF on the brain. In: *Anatomical Neuroendocrinology,* edited by W. E. Stumpf and L. D. Grant, pp. 290–297. Karger, Basel.

22. Knobil, E., and Sawyer, W. H., editors (1975): *The Pituitary Gland and Its Neuroendocrine Control, Part 1. Handbook of Physiology, Section 7, Volume 4,* Waverly Press, Baltimore.

23. Kostrzewa, R. M., Kastin, A. J., and Spirtes, M. A. (1975): α-MSH and MIF-I effects on catecholamine levels and synthesis in various rat brain areas. *Pharmacol. Biochem. Behav.,* 3:1017–1023.

24. Krivoy, W. A., Zimmermann, E., and Lande, S. (1974): Facilitation of development of resistance to morphine analgesia by desglycinamide[9]-lysine vasopressin. *Proc. Natl. Acad. Sci. USA,* 71:1852–1856.

25. Kruse, H., van Wimersma Griedanus, Tj. B., and deWied, D. (1977): Barrel rotation induced by vasopressin and related peptides in rats. *Pharmacol. Biochem. Behav.,* 7:311–313.

26. Lal, H. (1976): Narcotic dependence, narcotic action and dopamine receptors. *Life Sci.,* 17:483–496.

27. Lande, S., Flexner, J. B., and Flexner, L. B. (1972): Effect of corticotropin and desglycinamide[9]-lysine vasopressin on suppression of memory by puromycin. *Proc. Natl. Acad. Sci. USA,* 69:558–560.

28. Lauson, H. D. (1974): Metabolism of the neurohypophyseal hormones. In: *Handbook of Physiology, Section 7, Volume 4,* edited by E. Knobil and W. H. Sawyer, pp. 287–393. Waverly Press, Baltimore.

29. LeBlanc, A. E., and Cappell, H. (1976): Tolerance as adaptation: Interactions with behavior and parallels to other adaptive processes. In: *Alcohol and Opiates, Neurochemical and Behavioral Mechanisms,* edited by K. Blum, pp. 65–77. Academic Press, New York.

30. Legros, J., Gilot, P., Seron, X., Claessens, J., Adam, A., Moeglen, J. M., Audibert, A., and Berchier, P. (1978): Influence of vasopressin on learning and memory. *Lancet,* 1:41–42.

31. Nair, R. M. G., Kastin, A. J., and Schally, A. V. (1971): Isolation and structure of hypothalamic MSH release-inhibiting hormone. *Biochem. Biophys. Res. Commun.,* 43:1376–1381.

32. Nair, R. M. G., Redding, T. W., Kastin, A. J., and Schally, A. V. (1973): Site of inactivation of melanocyte-stimulating hormone-release-inhibiting hormone by human plasma. *Biochem. Pharmacol.,* 22:1915–1919.

33. Plotnikoff, N. P., and Kastin, A. J. (1974): Pharmacological studies with a tripeptide, prolyl-leucyl-glycine amide. *Arch. Int. Pharmacodyn. Ther.,* 211:211–224.

34. Rainbow, T. C., Flexner, J. B., Flexner, L. B., Hoffman, P. L., and Walter, R. (1979): Distribution, survival and biological effects in mice of a behaviorally active, enzymatically stable

peptide: Pharmacokinetics of cyclo(Leu-Gly) and puromycin-induced amnesia. *Pharmacol. Biochem. Behav.,* 10:787–793.

35. Ritzmann, R. F., Walter, R., and Bhargava, H. N. (1979): Blockade of narcotic-induced dopamine receptor super-sensitivity by cyclo(Leu-Gly). *Proc. Natl. Acad. Sci. USA,* 76:5997–5998.

36. Ritzmann, R. F., Walter, R., and Bhargava, H. N. (1980): Effects of Pro-Leu-Gly-NH₂ (MIF) on the central nervous system responses to morphine. In: *Neuropeptides and Neural Transmission,* edited by C. Ajmone-Marsan and W. Z. Traczyk, pp. 351–357. Raven Press, New York.

37. Roche, K. E., and Leshner, A. I. (1979): ACTH and vasopressin treatments immediately after a defeat increase future submissiveness in male mice. *Science,* 204:1343–1344.

38. Schmidt, W. K., Holaday, J. W., Loh, H. H., and Way, E. L. (1978): Failure of vasopressin and oxytocin to antagonize acute morphine nociception or facilitate narcotic tolerance development. *Life Sci,* 23:151–158.

39. Shlank, H., and Walter, R. (1972): Enzymatic cleavage of post-proline peptide bonds: Degradation of arginine vasopressin and angiotensin II. *Proc. Soc. Exp. Biol. Med.,* 141:452–455.

40. Smith, A. A., Karmen, M., and Gavitt, J. (1966): Blocking effect of puromycin, ethanol and chloroform on the development of tolerance to an opiate. *Biochem. Pharmacol.,* 15:1877–1879.

41. Tabakoff, B., and Ritzmann, R. F. (1977): The effects of 6-hydroxydopamine on tolerance to and dependence on ethanol. *J. Pharmacol. Exp. Ther.,* 203:319–331.

42. van Ree, J. M., Bohus, B., Versteeg, D. H. G., and de Wied, D. (1978): Neurohypophyseal principles and memory processes. *Biochem. Pharmacol.,* 27:1793–1800.

43. van Ree, J. M., and de Wied, D. (1976): Prolyl-leucyl-glycinamide (PLG) facilitates morphine dependence. *Life Sci.,* 19:1331–1340.

44. van Wimersma Greidanus, Tj. B., Bohus, B., and de Wied, D. (1975): The role of vasopressin in memory processes. In: *Progress in Brain Research, Vol. 42,* edited by W. H. Gispen, Tj. B. van Wimersma Greidanus, B. Bohus, and D. deWied, pp. 135–141. Elsevier, Amsterdam.

45. Versteeg, D. H. G., Tanaka, M., DeKloet, E. R., van Ree, J. M., and deWied, D. (1978): Prolyl-leucyl-glycinamide (PLG): Regional effects on α-MPT-induced catecholamine disappearance in rat brain. *Brain Res.,* 143:561–566.

46. Voith, K. (1977): Synthetic MIF analogues. II. Dopa potentiation and fluphenazine antagonism. *Arzneim. Forsch.,* 27:2290–2293.

47. Walter, R., Griffiths, E. C., and Hooper, K. C. (1973): Production of MSH-release-inhibiting hormone by a particulate preparation of hypothalami: Mechanisms of oxytocin inactivation. *Brain Res.,* 60:449–457.

48. Walter, R., Hoffman, P. L., Flexner, J. B., and Flexner, L. B. (1975): Neurohypophyseal hormones, analogs and fragments: Their effect on puromycin-induced amnesia. *Proc. Natl. Acad. Sci. USA,* 72:4180–4184.

49. Walter, R., Neidle, A., and Marks, N. (1975): Significant differences in the degradation of Pro-Leu-Gly-NH₂ by human serum and that of other species. *Proc. Soc. Exp. Biol. Med.,* 148:98–103.

50. Walter, R., Ritzmann, R. F., Bhargava, H. N., Rainbow, T. C., Flexner, L. B., and Krivoy, W. A. (1978): Inhibition by Z-Pro-D-Leu of development of tolerance to and physical dependence on morphine in mice. *Proc. Natl. Acad. Sci. USA,* 75:4573–4576.

51. Walter, R., Ritzmann, R. F., Bhargava, H. N., and Flexner, L. B. (1979): Prolyl-leucyl-glycinamide, cyclo (leucylglycine) and derivatives block development of physical dependence on morphine in mice. *Proc. Natl. Acad. Sci. USA,* 76:518–520.

52. Walter, R., Schwartz, I. L., Darnell, J. H., and Urry, D. W. (1971): Relation of the conformation of oxytocin to the biology of neurohypophyseal hormones. *Proc. Natl. Acad. Sci. USA,* 68:1355–1359.

53. Walter, R., and Simmons, W. H. (1977): Metabolism of neurohypophyseal hormones: Considerations from a molecular viewpoint. In: *Neurohypophysis,* edited by A. M. Moses and L. Share, pp. 167–188. Karger, Basel.

54. Walter, R., van Ree, J. M., and de Wied, D. (1978): Modification of conditioned behavior of rats by neurohypophyseal hormones and analogues. *Proc. Natl. Acad. Sci. USA,* 75:2493–2496.

55. Way, E. L., Loh, H. H., and Shen, F. (1969): Simultaneous quantitative assessment of morphine tolerance and physical dependence. *J. Pharmacol. Exp. Ther.,* 167:1–8.

56. Yamashiro, D., Tseng, L.-F., Doneen, B. A., Loh, H. H., and Li, C. H. (1977): β-Endorphin: Synthesis and morphine-like activity of analogs with D-amino acid residues in positions 1, 2, 4 and 5. *Int. J. Pept. Protein Res.,* 10:159–166.

Polypeptide Hormones, edited by
R. F. Beers, Jr. and E. G. Bassett.
Raven Press, New York © 1980.

30. Clinical Studies with Human β-Endorphin

Don H. Catlin, *David A. Gorelick, *Robert H. Gerner,
Ka Kit Hui, and **Choh Hao Li

Departments of Pharmacology and Medicine and *Psychiatry, Center for Health Sciences,
University of California at Los Angeles, Los Angeles, California 90024; and **Hormone
Research Laboratory, University of California, San Francisco, California 94143

INTRODUCTION

β-Endorphin is an untriakontapeptide with opiate-like activity that has recently been isolated from human pituitaries (18) and detected in human cerebrospinal fluid (CSF) (12) and plasma (22,24). The sequence of amino acids in β-endorphin is identical to positions 61–91 of β-lipotropin (β-LPH), a polypeptide that was isolated from ovine pituitary glands by Li and associates in 1964 (17).

Three basic approaches have been used to elucidate the function of endorphins in man: (a) blockade of the putative opiate receptors with a narcotic antagonist such as naloxone, (b) characterization of a change in the amount or concentration of endorphin in body tissues and fluids that result from or are associated with various stimuli and disease states, and (c) stimulation of endorphin systems by administering endorphins. Studies utilizing these research strategies have been reviewed (7,9,16,25), and suggest that endorphins may play a role in a wide variety of conditions including narcotic addiction, mental illness, obesity, and pain.

Clinical trials have been initiated with β-endorphin (2,3,6,10,14,26), [Des-Tyr¹]-γ-endorphin (β-LPH$_{62-77}$) (28), and FK 33–824, a synthetic analog of methionine-enkephalin (29). All three substances have been reported to ameliorate the symptoms of schizophrenia (13,14,28), and β-endorphin may also have a favorable effect in depression (2,14) and heroin withdrawal (26).

Initial clinical trials with most new drugs are conducted with an open design. The rationale for this is the large number of variables (e.g., dose, route of administration, and side effects) that must be studied before a double-blind study can be properly designed. In addition, if efficacy cannot be demonstrated in an open design, then there is no point in proceeding with more complicated studies. Our initial trials (3,4) and unpublished experience with β-endorphin established that there was no serious toxicity at doses up to 30 mg and that there may be efficacy in the treatment of methadone withdrawal. From the point of view of experimental design, our most important early finding was that an intravenous bolus dose of β-endorphin produced transient, mild side effects such as paresthesias and abdominal pressure. This meant that a double-blind design would be very difficult to carry out unless an active placebo were included, or unless some other type of administration procedure were utilized. Therefore, we discontinued bolus doses and began to administer β-endorphin by intravenous infusion, using a constant rate infusion pump calibrated to deliver the scheduled dose over 30 min. This technique has been satisfactory for carrying out the next phase of our studies. In this chapter we summarize our results on the physiological, behavioral, and hormonal effects of β-endorphin in eight depressed subjects and four subjects withdrawing from methadone.

MATERIALS AND METHODS

Synthetic human β-endorphin (19) was dissolved in normal saline and infused into a peripheral vein in a volume of 5 to 10 ml with a constant rate Harvard infusion pump. The subjects were eight depressed psychiatric patients and four subjects who had been maintained on 40 to 80 mg of methadone for at least 2 years. Written, informed consent was obtained from all subjects. The psychiatric diagnosis was according to the American Psychiatric Association Diagnostic and Statistical Manual III, draft of January 15, 1978. The diagnoses were: major depressive disorder, recurrent ($N = 5$); bipolar affective disorder, depressed ($N = 2$); schizoaffective disorder (affective-type), depressed ($N = 1$); and opioid dependence, continuous ($N = 4$). The average age of the eight depressed subjects (five females, three males) was 39.4 years (range 24 to 53). The range of ages of the methadone subjects (one female, three males) was 26 to 28 years.

The depressed subjects had not received any psychotropic drugs for 1 week before study, except for one subject who required a short-acting barbiturate for sleep. The methadone subjects were studied between 5 and 8 days after the abrupt discontinuation of methadone, that is, during the phase of acute methadone withdrawal (cf. 21). The four methadone subjects received diazepam (10 mg) for sleep. All subjects were studied in a randomized, double-blind, crossover design with each subject receiving placebo (saline) and β-endorphin. The mean crossover time was 5.4 days (range 1 to 8) for the depressed subjects, and 6 ($N = 2$) or 24 ($N = 2$) hr for the methadone subjects. The mean dose received by the depressed subjects was 8.0 mg/70 kg (range 4.3 to 10), and for the methadone subjects it was 8.5 mg/70 kg (range 5 to 14 mg).

All subjects were studied in at least two experimental sessions. As shown in Fig. 1, each session consisted of about 90 min divided into three consecutive 30-min periods (A, B, and C). Saline was administered during periods A and C, and during period B the subject received either β-endorphin or saline, according to the randomization schedule. The duration of period B varied between 29 and 35 min, depending on the volume to be infused and the rate adjustment on the pump. Blood was drawn from an indwelling venous catheter inserted

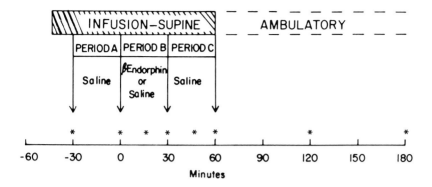

FIG. 1. Schematic diagram depicting the time course of an experimental session. Time 0 was defined as the onset of period B. Measurements designated as baseline refer to the time period −30 to 0 min (period A).

in the arm that was not receiving the infusion. Other aspects of the protocol, including the telemetry system for measuring heart rate and respiratory rate, have been described (3). The concentration of β-endorphin in plasma was determined by radioimmunoassay (RIA) (23). Other hormones were assayed by RIA in the laboratory of Robert T. Rubin and R. E. Poland at Harbor-UCLA Medical Center. Except as noted, the data analysis was based on the 0 to +60 min area under the curve (AUC) determined by the trapezoid rule and utilizing difference scores from the saline infusion baseline (period A). All p values given are two-tailed.

PLASMA LEVELS OF β-ENDORPHIN

Figure 2 shows the plasma concentration versus time curves for two subjects who received a typical 30-min infusion of β-endorphin. The mean concentrations of β-endorphin in plasma obtained from normal subjects is reported to be 5.8 pg/ml (22) and 21 pg/ml (30). These values are markedly lower than the levels of 300 to 500 ng/ml that are achieved by the end of the 30-min infusion of β-endorphin. Figure 2 also shows that after the infusion is complete, the decline in plasma levels is biphasic. The half-life of the latter phase of the curve is about 15 min.

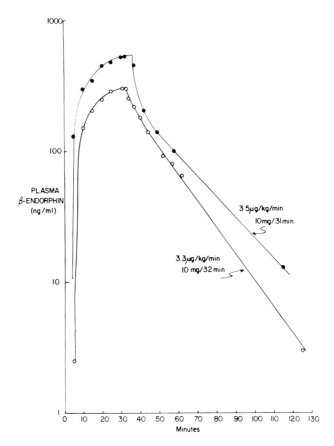

FIG. 2. Concentration of β-endorphin in plasma of two depressed subjects during and after the infusion of 10 mg of β-endorphin. The rates and duration of the infusions differed slightly in the two subjects.

HORMONAL EFFECTS

Prolactin

Animal studies have shown that β-endorphin increases plasma levels of prolactin (e.g., 5,24). This effect is presumably mediated by opiate receptors, since specific opiate antagonists (naloxone and naltrexone) block the opiate-induced release of prolactin (5,8,24). In man, two uncontrolled studies have found increased serum prolactin in two cancer pain patients (6), and in two psychiatric patients (15) after intravenous β-endorphin (3 to 10 mg). This is consistent with the fact that morphine (27) increases serum prolactin in man. As shown in Fig. 3, we found that β-endorphin increased serum prolactin in the depressed subjects ($p < 0.01$) and the withdrawing methadone addicts ($p < 0.05$). The time course of the β-endorphin effect depicts an increase 15 min after the initia-

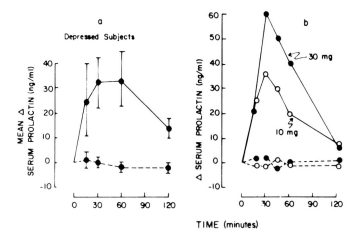

FIG. 3. a: Mean change in serum prolactin in six depressed subjects receiving 4.3 to 10 mg/70 kg of β-endorphin. Each data point is the mean (±SEM) change in serum prolactin compared with the baseline. β-Endorphin was infused at a constant rate between 0 and 30 min (●————●). Corresponding control infusion of saline is indicated by (●- - - -●). **b:** β-endorphin dose-serum prolactin response curves during and after infusion of 30 mg/70 kg (●————●) and 10 mg/70 kg (○————○) in a subject withdrawing from methadone. Each data point is the mean change in serum prolactin compared with the baseline. Corresponding control infusions of saline are indicated by (●----●) and (○----○).

tion of the 30-min β-endorphin infusion, a broad peak between 30 and 60 min, and levels returning toward baseline after 120 min. The prolactin response was dose-dependent in two addicts who received two different doses of β-endorphin (Fig. 3). Since there are no reports indicating that the narcotic antagonists block the β-endorphin-induced release of prolactin in man, it remains to be determined whether or not this effect is mediated by opiate receptors.

Growth Hormone

β-Endorphin also increases serum growth hormone (GH) in rats (see ref. 24), and morphine increased GH in man (27). Our subjects did not demonstrate an increase in GH; in fact, there was a trend in the direction of a decrease in serum GH for the depressed subjects.

PHYSIOLOGICAL EFFECTS

Respiration and Pupil Diameter

Two of the most consistent effects of morphine in man are respiratory depression and pupillary constriction. We have not observed pupillary constriction in our subjects, although Su et al. (26) report pupillary constriction after intravenous β-endorphin in withdrawing heroin addicts. We also did not detect a significant change in respiratory rate in six of the depressed subjects. Methadone withdrawal is characterized by tachypnea and increased respiratory rates, and β-endorphin decreased the rate toward normal ($p = 0.06$). Su et al. (26) also report a decrease in respiratory rate in withdrawing heroin addicts.

Blood Pressure and Heart Rate

Most studies report either no consistent effect of morphine on blood pressure (e.g., 31) or a slight decrease (1). The eight depressed subjects experienced a mean decrease of 5 mm Hg in systolic blood pressure at the +15 and +30 min time points; however, this decrease was not significant ($p = 0.10$). β-Endorphin produced no change in systolic blood pressure in the withdrawing addicts ($p = 0.3$). Other clinical studies have not reported an effect of β-endorphin on blood pressure (2,6).

Morphine does not cause a change in heart rate in man (1,31). β-Endorphin produced a biphasic effect on heart rate in the depressed subjects (Fig. 4). During the first 10 min of infusing β-endorphin, the rate increased (t-test, $p = 0.029$), followed by a steady decline between 10 and 60 min. In the subjects withdrawing from methadone, the initial increase in rate was not observed; however, compared with placebo, the rate was lower at 50 min ($p = 0.03$) and 60 min ($p < 0.01$). Thus, in both the depressed and methadone withdrawing subjects there was a postinfusion decrease in heart rate. Angst et al. (2) also reported a decrease in heart rate after β-endorphin.

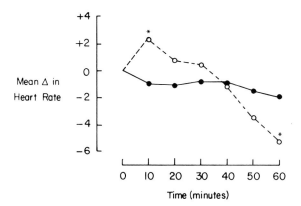

FIG. 4. Change in heart rate in eight depressed subjects during (0–30 min) and after infusion of 4.3–10 mg/70 kg of β-endorphin (○----○) or saline (●———●). Each data point is the mean change compared to preinfusion baseline. *, β-endorphin and saline responses differ at $p < 0.05$ by t-test.

BEHAVIORAL EFFECTS IN DEPRESSION

There are some clinical data supporting a role for endorphins in affective disorders. During acute episodes of mania the concentration of endorphins is increased in cerebrospinal fluid (20). Janowsky et al. (11) found that naloxone attenuated the signs and symptoms of mania in a small group of subjects with bipolar affective disorder. Using a single-blind experimental design, Kline et al. (14) administered β-endorphin (1.5–9 mg i.v., bolus) to three patients with unipolar depression and reported symptomatic improvement lasting several days in two patients. Angst et al. (2) administered up to 10 mg i.v. of β-endorphin to two unipolar and four bipolar depressed females in an open design; two bipolar patients and one unipolar patient switched into hypomania within a few hours of injection. The other three patients also had an acute antidepressant episode that was sustained for several days in two patients.

We collected behavioral data in eight depressed patients given 1.5 to 10 mg of β-endorphin. Data were collected along three time scales: acute, subacute, and chronic. Acute data was collected every 30 min during the period of infusion. This consisted of patient self-ratings on visual-analog scales, an adjective check-list, and the Beck depression scale. Subacute behavioral data was collected 1 hr before and 2 hr after each infusion session by an experienced, blind psychiatrist or psychologist (same rater for each subject) using the NIMH 15-point Physician's Rating Scale. Chronic behavioral data consisted of daily nurse's ratings using the modified Brief Psychiatric Rating Scale (BPRS) and daily patient self-ratings. β-Endorphin did not exert a robust anti-depressant effect on any of the time scales. There was, however, a tendency to greater improvement ($p = 0.09$) after β-endorphin than after placebo on the overall physician's rating scale (subacute time scale) and the depression subscale ($p = 0.09$), but not on the talkativeness subscale. There was no evidence of a hypomanic response in any subject, and there was no effect on the acute time scale (patient self-ratings) or on the chronic scale (BPRS and patient self-ratings).

We believe these results should be interpreted as consistent with the hypothesis that β-endorphin has beneficial effects in depression. Our inability to demonstrate statistically significant improvement ($p \leqslant 0.05$) may be due to the small size of the sample, the inclusion of subjects representing different subgroups of affective illness, or the use of a single administration with a limited range of doses. Future clinical trials will need to focus on these issues and the important general problem of improving techniques for measuring the effects of psychoactive substances in man.

SUMMARY

At the current stage of our investigation it is clear that intravenous infusions of β-endorphin produce hormonal and physiological effects in man. It is evident from Fig. 2 that the β-endorphin plasma concentrations achieved during the infusions are far in excess of baseline levels of endogenous β-endorphin; therefore, the observed effects are pharmacological rather than physiological. Furthermore, the effects described herein pertain only to the two disease states represented by the subjects. The results cannot be generalized to other populations, nor to other dosage regimens. The different effects in depressed subjects and methadone withdrawing subjects are readily explained in terms of the marked differences in physiological states that characterize these two diseases.

The increase in serum prolactin levels observed in both the depressed patients and the withdrawing addicts, and the decrease in respiratory rate in the latter group, are typical of the effects of narcotics. However, we have not observed other narcotic effects such as respiratory depression (in depressed subjects) and meiosis. However, respiratory depression by narcotics has not been specifically demonstrated in depressed subjects. Our inability to detect an effect on respiratory rate in depressed subjects could be due to (a) insensitive measurement methods, (b) insufficient dose, or (c) the lack of an effect of intravenous β-endorphin on this variable. The decrease in systolic blood pressure observed in the depressed group is compatible with the effects of other narcotics. However, the biphasic heart rate response in depressed subjects is not a typical opiate-like effect.

The overall pattern of results indicates a similarity between the effects of β-endorphin and morphine, but complete pharmacological equivalence has not been demonstrated. The selection of morphine as a prototype opioid is based on the extensive human data existing for this opiate. It should be noted, however, that other opioids have a different spectrum of clinical effects. Thus, the pattern of opiate-like effects produced by β-endorphin might more closely resemble those produced by an opioid other than morphine. Direct comparisons of the effects of morphine and other opioids with β-endorphin are needed to resolve this point. Two related issues are whether or not the observed β-endorphin effects are mediated by opiate receptors, and whether or not the effects in normal subjects will be similar to those found in depressed subjects. Both of the questions will also require additional research.

ACKNOWLEDGMENTS

We thank Drs. Robert T. Rubin and Russell E. Poland for growth hormone and prolactin analyses and P. Stern, C. Rimlinger, and F. Lee for technical assistance. Supported in part by USPHS grants DA-01006 (D. H. Catlin), MH-30245 (C. H. Li), RR-865 (UCLA Clinical Research Center), and RR-05756 (R. H. Gerner).

REFERENCES

1. Alderman, E. L., Barry, W. H., Graham, A. F., and Harrison, D. C. (1972): Hemodynamic effects of morphine and pentazocine differ in cardiac patients. *N. Engl. J. Med.,* 287:624–627.

2. Angst, J., Autenrieth, V., Brem, F., Koukkou, M., Meyer, H., Stassen, H. H., and Storck, U. (1979): Preliminary results of treatment with β-endorphin in depression. In: *Endorphins in Mental Health Research,* edited by E. Usdin, W. E. Bunney, Jr., and N. S. Kline, pp. 518–528. Macmillan, London.

3. Catlin, D. H., Hui, K. K., Loh, H. H., and Li, C. H. (1977): Pharmacologic activity of β-endorphin in man. *Commun. Psychopharmacol.,* 5:493–500.

4. Catlin, D. H., Hui, K. K., Loh, H. H., and Li, C. H. (1978): β-Endorphin: Subjective and objective effects during acute narcotic abstinence in man. In: *Advances in Biochemical Psychopharmacology, Vol. 18,* edited by E. Costa and M. Trabucchi, pp. 341–350. Raven Press, New York.

5. Dupont, A., Cusan, L., Labrie, F., Coy, D. H., and Li, C. H. (1977): Stimulation of prolactin release in the rat by intraventricular injection of β-endorphin and methionine-enkephalin. *Biochem. Biophys. Res. Commun.,* 75:76–82.

6. Foley, K. M., Inturrisi, C. E., Kourides, I. A., Kaiko, R. F., Posner, J. B., Houde, R. W., and Li, C. H. (1978): Intravenous (iv) and intraventricular (ivt) administration of beta-endorphin (β_H-EP) in man: Safety and disposition. In: *Characteristics and Function of Opioids,* edited by J. M. van Ree and L. Terenius, pp. 421–422. Elsevier/North-Holland, Amsterdam.

7. Goldstein, A. (1978): Endorphins: Physiology and clinical implications. *Ann. N.Y. Acad. Sci.,* 311:49–58.

8. Grandison, L., and Guidotti, A. (1977): Regulation of prolactin release by endogenous opiates. *Nature,* 270:357–359.

9. Guillemin, R. (1977): Endorphins, brain peptides that act like opiates. *N. Engl. J. Med.,* 296:226–227.

10. Hosobuchi, Y., and Li, C. H. (1979): Demonstration of the analgesic activity of human β-endorphin in six patients. In: *Endorphins in Mental Health Research,* edited by E. Usdin, W. E. Bunney, Jr., and N. S. Kline, pp. 529–534. MacMillan, London.

11. Janowsky, D., Judd, L., Huey, L., Roitman, N., Parker, D., and Segal, D. (1978): Naloxone effects on manic symptoms and growth-hormone levels. *Lancet,* 2:320.

12. Jeffcoate, W. J., McLoughlin, L., Hope, J., Rees, L. H., Ratter, S. J., Lowry, P. J., and Besser, G. M. (1978): β-Endorphin in human cerebrospinal fluid. *Lancet,* 2:119–121.

13. Jorgensen, A., Fog, R., and Veilis, B. (1979): Synthetic enkephalin analogue in treatment of schizophrenia. *Lancet,* 1:935.

14. Kline, N. S., Li, C. H., Lehmann, H. E., Lajtha, A., Laski, E., and Cooper, T. (1977): β-Endorphin-induced changes in schizophrenic and depressed patients. *Arch. Gen. Psychiatry,* 34:1111–1113.

15. Lehmann, H., Nair, N. P. V., and Kline, N. S. (1979): β-Endorphin and naloxone in psychiatric patients: Clinical and biological effects. *Am. J. Psychiatry,* 136:762–766.

16. Li, C. H. (1977): β-endorphin: A pituitary peptide with potent morphine-like activity. *Arch. Biochem. Biophys.,* 183:592–604.

17. Li, C. H., Barnafi, L., Chrétien, M., and Chung, D. (1965): Isolation and amino acid sequence of β-LPH from sheep pituitary glands. *Nature,* 208:1093–1094.

18. Li, C. H., Chung, D., and Doneen, B. A. (1976): Isolation, characterization and opiate activity of β-endorphin from human pituitary glands. *Biochem. Biophys. Res. Commun.,* 72:1542–1545.

19. Li, C. H., Lemaire, S., Yamashiro, D., and Doneen, B. A. (1976): The synthesis and opiate activity of β-endorphin. *Biochem. Biophys. Res. Commun.,* 71:19–25.

20. Lindstrom, L. H., Widerlob, E., Gunne, L.-M., Wahlstrom, A., and Terenius, L. (1978): Endorphins in human cerebrospinal fluid: Clinical correlations to some psychotic states. *Acta Psychiatr. Scand.,* 57:153–164.

21. Martin, W. R., Jasinski, D. R., Haertzen, C. A., Kay, D. C., Jones, B. E., Mansky, P. A., and Carpenter, R. W. (1973): Methadone: A Reevaluation. *Arch. Gen. Psychiatry,* 28:286–292.

22. Nakao, K., Nakai, Y., Oki, S., Horii, K., and Imura, H. (1978): Presence of immunoreactive β-endorphin in normal human plasma. A concomitant release of β-endorphin with adrenocorticotropin after metyrapone administration. *J. Clin. Invest.,* 62:1395–1398.

23. Rao, A. J., and Li, C. H. (1977): Immunochemical investigations of human pituitary β-lipotropin. *Int. J. Pept. Protein Res.,* 10:167–171.

24. Rivier, C., Vale, W., Ling, N., Brown, M., and Guillemin, R. (1977): Stimulation *in vivo* of the secretion of prolactin and growth hormone by β-endorphin. *Endocrinology,* 100:238–241.

25. Snyder, S. H. (1979): Clinical relevance of opiate receptor and opioid peptide research. *Nature,* 279:13–14.

26. Su, C.-Y., Lin, S.-H., Wang, Y.-T., Li, C. H., Hung, L. H., Lin, C. S., and Lin, B. C. (1978): Effects of β-endorphin on narcotic abstinence syndrome in man. *J. Formosan Med. Assoc.,* 77:133–142.
27. Tolis, G., Hickey, J., and Guyda, H. (1975): Effects of morphine on serum growth hormone, cortisol, prolactin and thyroid stimulating hormone in man. *J. Clin. Endocrinol. Metab.,* 41:797–800.
28. Verhoeven, W. M. A., van Praag, H. M., van Ree, J. M., and de Wied, D. (1979): Improvement of schizophrenic patients treated with [Des-Tyr¹]-γ-endorphin (DTγE). *Arch. Gen. Psychiatry,* 36:294–298.
29. von Graffenried, B., del Pozo, E., Roubicek, J., Krebs, E., Poldinger, W., Burmeister, P., and Kerp, L. (1978): Effects of the synthetic enkephalin analogue FK 33–824 in man. *Nature,* 272:729–730.
30. Wardlaw, S. L., and Frantz, A. G. (1979): Measurement of β-endorphin in human plasma. *J. Clin. Endocrinol. Metab.,* 48:176–180.
31. Zelis, R., Mansour, E. J., Capone, R. J., and Mason, D. T. (1974): Cardiovascular effects of morphine: The peripheral capacitance and resistance vessels in human subjects. *J. Clin. Invest.,* 54:1247–1258.

Polypeptide Hormones, edited by
R. F. Beers, Jr. and E. G. Bassett.
Raven Press, New York © 1980.

31. Discussion

Moderator: Choh Hao Li

H. O. J. Collier: I would like to make a few comments. Dr. Ramachandran, I found very interesting the lack of correspondence between potency in increasing cyclic AMP levels and in releasing corticosteroid.

Now, it seems to me a very parallel situation to that of opioids in which cyclic AMP formation and adenylate cyclase are inhibited, and opioids bind to the opiate receptor but at much lower concentrations when they inhibit adenylate cyclase; but, nonetheless in a group of opioids, there is a good correlation between potency in the two effects in the order in which they act.

Have you tried the group of peptides having adenylate cyclase inhibitor activity to see if there is a correlation?

I suggest this because in the NG108–15 neuroblastoma × glioma hybrid cell, the cyclic AMP response and the binding to opiate receptor correlate very well. Might the effects seen in other preparations be artifactual?

J. Ramachandran: We have done a lot of structure-function studies, as we had many ACTH analogs. Our initial aim was to look at the relationship between steroidogenesis and cyclic AMP. During our 1973 to 1976 studies, we observed there was no correlation.

Two years ago, at the International Congress of Endocrinology, we reported that many of these ACTH analogs were capable of stimulating maximal steroid production, but their ability to stimulate cyclic AMP production varied from 0 to 100%.

H. O. J. Collier: There is a certain degree of confusing results with a whole group of peptides that raise the question whether Dr. Hoffman can recommend an easily accessible, inactive peptide as control because of this confusion.

There was also a second point that I would like to make on this, and that concerns the observation of A. Herz' group on withdrawal effects—some are dominant, some are recessive. If you increase the dominant effect, you may suppress a recessive effect. Apparently you get the repression of withdrawal if you are observing only the recessive effect. But you might, in fact, get an enhancement of the dominant withdrawal effect that you might not be observing.

Dr. Hoffman, would you care to comment?

P. L. Hoffman: We looked at the effects of oxytocin and found none. Would you repeat the second question?

H. O. J. Collier: The second question concerned dominance and recessive withdrawal effects that, if you are observing a recessive withdrawal effect, may be reduced. That may not indicate dependence because, having observed a dominant effect, it might have been increased because the increase in dominant effect suppresses the recessive effect. So, unless you observed a large variety of withdrawal effects, it may be misleading.

P. L. Hoffman: I agree with that. There is only a limited number you can examine at one time but you do have to look at a great number of compounds.

P. H. Seeburg: Dr. Ramachandran, with high specific radioactivity of the ACTH with which you worked, you are in a beautiful position to look at the fate of the hormone inside the cell. Have you done any studies of this sort?

J. Ramachandran: No, we have not done these internal visual studies as yet. We hope to do this with photo-labeled materials.

J. E. Villarreal: Dr. Catlin, how does the response to β-endorphin compare with the standard response to an intravenous infusion of morphine, resulting in constipation, dizziness, pupillary effects, etc.?

D. H. Catlin: If you run down the list of typical opiate effects, you find that in some places there is agreement. In some places there is lack of agreement. For example, we have looked for pupillary constriction and we have not observed it.

Now, this could very well be because of the sensitivity of our measurement devices. We have not used sophisticated pupillography. We have used a ruler with holes punched in it. So we are reluctant to conclude, for example, that there is no pupillary constriction until a greater range of doses are explored and until better methods are brought to bear on that particular question. Constipation has not been a problem. The effect on blood pressure is consistent with morphine-like effects. The effect on respiration in the addicts is what you would expect, but again, we have not seen respiratory depression in the psychiatric patients.

I know of no study that is analogous to infusion of morphine over a 30-min period of time. Our results only pertain to the populations that we have studied.

As a last point on this, I think we confine it to a comparison with morphine as we know from the studies of Martin et al. at Lexington, and the receptor studies of others that there are at least three types of receptors and more than one type of agonist. Further, one agonist may alter blood pressure in one direction and a second in another. So I think it remains an open question.

K. A. Folkers: I would like to ask both Dr. Li and Dr. Raiti a question.

Many investigators have worked on the synthesis of fragments of HGH. Have any of these totally synthetic fragments been adequately demonstrated to have meaningful biological activity *in vivo?*

C. H. Li: You mentioned about fragments? The *in situ* fragments on the COOH-terminal fragments are not very active. As you know, about 6% is active as HGH. But when you combine with the actual 134, is fully active.

K. A. Folkers: I didn't mean the combination.

C. H. Li: The fragment has about 20% the activity of HGH.

Question: In vivo?

Dr. Li: In vivo and *in vitro.* Responsivity in the TP test is *in vivo.* The "kitchen cup test" is also *in vivo.*

K. A. Folkers: Is the synthetic fragment of HGH or BGH generally accepted as having meaningful biological activity in the rat or other species?

S. Raiti: About 10 years ago, Sonnenberg's group at the Sloan-Kettering Institute made and tested varying numbers of these fragments of BGH. They were able to demonstrate acute biological activities in terms of metabolic balance studies, sodium, nitrogen balance—things of that nature. But when they used them long-term in patients, they were really not able to determine any kind of real, sustained biological effects.

E. Gross: Dr. Raiti, you have said what I wanted to ask you to say. Now, to which extent did Marty Sonnenberg have synthetic fragments? That is really what Dr. Folkers wants to know. Marty has mentioned that, to the best of my information, he wanted us to make a fragment but he seems to have dropped the project, at least for the time being.

C. H. Li: I think I can say this: The BGH fragment is not active; but the HGH fragment is active.

K. A. Folkers: I was speaking particularly on the point of a totally synthesized fragment, not a fragment obtained by degradation, and with the human sequence.

C. H. Li: The 1–134 fragment of HGH we were talking about has not yet been synthesized. The 95–136 fragment of HGH was synthesized by Dr. Blake in 1974, but it was shown to have little growth-promoting activity.

K. A. Folkers: So, that as of today there is no known synthesized fragment of the HGH having acceptable *in vivo* activity?

C. H. Li: Correct.

K. A. Folkers: So it is still a challenge.

C. H. Li: Right.

J. M. Nolin: Let me go back to ACTH for a minute, if I may. I originally wanted to ask Dr. Ramachandran if he would care to speculate on the role of the incorporation of ACTH by the adrenal cortex target cells—what role it might play in the mechanism of action of ACTH—but I think I had better change that question into a comment in view of a previous question and Dr. Ramachandran's answer.

We have been studying uptake of ACTH-(1–24) in the adrenal cortex. We find uptake by fasciculata cells exclusively in the cytoplasm, but uptake by glomerulosa cells in both nuclei and cytoplasm. At the moment, we are looking at it in terms of what role they may play in receptor movement and so on.

J. Ramachandran: As I already said, we have not looked at internalization, but recent work with insulin and EGF in isolated hepatocytes has shown convincingly that internalization is not necessary for the biological action.

If you block internalization with amines like methylamine, the stimulation of transport of sugars by insulin or of DNA synthesis by EGF are not affected. It was speculated that the internalization may be a mechanism necessary only for metabolism with hormone or, perhaps, regulation to lower the responsiveness of the target tissue.

We have to keep that possibility in mind, but it is not impossible that ACTH exerts an action at the internal site also; we have no information on that at this time.

J. Meinhofer: Dr. Catlin, is it possible at this time to evaluate the effects of β-endorphin in the narcotic response?

D. H. Catlin: Narcotic addiction?

J. Meinhofer: Yes.

D. H. Catlin: It has physiologic effects. The data on behavioral effects are still too preliminary to mention. Active difference in the depressed patients isn't as you would expect but we are not ready to make any conclusion about addiction. Clearly, this is an area that needs investigation. But addicts are difficult to work with and it requires complicated studies. The protocol is 10 days long and we have a number of subjects. We even tried the Miller protocol. It has taken quite a while to accumulate data that will fit into the experimental design and can be reported.

C. H. Li: Dr. Catlin, would you make a comment as to the results of Dr. Su's result in Taipei on the opium-heroin rather than the methadone addicts?

D. H. Catlin: Dr. Su used a placebo group, not a crossover design. I think he had four patients in the drug treatment group and four in the placebo group. He reported good results in terms of amelioration of the sickness in heroin addicts, and rather nice results with improvement in physiology and improvement in well-being.

L. Recant: Dr. Catlin, have you studied the blood sugar or insulin levels or glucagon levels during these β-endorphin infusions in view of Dr. Unger's observations, namely that β-endorphin does decrease somatostatin levels in the perfused pancreas and increase insulin and glucagon levels very strikingly?

D. H. Catlin: We have, to some extent, looked at this, but time limited the breadth of my talk.

B. W. Erickson: Dr. Hoffman, in view of the behavioral effects of chocolate, it would be useful if we had similar data on the cyclophenylalanine or its analogs. Have such studies been made?

P. L. Hoffman: No.

C. H. Li: Dr. Raiti, may I ask you a question about the extrasomatotropic effects of HGH?

S. Raiti: I am not familiar with any specific studies done in relation to that. What I referred to was the healing of fractures, but I think there were so few studies that really need to be explored.

C. H. Li: Why are they not undertaking such studies?

S. Raiti: We try to encourage the non-somatotropin use of HGH by inserting notes about its availability in various journals, but people just don't submit applications for it.

C. H. Li: If you had 20 g of β-endorphin in your hands, which type of patient would you like to use first, Dr. Catlin?

D. H. Catlin: Complicated question.

C. H. Li: Very simple question.

D. H. Catlin: I am trying to finesse it. It can be shown that β-endorphin has important effects in the depression illness; the scope of such therapy would be much broader. I think part of the rationale for working with patients going through withdrawal is that they are very sensitive to opiates. In these initial phases of our work, we are trying to get some valid evidence of activity and data on dose and range, so that in future studies we can really home in on questions of efficacy.

So if you put a gun at my head, I would run trials with the depressed population.

K. A. Folkers: During this session, somatomedin was mentioned, but I gained the impression that perhaps it may not have definite clinical promise, although I might have missed a point. Could it be that something is still missing in the somatomedin research which could be very important if clarified by future studies?

S. Raiti: The story of somatomedin is the KABI group in Sweden; in the last 10 years they have expended millions of dollars on somatomedin. They obtain it from human plasma and to the best of my knowledge, they have not determined the complete structure. If it is known, they haven't published it.

As far as we know, somatomedin is probably the intermediate between GH and tissues; there are few investigators who question its role in the growth-promoting activity of growth hormone.

K. A. Folkers: There is quite a bit of chemistry about somatomedin already available. There are two alternatives: Either wait until something meaningful can be synthesized from sequence data or take the naturally isolated material, which I presume would have some degree of potency, and conduct selective tests on it.

S. Raiti: It is hard to get the naturally occurring material from tons of plasma. Yields are in the range of 10 to 100 mg.

C. H. Li: Even if you had a gram of somatomedin, it does not promote growth *in vivo*—only GH promotes growth.

S. Raiti: If what you say is correct, Stanley Ellis is probably correct in stating that the phenomenon that was seen with somatomedin is most likely an indirect effect.

C. H. Li: Dr. Raiti, how many pituitary patients have been treated with HGH?

S. Raiti: It is very hard to give that kind of estimate. In terms of actual numbers, I can say we have no waiting list, and haven't had one for some time. We have removed all the restrictions such as the 5-foot rule and limiting administration of it to a period of 8 months. We have enough to treat all the patients that come to see us.

We are currently treating about 1,600 patients a year and that is more than any country is able to do. We estimate that about 130 patients are buying HGH from KABI.

J. E. Villarreal: There are some reports in the European literature of the anti-depressant effects of morphine. The use of morphine and morphine analogs in depressed patients has the unfortunate consequence of tolerance and addiction. Is this the case for β-endorphin, Dr. Catlin?

D. H. Catlin: Again, that is a complicated question. Many of those studies are really anecdotal.

In discussing an anti-depressant effect, we must differentiate it as a true pharmacological effect versus the euphoric effect that most people get after taking morphine or heroin. In addition, there is the whole issue of the measurement of depression: How do you actually measure depression? How do you measure improvement? The methods are difficult. As you know, many depressed patients have responded to a placebo, so it is a tall order to show efficacy in depression.

D. H. Gelfand: Dr. Catlin, would you predict that schizophrenic patients who have been given β-endorphin improved, when those given naloxone would get worse?

D. H. Catlin: Are you asking what I think the effects of naloxone would be, whether naloxone will block the effects of β-endorphin? Presumably they will, but much depends on other factors. We don't have any data on that specific question.

As you know, there is much data on the use of naloxone in schizophrenic and depressed patients. We can easily find a paper which will support any point of view on this.

Polypeptide Hormones, edited by
R. F. Beers, Jr. and E. G. Bassett.
Raven Press, New York © 1980.

32. Introduction to Section E: Gastrointestinal Hormones

Stephen R. Bloom

Royal Postgraduate Medical School, Hammersmith Hospital, London W12 0HS, England

Pavlov made a fundamental contribution by recognizing the importance of control of digestion by the local innervation. Unfortunately, his concepts were eclipsed by the dramatic findings of Bayliss and Starling that an extract of duodenal mucosa would do everything that Pavlov's nerves were supposed to. The term "hormone" was coined to describe the new concept of secretin and other such chemical messengers acting via the bloodstream. Our understanding of the endocrine system, when the cells were gathered as glands, advanced rapidly, as it was possible to show deficiency syndromes by gland extirpation and the effects of hormonal excess by injecting gland extracts. In contrast, the understanding of gastrointestinal endocrinology proceeded extremely slowly, primarily because the gastrointestinal endocrine cells are widely scattered down the gut and the many hormones have an overlapping distribution. The gut is indeed an excellent example of the nature of the "diffuse endocrine system" that is present throughout the body and whose total mass is considerably greater than that of the glandular endocrine system. The fundamental difference between these two entities is that the glandular endocrine system responds to a single stimulus (e.g., the blood calcium concentration in a single arteriole going to the parathyroid gland) whereas the diffuse endocrine system responds to a diffuse and discontinuous stimulus (e.g., a MacDonald's hamburger swallowed unchewed during a lunch hour conversation with one's divorce lawyer). The endocrine cells of the gut have to produce an accurate integrated signal reflecting the total food input and produce an appropriate secretion of digestive juices and adjustment of metabolism. Progress was thus delayed by the technical difficulty of purifying the scattered hormone peptides from extracts containing a billionfold greater concentration of extraneous matter. It was only when the methodology of protein purification was very greatly improved that the task could be achieved. In 1961 secretin was finally purified and purifications of other hormonal peptides have followed with increasing speed. Once the peptide was purified its pharmacology could be studied. Antibodies could also be raised to allow both measurement by radioimmunoassay and tissue localization by immunocytochemistry.

Thirteen neurohormonal peptides are generally recognized as present in the gut and are shown in Table 1. Many other peptides, e.g., TRH, chymodenin, and vasopressin have been described, but their presence and quantities have not been generally agreed on. The investigation of the gut hormonal peptides led directly to the finding, now receiving so much emphasis, of regulating peptides that are present both in the central nervous system (CNS) and the periphery. These substances, which may be found in both nerves and endocrine cells, emphasize the unity of the body's control system and help resolve the original dispute between Pavlov and Bayliss and Starling. Both were right, as all physiological systems are regulated by both nerves and circulating hormones. In addition, a single peptide, for example, cholecystokynin, can have a role both as a neurotransmitter and as a circulating hormone.

In the last few years the ready availability of relatively cheap synthetic peptide hormones has allowed many more research workers to investigate their function. Added impetus has been given by the great importance of peptidergic neurotransmitters in control of the CNS, where they seem to be of fundamental relevance in the regulation of the slower functions, such as alertness, mood, and sexual drive. It is now clear that the action of a hormone can no longer be considered in isolation from neural control, and nowhere is this better illustrated than in the gut. Not only are the endocrine cells themselves influenced by neural connec-

TABLE 1. *An indication of possible functions of established gut neurohormonal peptides*

Peptide	Location	Mode	Possible action
Gastrin	Antrum, upper small intestine	Hormonal	Stimulate gastric acid, trophic to mucosa
Pancreatic polypeptide	Pancreas	Hormonal	Inhibit pancreatic enzyme and gall bladder contraction
Secretin	Duodenum and jejunum	Hormonal	Stimulate pancreatic bicarbonate
Cholecystokinin-pancreozymin	Small intestine	Hormonal	Stimulate pancreatic enzyme and gall bladder contraction
Motilin	Small intestine	Hormonal	Stimulate upper GI motor
Gastric inhibitory peptide	Small intestine	Hormonal	Insulinotrophic
Neurotensin	Ileum	Hormonal	Inhibit gastric motor
Enteroglucagon	Ileum and colon	Hormonal	Trophic to enterocyte
Somatostatin	All areas, esp. upper GI and pancreas	Local hormone	Inhibit secretion and contraction
Vasoactive intestinal polypeptide	All areas	Neurotransmitter	Secretomotor, vasodilator and smooth muscle relaxant
Substance P	All areas	Neurotransmitter	Smooth muscle contraction, pain
Enkephalin	All areas	Neurotransmitter	Inhibition, secretion, and motor effects
Bombesin	All areas	Neurotransmitter	Secretomotor

tions, but so in addition are the target tissues. The old definition of a hormone as something that acted via the circulation is no longer appropriate, as the same substance is very frequently also present in nerves. Nonetheless, for the investigator the difference remains real, as measurement of circulating substances is far easier and their function can be mimicked by infusions. Thus, the hormonal role of regulating peptides is likely to be elucidated earlier than is their importance when acting as neurotransmitters. This section has therefore addressed itself to several fundamental problems of the regulating peptides acting in their hormonal mode: first, the heterogeneity of the peptide hormones which so greatly complicates their accurate measurement; second, the distribution and tissue localization that gives us fundamental information on the likely role of each substance; and third, the interaction with cellular receptors and their structure-activity relationships. Finally, the possible physiological effects of the peptides, both centrally and peripherally, are considered.

Polypeptide Hormones, edited by
R. F. Beers, Jr. and E. G. Bassett.
Raven Press, New York © 1980.

33. Gastrointestinal Hormones: Nature and Heterogeneity

G. J. Dockray

Physiological Laboratory, University of Liverpool, Liverpool L69 3BX, England

INTRODUCTION

Present interest in the biologically active peptides of the gut owes much to the chemical advances of the 1950s and 1960s that led to the isolation and elucidation of structure of gastrin, secretin, and cholecystokinin (CCK). The full chemical characterization of these hormones brought to a climax decades of speculation that had been initiated with the discovery of gastrin and secretin in the early years of the century and of CCK (and pancreozymin) somewhat later (17). The subsequent availability of pure natural and synthetic peptides made possible the development of specific antisera and the application of these in immunohistochemical and radioimmunoassay (RIA) studies. The results of such studies have established the origin of gut hormones in discrete mucosal endocrine cells, and have permitted their estimation in blood, and so provided a foundation for interpreting the physiological and clinical significance of these hormones. In addition, in the last few years a number of other active peptides have been recognized as originating in the gut. Some of these have been isolated from side fractions during the purification of the main gut hormones, whereas others have so far only been identified by RIA or immunohistochemistry.

Several quite unexpected findings have emerged from these recent studies that, taken as a whole, serve to challenge long-standing ideas on the organization of the gut endocrine system and its relationships to other control systems in the body. First, it has become clear that many of the active peptides of the gut are related both to each other and to other non-gut peptides by similarities in sequence. These similarities almost certainly reflect a shared evolutionary history of the molecules in question, and so draw attention to the importance of considering the phylogenetic relationships of the gut hormones in a context broader than that of digestive physiology alone (10). Second, some of the hormonal and related peptides of the gut have been shown to exist in several molecular forms. This heterogeneity can be expressed either in terms of different forms varying in chain length, or as different peptides modified at one or more residues in the chain. So, for example, although it is convenient to speak of gastrin as if it were a single molecular entity, we are in reality dealing with a number of different molecular forms that vary in their distribution and biological properties. Third, it is now clear that many of the active peptides found in gut extracts arise not from mucosal endocrine cells, but rather from the nerves of the enteric plexuses, whereas others occur in both nerves and endocrine cells. The active peptides in a crude extract might, therefore, represent either gut hormones, or gut neurotransmitters (or both). It is also relevant to note here the possibility of other modes of control, notably paracrine mechanisms, that might be defined as the diffusion of active substances through the extracellular space from their cells of origin to their targets. Clearly, interpreting the physiological significance of the responses evoked by intravenous administration of gut extracts, or even pure peptides, can never again be as simple as when Bayliss and Starling (1) carried out their classic experiments that elucidated the role of secretin in controlling the flow of pancreatic juice. The problems do not end here, however, since several gut hormones are now known to occur elsewhere in the body, particularly in the central nervous system (CNS), where they presumably function as neurotransmitters or neuromodulators. This particular point has far reaching implications in that it emphasizes that the gut hormones are not an isolated system, but instead need to be considered in conjunction with other systems far removed from the gastrointestinal tract.

HORMONAL FAMILIES

The available structural data allow us to identify at least four groups or families of peptides that are related by sequence similarities. This scheme is certain to require modification as more peptides are sequenced; new families might emerge and the interrelationships of existing families become clearer. The different groups of peptides are generally thought to have arisen by duplication of an ancestral gene followed by divergence through point mutation (7,10). Each group contains at least one peptide that occurs in both gut endocrine cells and central or peripheral nerves. This dual distribution may simply be an illustration of biological conservation, whereby a particular molecule has been put to use in different control systems by changes in the patterns of gene expression in different cells (10). An alternative view, favored by Pearse (33), is that there is a common developmental and phylogenetic origin of peptide-producing endocrine cells and nerves, but as yet there is little direct evidence from experimental embryology to support this idea.

Gastrin and Cholecystokinin

The chemistry of gastrin and cholecystokinin has been reviewed many times (18,19,29). The main forms of gastrin isolated from pyloric antral mucosa or gastrinoma tumors are peptides of 17 and 34 amino acid residues (G17 and G34, respectively). The two forms of CCK isolated from hog duodenum are peptides of 33 and 39 residues (CCK33 and CCK39), respectively). In addition, the COOH-terminal octapeptide (CCK8) of CCK has recently been isolated from sheep brain (11). The similarity in sequence of CCK and gastrin is limited to an identical COOH-terminal pentapeptide amide (Table 1), and an adjacent tyrosine residue that is sulfated in CCK (seventh position from the COOH-terminus) and may or may not be sulfated in gastrin (sixth position from the COOH-terminus). The conservation of the COOH-terminal regions of gastrin and CCK can be directly related to the fact that these sequences are essential for biological activity; mid- and NH2-terminal regions of the two hormones are less important in determining biological activity and are less well conserved (10). The COOH-terminal tetrapeptide is the minimal fragment of both hormones needed for appreciable biological activity. The potency of COOH-terminal fragments of gastrin for stimulation of acid secretion increases with chain length up to about seven residues; there is no requirement for sulfation of the tyrosine for gastrin-like activity. In contrast, the potency of CCK for its main targets (gallbladder and pancreas) is dependent both on the sulfation of the tyrosine and its position; desulfation and shifting the sulfated tyrosine away from the seventh position from the COOH-terminus lowers potency markedly (44).

Peptides with biological and immunochemical properties closely resembling CCK8 occur widely throughout the vertebrates. They are present, for example, in the lampreys, which are living representatives of the earliest vertebrate group, the Agnatha (7,10). Some CCK-like peptides, e.g., cerulein, also occur in high concentrations in specialized dermal glands in certain amphibians, e.g., *Xenopus laevis*. Taken together, these observations provide further evidence for the highly conserved nature of the COOH-terminal portion of CCK. In all vertebrates so far studied, CCK8-like peptides occur in high concentrations in both gut and brain. The dual distribution of CCK-like peptides in nerves and endocrine cells is therefore likely to be of great antiquity. Most intestinal CCK is localized in endocrine cells of the mucosa, but there are also significant amounts of CCK8-like activity in the myenteric plexus, particularly in jejunum and ileum (13). In contrast, gastrin-like peptides are localized mainly in the antral mucosal endocrine cells, although small amounts occur in pituitary also (35). We have not been able to confirm the report by Uvnas-Wallensten et al. (42) of G17-like immunoreactivity in the vagus nerve; instead, we have found in dog vagus

TABLE 1. *COOH-terminal sequences of gastrin and CCK*[a]

| Gastrin | -Glu-Glu -Ala-Tyr -Gly-Trp-Met-Asp-Phe-NH2 |
| CCK | -Arg-Asp-Tyr-Met-Gly-Trp-Met-Asp-Phe-NH2 |

[a] The two main forms of gastrin (G17 and G34) are extended at the NH2-terminus as peptides of 17 and 34 residues. CCK33 and CCK39 are also extended at the NH2-terminus to give peptides of 33 and 39 residues. In CCK, the tyrosine is always sulfated; G17 and G34 each occur in two forms differing in the presence or absence of a sulfate on the tyrosine.

small amounts of immunoreactivity resembling CCK8 that accumulated proximally after ligation of the nerve (R. A. Gregory, H. J. Tracy, and G. J. Dockray, *unpublished observations*).

Much of the recent progress in understanding the physiology, pathophysiology, and cellular distribution of gastrin can be attributed to the availability of reliable RIA methods. Gastrin RIAs usually employ antisera specific for the COOH-terminus of the molecule. These antisera frequently cross-react to some extent with CCK and the relative immunochemical potencies of gastrin and CCK always need to be rigorously established. The importance of this point is illustrated by the fact that the original report of gastrin-like immunoreactivity in brain (43) was later shown to be due to cross-reacting CCK8 (6,11,34). Antisera specific for the NH₂-terminal regions of gastrin and CCK offer the capacity for specific estimation of these substances (Fig. 1). Such antisera tend to show species specificity and this may limit their use; they may also cross-react with inactive NH₂-terminal fragments of gastrin or CCK (9). Recently we used an antiserum specific for the NH₂-terminus of G34 in structural studies of this peptide. Porcine G34 synthesised by Kenner and co-workers according to the sequence proposed by Harris was found to have only a trace amount of activity with this antiserum compared with natural porcine G34. Subsequently, Hood proposed an alternative sequence for porcine G34 that differed from the original

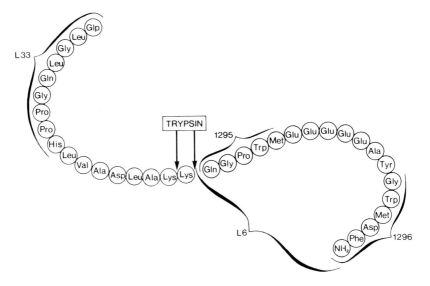

FIG. 1. Sequence of porcine G34 showing specificity of different antisera. Trypsin cleaves lysines at position 16 and 17 to yield G17 (COOH-terminal fragment) and a biologically inactive NH₂-terminal fragment. COOH-terminal specific antisera like 1296 cross-react with both G17 and G34; NH₂-terminal-specific antisera like L33 cross-react with G34 and the inactive NH₂-terminal tryptic peptide. Note that L33 cross-reacts weakly with synthetic peptides with the originally proposed G34 structure (His⁷ Pro⁹); synthetic G34 with the revised sequence (Pro⁷ His⁹) has full immunochemical potency compared with natural porcine G34. (From ref. 9.)

sequence in the inversion of His[7]-Pro[8]-Pro[9] for Pro[7]-Pro[8]-His[9]. Synthetic G34 with the revised sequence was fully active with the NH_2-terminal-specific antiserum (9). The use of highly specific antisera, therefore, allowed us first to identify a possible error in sequence, and then to select between two alternative sequences.

Recently, Rehfeld and Larsson (36) described a factor with immunochemical properties resembling those of the COOH-terminal tetrapeptide of gastrin and CCK. This factor was reported to occur in high concentrations throughout the gut and brain, i.e., in all tissues producing either gastrin or CCK. The precise identity of this material has not yet been established by isolation and sequencing, and at the time of writing its physiological significance is far from clear.

Secretin and Glucagon

Similarities in the sequence of secretin, glucagon, vasoactive intestinal polypeptide (VIP), and gastric inhibitory polypeptide (GIP) are apparent when these peptides are aligned from the NH_2-terminus (28). Only a single residue (Phe[6]) is common to all four peptides. Certain fragments of secretin (and VIP) retain some of the biological properties of the whole molecule on the exocrine pancreas, but there are no clear-cut active fragments such as distinguish the COOH-terminal regions of gastrin and CCK (16). Similarities in the sequences of secretin, glucagon, VIP, and GIP do, however, tend to be more common in the NH_2-terminal than in the COOH-terminal regions, and it seems plausible to suppose that the NH_2-terminal regions are well conserved because they are of particular biological importance. In the case of glucagon and VIP, there is good evidence of strong selective pressures maintaining the amino acid sequence. Thus, avian and mammalian glucagons differ in only one or two residues out of 29, and avian and mammalian VIPs differ in only 4 to 28 residues (7,10). There are probably other members of this family waiting to be discovered. One such peptide—porcine intestine, histidine NH_2-terminus, isoleucine amide COOH-terminus (PIHIA)—has recently been described by Mutt (28).

On present evidence, secretin and GIP are located primarily in intestinal endocrine cells (39). In mammals, glucagon occurs mainly in α islet cells of the pancreas, but larger peptides that cross-react in some glucagon RIAs occur in gut endocrine cells. VIP is virtually ubiquitous. In the gut, it is found in mucosal endocrine cells and in enteric nerves; it also occurs in nerves of the urinogenital tract and in brain (2,23). At least three variants of VIP have been found by RIA. In human colon, these occur primarily in the mucosal layers, whereas a peptide with the properties of authentic VIP predominates in extracts of the muscle layers and probably originates from the myenteric plexus (5). In some tissues, e.g., rat jejunum, the variants may be the predominant form of VIP (13). The VIP variants cross-react with NH_2-terminal-specific VIP antisera that show negligible immunoreactivity with secretin and glucagon; the variants can be separated from VIP by fractionation on CM-Sephadex when they emerge before authentic VIP, indicating that they are less positively charged; on gel filtration they co-elute with authentic VIP. It is not yet clear whether these variants are distinct peptides closely related in sequence to VIP, or whether they are fragments or metabolites of VIP.

Substance P and Bombesin

A number of peptides of gut, brain, and other tissues have been shown to terminate in -Leu-Met-NH_2, and this sequence serves as the reference point for this family (Table 2). The main mammalian representative of the group is substance P; this was recognized as being present in both gut and brain as early as 1931, but it was only isolated and sequenced relatively recently (4). Other members of the group include the amphibian skin gland peptides, physalemin and bombesin, as well as eledoisin from the salivary glands of cephalopod molluscs. Neurotensin has been isolated from mammalian brain and gut (3), and shares with substance P a common dipeptide sequence in its NH_2-terminal portion, and a COOH-terminal leucine that matches the penultimate leucine in substance P. Neurotensin lacks the COOH-terminal methionine amide and so is an atypical member of the group. Amphibian skin peptides with phenylalanine in the penultimate position are also known, e.g., litorin and ranatensin. These closely resemble bombesin in other parts of the chain. The structural similarities uniting this group are clearly less convincing than those for the gastrin and secretin families, and will certainly need reviewing in the future. It is worth noting that chicken secretin also terminates in -Leu-Met-NH_2, but for present purposes this peptide is best considered with the secretin-glucagon group.

Extracts of mammalian gut and brain cross-react in specific bombesin RIAs (15,45). Also, McDonald et al. (25) have reported the isolation of a peptide from the non-antral stomach of pigs that has one of the most striking actions of bombesin, i.e., stimulation of gastrin release. On this evidence, it seems likely that there is a counterpart of the amphibian skin peptide bombesin in the mammalian gut. Fractionation of rat stomach by gel filtration separates two main peaks of material with bombesin-like immunoreactivity (BLI) (Fig. 2). One of these co-elutes with the amphibian peptide; the other elutes earlier and so is probably a larger peptide (45). The former material accounts for most BLI in brain and throughout the small and large intestines. Immunocytochemical studies indicate that in rat gut, BLI is localized in nerves of the myenteric plexus

TABLE 2. *Substance P and bombesin-related peptides*

Substance P	Arg-Pro-Lys-Pro-Gln-Gln-Phe-Phe-Gly-Leu-Met-NH_2
Neurotensin	Glp-Leu-Tyr-Glu-Asn-Lys-Pro-Arg-Arg-Pro-Tyr-Ile-Leu
Physalemin	Glp-Ala-Asp-Pro-Asn-Lys-Phe-Tyr-Gly-Leu-Met-NH_2
Eledoisin	Glp-Pro-Ser-Lys-Asp-Ala-Phe-Ile-Gly-Leu-Met-NH_2
Bombesin	Glp-Gln-Arg-Leu-Gly-Asn-Gln-Trp-Ala-Val-Gly-His-Leu-Met-NH_2
Litorin	Glp-Gln-Trp-Ala-Val-Gly-His-Phe-Met-NH_2

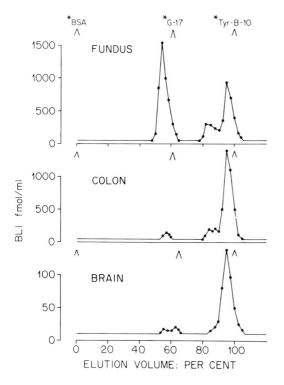

FIG. 2. Immunoreactive bombesin-like peptides separated by gel filtration on Sephadex G50. Extracts were prepared from gastric fundus, colon, and brain of rats by boiling tissues in 0.6% acetic acid, and centrifuging. BLI was estimated by radioimmunoassay, using an antiserum to synthetic bombesin and Tyr¹ bombesin COOH-terminal decapeptide labeled with ¹²⁵I. In this assay the structurally related peptide substance P has less than 0.01% immunochemical potency relative to bombesin. (From ref. 45.)

and gastric mucosa (13). In the rat, there do not appear to be bombesin-like peptides in gut mucosal endocrine cells. However, in other species, notably amphibians and birds, gastric mucosal endocrine cells containing bombesin-like peptides are plentiful (13). In mammals, substance P occurs in both mucosal enterochromaffin cells and central and peripheral nerves.

Increasing attention is being given to the role of substance P as a central neurotransmitter, and, for example, there is evidence for a role as a neurotransmitter at sensory neurones in the dorsal horn (32). In contrast, the role of substance P in the gut is still poorly understood. Moreover, as yet the roles of neurotensin and bombesin in the gut also remain ill-defined. The intravenous injection of bombesin stimulates gastrin release, and since there are bombesinergic nerve fibers in the antral mucosa it is conceivable that bombesin functions as a neurotransmitter mediating gastrin release. Intravenous bombesin also increases the frequency, and decreases the amplitude, of pacesetter potentials in intestinal smooth muscle, and so presumably bombesin-like peptides in the myenteric plexus might control motility in the gut (15).

Insulin

In lower chordates and some molluscs, insulin-like immunoreactivity has been localized to gut mucosa endocrine-like cells (see refs. 7,10). These observations, together with the embryological evidence indicating that pancreatic β-cells emerge as an outgrowth of the duodenum, firmly place insulin as a member of the gut endocrine system. Insulin has also been found in brain (20), and so can be included in the growing list of gut-brain peptides as well. Recently, several other peptides with structures related to that of insulin, or its precursor proinsulin, have been characterized. One of these, relaxin, has been isolated from pig ovary (21,38). Relaxin stimulates relaxation of the pubic symphysis, and dilatation and softening of the cervix to facilitate passage of the young at birth. Relaxin consists of two chains, A and B, of 22 and 30 residues, respectively, linked by disulfide bonds in the same position as those in insulin, and also shows other, although rather limited, homologies with insulin (21,38). A third member of the insulin family is one of the serum insulin-like growth factors that are not suppressed by insulin antibodies. These factors account for at least some of the growth-promoting actions of serum on cells in culture, although their physiological role and cells of origin remain obscure. One of these growth factors has been characterized as a single-chain peptide of 70 residues cross-linked by three disulfide bridges and bearing homologies with the single-chain precursor of insulin, proinsulin (37). There may also be structural homologies between proinsulin and other growth factors, notably nerve growth factor isolated from mouse submaxillary glands.

Others

Many of the gut peptides that have been isolated or identified can be placed in one or other of the main families. However, there remain some peptides with no obvious affinities. Among these are motilin, somatostatin, and pancreatic polypeptide (PP). Almost certainly these peptides are produced initially as large precursor molecules and clues to their biological relationships may well be found in their precursors. They may even share precursors with other active peptides. The evidence suggesting that corticotropin, the melanotropins, β-lipotrophin, and the endorphins are all produced from a common precursor according to different post-translational processing pathways, provides an obvious model system for explaining this type of relationship (24,30). The reports of corticotrophin and enkephalin immunoreactivity in the gut also make this system directly relevant to the present considerations (22).

The presence of apparently homologous peptides in tissues as different as ovary, gut, and brain suggests a previously unsuspected degree of uniformity in the organization of the molecular messengers as hormones and neurotransmitters. It also emphasizes that neither the gut endocrine system, nor any other single control system, can be considered on its own. Studies on the mechanisms involved in synthesis, storage, release, and mode of action of gut hormones are likely to have implications for the study of these peptides in the CNS, and vice versa.

HETEROGENEITY

It is useful to identify two types of heterogeneity in hormonal and related peptides. The first is characterized by the existence of different forms of a substance varying in chain length, the second by peptides of similar chain length differing in modifications to a particular residue. The point is readily illustrated by reference to gastrin. The sequence of G17 corresponds to that of the COOH-terminal heptadecapeptide of G34. Minute amounts of other, still larger, forms of gastrin have been described in tissue extracts, but these have not been fully characterized although they may well correspond to peptides extended at the NH_2-terminus of G34. In addition, both G34 and G17 exist in two forms, depending on whether or not the tyrosine residue in the COOH-terminal part of the molecule is sulfated (19). Other types of modification that might conceivably account for the second type of heterogeneity could include glycosylated and N-acetylated variants, and the presence or absence of COOH-terminal amides; such variants have been described from some pituitary hormones, but not as yet for gut peptides.

Biosynthetic Significance

Both types of heterogeneity are presumed to arise from modifications of the primary product of mRNA translation. In this sense, the multiple forms of gut hormones are distinct from isoenzymes, and from the different forms of peptides like the enkephalins, which differ in primary sequence and presumably have different structural genes. In the case of gastrin, CCK, and glucagon, the forms differing in chain length also differ in biological properties so that the factors governing the rates of synthesis and secretion of different forms are of clear physiological importance. The biosynthesis of other peptides (insulin, parathyroid hormone, corticotrophin, etc.) has in the past been successfully studied by following the incorporation of radiolabeled amino acids in pulse chase experiments (40). However, these methods have so far proved unrewarding for gut hormones like gastrin (G. J. Dockray, *unpublished observations*). In part this is probably due to the low rates of synthesis of gut peptides. Thus, antral G-cells store sufficient gastrin for at least 10 normal meal responses. Also, the gut endocrine cells are a minority population and are surrounded by other cell types (mucous, pepsinogen, etc.) with particularly high rates of protein turnover. The rate of incorporation of labeled amino acids into gut hormones is therefore expected to be low compared with that into other secretory proteins in the same tissue. In addition, gastrin synthesis in some species is obviously closely linked with the digestive cycle. For example, in rats starved for 2 or 3 days, serum and antral concentrations of gastrin are markedly reduced (27).

The nature of the physiological stimuli for gastrin synthesis are unknown and so there are obvious difficulties in trying to study gastrin biosynthesis *in vitro* when the tissues are isolated from these stimuli. Such problems are not of course unsurmountable, but nevertheless they have prompted the development of alternative approaches to the study of biosynthetic mechanisms. One of these has been the detailed analysis of the interrelationships of different molecular forms. If, as seems plausible, G17 is a product of trypsin-like cleavage of G34 then one might predict the existence of equimolar amounts of G17 and an NH_2-terminal fragment of G34. The NH_2-terminal fragment would not be biologically active but might cross-react with antibodies specific for the NH_2-terminus of G34 (Fig. 1). We raised such antibodies in rabbits immunized with G34 and were able to show that, in the antral mucosa of pig, there were indeed equimolar amounts of G17 and a molecule with the properties of the NH_2-terminal tryptic peptide of G34 (14). Further, we showed in immunohistochemical studies that both G17 and the NH_2-terminal antigenic determinant of G34 were present in the same cells (14). We have recently found a second factor, designated big gastrin III (BGIII), in hog antral extracts that cross-reacts with NH_2-terminal-specific G34 antibodies, but not with COOH-terminal-specific antibodies (18). This factor elutes from Sephadex G50 gel filtration columns in a similar position to G34, suggesting roughly similar molecular size; on ion-exchange chromatography (AE cellulose), BGIII eluted after G34 but before G17, indicating that it might be more acidic than G34 (Fig 3).

Structural studies on BGIII are presently in progress. Preliminary results suggest that after digestion with typsin, a COOH-terminal fragment is released that has an amino acid composition that includes all the residues in G17. One interesting possibility is that BGIII consists of G34 extended at the COOH-terminus, possibly by a glycine residue. A COOH-terminal amide is commonly found in active peptides, and in the case of gastrin and CCK is essential for biological activity. Melittin, a peptide from bee venom, also terminates in a COOH-terminal amide. Suchanek and Kreil (41) have shown that translation in a cell-free system of the mRNA for melittin yields a precursor terminating not in glutaminamide but rather in glutamylglycine. The mechanism of formation of the COOH-terminal amide in melittin might therefore be via substitution of glycine with ammonia, and a similar mechanism could apply in the biosynthesis of the COOH-terminal amide in gastrin.

Recently, Noyes et al. (31) initiated a promising approach to the study of gastrin biosynthesis that should also be applicable to other peptides of known sequence that have low rates of synthesis. These authors prepared an oligonucleotide corresponding to the unique 4–7 sequence of G17 and used this as a primer for synthesis of cDNA from hog antral mRNA. The nucleotide sequence of cDNA corresponded to the sequence of the NH_2-terminal region of G34, and was extended to reveal a pair of arginine residues preceding the G34 sequence. The size of mRNA coding for gastrin was estimated to be 110–140 residues.

There is ample evidence to indicate that for many peptide hormones, including insulin, parathyroid hormone, and corticotrophin, large precursors are cleaved

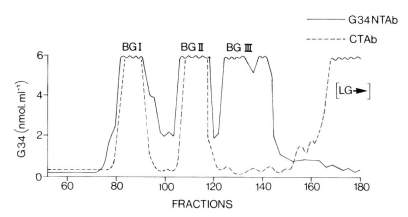

FIG. 3. Fractionation of a partially purified preparation of G34 from hog antral mucosa on aminoethyl cellulose, using a gradient of triethylamine carbonate from 0.05 M pH 6.4 to 0.5 M pH 7.4. Radioimmunoassay of the column eluates was carried out using two antisera: a COOH-terminal specific antiserum, 1296 (CT Ab) which reveals unsulfated G34 (BGI), sulfated G34 (BGII) and G17 (LG), and an NH$_2$-terminal-specific antiserum, L33 (G34NTAb) which reveals an additional form, BGIII. (From ref. 18.)

at the site of two consecutive basic residues to yield the active peptide. The presence of two lysines at the site of cleavage of G34 that yields G17 is therefore circumstantial evidence for a product-precursor relationship of G34 and G17. Similarly, the proposed pair of arginine residues preceding the sequence of G34 supports the notion of a still larger biosynthetic precursor of G34 (31). The sequence of consecutive basic residues is readily cleaved by trypsin, and although the enzymes involved in intracellular conversion of hormonal precursors remain poorly defined, they are generally thought to be trypsin-like. In this regard it is striking, therefore, that the cleavage point in CCK33 that gives CCK8 is a single basic residue (arginine) rather than a pair. Moreover, the next residue is aspartic acid, and this particular bond is particularly resistant to tryptic digestion. Thus, although there is no reason at present to doubt that CCK33 or some other larger form of CCK is cleaved to give CCK8, the mechanism of conversion would appear to be distinct from that for other peptide hormones.

Tissue Variation in the Distribution of Molecular Forms

There are several examples of tissue differences in the distribution of various molecular forms of gut hormones. Thus, in all species so far examined, over 95% of antral gastrin is attributable to G17, and G34 is always a minor component. In many species, duodenal gastrin is negligible, but in man duodenal gastrin concentrations are 10 to 20% those in antrum and G34 accounts for over 50% of total immunoreactivity (12). There are also small amounts of gastrin (1–5% antral concentrations) in hog pituitary, and again G34 accounts for over half of the total activity (35). It seems probable that in duodenum and pituitary there is incomplete conversion of G34 to G17.

The factors determining the rates of conversion and secretion of G17 and G34 are of physiological importance, since these peptides differ in biological activity. Thus, G34 is cleared about five times less rapidly than G17 (44), so that, although it is a minor component in antral mucosa, it accounts for a much higher proportion of circulating gastrin concentration. In fact, the relative contribution of G34 to total serum gastrin is even higher than that predicted from tissue concentrations and clearance rates (12), possibly due to preferential release from antral G-cells. The potency of G34 for acid secretion is about one-fifth that of G17 when expressed in terms of concentrations in blood needed for a particular rate of acid secretion. Thus, although G17 may account for less than half total circulating gastrin, it accounts for over 75% of circulating biological activity. In patients with duodenal and gastric ulcers there are increased concentrations of total immunoreactive gastrin, but most of this increase is due to G34 (12), so that circulating gastrin biological activity is only slightly increased. The reasons for the relatively higher amounts of G34 in peptic ulcer remain uncertain.

Considerations similar to those discussed for gastrin may well apply to glucagon (26), CCK, and perhaps other gut hormones. For example, in gut, CCK8 and larger forms like CCK33 occur in approximately equal concentrations. In contrast, in cerebral cortex there are relatively high concentrations of CCK8, but larger molecular forms account for only a small amount of total immunoreactive CCK (8,13). Again, the differences can be attributed to different rates of conversion. Both CCK8 and CCK33 are biologically active. However, CCK33 is thought to be less susceptible to hepatic degradation than CCK8, and so after release from the intestine probably makes a relatively greater contribution to total circulating CCK.

REFERENCES

1. Bayliss, W. M., and Starling, E. H. (1902): The mechanism of pancreatic secretion. *J. Physiol. (Lond.),* 28:325–353.
2. Bryant, M. G., Bloom, S. R., Polak, J. M., Albuquerque, R. H., Modlin I., and Pearse, A. G. E. (1976): Possible dual role for vasoactive intestinal peptide as gastrointestinal hormone and neurotransmitter substance. *Lancet,* 1:991–993.
3. Carraway, R., and Leeman, S. E. (1974): The amino acid sequence, chemical synthesis and radioimmunoassay of neurotensin. *Fed. Proc.,* 33:548 (Abstr. 811).
4. Chang, M. M., and Leeman, S. E. (1970): Isolation of a sialogogic peptide from bovine hypothalamus and its characterization as substance P. *J. Biol. Chem.,* 245:4784–4790.
5. Dimaline, R., and Dockray, G. J. (1978): Multiple immunoreactive forms of vasoactive intestinal peptide in human colonic mucosa. *Gastroenterology,* 75:387–392.
6. Dockray, G. J. (1976): Immunochemical evidence of cholecystokinin-like peptides in brain. *Nature,* 264:568–570.
7. Dockray, G. J. (1977): Molecular evolution of gut hormones: Application of comparative studies on the regulation of digestion. *Gastroenterology,* 72:344–358.
8. Dockray, G. J. (1977): Immunoreactive component resembling cholecystokinin octapeptide in intestine. *Nature,* 270:359–361.

9. Dockray, G. J. (1979): Immunochemistry of gastrin and cholecystokinin: Development and application of region specific antisera. In: *Gastrins and the Vagus,* edited by J. F. Rehfeld and E. Amdrup, pp. 73–83. Academic Press, London.

10. Dockray, G. J. (1979): Comparative biochemistry and physiology of gut hormones. *Annu. Rev. Physiol.,* 41:83–95.

11. Dockray, G. J., Gregory, R. A., Hutchinson, J. B., Harris, J. I., and Runswick, M. J. (1978): Isolation, structure and biological activity of two cholecystokinin octapeptides from sheep brain. *Nature,* 274:711–713.

12. Dockray, G. J., and Taylor, I. L. (1978): Different forms of gastrin in peptic ulcer. In: *Gastrointestinal Hormones and Pathology of the Digestive System,* edited by M. I. Grossman, V. Speranza, N. Basso, and E. Lezoche, pp. 91–96. Plenum Press, New York.

13. Dockray, G. J., Vaillant, C., Dimaline, R., Hutchison, J. B., and Gregory, R. A. (1979): Characterization of molecular forms of cholecystokinin, vasoactive intestinal polypeptide and bombesin-like immunoreactivity in nerves and endocrine cells. In: *Hormone Receptors in Digestion and Nutrition,* edited by G. Rosselin, P. Fromageot, and S. Bonfils, pp. 501–511. Elsevier/North-Holland, Amsterdam.

14. Dockray, G. J. Vaillant, C., and Hopkins, C. R. (1978): Biosynthetic relationships of big and little gastrins. *Nature,* 273:770–772.

15. Erspamer, V., Melchiorri, P., Falconieri Erspamer, C., and Negri, L. (1978): Polypeptides of the amphibian skin active on the gut and their mammalian counterparts. In: *Gastrointestinal Hormones and Pathology of the Digestive System,* edited by M. I. Grossman, V. Speranza, N. Basso, and E. Lazoche, pp. 51–64. Plenum Press, New York.

16. Gardner, J. D. (1979): Regulation of pancreatic exocrine function *in vitro:* Initial steps in the actions of secretagogues. *Annu. Rev. Physiol.,* 41:55–66.

17. Gregory, R. A. (1977): The gastrointestinal hormones: An historical review. In: *The Pursuit of Nature,* edited by A. L. Hodgkin et al., pp. 105–132. Cambridge University Press, Cambridge.

18. Gregory, R. A. (1979): Some aspects of the structure of gastrin and gastrin-like forms and fragments in gut and brain. In: *Gastrins and the Vagus,* edited by J. F. Rehfeld and E. Amdrup, pp. 47–55. Academic Press, London.

19. Gregory, R. A., and Tracy, H. J. (1975): The chemistry of the gastrins: Some recent advances. In: *Gastrointestinal Hormones,* edited by J. C. Thompson, pp. 13–24. University of Texas Press, Austin.

20. Havrankova, J., Schmechel, D., Roth, J., and Brownstein, M. (1978): Identification of insulin in rat brain. *Proc. Natl. Acad. Sci. USA,* 75:5737–5741.

21. James, R., Niall, H., Kwok, S., and Bryant-Greenwood, G. (1977): Primary structure of porcine relaxin: Homology with insulin and related growth factors. *Nature,* 267:544–546.

22. Larsson, L.-I. (1979): Peptides of the gastrin cell. In: *Gastrins and the Vagus,* edited by J. F. Rehfeld and E. Amdrup, pp. 5–14. Academic Press, London.

23. Larsson, L.-I., Fahrenkrug, J., Schaffalitzky de Muckadell, O., Sundler, F., Hakanson, R., and Rehfeld, J. F. (1976): Localization of vasoactive intestinal polypeptide (VIP) to central and peripheral neurones. *Proc. Natl. Acad. Sci. USA,* 73:3197–3200.

24. Mains, R. E., Eipper, B. A., and Ling, N. (1977): Common precursor to corticotrophins and the endorphins. *Proc. Natl. Acad. Sci. USA,* 74:3014–3018.

25. McDonald, T. J., Nilsson, G., Vagne, M., Ghatei, M., Bloom, S. R., and Mutt, V. (1978): A gastrin releasing peptide from the porcine non-antral gastric tissue. *Gut,* 19:767–774.

26. Moody, A. J., Jacobsen, H., and Sundby, F. (1978): Gastric glucagon and gut glucagon-like immunoreactants. In: *Gut Hormones,* edited by S. R. Bloom, pp. 369–378. Churchill Livingstone, Edinburgh.

27. Mortensen, N. J. McC., Morris, J. F., and Owens, C. (1979): Gastrin and the ultra-structure of G cells in the fasting rat. *Gut,* 20:41–50.

28. Mutt, V. (1978): Progress in intestinal hormone research. In: *Gastrointestinal Hormones and Pathology of the Digestive System,* edited by M. I. Grossman, V. Speranza, N. Basso, and E. Lezoche, pp. 133–146. Plenum Press, New York.

29. Mutt, V. (1979): Chemistry of the cholecystokinins. In: *Gastrins and the Vagus,* edited by J. F. Rehfeld and E. Amdrup, pp. 57–71. Academic Press, London.

30. Nakanishi, S., Inoue, A., Kita, T., Nakamura, M., Chang, A. C. Y., Cohen, S. N., and Numa, S. (1979): Nucleotide sequence of cloned cDNA for bovine corticotrophin-β-lipotropin precursor. *Nature,* 278:423–427.

31. Noyes, B. E., Mevarech, M., Stein, R., and Agarwal, K. L. (1979): Detection and partial sequence analysis of gastrin mRNA by using an oligodeoxynucleotide probe. *Proc. Natl. Acad. Sci. USA,* 76:1770–1774.

32. Otsuka, M., and Takahashi, T. (1977): Putative peptide neurotransmitters. *Annu. Rev. Pharmacol.,* 17:425–439.

33. Pearse, A. G. E. (1976): Peptides in brain and gut. *Nature,* 262:92–94.

34. Rehfeld, J. F. (1978): Immunochemical studies on cholecystokinin: II. Distribution and molecular heterogeneity in the central nervous system and small intestine of man and hog. *J. Biol. Chem.,* 253:4022–4030.

35. Rehfeld, J. F. (1978): Localization of gastrins to neuro- and adenohyophysis. *Nature,* 271:771–773.

36. Rehfeld, J. F., and Larsson, L.-I. (1979): The predominant antral gastrin and intestinal cholecystokinin is the common COOH-terminal tetrapeptide amide. In: *Gastrins and the Vagus,* edited by J. F. Rehfeld and E. Amdrup, pp. 85–94. Academic Press, London.

37. Rinderknecht, E., and Humbel, R. E. (1978): The amino acid sequence of human insulin-like growth factor I and its structural homology with proinsulin. *J. Biol. Chem.,* 253:2769–2776.

38. Schwabe, C., and McDonald, J. K. (1977): Relaxin: A disulfide homolog of insulin. *Science,* 197:914–915.

39. Solcia, E., Polak, J. M., Pearse, A. G. E., Forssmann, W. G., Larsson, L. I., Sundler, F., Lechago, J., Grimelius, L., and Grossman, M. I. (1978): Lausanne 1977 classification of gastroenteropancreatic endocrine cells. In: *Gut Hormones,* edited by S. R. Bloom, pp. 40–48. Churchill Livingstone, Edinburgh.

40. Steiner, D. F. (1976): Peptide hormone precursors: Biosynthesis, processing and significance. In: *Peptide Hormones,* edited by J. A. Parsons, pp. 49–64. Macmillan, London.

41. Suchanek, G., and Kreil, G. (1977): Translation of melittin messenger RNA *in vitro* yields a product terminating with glutamylglycine rather than with glutaminamide. *Proc. Natl. Acad. Sci. USA,* 74:975–978.

42. Uvnas-Wallensten, K., Rehfeld, J. F., Larsson, L.-I., and Uvnas, B. (1977): Hetpadecapeptide gastrin in the vagal nerve. *Proc. Natl. Acad. Sci. USA,* 73:5707–5710.

43. Vanderhaeghen, J. J., Signeau, J. C., and Gepts, W. (1975): New peptide in vertebrate CNS reacting with antigastrin antibodies. *Nature,* 257:604–605.

44. Walsh, J. H., and Grossman, M. I. (1975): Gastrin. *N. Engl. J. Med.,* 292:1324–1332.

45. Walsh, J. H., Wong, H., and Dockray, G. J. (1979): Bombesin-like peptides in mammals. *Fed. Proc.,* 38:2315–2319.

Polypeptide Hormones, edited by
R. F. Beers, Jr. and E. G. Bassett.
Raven Press, New York © 1980.

34. Gastrointestinal Hormones: Distribution and Tissue Localization

J. M. Polak and S. R. Bloom

*Departments of Histochemistry and Medicine, Royal Postgraduate Medical School,
London W12 0HS, England*

INTRODUCTION

The discovery of secretin in the duodenum by Bayliss and Starling in 1902
(3) initiated, under the new term "hormone," the revolutionary concept of
"chemical messengers" transported to distant organs by the blood. In spite of
the nonglandular nature of the duodenum, endocrinology was subsequently almost exclusively understood to be "glandular" endocrinology, with ductless
glands (e.g., thyroid and pituitary) producing most of the circulating hormones.
However, the discovery of more peptide hormones in the gut introduced another
aspect of endocrinology, that of a nonglandular or "diffuse" endocrine organ.

Although a number of the known peptides were originally extracted from
the gut, it is now well established that gut hormones are present in many other
organs in both endocrine cells and nerves (e.g., lung, urogenital tract, and salivary
glands). However, because more of them are produced in the gut than anywhere
else, the peptides of this newly discovered diffuse neuroendocrine system are
often included in the general term "gut hormone."

TECHNOLOGY

Two immunological procedures, radioimmunoassay (RIA) and immunocytochemistry, used in combination, have provided the most suitable approach to
the study of the distribution and tissue localization of the "gut" hormones.

RIA supplies information on the molecular forms and absolute quantities
of hormones in blood and tissue. Immunocytochemistry is, so far, the most
valuable method of obtaining information regarding the precise tissue localization
(29) of a hormone in cells and/or nerves. However, a number of problems
must be overcome to develop this technique into a useful tool. These mainly
concern *fixation* and *specificity.*

Fixation

Peptide hormones are soluble in water and, therefore, may be dissolved during
immunostaining. It is thus necessary to use a fixative that can render the peptides

in the tissue insoluble while retaining their antigenicity. Although classic cross-linking agents, such as the conventional aldehyde fixatives, are useful in some cases, a wider range of successful immunostaining is currently obtained by the use of two other cross-linking agents, *p*-benzoquinone and diethylpyrocarbonate, either in solution or in vapor form (31).

Specificity

Antibodies to peptide hormones are raised by immunization with a complex immunogen. This is composed of the pure small peptide coupled to a larger molecule (e.g., bovine serum albumin, thyroglobulin, and hemocyanin) by a cross-linking agent (e.g., carbodiimide and glutaraldehyde). The immunogen is then mixed with an adjuvant (e.g., tubercle bacilli) and injected into the receiving animal. The antisera produced will be heterospecific, containing a mixed population of antibodies to the various components of the immunogen.

In the RIA system this is not a problem, as the technique is based on competition between the specific radiolabeled peptide and the peptide present in blood and tissue for binding sites on the corresponding antibody present in the serum. However, antibody heterogeneity can be a problem in immunocytochemistry, which depends for its success on the specificity of binding of the desired serum antibodies to one of the numerous antigens present in the tissue. There are several ways of ensuring specificity of immunocytochemical staining. One of the main requirements is for exceedingly avid antibodies of high titer, which allows the antiserum to be diluted to its maximal extent, thus removing minor subpopulations of unwanted antibodies. Rigorous washing will remove weakly attached antibodies. Immunoaffinity absorption can be used as a means of purifying antibodies for immunocytochemistry, but complete prevention of the immunostaining by preabsorption of the antibody with a small quantity of the corresponding pure antigen is a necessary precaution to establish specificity.

A new technique for obtaining monospecific (monoclonal) antibodies has recently been developed. This involves cloning hybrid myeloma cells (immunoglobulin-producing myeloma cells with spleen T-lymphocytes of the immunized animal) and, in the not too distant future, this system for programmed antibody production will further ensure specificity in immunocytochemistry (26).

TRIPARTITE FUNCTION OF THE DIFFUSE NEUROENDOCRINE SYSTEM

It has recently become evident that "gut" hormones are localized in both endocrine/paracrine cells and in nerves of the autonomic nervous system (34). In addition, it is now recognized that many peptide hormones do not behave in the classic manner (transport by the circulation to distant target organs), but instead act locally after release from either paracrine cells or nerve terminals (35). Thus, a single peptide can have a tripartite set of actions: as a local (paracrine) hormone, as a classic circulating hormone, and/or as a neurotransmitter/ neuromodulator.

We shall now discuss the individual hormones, dividing them into three groups: circulating hormones, local hormones, and peptidergic neurotransmitters.

HORMONES ACTING VIA THE CIRCULATION

Hormones acting via the circulation are produced and secreted by endocrine (APUD) cells of the gastrointestinal mucosa, which are shown by conventional histological staining as clear (poorly stained) cells intermingled with nonendocrine elements. Some histological methods for secretory granules, such as lead hematoxylin or silver impregnation, demonstrate them well (17). However, immunocytochemistry, using highly specific antibodies, has become the most reliable and accurate method for the study of the precise cellular localization and functional characteristics of the various gut hormones. In addition, several refinements of the immunocytochemical procedure, [e.g., serial semithin/thin sectioning technique (41), double staining after elution of the primary antibody (46), and the simultaneous use of two different antisera (3)] have recently allowed the full characterization of the various hormone-producing cells. Some ultrastructural features of the cells are of excellent diagnostic value, especially the presence of electron-dense secretory granules of characteristic size, density, limiting membrane, and halo. In addition to the secretory granules, a luminal tuft of microvilli and intracytoplasmic microfilaments can often be distinguished (Fig. 1). These features alone often allow a fairly accurate identification to be made. The criteria for the electron microscopic classification of the APUD cells are continually being refined and improved, the latest system being the Lausanne classification (45).

The ultrastructural appearance of these cells has led to their interpretation as modified neural elements with a receptor surface (microvilli), (neuro)secretory granules, and microfilaments for their intracytoplasmic transport.

Gut Hormones

Eight circulating gut hormones are recognized at present. By their distribution throughout the gut, they can be subdivided into three major anatomical areas of origin; stomach, upper intestine, and lower intestine (Table 1).

Gastrin

Gastrin is present in blood and tissue in numerous molecular forms, the two main ones being composed of 17 (G17) and 34 (G34) amino acids. Gastrin is found mostly in the antrum (Fig. 2), where the predominant form is G17.

The cell of origin is the well-established antral G (AG) cell, with classic flocculent granules, 360 ± 56 nm (range, 160 to 410 nm) in diameter (14).

Gastrin is also found in considerable quantities in the upper small intestine, where it is produced by the recently described intestinal gastrin (IG) cell with

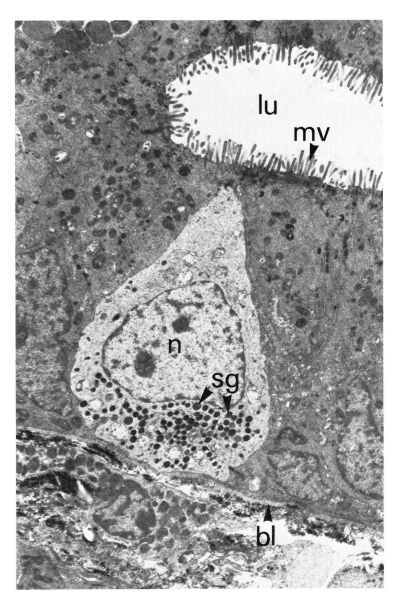

FIG. 1. Electron micrograph of endocrine cells in human duodenum. Section was fixed by glutaraldehyde and osmium and stained with uranyl acetate/lead citrate. n, nucleus; sg, secretory granules; bl, basal lamina; mv, microvilli; lu, lumen. ×6,375.

TABLE 1. Gut hormones: chemistry and distribution

Function and peptide	Stomach		Upper gut			Lower gut		Pancreas	M.W.	No. of amino acids	Granule size (nm ± SD)
	Fundic	Anterior	Duodenum	Jejunum	Ileum	Colon					
Circulating hormone											
Gastrin (G17)		+	+						2,100	17	360 ± 56
Gastrin (G34)		+	+	+					3,800	34	175 ± 32
Secretin			+	+					3,073	27	240 ± 32
Motilin			+	+					2,700	22	180 ± 24
CCK			+	+	+				3,883	34	250 ± 17
GIP		+	+	+					5,105	43	350 ± 24
EG (enteroglucagon)					+	+			1,673	13	210 ± 26
Neurotensin				+	+						300 ± 39
PP (pancreatic polypeptide)							+		4,273	36	200 ± 22
Local/paracrine											
Somatostatin	+	+	+	+	+	+			1,639	14	310 ± 46
Neurotransmitter											
VIP	+	+	+	+	+	+			3,326	28	
Substance P	+	+	+	+	+	+			1,347	11	
Bombesin	+	+	+	+	+	+			1,620	14	
Leu-enkephalin	+	+			+	+			556	5	
Met-enkephalin	+	+	+	+	+	+			574	5	

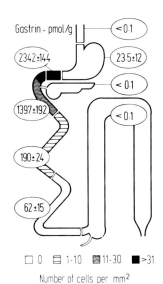

FIG. 2. Map showing the distribution of gastrin in the human gut.

small (175 ± 26 nm; range, 90 to 220 nm), dense secretory granules (Fig. 3) (14). The predominant molecular form of intestinal gastrin is G34.

Secretin

Secretin is a 27-amino acid peptide present in the upper intestine and produced by the S cell of the electron microscopic classification, containing secretory granules of small or intermediate size (240 ± 32 nm; range, 180 to 290 nm).

Cholecystokinin

CCK is a 34-amino acid peptide sharing with gastrin the five COOH-terminal amino acids. It is found in tissue and in circulation in many molecular forms of variable biological activity. It is localized in the upper small intestine (Fig. 4) in a separate and well-characterized cell type, the I cell of the ultrastructural classification, containing intermediately sized secretory granules, (350 ± 17 nm; range, 230 to 270 nm), hence the name of the cell (13).

Glucose-Dependent Insulinotropic Polypeptide

Glucose-dependent insulinotropic polypeptide (GIP) is a 43-amino acid peptide extractable principally from the upper intestine (Fig. 5). It is produced by the K cells of the electron microscopic classification which display rather large (350 ± 24 nm; range, 360 to 400 nm), round, secretory granules with tightly fitting membranes and dense cores (Fig. 6) (12).

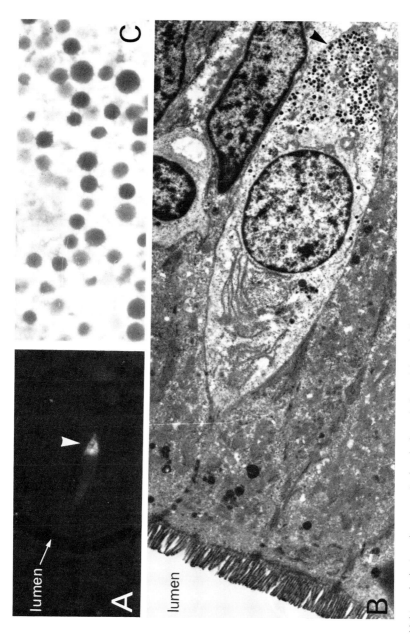

FIG. 3. Light and electron immunocytochemical rendering of intestinal gastrin cells by the semithin/thin method. **A:** A 1 μ-section of human intestine marked with *white arrow*; ×630. **B:** Serial thin (800 nm) section showing intestinal gastrin cells almost reaching the lumen; ×4,050. **C:** Higher magnification to show details of secretory granules; ×27,000.

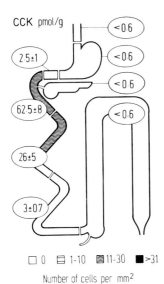

FIG. 4. Map showing the distribution of CCK in the human gut.

Motilin

Motilin was originally extracted from the upper small intestine in a single molecular form as a 22-amino acid peptide. It has, however, recently been found to be present in blood and tissue in two molecular forms, only one of which elutes during gel chromatography at the same level as pure natural motilin, the other being of a larger size. The use of antibodies specific to the NH_2-

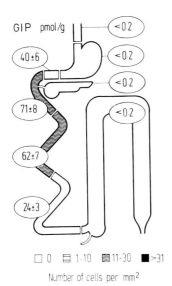

FIG. 5. Map showing the distribution of GIP in the human gut.

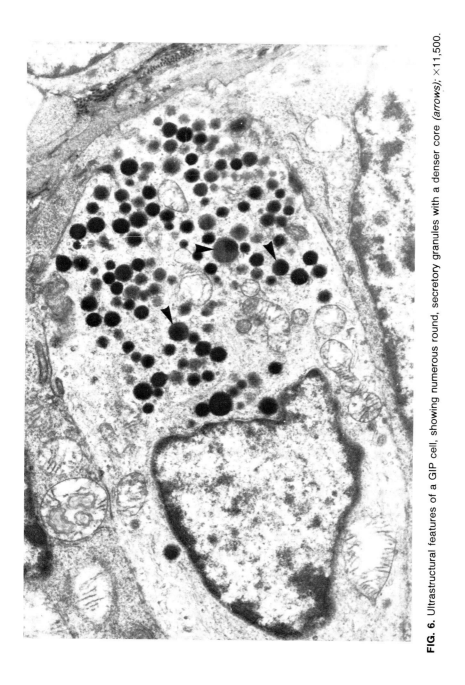

FIG. 6. Ultrastructural features of a GIP cell, showing numerous round, secretory granules with a denser core (arrows); ×11,500.

and COOH-terminal regions of the molecule indicates that the larger form is mostly detected by the use of NH$_2$-terminally directed antibodies and is present mainly in one type of enterochromaffin cell of the small intestine (Fig. 7). The smaller form is detected by COOH-terminally directed antibodies and is mostly

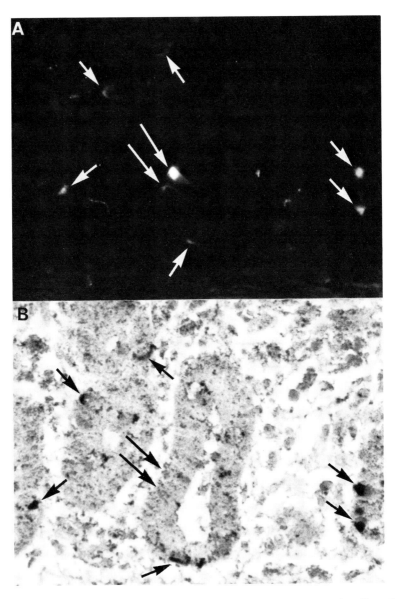

FIG. 7. Human duodenal mucosa stained with COOH- and NH$_2$-terminal directed motilin antibodies showing reactive argentaffin *(small arrow)* and non-argentaffin *(large arrow)* cells by **A:** immunofluorescence and **B:** silver impregnation (argentaffin) of the same section; ×129.

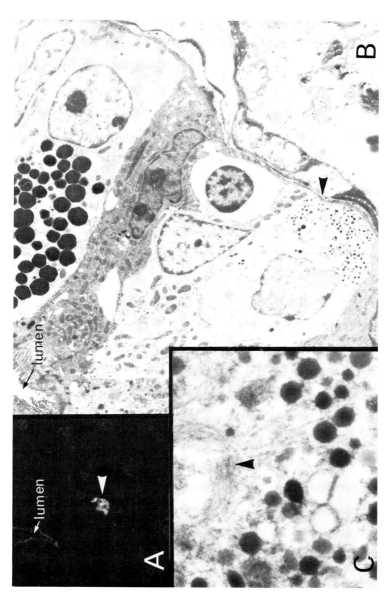

FIG. 8. Light and electron immunocytochemical rendering of the motilin cell by the semithin/thin method. **A:** A 1 μm section with cell marked by *arrow;* ×5,950. **B:** A serial thin (800 nm) section showing its electron microscopic characteristics. **C:** More details of the motilin cell. Microfilaments marked with *arrow;* ×29,750.

present in a non-enterochromaffin cell type of the upper gut, which contains small secretory granules (37). This cell, now known as the M cell, was previously included in the heterogeneous group of D_1 cells. (EC: 300 ± 60 nm; range, 175 to 360 nm. M: 189 ± 24 nm, range 160 to 190 nm) (Fig. 8).

Enteroglucagon

Enteroglucagon is the name given to a glucagon-like immunoreactive material found predominantly in the lower intestine (Fig. 9) and known to be produced by endocrine-like cells that contain large (210 ± 26 nm; range, 170 to 250 nm), round, dense, secretory granules surrounded by a tightly fitting membrane (38). Immunocytochemical staining often reveals that the enteroglucagon cells as well as their luminal microvilli are provided with basally located, elongated processes (Fig. 10).

Neurotensin

Neurotensin is an 11-amino acid peptide almost exclusively present in the ileal mucosa (42), in characteristic endocrine-like cells containing the largest type of secretory granules (300 ± 39 nm; range, 170 to 350 nm).

Pancreatic Polypeptide

Pancreatic polypeptide (PP) is a 36-amino acid peptide localized almost exclusively to the pancreas. The PP cell show rather irregular membrane-bound secretory granules of an average size of 200 ± 22 nm).

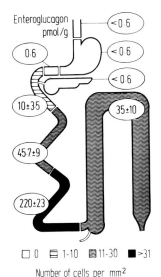

FIG. 9. Map showing the distribution of enteroglucagon in the human gut.

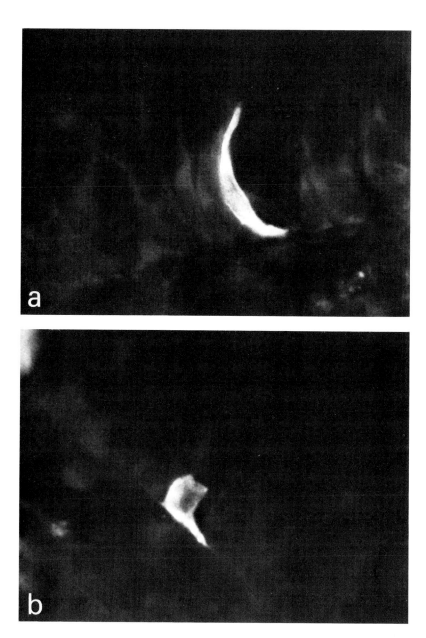

FIG. 10. Immunofluorescent glucagon cells in human colon. **a:** Cell extends from basal lamina to lumen; **b:** Cell process extending along basal lamina; ×770.

LOCAL (PARACRINE) HORMONES

Somatostatin and Its Pathologies

Somatostatin, an ideal example of the paracrine hormone group, is a 14-amino acid peptide originally extracted from the hypothalamus during the search for the factor responsible for the control of release of growth hormone (10). Large quantities of somatostatin were later found in the gut and pancreas (40). Immunocytochemical techniques localize somatostatin to the D cells of the gut and pancreas (40), which are characterized by the presence of large (310 ± 46 nm; range, 260 to 270 nm), round, and uniform secretory granules (45). In addition, these techniques often show the cells to be provided with elongated processes that may terminate in a bulbous swelling on another endocrine/exocrine cell (Fig. 11). This structural feature may provide support for the postulated role of somatostatin as a local hormone (acting in the neighborhood of its release).

Somatostatin is a powerful inhibitory factor for the release of all the gut hormones as well as a controlling agent for a number of gastrointestinal functions (7). It is therefore possible that somatostatin malfunction plays an important role in gastrointestinal and pancreatic diseases. Antral somatostatin deficiency has lately been suggested (18,36) as one of the many factors involved in the etiopathogenesis of duodenal ulceration.

A significant somatostatin deficiency has recently been found in the pancreas of children with intractable hypoglycemia, hyperinsulinism, and insulin cell hyperplasia (nesidioblastosis). The shortage of somatostatin evidently leads to lack of control of the excessive insulin release.

In numerous cases, somatostatin has been found to suppress successfully the hormone release from functioning tumors of the pancreas (insulinomas, VIPomas, glucagonomas, and gastrinomas). Some of these cases are refractory, however. This can now be explained by the positive finding that these particular tumors already contain abnormally high amounts of somatostatin (9).

PEPTIDERGIC NEUROTRANSMITTERS

Immunochemistry has recently demonstrated the presence of gut peptides in nerves of the autonomic innervation. This supports the concept of a third part of the autonomic nervous system in addition to the former cholinergic and adrenergic divisions (15,34). The additional noncholinergic, nonadrenergic component was considered by Burnstock to be "purinergic" (15,16) on the basis of neurophysiological and histochemical studies and to be "peptidergic" by Baumgarten and co-workers on the basis of their ultrastructural findings (2).

Immunocytochemical techniques readily demonstrate fine beaded, peptide-containing nerve fibers. However, the demonstration of neuronal cell bodies is difficult, as the peptides produced in the soma are rapidly transported to the

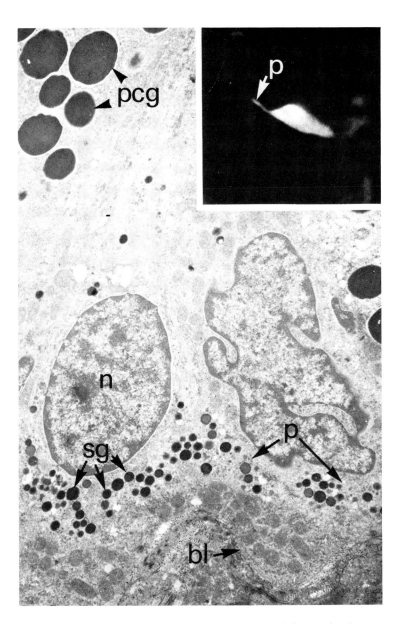

FIG. 11. Electron micrograph of somatostatin (D) cell in human jejunum showing processes extending from basal part of cell. Modified Karnovsky's fixation and uranyl acetate/lead citrate stain; n, nucleus of somatostatin cell; sg, somatostatin cell secretory granules; p, cell process; bl, basal lamina; pcg, paneth cell granules. ×8,925. **Inset** shows immunofluorescent somatostatin cell displaying a similar cell process, p. ×455.

nerve fibers and terminals. To retain the peptide in the cell bodies, it is often necessary to use some kind of transport inhibitor such as colchicine or vinblastine, *in vivo*, prior to immunostaining, but this can be a rather drastic pharmacological procedure.

To overcome this problem, an alternative method has recently been employed. This is based on the use of cultures of the submucous and myenteric plexuses of the gut wall and the demonstration by immunocytochemical methods of nerve fibers outgrown from the cultured cell bodies (23). Using this technique, the intrinsic origin of the gut peptidergic innervation [vasoactive intestinal polypeptide (VIP), substance P, and enkephalin] has conclusively been shown.

This has been further supported by the successful immunostaining of all these neuropeptides after extrinsic denervation of the gut wall (23).

Substance P

Substance P was the first peptide to be found in both the brain and the gut. It was discovered by von Euler and Gaddum (49) while they were working on the distribution of acetylcholine in the gut. It was originally described as a potent hypotensive and gut contractile peptide and later identified with the sialogenic peptide described by Leeman and co-workers (25).

Substance P is an 11-amino acid peptide present along the entire length of the gut and localized to an intrinsic system of nerve fibers with cell bodies in the gut wall. Substance P is also well represented outside the gut. In the lung, it is found in fine nerve fibers around the bronchi, bronchioles, vessels, and alveolar walls. A rich supply of substance P nerves is found along the entire length of the ureter, innervating the muscle, submucosa, and adventitia (Fig. 12). Parallel electron microscopic studies reveal the presence of numerous neurosecretory granules that are larger and more dense than those classically described as adrenergic or cholinergic. In the genital tract and skin, substance P is found in close contact with the epithelial layers. This localization supports its postulated role as a putative sensory neurotransmitter (28).

Bombesin

Bombesin is a 14-amino acid peptide originally extracted from the discoglossid frog *Bombina bombina* by Erspamer and co-workers (19). It is part of the wide group of amphibian skin peptides with counterparts in man and other mammals. Bombesin is present in the brain, lung, and gut (39) (Fig. 13), where immunocytochemical techniques localize it to both nerves (gut and brain) and APUD cells (amphibian and avian gut, clear cells of the bronchial epithelium).

Enkephalins

The enkephalins, leucine- and methionine-enkephalin, are two pentapeptides that differ only at their COOH-terminal end (24). They are both present in

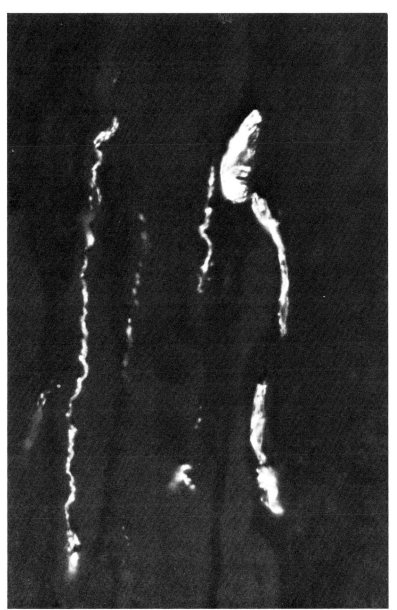

FIG. 12. Nerves containing substance P-like immunoreactivity in the muscle coat of guinea pig ureter; ×454.

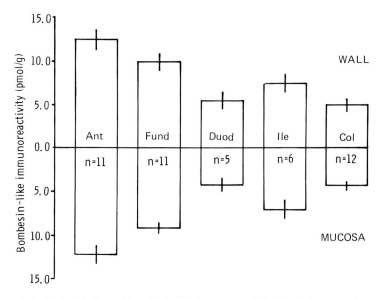

FIG. 13. Distribution of bombesin-like immunoreactivity in the human gut.

man and other mammals, the ratio of methionine- to leucine-enkephalin being approximately 4 to 1. The enkephalins are also chemically related to a larger group of peptides that, because of their opioid actions, are all included under the generic term "endorphins" (22). The enkephalins are the smallest of this group. The larger endorphins are found in the brain and pituitary, whereas the enkephalins, in addition to their separate localization in the brain, are also found in the gut and sympathetic tissue, including the type I cells of the carotid body. In the gut, they are mostly present in the autonomic innervation with cell bodies intrinsic to the gut wall.

Vasoactive Intestinal Polypeptide

Vasoactive intestinal polypeptide (VIP) is a 28-amino acid peptide originally extracted from the gastrointestinal tract (43) and later found in similar significant quantities in the brain (11), pancreas (33), pituitary (47), salivary gland (50), upper respiratory tract (44), and urogenital tract (5). Immunocytochemical examination reveals that its principal localization is in fine nerve fibers (Fig. 14) that, in the periphery, form part of the autonomic peptidergic innervation. The obvious actions of VIP as a secretory agent, muscle relaxant, and vasodilatory substance (43) correlate well with its presence (Fig. 15) in nerve fibers, which run in close proximity to secretory structures (gut mucosa, pancreatic islets, and endometrium), smooth muscle (ureter, gut wall, and myometrium), and blood vessels of most organs where VIP is found.

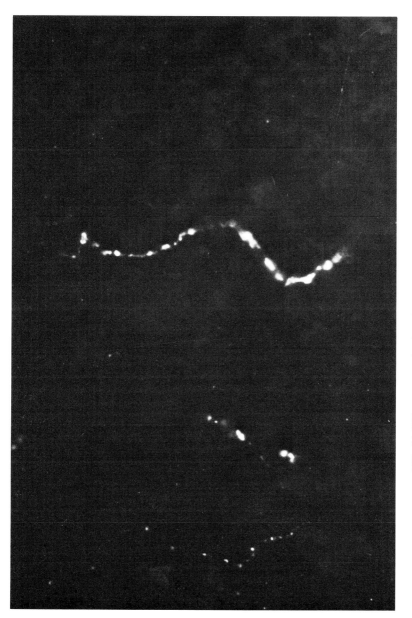

FIG. 14. VIP nerve running in submucosa of human colon; ×468.

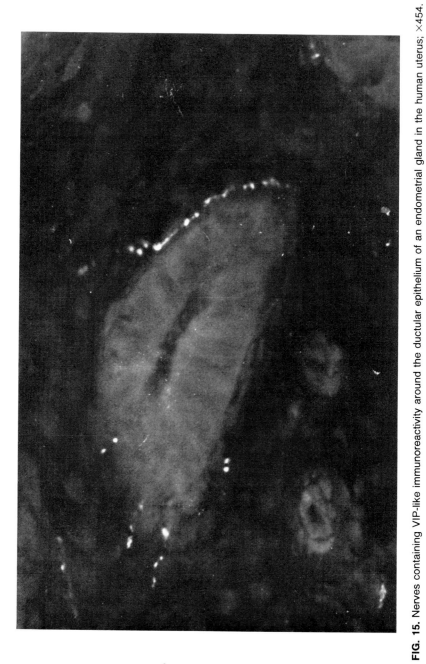

FIG. 15. Nerves containing VIP-like immunoreactivity around the ductular epithelium of an endometrial gland in the human uterus; ×454.

TUMOR PATHOLOGY

The agent responsible for the clinical features of the Verner-Morrison syndrome (48) remained unknown until 1973. VIP was then found to be present in large quantities in both the tumor tissue (usually pancreatic) and the circulation (8). The Verner-Morrison syndrome has since been recognized as the VIPoma syndrome and most of its clinical features have now been experimentally reproduced by intravenous injections of large quantities of VIP (27).

NON-TUMOR PATHOLOGY

A marked decrease in the gut VIP content has recently been shown in diseases such as Hirschprung's disease (4), Chagas' disease (6), and idiopathic esophageal achalasia which primarily involve degeneration or absence of the neuronal cell bodies of the gut autonomic innervation. In contrast, a marked increase in VIP levels in neuronal cell bodies and fibers of the wall has lately been noted in areas of the gut affected by inflammatory bowel disease, especially Crohn's disease (32) (Fig. 16).

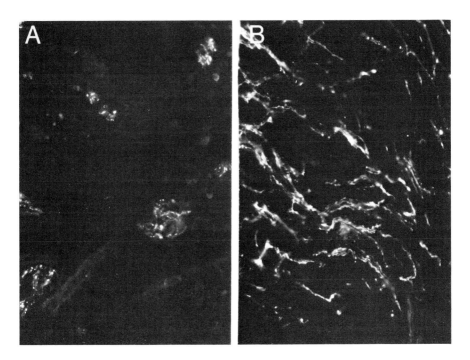

FIG. 16. VIP nerves **(A)** in submucosa of normal human colon and **(B)** in similar area in colon of a patient with Crohn's disease; ×273.

CONCLUSIONS

The number of "gut hormones" has grown rapidly in the last decade. Some of them were originally extracted from the gut, whereas others were found first in the brain. It has lately become evident that these peptides are not confined to the tissues where they were first discovered, but are far more widely distributed throughout the body. This aspect of their distribution and the information provided by their immunocytochemical localization in endocrine and neural elements indicates that they play an important controlling role in a number of functions and emphasizes the unity of the two key regulatory systems, the neural and endocrine systems. This was already pointed out, on the basis of his original observations, by Feyrter (20), who described the presence of a "clear cell" system or "diffuse endocrine system" with mainly local or paracrine actions. Pearse, in his seminal APUD concept (30), emphasized the functional unity of Feyrter's (20) diffuse endocrine system and postulated a common neuroectodermal origin for its components. Fujita (21) with his ultrastructural studies has recently further supported Pearse's observations, suggesting the unifying name of "paraneurons" for the members of this diffuse neuroendocrine system.

Studies on the gut distribution and tissue localization of the hormones and neuropeptides have led to the realization that they all have a circumscribed—although overlapping—distribution and are produced by well-characterized types of cell or neuron. Modern techniques of gut neuroendocrine pathology will soon permit the better understanding of gastrointestinal diseases.

ACKNOWLEDGMENTS

This research was generously supported by grants from the Council of Tobacco Research (USA), the Medical Research Council, and Janssen Pharmaceuticals.

REFERENCES

1. Arimura, A., Sato, H., Dupont, A., Nishi, N., and Schally, A. V. (1975): Somatostatin: Abundance of immunoreactive hormone in rat stomach and pancreas. *Science,* 189:1007–1009.
2. Baumgarten, H. G., Holstein, A. F., and Owman, C. H. (1970): Auerbach's plexus of mammals and man: Electron microscopical identification of three different types of neuronal processes in myenteric ganglia of the large intestine from rhesus monkeys, guinea-pigs and man. *Z. Zellforsch.,* 106:376–397.
3. Bayliss, W. M., and Starling, E. H. (1902): The mechanism of pancreatic secretion. *J. Physiol. (Lond.),* 28:325–353.
4. Bishop, A. E., Lake, B., and Polak, J. M. (1979): Abnormalities of the peptidergic nerves in Hirschprung's disease. *Handbook, July 1979 Meeting of the Pathological Society of Great Britain.*
5. Bishop, A. E., Polak, J. M., and Bloom, S. R. (1979): Vasoactive intestinal polypeptide innervation of the genital tract of women. *J. Endocrinol.,* 80:33–34.
6. Bishop, A. E., Polak, J. M., Long, R. G., and Bloom, S. R. (1979): Chagas disease: Decrease of VIP and substance P in the gut. *Handbook, July 1979 Meeting of the Pathological Society of Great Britain.*
7. Bloom, S. R. (1978): Somatostatin and gut. *Gastroenterology,* 75:145–147.

8. Bloom, S. R., Polak, J. M., and Pearse, A. G. E. (1973): Vasoactive intestinal peptide and the watery diarrhoea syndrome. *Lancet,* 2:14–16.

9. Bloom, S. R., Polak, J. M., and West, A. M. (1978): Somatostatin content of pancreatic endocrine tumours. *Metabolism,* 27:1235–1238.

10. Brazeau, P., Vale, W., Burgus, R., Ling, N., Butcher, M., Rivier, J., and Guillemin, R. (1973): Hypothalamic polypeptide that inhibits the secretion of immunoreactive pituitary growth hormone. *Science,* 179:77–79.

11. Bryant, M. G., Bloom, S. R., Polak, J. M., Albuquerque, R. H., Modlin, I., and Pearse, A. G. E. (1976): Possible dual role for vasoactive intestinal peptide gastrointestinal hormone and neurotransmitter substance. *Lancet,* 1:991–993.

12. Buchan, A. M. J., Polak, J. M., Capella, C., Solcia, E., and Pearse, A. G. E. (1978): Electron immunocytochemical evidence for the K cell: Localization of gastric inhibitory polypeptide (GIP) in man. *Histochemistry,* 56:37–44.

13. Buchan, A. M. J., Polak, J. M., Solcia, E., Capella, C., Hudson, D., and Pearse, A. G. E. (1978): Electroimmunocytochemical evidence for the human intestinal I cell as the source of CCK. *Gut,* 19:403–407.

14. Buchan, A. M. J., Polak, J. M., Solcia, E., and Pearse, A. G. E. (1979): Localization of intestinal gastrin in a distinct endocrine cell type. *Nature,* 277:138–140.

15. Burnstock, G. (1972): Purinergic nerves. *Pharmacol. Rev.,* 24:509–581.

16. Burnstock, G., Campbell, G., and Rand, M. J. (1966): The inhibitory innervation of the taenia of the guinea pig caecum. *J. Physiol. (Lond.),* 182:504–526.

17. Capella, C., Solcia, E., Frigerio, B., and Buffa, R. (1976): Endocrine cells of the human intestine: An ultrastructural study. In: *Endocrine Gut and Pancreas,* edited by T. Fujita, pp. 43–59. Elsevier, Amsterdam.

18. Chayvialle, J. A. P., Descos, F., Bernard, C., Martin, A., Barbe, C., and Partensky, C. (1978): Somatostatin in mucosa of stomach and duodenum in gastroduodenal disease. *Gastroenterology,* 75:13–19.

19. Erspamer, V., and Melchiorri, P. (1973): Active polypeptides of the amphibian skin and their synthetic analogues. *Pure Appl. Chem.,* 35:463–494.

20. Feyrter, F. (1938): Uber diffuse endokrine epitheliale Organe. *Zentralbl. Inn. Med.,* 59:545.

21. Fujita, T., and Kobayashi, S. (1977): Structure and function of gut endocrine cells. *Int. Rev. Cytol. (Suppl).,* 6:187–227.

22. Guillemin, R. (1978): Peptides in the brain: The new endocrinology of the neuron. *Science,* 202:390–402.

23. Jessen, K. R., Polak, J. M., Van Noorden, S., Bryant, M. G., Bloom, S. R., and Burnstock, G. (1979): A new approach to the demonstration of the enteric plexus origin of peptide-containing nerves by immunocytochemistry and radioimmunoassay. *Gastroenterology,* 76:1161 (Abstr.).

24. Kosterlitz, H. W., and Hughes, J. (1975): Some thoughts on the significance of enkephalin, the endogenous ligand. *Life Sci.,* 17:91–96.

25. Leeman, S. E., and Hammerschlag, R. (1967): Stimulation of salivary secretion by a factor extracted from hypothalamic tissue. *Endocrinology,* 81:803–810.

26. Melchers, F. (1978): Lymphocyte hybridomas. *Curr. Top. Microbiol. Immunol.,* 81:R9–R23.

27. Modlin, I. M., Bloom, S. R., and Mitchell, S. J. (1977): Role of VIP in diarrhoea. *Gut,* 18:A418–A419.

28. Mroz, E. A., and Leeman, S. E. (1977): Substance P. *Vitam. Horm.,* 35:209–276.

29. Nakane, P. K. (1968): Simultaneous localization of multiple tissue antigens using the peroxidase-labelled antibody method: A study on pituitary glands and the rat. *J. Histochem. Cytochem.,* 16:557–560.

30. Pearse, A. G. E. (1969): The cytochemistry and ultrastructure of polypeptide hormone-producing cells of the APUD series, and the embryologic, physiologic and pathologic implications of the concept. *J. Histochem. Cytochem.,* 17:303–313.

31. Pearse, A. G. E., and Polak, J. M. (1975): Bifunctional reagents as vapour- and liquid-phase fixatives for immunohistochemistry. *Histochem. J.,* 7:179–186.

32. Polak, J. M., Bishop, A. E., and Bloom, S. R. (1978): The morphology of VIPergic nerves in Crohn's disease. *Scand. J. Gastroenterol.,* 13(S49):144.

33. Polak, J. M., Bishop, A. E., Bloom, S. R., Buchan, A. M., and Timson, C. M. (1978): The VIPergic innervation of the pancreas. *Scand. J. Gastroenterol.,* 13(S49):145.

34. Polak, J. M., and Bloom, S. R. (1978): Peptidergic nerves of the gastrointestinal tract. *Invest. Cell Pathol.,* 1:301–326.

35. Polak, J. M., and Bloom, S. R. (1978): Peptidergic innervation of the gastrointestinal tract. In: *Gastrointestinal Hormones and Pathology of the Digestive System,* edited by M. Grossman, V. Speranza, N. Basso, and E. Lezoche, pp. 27–49. Plenum Press, New York.

36. Polak, J. M., Bloom, S. R., Bishop, A. E., and McCrossan, M. V. (1978): D cell pathology in duodenal ulcers and achlorhydria. *Metabolism,* 27(S1):1239–1242.

37. Polak, J. M., and Buchan, A. M. J. (1979): Motilin immunocytochemical local section indicates possible molecular heterogeneity or the existence of a motilin family. *Gastroenterology,* 76:1065–1066.

38. Polak, J. M., Bloom, S. R., Coulling, I., and Pearse, A. G. E. (1971): Immunofluorescent localization of enteroglucagon cells in the gastrointestinal tract of the dog. *Gut,* 12:311–318.

39. Polak, J. M., Ghatel, M. A., Wharton, J., Bishop, A. E., Bloom, S. R., Solcia, E., Brown, M. R., and Pearse, A. G. E. (1978): Bombesin-like immunoreactivity in the gastrointestinal tract, lung and central nervous system. *Scand. J. Gastroentol.,* 13(S49):148.

40. Polak, J. M., Pearse, A. G. E., Grimelius, L., Bloom, S. R., and Arimura, A. (1975): Growth-hormone releasing inhibiting hormone (GH-RIH) in gastrointestinal and pancreatic D cells. *Lancet,* 1:1220–1222.

41. Polak, J. M., Pearse, A. G. E., and Heath, C. M. (1975): Complete identification of endocrine cells in the gastrointestinal tract using semithin-thin sections to identify motilin cells in human and animal intestine. *Gut,* 16:225–229.

42. Polak, J. M., Sullivan, S. M., Bloom, S. R., Buchan, A. M. J., Facer, P., Brown, M. R., and Pearse, A. G. E. (1977): Specific localization of neurotensin to the N cell in human intestine by radioimmunoassay and cytochemistry. *Nature,* 270:183–184.

43. Said, S. I. (1978): VIP overview. In: *Gut Hormones,* edited by S. R. Bloom, pp. 465–468. Churchill Livingstone, Edinburgh.

44. Said, E. E., and Mutt, V. (1969): Long-acting vasodilator peptide from lung tissue. *Nature,* 224:699–700.

45. Solcia, E., Polak, J. M., Pearse, A. G. E., Forssmann, W. G., Larsson, L. I., Sundler, F., Lechago, J., Grimelius, L., and Grossman, M. I. (1978): Lausanne 1977 classification of gastroenteropancreatic endocrine cells. In: *Gut Hormones,* edited by S. R. Bloom, pp. 40–48. Churchill Livingstone, Edinburgh.

46. Tramu, G., Pillez, A., and Leonardelli, J. (1978): An efficient method of antibody elution for the successive or simultaneous localization of two antigens by immunocytochemistry. *J. Histochem. Cytochem.,* 26:322–324.

47. Van Noorden, S., Polak, J. M., Bloom, S. R., and Bryant, M. G. (1979): Vasoactive intestinal polypeptide in the pituitary pars nervosa. *Neuropathol. Appl. Neurobiol.,* 5:149–153.

48. Verner, J. V., and Morrison, A. B. (1974): Endocrine pancreatic islet disease with diarrhoea. *Arch. Intern. Med.,* 133:492–500.

49. von Euler, U. S., and Gaddum, J. H. (1931): An unidentified depressor substance in certain tissue extracts. *J. Physiol. (Lond.),* 72:74–87.

50. Wharton, J., Polak, J. M., Bryant, B. G., Van Noorden, S., and Bloom, S. R. (1979): Vasoactive intestinal polypeptide (VIP)-like immunoreactivity in salivary glands. *Life Sci.,* 25:273–280.

Polypeptide Hormones, edited by
R. F. Beers, Jr. and E. G. Bassett.
Raven Press, New York © 1980.

35. Receptors Mediating the Actions of Gastrointestinal Peptides and Other Secretagogues on Pancreatic Acinar Cells

Robert T. Jensen and Jerry D. Gardner

Digestive Diseases Branch, National Institute Arthritis, Metabolism, and Digestive Diseases, National Institutes of Health, Bethesda, Maryland 20205

INTRODUCTION

In pancreatic acinar cells there appear to be two mechanisms by which secreta-gogues can increase enzyme secretion [(Fig. 1); see also ref. 22]. One mechanism involves binding of the secretagogue to receptors on the outer surface of the plasma membrane, release of intracellular calcium and, after a series of presently undefined steps, stimulation of enzyme secretion. The other mechanism involves binding of the secretagogue to receptors on the outer surface of plasma membrane, activation of adenylate cyclase on the inner surface of the plasma membrane, increased cellular cyclic AMP, activation of cyclic AMP-dependent protein kinase and, after a series of undefined steps, stimulation of enzyme secretion. The initial steps in these two pathways are functionally distinct. Secre-

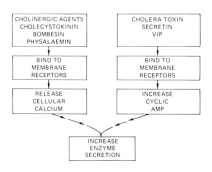

FIG. 1. Outline of the initial steps in the action of secretagogues on pancreatic acinar cells.

Editorial note: The spelling of cerulein and physalemin is in accordance with *Dorland's Medical Dictionary,* 25th ed. The investigators who isolated these substances designate them caerulein and physalaemin.

tagogues that cause release of cellular calcium do not increase cyclic AMP and do not alter the increase in cyclic AMP caused by other secretagogues. Similarly, secretagogues that increase cellular cyclic AMP do not alter calcium transport and do not alter the increase in calcium outflux caused by other secretagogues. Although these two biochemical pathways by which secretagogues increase pancreatic enzyme secretion are separate during their initial steps, they interact at some presently unknown, later step to cause "potentiation" of enzyme secretion. That is, the increase in enzyme secretion caused by a secretagogue that promotes release of cellular calcium in combination with a secretagogue that elevates cellular cyclic AMP is substantially greater than the sum of the increase caused by each secretagogue acting alone. In contrast, the increase in enzyme secretion caused by a maximally effective concentration of two secretagogues, each of which has the same mode of action, is the same as the increase caused by the more effective secretagogue alone.

SECRETAGOGUES THAT CAUSE
RELEASE OF INTRACELLULAR CALCIUM

As is illustrated in Table 1, the various secretagogues that increase enzyme secretion by causing release of cellular calcium can be subdivided on the basis of the particular class of receptors with which they interact. These different classes of receptors can be identified by using specific competitive antagonists (e.g., atropine to identify muscarinic cholinergic receptors) or by measuring binding of a radiolabeled ligand (e.g., ^{125}I-[Tyr^4]bombesin to identify bombesin receptors).

Cholecystokinin and Structurally Related Peptides

Cholecystokinin (CCK) is a peptide that was originally isolated and purified from hog upper small intestine and found to contain 33 amino acid residues (36–40). In the course of investigating the structure of CCK, Mutt and Jorpes (39) detected a peptide that differed from CCK in that although it was retained by a CM-cellulose column, it was eluted by 0.2 M but not by 0.02 M ammonium bicarbonate. This peptide, which has been termed "CCK variant," possesses 39 amino acids. The COOH-terminal 33-amino acid residues are identical to those of CCK_{33} and the NH$_2$-terminal hexapeptide sequence is Tyr-Ile-Gln-Gln-Ala-Arg (38). There are also two other naturally occurring peptides that are structurally similar to CCK. Cerulein is a decapeptide originally isolated from the skin of an Australian hylid frog, *Hyla caerulea* (2,20,21), and seven of the eight COOH-terminal amino acids in cerulein are identical to those in the COOH-terminal octapeptide of CCK (Fig. 2). CCK and gastrin are structurally similar in that they share an identical COOH-terminal pentapeptide amide (Fig. 2).

The intrinsic biological activity of CCK resides in the COOH-terminal portion

TABLE 1. *Receptors that mediate the action of those pancreatic secretagogues that act by increasing calcium outflux*

Class of receptors	Receptors interact with	Region of intrinsic biological activity[a]	Competitive antagonist	Used to examine binding
CCK	CCK Cerulein Gastrin	COOH-terminal tetrapeptide	Butyryl cyclic GMP	[³H]Cerulein ?
Bombesin	Bombesin Litorin Ranatensin Alytesin	COOH-terminal hexapeptide	None known	¹²⁵I-[Tyr⁴]Bombesin
Physalemin	Physalemin Substance P Eledoisin Kassinin	COOH-terminal pentapeptide	None known	¹²⁵I-Physalemin
Cholinergic	Muscarinic cholinergic agonists	—	Muscarinic cholinergic antagonists	[³H]QNB ?

[a] Referring to the smallest portion of the molecule that retains biological activity.

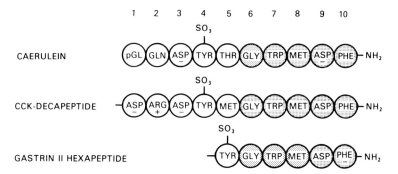

FIG. 2. Amino acid sequences of cerulein, the COOH-terminal decapeptide of cholecystokinin (CCK), and the COOH-terminal hexapeptide of gastrin II. *Shaded circles* indicate amino acids that are identical.

of the molecule and all of the COOH-terminal fragments and analogs of CCK studied to date are equal in efficacy to CCK but have different potencies (9,10, 27,37,45,53,54). The smallest fragment of CCK that possesses full biological activity is the COOH-terminal tetrapeptide. The COOH-terminal octapeptide and heptapeptide of CCK as well as cerulein are approximately 10 times more potent than native CCK, whereas COOH-terminal fragments of CCK possessing 10 or more amino acids (including CCK variant) have the same potencies as does CCK. Gastrin and the COOH-terminal hexapeptide of CCK are approximately 100 times less potent than CCK. Although removing the sulfate moiety from the tyrosine in gastrin does not alter its potency or efficacy, removing the sulfate moiety from the tyrosine in CCK causes a 500-fold reduction in its potency. The effects of other structural modifications of the COOH-terminal portion of CCK on biological activity are summarized elsewhere (9,10,45,47).

The findings that the COOH-terminal octapeptide and heptapeptide of CCK are more potent than native CCK raises the possibility that CCK and CCK-variant are "pro-hormones" (analogous to pro-insulin and proparathyroid hormone). That is, a COOH-terminal fragment, such as the octapeptide, may be the predominant biologically active form of the peptide that is present in the circulation and that exerts the biological effects conventionally attributed to CCK. Alternatively, CCK or its variant may be released into the circulation and degraded (by enzymes in plasma or certain tissues) to a smaller, more biologically active form. Although answers to these questions will have to await identification and characterization of the form(s) of CCK in plasma, CCK appears to be unique among the various peptide hormones in that a fragment is at least 10 times more potent than the molecule conventionally referred to as the hormone.

In general, the structural requirements for occupation of a peptide hormone receptor are quite stringent in that only other peptides will bind to the hormone receptor and the peptides that do bind are usually fragments of the hormone or analogs with a similar chemical structure. One striking exception to this general pattern occurs with the opiate receptors (31,55). These receptors can interact not only with peptides (the enkephalins) but also with morphine and structurally related alkaloid compounds. A second apparent exception to the general principle that only peptides will bind to peptide hormone receptors is the finding that butyryl derivatives of cyclic GMP will competitively antagonize the action of CCK and structurally related peptides on pancreatic acinar cells (47). These derivatives of cyclic GMP are specific for the action of peptides that interact with the CCK receptor since butyryl derivatives of cyclic GMP do not alter the actions of other pancreatic secretagogues such as bombesin, physalemin, cholinergic agents, secretin, vasoactive intestinal peptide (VIP), or A23187 (47). In competitively inhibiting the action of CCK $N^2,O^{2'}$-dibutyryl cyclic GMP is more potent than the $O^{2'}$-monobutyryl derivative which, in turn, is more potent than N^2-monobutyryl cyclic GMP (47). Native cyclic GMP at concentrations as high as 10 mM does not alter the action of CCK or structurally related peptides (47).

Studies of binding of [³H]cerulein to intact pancreatic acinar cells and to purified plasma membranes from acinar cells have identified a class of binding sites than interact with CCK, cerulein, and gastrin as well as fragments and analogs of these peptides but not with other pancreatic secretagogues (15–19, 50,51). The relative potencies with which various peptides inhibit binding of [³H]cerulein are similar to those with which they produce functional changes in intact cells or isolated plasma membranes. For a given peptide, however, its potency for inhibiting binding of [³H]cerulein is 10 to 100 times less than its potency for increasing enzyme secretion. This wide discrepancy may be attributable to the studies having been performed under different incubation conditions and with different tissue preparations. This discrepancy may also reflect the presence of spare receptors or multiple functional states of the receptor as suggested by the authors. These discrepancies as well as others (see ref. 23 for discussion) may also indicate that the sites to which [³H]cerulein binds are not the sites with which the peptide interacts to cause calcium release and amylase secretion from pancreatic acinar cells. Obviously, additional studies are needed to establish fully the significance of [³H]cerulein binding to pancreatic acinar cells.

Bombesin and Structurally Related Peptides

A second class of membrane receptors that cause release of cellular calcium are those that interact with bombesin, alytesin, ranatensin, and litorin (Table 1). These peptides were initially isolated from amphibian skin and are named after the frog from which they were derived (20,21). For example, bombesin was isolated from the skin of *Bombina bombina*. These peptides, however, are not unique to amphibians because bombesin-like immunoreactivity has been found in mammalian tissues (20,21).

Like members of the CCK family of peptides, the terminal carboxyl moiety of bombesin, alytesin, ranatensin, and litorin is amidated (Fig. 3). Furthermore, in the COOH-terminal octapeptide portion of each of these amphibian peptides there are seven identical amino acids, and both bombesin and alytesin contain a penultimate leucine residue, whereas both ranatensin and litorin contain a penultimate phenylalanine residue (Fig. 3).

The intrinsic biological activity of bombesin and structurally related peptides is a property of the COOH-terminal portion of the molecule, and the COOH-terminal nonapeptide of bombesin has the same potency and efficacy as does the native tetradecapeptide (18,48). Shorter COOH-terminal fragments of bombesin still possess full intrinsic biological activity, but their potencies are less than that of native bombesin. The region of the bombesin molecule that possesses intrinsic biological activity also determines the affinity of the peptide for its receptor. Of the fragments and analogs of bombesin that have been tested, none has been found to occupy the receptor and not cause a full biological response (18,34,35,48). Thus, there is no known competitive antagonist of the action of bombesin and related peptides.

Receptors for bombesin and related peptides can be identified by measuring binding of ^{125}I-[Tyr^4]bombesin (Table 1). Binding of ^{125}I-labeled [Tyr^4]bombesin is saturable, temperature-dependent, and reversible, and reflects interaction of the labeled peptide with a single class of binding sites on the plasma membrane of pancreatic acinar cells (34). Each acinar cell possess approximately 5,000 binding sites, and binding of the tracer to these sites can be inhibited by bombesin, alytesin, ranatensin, and litorin but not by other pancreatic secretagogues such as CCK, physalemin, secretin, VIP, or cholinergic agents (34). With bombesin, alytesin, ranatensin, and litorin there is a close correlation between the relative potencies with which the peptides inhibit binding of ^{125}I-[Tyr^4]bombesin and

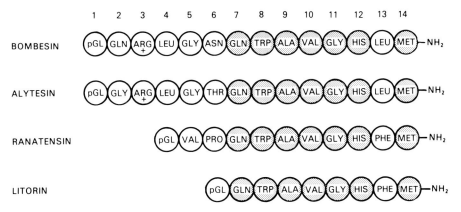

FIG. 3. Amino acid sequences of bombesin, alytesin, ranatensin, and litorin. *Shaded circles* indicate amino acids that are identical.

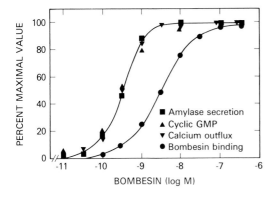

FIG. 4. Dose-response curves for bombesin binding and the bombesin-induced increases in calcium outflux, cyclic GMP, and amylase secretion in dispersed pancreatic acini. (From ref. 34.)

their relative potencies for causing changes in cell function (34). For a given peptide, however, a 10-fold higher concentration is required for half-maximal inhibition of binding than for half-maximal stimulation of enzyme secretion, calcium outflux, or cellular accumulation of cyclic GMP (Fig. 4). Thus, in pancreatic acinar cells occupation of approximately 25% of the receptors by bombesin, alytesin, ranatesin, litorin or a fragment or structural analog is sufficient to cause maximal changes in calcium outflux, cyclic GMP, and amylase secretion (34,35).

Physalemin and Structurally Related Peptides

A third class of membrane receptors that cause release of cellular calcium are those that interact with physalemin, substance P, eledoisin, and kassinin (Table 1). Physalemin and kassinin were originally isolated from frog skin, whereas eledoisin was originally isolated from the posterior salivary gland of a mollusc (1,20,21). Substance P was originally isolated from mammalian brain and gastrointestinal mucosa (57), and has been found subsequently in spinal cord (13,56), dorsal ganglia (13,56) and plasma (44,58) as well as enterochromaffin cells in intestinal mucosa (32,43,46).

Physalemin, substance P, eledoisin, and kassinin each resemble bombesin and its naturally occurring analogs in that the COOH-terminal residue is methionine amide (Fig. 5). Physalemin, substance P, eledoisin, and kassinin also have a similar COOH-terminal pentapeptide sequence in which four of five amino acids are in the same position in each peptide (Fig. 5).

Like the CCK-related peptides and the bombesin-related peptides, the intrinsic biological activity of physalemin and structurally related peptides is a property of the COOH-terminal region of the molecule (5–7). The smallest COOH-terminal fragment of physalemin that has been examined and found to retain biological activity is the pentapeptide. Eledoisin is approximately 50% more effective than physalemin or substance P in stimulating pancreatic enzyme secretion (33) and

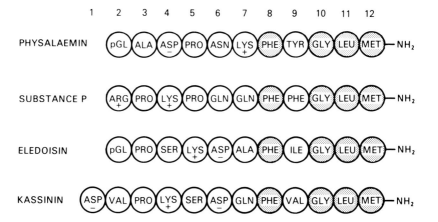

FIG. 5. Amino acid sequences of physalemin, substance P, eledoisin, and kassinin. *Shaded circles* indicate amino acids that are identical.

physalemin and eledoisin have also been found to have different efficacies for producing hypotension *in vivo* and contraction of large intestine, small intestine, and rat uterus *in vitro* (5–7). These findings raise the possibility that a peptide exists or can be synthesized that will be able to occupy the receptor but that will be devoid of intrinsic biological activity. These findings also suggest that with physalemin and related peptides, the portion of the molecule that possesses intrinsic biological activity is not congruent with the region of the molecule that influences the affinity of the peptide for its receptor.

Receptors for physalemin and related peptides can be identified by measuring binding of ^{125}I-physalemin (Table 1). Binding of labeled physalemin to pancreatic acinar cells is saturable, temperature-dependent, and reversible, and reflects interaction of the labeled peptide with a single class of binding sites on the plasma membrane of pancreatic acinar cells (33). Each acinar cell possesses approximately 500 binding sites, and binding of the tracer to these sites can be inhibited by physalemin, substance P, eledoisin, and kassinin but not by other pancreatic secretagogues such as bombesin, CCK, secretin, VIP, or cholinergic agents (33). With physalemin, substance P, eledoisin, and kassinin there is a close correlation between their relative potencies for inhibiting of binding of ^{125}I-physalemin and those for causing changes in cell function (33). For a given peptide, however, a threefold higher concentration is required for half-maximal inhibition of binding than for half-maximal stimulation of enzyme secretion or calcium outflux (33). Thus, in pancreatic acinar cells occupation of approximately 45% of the receptors by physalemin, substance P, eledoisin, kassinin, or a fragment or structural analog is sufficient to cause maximal changes in cell function. Furthermore, physalemin, a peptide isolated from amphibian skin, can be radiolabeled and used to examine directly the function of receptors which in mammals probably mediates the action of substance P.

Muscarinic Cholinergic Agents

In addition to receptors for gastrointestinal peptides, pancreatic acinar cells also possess receptors that interact with muscarinic cholinergic agents (Table 1). This class of receptors can be identified by the abilities of atropine and other muscarinic antagonists to competitively inhibit the actions of acetylcholine and other cholinergic agonists (27,47). Radiolabeled quinuclidinyl benzilate, [^{3}H]QNB, has been used to examine the interaction of various agents with muscarinic cholinergic receptors in several different tissues; however, no such studies using the pancreas have been reported in detail.

SECRETAGOGUES THAT INCREASE CELLULAR CYCLIC AMP

As illustrated in Table 2, the various secretagogues that increase cyclic AMP in pancreatic acinar cells can be subdivided on the basis of the particular class of receptors with which they interact. These different classes of receptors can be identified by using specific competitive antagonists and by measuring binding of a radiolabeled ligand.

Secretin and VIP

Secretin is a heptacosapeptide (41) originally isolated from the upper small intestine (3) and is the substance for which the term "hormone" was coined (4). VIP is an octacosapeptide (also isolated from upper small intestine) that was initially named for its ability to produce a decrease in blood pressure after intravenous injection in dogs (8,42,52). VIP and secretin have a similar spectrum of biological activities that reflect the similarities in their molecular structure (Fig. 6). Like the peptides related to CCK, bombesin, and physalemin, both secretin and VIP possess a COOH-terminal amide (Fig. 6). VIP and secretin share nine amino acid identities. Eight of these identities are in the NH$_2$-terminal region; one is in the COOH-terminal region (Fig. 6). VIP and secretin also share 10 amino acids that, although not identical, confer a similar chemical atmosphere on the molecule. Of these 10 amino acid similarities, three are in the NH$_2$-terminal region and seven are in the COOH-terminal region (Fig. 6).

In contrast to those peptides that increase calcium release from acinar cells and have their intrinsic biological activity in the COOH-terminal portion of the molecule, in VIP and secretin the intrinsic biological activity resides in the NH$_2$-terminal portion of the molecule (14,49). For example, secretin$_{1-14}$ has an efficacy equal to that of native secretin, whereas secretin$_{5-27}$ and secretin$_{14-27}$ have efficacies less than 2% of that of secretin (14,24–26,29,49). Although COOH-terminal partial sequences of VIP and secretin have little or no intrinsic biological activity, these peptides are able to interact with the receptors for VIP and secretin, and therefore, function as competitive antagonists (14,24–26,29,49). Both the NH$_2$-terminal and the COOH-terminal regions of VIP and

TABLE 2. *Receptors that mediate the action of those pancreatic secretagogues that act by increasing cyclic AMP*

Class of receptors	Receptors interact with	Region of intrinsic biological activity	Competitive antagonist	Used to examine binding
VIP-preferring	VIP, secretin	NH_2-terminal tetrapeptide[a]	Secretin$_{5-27}$ Secretin$_{14-27}$ VIP$_{14-28}$	^{125}I-VIP
Secretin-preferring	Secretin, VIP	NH_2-terminal tetrapeptide[a]	Secretin$_{5-27}$ Secretin$_{14-27}$ VIP$_{14-28}$	^{125}I-VIP ^{125}I-Secretin
Cholera toxin	Cholera toxin	A$_1$ Subunit	Choleragenoid	^{125}I-Cholera toxin

[a] Although secretin$_{1-14}$ possesses biological activity, secretin$_{5-27}$ has only 2% of the intrinsic biological activity of secretin$_{1-27}$. This suggests that the smallest portion of the molecule that possesses biological activity is probably less than secretin$_{1-14}$ (e.g., the NH_2-terminal tetrapeptide).

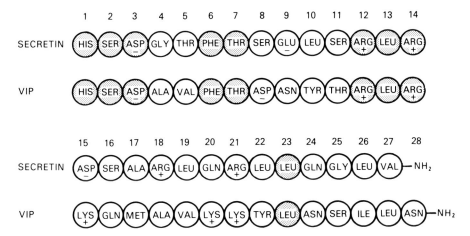

FIG. 6. Amino acid sequences of secretin and vasoactive intestinal peptide (VIP). *Shaded circles* indicate amino acids that are identical.

secretin influence the affinity of the peptide for its receptors (14,24–26,29,49). For example, the affinities of secretin$_{1-14}$ and secretin$_{14-27}$ for the secretin receptors are approximately 1,000-fold less than the affinity of secretin for these same receptors. Finally, one feature of VIP and secretin that distinguishes them from the other peptides that stimulate pancreatic enzyme secretion is that, to date, no fragment of either peptide has been found to be as potent as the native molecule.

The receptors that interact with VIP and secretin can be distinguished by measuring binding of ^{125}I-VIP or ^{125}I-secretin or by using those COOH-terminal fragments of secretin or VIP which function as competitive antagonists (Table 2). Binding of ^{125}I-VIP to pancreatic acinar cells is inhibited by VIP and by secretin but not by other secretagogues such as CCK, bombesin, physalemin, or cholinergic agents. COOH-terminal fragments of secretin or VIP competitively antagonize the effects of VIP and secretin on pancreatic acinar cells but do not alter the actions of other secretagogues (14,24–26,29,49).

Pancreatic acinar cells possess two functionally distinct classes of receptors, each of which interacts with VIP and secretin to cause activation of adenylate cyclase and increased cellular cyclic AMP. The distinguishing features of these two classes of receptors are given in Table 3.

Studies of binding of ^{125}I-VIP to pancreatic acinar cells have shown that one class of receptors has a high affinity for VIP (K_d 0.7 nM) and a low affinity for secretin (K_d 8 μM). Each acinar cell possesses 9,000 of these VIP-preferring receptors (14). The affinity of secretin$_{5-27}$ for these receptors (K_d 6 μM) is approximately the same as that of native secretin. In secretin$_{5-27}$, replacing the aspartic acid residue in position 15 by its carboxamide derivative, [Asn^{15}]secretin$_{5-27}$, or by lysine, [Lys^{15}]secretin, causes an eightfold increase in the apparent affinity

TABLE 3. *Characteristics of VIP-preferring receptors and secretin-preferring receptors on pancreatic acinar cells*

	VIP-Preferring receptors	Secretin-preferring receptors
Number of sites per acinar cell	9,000	135,000
	K_d [a]	
VIP	0.7 nM	82 nM
Secretin	8 μM	0.2 nM
Secretin$_{5-27}$	6 μM	0.2 μM
[Asn^{15}]Secretin$_{5-27}$	0.8 μM	0.2 μM
[Lys^{15}]Secretin$_{5-27}$	0.8 μM	1.2 μM
Maximal increase in cyclic AMP	10-fold	60- to 90-fold
Response	Increase amylase secretion	Not known

[a] K_d is the concentration of the peptide required to occupy 50% of the receptors.

of the peptide for the VIP-preferring receptors (29). Thus, the absence of an acidic residue in position 15 of secretin$_{5-27}$ is sufficient to increase the apparent affinity of the peptide for the VIP-preferring receptors and the presence of a basic lysyl residue does not cause a further increase in the apparent affinity of the peptide. Since VIP has lysine in position 15, one might anticipate that in secretin$_{5-27}$ replacing the aspartic acid in position 15 by lysine would make the peptide more VIP-like. This is, in fact, what occurs; however, the increased affinity of the substituted peptide appears to result from the removal of the negatively charged aspartic acid rather than the addition of the positively charged lysine (29).

Occupation of the VIP-preferring receptors by VIP causes a 10-fold increase in cellular cyclic AMP (Table 3) and a corresponding increase in enzyme secretion (Fig. 7). Although the increase in enzyme secretion caused by secretin is also mediated by the VIP-preferring receptors (29), occupation of these receptors by secretin does not cause a detectable increase in cellular cyclic AMP (26,29,49). This failure to detect an effect of secretin on cyclic AMP occurs because the increase in cyclic AMP (approximately 90-fold increase) caused by secretin acting through the secretin-preferring receptors obscures the increase in cyclic AMP caused by secretin acting through the VIP-preferring receptors (29).

As occurs with bombesin-related peptides (Fig. 4), the dose-response curve for VIP-stimulated enzyme secretion is to the left of the dose-response curve that describes occupation of the VIP-preferring receptors by VIP (Fig. 7, *left panel*). However, in contrast to results obtained with bombesin-related peptides (Fig. 4), with VIP the dose-response curve for the increase in the mediator (cyclic AMP) is not significantly different from the dose-response curve for occupation of VIP-preferring receptors (Fig. 7, *left panel*). Thus, with VIP and with bombesin, maximal stimulation of enzyme secretion occurs when only a fraction of the receptors are occupied by the secretagogue. With bombesin, this "spareness" is at the receptor level because the dose-response curves for the changes that are thought to mediate the action of bombesin on enzyme secretion are the same as those for bombesin-stimulated enzyme secretion (Fig. 4). With VIP, however, this "spareness" is at the level of cyclic AMP because submaximal changes in cyclic AMP are sufficient to cause maximal changes in enzyme secretion (Fig. 7, *left panel*). Results similar to those illustrated in that figure have also been obtained with cholera toxin (28). Additional evidence that in response to VIP interacting with the VIP-preferring receptors, acinar cells can produce more cyclic AMP than is necessary for maximal stimulation of enzyme secretion comes from studies using a competitive antagonist of the action of VIP. As illustrated in Figure 7, *right panel,* the dose-response curve for the inhibition of VIP-stimulated enzyme secretion by [Asn^{15}]secretin$_{5-27}$ is to the right of that for inhibition of the VIP-induced increase in cyclic AMP and that for inhibition of VIP binding. Thus, the antagonist does not alter VIP-stimulated enzyme secretion until VIP binding and VIP-stimulated cyclic AMP are reduced by more than 30% (Fig. 7, *right panel*).

Studies of binding of ^{125}I-VIP have also shown that pancreatic acinar cells possess a class of receptors that has a high affinity for secretin (K_d 0.2 nM) and a low affinity for VIP (K_d 82 nM). Each acinar cell possesses 135,000 of these secretin-preferring receptors (14). In contrast with the VIP-preferring receptors, for which secretin and for secretin$_{5-27}$ have the same affinities, the affinity of secretin for the secretin-preferring receptors is 1,000 times greater

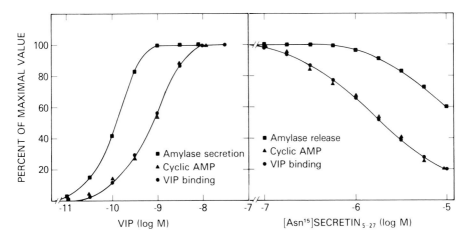

FIG. 7. Left: Dose-response curve for VIP binding to VIP-preferring receptors and the VIP-induced increases in cyclic AMP and amylase secretion in dispersed pancreatic acini. **Right:** Effect of [Asn^{15}]secretin$_{5-27}$ on VIP binding to VIP-preferring receptors and on the VIP-induced increases in cyclic AMP and amylase secretion in dispersed pancreatic acini. (From ref. 29.)

than the affinity of secretin$_{5-27}$ for these same receptors (Table 3). Moreover, in secretin$_{5-27}$ replacing the aspartic acid residue in position 15 by asparagine, [Asn^{15}]secretin$_{5-27}$, does not alter the affinity of the peptide for the secretin-preferring receptors, whereas replacement by lysine, [Lys^{15}]secretin$_{5-27}$, causes a sixfold reduction in the apparent affinity of the peptide for these receptors (29). Thus, the *absence* of a basic residue in position 15 of secretin$_{5-27}$ is sufficient to increase the affinity of the peptide for the secretin-preferring receptors and the presence of an acidic aspartyl residue does not cause a further increase in the apparent affinity of the peptide. Furthermore, although the VIP-preferring receptors differ from the secretin-preferring receptors in their abilities to distinguish between secretin$_{5-27}$ and its derivatives, each class of receptors displays the somewhat surprising characteristic that the affinities for secretin$_{5-27}$ and its analogs are influenced primarily by the *absence* of a particular charge in position 15 but not by the presence of the opposite charge (29). Occupation of the secretin-preferring receptors by VIP or secretin causes a 60- to 90-fold increase in cellular cyclic AMP (Table 3); however, what cellular function, if any, is altered as a consequence of this increase in cyclic AMP is not known (29). The lack of an accompanying increase in enzyme secretion may reflect compartmentalization of cellular cyclic AMP such that the increase in the cyclic nucleotide is not in the appropriate compartment to increase enzyme secretion. Another possibility is that each pancreatic acinar cell possesses one but not both classes of receptors and that in the cells possessing secretin-preferring receptors, enzyme secretion is not increased by cyclic AMP.

Cholera Toxin

Cholera toxin is a protein with a molecular weight of about 83,000 and is composed of three subunits (see review, ref. 30). The B subunit, also referred to as "choleragenoid" or "aggregated B subunit," has a molecular weight of approximately 54,000 and is thought to be composed of 4 to 6 identical monomers. The A$_1$ subunit has an apparent molecular weight of 23,000, whereas the A$_2$ subunit has a molecular weight of about 6,000. A simplified view of the functions of the different portions of the cholera toxin molecule is that the B subunit, which has no intrinsic biological activity, binds to monosialogangliosides on the outer surface of the plasma membrane. The A$_2$ subunit in some unknown way facilitates the passage of the A$_1$ subunit across the membrane, where the A$_1$ subunit causes activation of adenylate cyclase.

In pancreatic acinar cells, receptors for cholera toxin can be identified by measuring binding of ^{125}I-cholera toxin (Table 2) and there is a good correlation between the ability of native toxin to inhibit binding of ^{125}I-cholera toxin and the ability of the toxin to activate adenylate cyclase and increase cellular cyclic AMP (28). Other pancreatic secretagogues do not inhibit binding of ^{125}I-cholera toxin (28). The relationship between binding of cholera toxin and its abilities to increase cyclic AMP and enzyme secretion is similar to that for VIP acting through the VIP-preferring receptors (29). That is, with cholera toxin, submaximal changes in cellular cyclic AMP are sufficient to cause maximal stimulation of enzyme secretion (28).

Choleragenoid, which has the ability to interact with the cholera toxin binding sites but which has no intrinsic biological activity, functions as a competitive antagonist of the action of cholera toxin (Table 2).

Recent studies of the mechanism of action of cholera toxin indicate that, in contrast with other agonists that activate adenylate cyclase, binding of the toxin molecule per se is not sufficient to elicit activation of adenylate cyclase (30). Since a portion of the toxin molecule must traverse the plasma membrane to activate adenylate cyclase, it is not appropriate to think of the membrane structures to which the toxin initially binds in the same way that one thinks of a receptor for hormones or neurotransmitters. Another important difference between cholera toxin and other agonists that activate adenylate cyclase is that cholera toxin (and the A_1 subunit in particular) appears to possess enzymic activity and this activity activates adenylate cyclase by catalyzing the ADP ribosylation of a regulatory component of the cyclase system (30). Finally, activation of adenylate cyclase by cholera toxin appears to involve a toxin-induced inhibition of the breakdown of GTP and this gives rise to a "persistently activated state" of adenylate cyclase (11,12). Hormones and neurotransmitters, on the other hand, appear to activate adenylate cyclase by enhancing the activation of adenylate cyclase caused by GTP (11,12). These actions can account for the ability of cholera toxin to potentiate the increase in cellular cyclic AMP or activation of adenylate cyclase caused by hormones or neurotransmitters in a number of different tissues (30) including pancreatic acinar cells (28).

ACKNOWLEDGMENT

We thank Mary Ernst for preparing this manuscript for publication.

REFERENCES

1. Anastasi, A., Erspamer, V., and Cei, J. M. (1964): Isolation and amino acid sequence of physalaemin, the main active polypeptide of the skin of *Physalaemus fuscumaculatus. Arch. Biochem. Biophys.,* 108:341–348.
2. Anastasi, A., Erspamer, V., and Endean, R. (1968): Isolation and amino acid sequence of caerulein, the active decapeptide of the skin of *Hyla caerulea. Arch. Bhiochem. Biophys.,* 125:57–68.
3. Bayliss, W. M., and Starling, E. H. (1902): The mechanism of pancreatic secretion. *J. Physiol. (Lond.),* 28:325–353.
4. Bayliss, W. M., and Starling, E. H. (1904): The chemical regulation of the secretory process. *Proc. R. Society,* 73:310–322.
5. Bernardi, L., Bosisio, G., Chillemi, F., DeCaro, G., De Castiglione, R., Erspamer, V., Glaesser, A., and Goffredo, O. (1964): Synthetic peptides related to eledoisin. *Experientia,* 20:306–309.
6. Bernardi, L., Bosisio, G., Chillemi, F., DeCaro, G., DeCastiglione, R., Erspamer, V., Glaesser, A., and Goffredo, O. (1965): Synthetic peptides related to eledoisin. *Experientia,* 21:695–696.

7. Bernardi, L., Bosisio, G., Chillemi, F., DeCaro, G., DeCastiglione, R., Erspamer, V., and Goffredo, O. (1966): Synthetic peptides related to eledoisin. *Experientia,* 22:29–32.
8. Bodanszky, M., Klausner, Y. S., and Said, S. I. (1973): Biological activities of synthetic peptides corresponding to fragments of and to the entire sequence of the vasoactive intestinal peptide. *Proc. Natl. Acad. Sci. USA,* 70:382–384.
9. Bodanszky, M., Martinez, J., Priestley, G. P., Gardner, J. D., and Mutt, V. (1978): Cholecystokinin (pancreozymin). IV[I] Synthesis and properties of a biologically active analogue of the C-terminal 7-peptide with ε-hydroxynorleucine sulfate replacing tyrosine sulfate. *J. Med. Chem.,* 21:1030–1035.
10. Bodanszky, M., Natarajan, S., Hahne, W., and Gardner, J. D. (1977): Cholecystokinin-pancreozymin. III. Synthesis and properties of an analog of the C-terminal heptapeptide with serine-sulfate replacing tyrosine-sulfate. *J. Med. Chem.,* 20:1047–1050.
11. Cassel, D., Levkovitz, H., and Selinger, Z. (1977): The regulatory GTPase of turkey erythrocyte adenylate cyclase. *J. Cyclic Nucleotide Res.,* 3:393–406.
12. Cassel, D., and Selinger, Z. (1977): Mechanism of adenylate cyclase activation by cholera toxin: Inhibition of GTP hydrolysis at the regulatory site. *Proc. Natl. Acad. Sci. USA,* 74:3307–3311.
13. Chan-Palay, V., and Palay, S. L. (1977): Immunocytochemical identification of substance P cells and their process in rat sensory ganglia and their terminals in the spinal cord: Light microscopic studies. *Proc. Natl. Acad. Sci. USA,* 74:3597–3601.
14. Christophe, J. P., Conlon, T. P., and Gardner, J. D. (1976): Interaction of porcine vasoactive intestinal peptide with dispersed pancreatic acinar cells from the guinea pig. Binding of radioiodinated peptide. *J. Biol. Chem.,* 251:4629–4634.
15. Christophe, J., DeNeef, P., Deschodt-Lanckman, M., and Robberecht, P. (1978): The interaction of caerulein with the rat pancreas. II. Specific binding of [³H]caerulein on dispersed acinar cells. *Eur. J. Biochem.,* 91:31–38.
16. Deschodt-Lanckman, M., Robberecht, P., Camus, J. C., and Christophe, J. (1977): Wheat germ agglutinin inhibits basal- and stimulated-adenylate cyclase activity as well as the binding of [³H]caerulein to rat pancreatic plasma membranes. *J. Cyclic Nucleotide Res.,* 3:177–187.
17. Deschodt-Lanckman, M., Robberecht, P., Camus, J., and Christophe, J. (1978): The interaction of caerulein with the rat pancreas. I. Specific binding of [³H]caerulein on plasma membranes and evidence for negative cooperativity. *Eur. J. Biochem.,* 91:21–29.
18. Deschodt-Lanckman, M., Robberecht, P., DeNeef, P., Lammens, M., and Christophe, J. (1976): *In vitro* action of bombesin and bombesin-like peptides on amylase secretion, calcium efflux and adenylate cyclase activity in the rat pancreas. *J. Clin. Invest.,* 58:891–898.
19. Deschodt-Lanckman, M., Svoboda, M., Camus, J., and Robberecht, P. (1977): Regulation of the dissociation of [³H]caerulein from its pancreatic receptors: Evidence for negative cooperativity. In: *Hormonal Receptors in Digestive Tract Physiology,* edited by S. Bonfils, P. Fromageot, and G. Rosselin, pp. 325–326. North-Holland, Amsterdam.
20. Erspamer, V., and Melchiorri, P. (1973): Active polypeptides of the amphibian skin and their synthetic analogs. *Pure Appl. Chem.,* 35:463–494.
21. Erspamer, V., and Melchiorri, P. (1975): Actions of bombesin on secretions and motility of the gastrointestinal tract. In: *Gastrointestinal Hormones,* edited by J. C. Thompson, pp. 575–589. University of Texas Press, Austin.
22. Gardner, J. D. (1979): Regulation of pancreatic exocrine function *in vitro.* Initial steps in the action of secretagogues. *Annu. Rev. Physiol.,* 41:55–66.
23. Gardner J. D. (1979): Receptors for gastrointestinal hormones. *Gastroenterology,* 76:202–214.
24. Gardner, J. D., Conlon, T. P., and Adams, T. D. (1976): Cyclic AMP in pancreatic acinar cells: Effects of gastrointestinal hormones. *Gastroenterology,* 70:29–35.
25. Gardner, J. D., Conlon, T. P., Beyerman, H. C., and Van Zon, A. (1977): Interaction of synthetic 10-tyrosyl analogs of secretin with hormone receptors on pancreatic acinar cells. *Gastroenterology,* 73:52–56.
26. Gardner, J. D., Conlon, T. P., Fink, M. L., and Bodanszky, M. (1976): Interactions of peptides related to secretin with hormone receptors on pancreatic acinar cells. *Gastroenterology,* 71:965–970.
27. Gardner, J. D., Conlon, T. P., Klaeveman, H. L., Adams, T. D., and Ondetti, M. A. (1975): Action of cholecystokinin and cholinergic agents on calcium transport in isolated pancreatic acinar cells. *J. Clin. Invest.,* 56:366–375.
28. Gardner, J. D., and Rottman, A. J. (1979): Action of cholera toxin on dispersed acini from guinea pig pancreas. *Biochem. Biophys. Acta,* 585:250–265.

29. Gardner, J. D., Rottman, A. J., Natarajan, S., and Bodanszky, M. (1979): Interaction of secretin$_{5-27}$ and its analogues with hormone receptors on pancreatic acini. *Biochim. Biophys. Acta,* 583:491–503.
30. Gill, D. M. (1977): Mechanism of action of cholera toxin. In: *Advances in Cyclic Nucleotide Research, Vol. 8,* edited by P. Greengard and G. A. Robison, pp. 85–118. Raven Press, New York.
31. Goldstein, A. (1976): Opioid peptides (endorphins) in pituitary and brain. *Science,* 193:1081–1086.
32. Heitz, P., Polak, J. M., Timson, C. M., and Pearse, A. G. E. (1976): Enterochromatiffin cells as the endocrine source of gastrointestinal substance P. *Histochemistry,* 49:343–347.
33. Jensen, R. T., and Gardner, J. D. (1980): Interaction of physalaemin, substance P and eledoisin with specific membrane receptors on pancreatic acinar cells. *Proc. Natl. Acad. Sci. USA,* 76:5679–5683.
34. Jensen, R. T., Moody, T., Pert, C., Rivier, J. E., and Gardner, J. D. (1978): Interaction of bombesin and litorin with specific membrane receptors on pancreatic acinar cells. *Proc. Natl. Acad. Sci. USA,* 75:6139–6143.
35. Jensen, R. T., Rivier, J. E., and Gardner, J. D. (1979): Structural requirements for interaction of various peptides with bombesin receptors on pancreatic acinar cells. *Gastroenterology,* 76:1160.
36. Jorpes, E., and Mutt, V. (1966): Cholecystokinin and pancreozymin, one single hormone? *Acta Physiol. Scand.,* 66:196–202.
37. Jorpes, J. E., and Mutt, V. (1973): Secretin and cholecystokinin (CCK). In: *Secretin, Cholecystokinin, Pancreozymin and Gastrin,* edited by J. E. Jorpes and V. Mutt, pp. 1–177. Springer-Verlag, New York.
38. Mutt, V. (1976): Further investigations on intestinal hormonal polypeptides. *Clin. Endocrinol.,* 5(Suppl.):175s–183s.
39. Mutt, V., and Jorpes, J. E. (1968): Structure of porcine cholecystokinin-pancreozymin 1. Cleavage with thrombin and trypsin. *Eur. J. Biochem.,* 6:156–162.
40. Mutt, V., and Jorpes, E. (1971): Hormonal polypeptides of the upper intestine. *Biochem. J.,* 125:57–58.
41. Mutt, V., Jorpes, J. E., and Magnusson, S. (1970): Structure of porcine secretin. The amino acid sequence. *Eur. J. Biochem.,* 15:513–519.
42. Mutt, V., and Said, S. I. (1974): Studies of the porcine vasoactive intestinal octacosapeptide. *Eur. J. Biochem.,* 42:581–589.
43. Nilsson, G., Larsson, L. I., Hakanson, R., Brodin, E., Pernow, B., and Sundler, F. (1975): Localization of substance P-like immunoreactivity in mouse gut. *Histochemistry,* 43:97–99.
44. Nilsson, G., Pernow, B., Fischer, G. H., and Folkers, K. A. (1975): Presence of substance P-like immunoreactivity in plasma from man and dog. *Acta Physiol. Scand.,* 94:542–544.
45. Ondetti, M., Rubin, B., Engel, S. L., Plusec, J., and Sheehan, J. T. (1970): Cholecystokinin-Pancreozymin: Recent developments. *Am. J. Dig. Dis.,* 15:149–156.
46. Pearse, A. G. E., and Polak, J. M. (1975): Immunocytochemical localization of substance P in mammalian intestine. *Histochemistry,* 41:373–375.
47. Peikin, S. R., Costenbader, C. L., and Gardner, J. D. (1979): Actions of derivatives of cyclic nucleotides on dispersed acini from guinea pig pancreas: Discovery of a competitive antagonist of the action of cholecystokinin. *J. Biol. Chem.,* 254:5321–5327.
48. Rivier, J., and Brown, M. (1978): Bombesin, bombesin analogues, and related peptides: Effects on thermoregulation. *Biochemistry,* 17:1766–1771.
49. Robberecht, P., Conlon, T. P., and Gardner, J. D. (1976): Interaction of porcine vasoactive intestinal peptide with dispersed acinar cells from the guinea pig: structural requirements for effects of VIP and secretin on cellular cyclic AMP. *J. Biol. Chem.,* 251:4635–4639.
50. Robberecht, P., Deschodt-Lanckman, M., Camus, J., and Christophe, J. (1977): Specific binding and mode of action of caerulein on plasma membranes of rat pancreas. In: *Hormonal Receptors in Digestive Tract Physiology,* edited by S. Bonfils, P. Fromageot, and G. Rosselin, pp. 261–274. North-Holland, New York.
51. Robberecht, P., Deschodt-Lanckman, M., Morgat, J. L., and Christophe, J. (1978): The interaction of caerulein with the rat pancreas. 3. Structural requirements for *in vitro* binding of caerulein-like peptides and its relationship to increased calcium outflux, adenylate cyclase activation and secretion. *Eur. J. Biochem.,* 91:39–48.
52. Said, S. I., and Mutt, V. (1972): Isolation from porcine-intestinal wall of a vasoactive octacosapeptide related to secretin and to glucagon. *Eur. J. Biochem.,* 28:199–204.

53. Shelby, H. T., Gross, L. P., Lichty, P., and Gardner, J. D. (1976): Action of cholecystokinin and cholinergic agents on membrane-bound calcium in dispersed pancreatic acinar cells. *J. Clin. Invest.*, 58:1482–1493.

54. Sjodin, L., and Gardner, J. D. (1977): Effect of cholecystokinin variant (CCK_{39}) on dispersed acinar cells from guinea pig pancreas. *Gastroenterology*, 73:1015–1018.

55. Snyder, S. H. (1977): Opiate receptors in the brain. *N. Engl. J. Med.*, 296:266–271.

56. Takahashi, T., Kinishi, S., Powell, D., Leeman, S. W., and Otsuka, M. (1974): Identification of the motorneuron-depolarizing peptide in bovine dorsal root as hypothalmic Substance P. *Brain Research*, 73:59–69.

57. von Euler, U. S., and Gaddum, J. H. (1931): An unidentified depressor substance in certain tissue extracts. *J. Physiol. (Lond.)*, 72:74–87.

58. Yanaihara, N., Sato, H., Hirohashi, M., Sakagami, M., Yamamoto, K., Hashimoto, T., Yanaihara, N., Obe, K., and Kaneko, T. (1976): Substance P radioimmunoassay using *N*-tyrosyl-substance P and demonstration of the presence of substance P-like immunoreactivities in human blood and porcine tissue extracts. *Endocrinol. Jpn.*, 23:457–463.

Polypeptide Hormones, edited by
R. F. Beers, Jr. and E. G. Bassett.
Raven Press, New York © 1980.

36. Satiety Effect of Gastrointestinal Hormones

Gerard P. Smith

Department of Psychiatry, Cornell University Medical College, and Edward W. Bourne Behavioral Research Laboratory, New York Hospital, White Plains, New York 10605

INTRODUCTION

The function of gut hormones has been traditionally sought in their effects on smooth muscle and glands of the gastrointestinal tract. Recently, three other functions have been discovered. These are the effect of gut hormones on other endocrine glands (22), the trophic effect of gut hormones on the gut itself (9), and the effect of gut hormones on feeding behavior (25,26). Our laboratory has been concerned with the satiety effect of gut hormones. I shall review that work in this chapter and describe the questions we are now trying to answer.

The idea that gut hormones might act to inhibit food intake was first tested by N. F. Maclagan in 1937. Maclagan (19) showed that an extract of the small intestine inhibited food intake in rabbits. This extract was called enterogastrone by Kosaka and Lim (12) because it inhibited gastric secretion. Thirty years later, Schally and colleagues (23) reported that a more purified extract of entero-gastrone inhibited food intake in mice. This promising work with enterogastrone has not been pursued further.

In the 1950s and early 1960s, pancreatic glucagon was also shown to inhibit food intake in animals and man (21), but chronic administration of the hormone produced undesirable metabolic side effects (2,15,21).

In 1972, Gibbs and I began to investigate the effect of the available gut hormones on feeding behavior. We did this for two reasons—ignorance and utility. The ignorance concerned the physiological mechanisms for stopping feeding. The ignorance was total. Gastric distention and increased glucose utilization had been suggested as mechanisms for ending a meal, but the experimental evidence for them was not compelling. We thought that gut hormones should be tested for a satiety effect because they are released by the contact of ingested food with the muscosa of the stomach and intestine. This means that gut hormones are in the right place and are released at the right time to serve as a negative feedback signal for terminating a meal.

The utility we had in mind was a new form of therapy for human obesity. Since effective treatment was (and still is) not available, the discovery of a satiety effect for gut hormones would provide the first opportunity to test the therapeutic potential of a substance(s) that was part of the endogenous, physiological mechanism for short-term satiety.

METHODS

The sham-feeding rat (Fig. 1) has served as a useful preparation for assaying the satiety effect of gut hormones. Sham-feeding is accomplished by permitting an ingested liquid diet to drain out through a gastric cannula. When appropriate criteria are met, drainage of gastric contents is complete (13). The major advantage of the sham-feeding rat as a preparation for assaying satiety effects is that rats do not stop sham-feeding after 17 hr food deprivation (29). Thus, there are no false-positive satiety responses to test substances. The other advantages of the preparation are that (a) the surgery required to implant the gastric cannula is relatively simple, and (b) the fistula can be closed with a screw cap; this technique permits a sufficient period of normal feeding between tests to maintain the rats in good health.

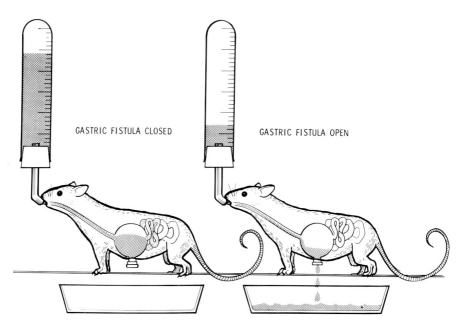

GASTRIC FISTULA CLOSED   GASTRIC FISTULA OPEN

FIG. 1. When the gastric fistula is closed, ingested liquid food enters the stomach, passes into the small intestine, and is absorbed. When the gastric fistula is open, ingested liquid food enters the stomach and immediately passes out the open fistula. The loss of ingested food out of the stomach is associated with sustained ingestion of large amounts of liquid diet. Such a process is called sham-feeding. (From ref. 26, with permission.)

RESULTS AND DISCUSSION

Satiety Effect of Cholecystokinin in Rats

An impure extract of cholecystokinin (CCK) and the synthetic COOH-terminal octapeptide of cholecystokinin (CCK-8) inhibited sham feeding (6,7,17). The magnitude of the inhibition was a function of the dose of CCK or CCK-8 and the route of administration (Fig. 2).

Desulfation of CCK-8 reduced the potency of CCK-8 for satiety about 10-fold (7,17). The decreased potency of desulfated CCK-8 is characteristic of the known biological actions of CCK (10). Therefore, the satiety effect is a new biological action of CCK.

Since the satiety effect has this important structural constraint, it suggests that the receptor for the satiety effect is similar to known CCK receptors. All of the CCK receptors that have been characterized are in peripheral visceral tissues (see Chapter 35). This suggests that CCK acts on receptors in a peripheral

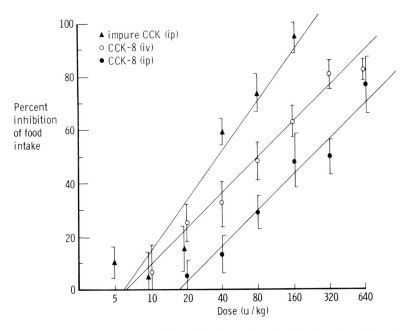

FIG. 2. Percent inhibition of sham-fed liquid diet in a 60-min test is a function of the dose of impure (20%) CCK and CCK-8. Points represent means and brackets represent SE for data from at least five rats tested at each dose. Note that (a) the slow intravenous infusion of CCK-8 is a more effective method of administration than intraperitoneal injection of CCK-8; and (b) the slope of the log dose-response line for impure CCK is to the left and significantly steeper than the log dose-response lines for impure CCK and CCK-8 suggests that the satiety effect of impure CCK is not entirely due to the CCK in the extract. (From ref. 17, with permission.)

visceral site to initiate the satiety effect. If this were true, then there must be some neural or hormonal pathway that connects the visceral site of CCK to the brain because it is axiomatic that the brain is necessary for all behavioral effects. The vagus nerve serves this function: Abdominal vagotomy markedly reduces or abolishes the satiety effect of CCK-8 (16,24). Since blockade of the visceral effects of vagal motor fiber(s) by atropine methylnitrate did not change the satiety effect of CCK-8 (G. P. Smith, *unpublished observations*), the critical lesion produced by abdominal vagotomy appears to be section of vagal sensory fibers. Although it is not clear which abdominal vagal sensory field must be lesioned, we know that the destruction of the vagal innervation of the liver is not necessary to block the satiety effect of CCK-8 (24).

The blockade by abdominal vagotomy of the satiety effect of CCK-8 is strong evidence that the satiety effect is initiated peripherally. The report of Nemeroff et al. (20) that the threshold for CCK-8 to inhibit tail-pinch induced feeding was lower when CCK was administered intraperitoneally than when CCK-8 was administered intracerebroventricularly is additional evidence for a peripheral site of action. However, the recent discovery of brain CCK (see Chapter 33) means that there are also central CCK receptors. It now becomes important to investigate the possible satiety and other behavioral effects of stimulation of these receptors by brain CCK and, perhaps, by intestinal CCK.

At this time, there are two reports that are consistent with a satiety effect produced by stimulation of brain CCK receptors. The first is that of Stern et al. (27). They demonstrated that cerulein, a decapeptide that is structurally similar to CCK-8 and that produces all the known biological effects of CCK, including satiety (6,27), inhibited the intake of solid food in 30 min tests when it was injected into the lateral cerebral ventricle or into the ventromedial hypothalmic nucleus (VMH). The threshold dose required for satiety after central administration was clearly less than the minimal dose required after peripheral administration. Stern et al. argued that the VMH was a specific site for the satiety effect of cerulein because (a) identical injections of cerulein into the lateral hypothalamus did not inhibit feeding; (b) a single dose of peripherally administered cerulein did not produce satiety in VMH-lesioned rats; and (c) there was an apparent increased uptake of ^{3}H-cerulein in the VM area after peripheral administration. This neat scheme requires further testing because Kulkoski et al. (14) failed to confirm it when they observed the usual satiety effect of peripherally administered CCK-8 in VMH-lesioned rats.

The second report that supports a satiety effect from stimulation of central CCK receptors is that of Maddison (18). He showed that administration of impure CCK into the lateral cerebral ventricle prolonged postprandial satiety. Since the satiety effect of impure CCK is not entirely due to the CCK in the extract (see Fig. 2), it will be necessary to reproduce Maddison's result with CCK-8 before considering it as evidence for a satiety effect of CCK acting on central receptors.

Satiety Effect of Cholecystokinin in Monkeys and Man

Gibbs and Falasco extended the satiety effect of CCK to the rhesus monkey. They demonstrated a dose-related inhibition of normal feeding (4) and of sham-feeding (Fig. 3; also ref. 3). The dose of CCK that abolished sham-feeding in the monkey did not produce toxic side effects such as retching, vomiting, diarrhea, or behavioral displays characteristic of pain or distress. In fact, after CCK administration, monkeys displayed postprandial behaviors that were similar to their normal postprandial behaviors. The lack of toxicity in monkeys complemented the failure of acute or chronic administration of CCK to produce signs of toxicity in rats (6).

Since CCK inhibited food intake in rats and monkeys in doses that did not produce toxicity, we collaborated with Kissileff and co-workers (11) to study the effect of CCK-8 in humans. Slow intravenous infusion of CCK-8 significantly decreased food intake in 12 lean men (Table 1). The effective dose was small, (approximately 31 ng/kg) and there was no significant toxicity. The reason(s) why CCK-8 worked under our conditions, but was ineffective under other conditions (8) is not clear.

We are attempting to replicate this acute inhibition of food intake in a group of moderately obese subjects. If CCK-8 inhibits food intake in these obese sub-

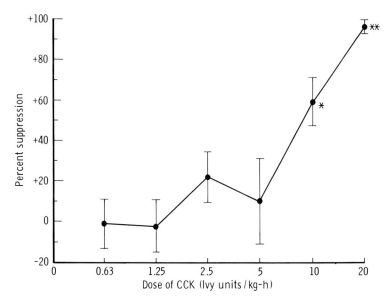

FIG. 3. Mean percent suppression (+SE) of sham intake over 60 min produced by intravenous infusion of CCK compared with intravenous infusion of saline in rhesus monkeys (n = 5 for all doses except the 0.63 dose for which n = 3). *, $p < 0.05$; **, $p < 0.005$; matched pairs t-test, one tailed. (From ref. 3, with permission.)

TABLE 1. *Inhibition of food intake by CCK-8 in lean men*[a]

Food intake		
Saline	CCK-8	Difference[b]
644	522	122 ± 50

[a] Intake of a liquified lunch of yogurt and fruit by 12 lean young men during intravenous infusion of saline and of CCK-8. The average dose of CCK-8 was 31 ng/kg. The intakes are the average of two tests in each subject done under double-blind conditions. Nine of 12 subjects ate less during CCK-8 infusions than during saline infusions and the difference in the amount eaten during the two kinds of infusion for the entire group was statistically significant ($p < 0.05$).
[b] SE indicated.

jects, then we will attempt to decrease body weight in them by chronic CCK-8 treatment.

Is the Satiety Effect a Physiological Function of CCK?

Two facts suggest that the satiety effect of exogenous CCK is a physiological function of CCK, i.e., that endogenous CCK released by contact of ingested food with the mucosa of the small intestine acts to inhibit feeding and elicit postprandial satiety. First, there is the consistent ability of CCK to produce satiety in rats, rabbits, sheep, monkeys, and humans (26). Second, a variety of food stimuli release endogenous CCK in several forms (see Chapter 33). However, these facts are only suggestive; they do not prove the physiological status of CCK. An adequate test of this question depends on the development of a reliable method for measuring circulating CCK. None exists (28). When one becomes available, it will be possible to measure the pattern of release of the various forms of CCK and compare the quantity released with the quantity of exogenous CCK required to produce satiety.

This methodological advance will constitute a necessary step in investigating the physiological status of the satiety effect of CCK, but it will not be sufficient because CCK is not the only physiological mechanism for short-term satiety. We know this from the fact that abdominally vagotomized rats satiate normally or more quickly than normal (depending on the test diet) even though abdominal vagotomy blocks the satiety effect of CCK-8. If CCK is not the only physiological mechanism for short-term satiety, CCK is likely to act with these other mechanisms. We have demonstrated such a synergism for satiety of CCK and the mechanisms (presumably neural) activated by the food-contingent stimuli of sham feeding (1). The existence of such synergism between the multiple mechanisms for short-term satiety complicates the test of the physiological status of any one of them until most or all of them are known and brought under experimental control. For these reasons, it will be difficult to settle the physiological status of the satiety effect of CCK in the near future.

Satiety Effect of Other Gut Hormones

We have tested four other gut hormones in the sham-feeding rat preparation. Gastrin, secretin, and gastric inhibitory polypeptide had no significant satiety effect over a 1,000-fold dose range. Bombesin, however, has recently been shown to have a potent and clear satiety effect without apparent toxicity (5). This effect of bombesin is now being investigated in the rhesus monkey.

SUMMARY

Gut hormones are released by ingested food. Thus, they could serve as mechanisms for short-term satiety. Of the five gut hormones we have tested, CCK and bombesin have a significant satiety effect. At the present time, the physiological status of these hormones in short-term satiety is uncertain and their therapeutic usefulness in the treatment of obesity has not been evaluated. But the fact that two gut hormones have a significant satiety effect suggests that further investigation of the effect of gut hormones on feeding behavior can dispel some of the ignorance surrounding the physiology of satiety and improve the treatment of human obesity.

ACKNOWLEDGMENTS

I thank Dr. J. Gibbs for his constant collaboration in our work and for his critical review of this manuscript. The research described was supported by National Institutes of Health grants AM 17240 and MH 15455, and by Research Scientist Development Awards MH 00149 and MH 70874.

REFERENCES

1. Antin, J., Gibbs, J., and Smith, G. P. (1978): Cholecystokinin interacts with pregastric food stimulation to elicit satiety in the rat. *Physiol. Behav.,* 20:67–70.
2. Ezrin, C., Salter, J. M., Ogryzlo, M. A., and Best, C. H. (1958): The clinical and metabolic effects of glucagon. *Can. Med. Assoc. J.,* 78:96–98.
3. Falasco, J. D., Smith, G. P., and Gibbs, J. (1979): Cholecystokinin suppresses sham feeding in the rhesus monkey. *Physiol. Behav.,* 23:887–890.
4. Gibbs, J., Falasco, J. D., and McHugh, P. R. (1976): Cholecystokinin decreased food intake in rhesus monkeys. *Am. J. Physiol.,* 230:15–18.
5. Gibbs, J., and Martin, C. F. (1979): Bombesin suppresses sham feeding in rats. *Soc. Neurosci. Abstr.,* 5:217.
6. Gibbs, J., Young, R. C., and Smith, G. P. (1973): Cholecystokinin decreases food intake in rats. *J. Comp. Physiol. Psychol.,* 84:488–495.
7. Gibbs, J., Young, R. C., and Smith, G. P. (1973): Cholecystokinin elicits satiety in rats with open gastric fistulas. *Nature,* 245:323–325.
8. Greenway, F. L., and Bray, G. A. (1977): Cholecystokinin and satiety. *Life Sci.,* 21:769–772.

9. Johnson, L. R. (1976): The trophic action of gastrointestinal hormones. *Gastroenterology,* 70:278–288.

10. Jorpes, J. E., and Mutt, V. (1973): Secretin and cholecystokinin (CCK). In: *Secretin, Cholecystokinin, Pancreozymin and Gastrin,* edited by J. E. Jorpes and V. Mutt, pp. 33–34. Springer-Verlag, New York.

11. Kissileff, H. R., Pi-Sunyer, F. X., Thornton, J., and Smith, G. P. (1979): Cholecystokinin-octapeptide (CCK-8) decreases food intake in man. *Am. J. Clin. Nutr.,* 32:939.

12. Kosaka, T., and Lim, R. K. S. (1930): Demonstration of the humoral agent in fat inhibition of gastric secretion. *Proc. Soc. Exp. Biol. Med.,* 27:890–891.

13. Kraly, F. S., Carty, W. J., and Smith, G. P. (1978): Effects of pregastric food stimuli on meal size and intermeal interval in the rat. *Physiol. Behav.,* 20:779–784.

14. Kulkosky, P. J., Breckenridge, C., Krinsky, R., and Woods, S. C. (1976): Satiety elicited by the C-terminal octapeptide of cholecystokinin-pancreozymin in normal and VMH-lesioned rats. *Behav. Biol.,* 18:227–234.

15. Lipsett, M. B., Engle, H. R., and Bergenstal, D. M. (1960): Effects of glucagon on plasma unesterified fatty acids and on nitrogen metabolism. *J. Lab. Clin. Med.,* 56:342–354.

16. Lorenz, D. N., and Goldman, S. A. (1978): Dependence of the cholecystokinin satiety effect on vagal innervation. *Soc. Neurosci. Abstr.,* 4:178.

17. Lorenz, D. N., Kreielsheimer, G., and Smith, G. P. (1979): Effect of cholecystokinin, gastrin, secretin and GIP on sham feeding in the rat. *Physiol. Behav.,* 23:1065–1072.

18. Maddison, S. (1977): Intraperitoneal and intracranial cholecystokinin depress operant responding for food. *Physiol. Behav.,* 19:819–824.

19. Maclagan, N. F. (1937): The role of appetite in the control of body weight. *J. Physiol. (Lond.)* 90:385–394.

20. Nemeroff, C. B., Osbahr, A. J., III, Bissette, G., Jahnke, G. Lipton, M. A., and Prange, Jr., A. J. (1978): Cholecystokinin inhibits tail pinch-induced eating in rats. *Science,* 200:793–794.

21. Penick, S. B., and Hinkle, L. E., Jr. (1961): Depression of food intake in healthy subjects by glucagon. *N. Engl. J. Med.,* 264:893–897.

22. Pfeiffer, E. F., Raptis, S., and Fussgänger, R. (1973): Gastrointestinal hormones and islet function. In: *Secretin, Cholecystokinin, Pancreozymin and Gastrin,* edited by J. E. Jorpes and V. Mutt, pp. 259–310. Springer-Verlag, New York.

23. Schally, A. V., Redding, T. W., Lucien, H. W., and Meyer, J. (1967): Enterogastrone inhibits eating by fasted mice. *Science,* 157:210–211.

24. Smith, G. P., and Cushin, B. J. (1978): Cholecystokinin acts at a vagally innervated abdominal site to elicit satiety. *Soc. Neurosci. Abstr.,* 4:180.

25. Smith, G. P., and Gibbs, J. (1976): Cholecystokinin and satiety: Theoretic and therapeutic implications. In: *Hunger: Basic Mechanisms and Clinical Implications,* edited by D. Novin, W. Wyrwicka, and G. Bray, pp. 349–355. Raven Press, New York.

26. Smith, G. P., and Gibbs, J. (1979): Postprandial satiety. In: *Progress in Psychobiology and Physiological Psychology, Vol. 8,* edited by J. M. Sprague and A. N. Epstein, pp. 199–242. Academic Press, New York.

27. Stern, J. J., Cudillo, C. A., and Kruper, J. (1976): Ventromedial hypothalamus and short-term feeding suppression by caerulein in male rats. *J. Comp. Physiol. Psychol.,* 90:484–490.

28. Straus, E. (1978): Radioimmunoassay of gastrointestinal hormones. *Gastroenterology,* 74:141–152.

29. Young, R. C., Gibbs, J. Antin, J., Holt, J., and Smith, G. P. (1974): Absence of satiety during sham-feeding in the rat. *J. Comp. Physiol. Psychol.,* 87:795–800.

Polypeptide Hormones, edited by
R. F. Beers, Jr. and E. G. Bassett.
Raven Press, New York © 1980.

37. Establishing the Physiology of Gastrointestinal Hormones

Stephen R. Bloom and Julia M. Polak

Royal Postgraduate Medical School, Hammersmith Hospital, London W12 0HS, England

INTRODUCTION AND GENERAL PRINCIPLES

The recognition of gut hormones is as old as the century. It is noteworthy, however, that in spite of now knowing the amino acid sequence, localization, and pharmacology, their physiological role is still to a considerable degree uncertain. This is thus an area of much current investigative activity. Obvious fundamental requirements prior to consideration of the physiological role of each new hormonal peptide are (a) its chemical nature, (b) its localization, and (c) its pharmacology. Each of these basic facts present difficulties. As illustrated earlier (Chapter 33), most hormonal peptides are present in multiple forms that may or may not have an identical spectrum of activity and nearly always differ in their potency. As described by Polak and Bloom (Chapter 34), while the tissue localization is in agreement for many peptides, there is still active controversy concerning others. In addition, many substances exist both in nerves and in cells, which implies that their physiological role may vary with their location. Finally, for almost every peptide being considered, there is inadequate pharmacological data. This is partly because the subject is relatively new and there has been insufficient time to explore all investigative avenues and partly because until recently the supply of the peptides was very limited. Advances in our ability to produce relatively cheap synthetic peptides of chain length up to 20 amino acids has circumvented this problem for many hormones, but, for example, glucose-dependent insulinotropic peptide (GIP) and the larger forms of gastrin and cholecystokinin (CCK) are still available only from natural sources and therefore in small quantities. Indeed, most of the larger forms of hormones have not been isolated and so their actions cannot be tested. Uniquely of the recognized gut hormones, no form of enteroglucagon (glucagon-like immunoreactivity of intestinal origin) has been purified in sufficient quantities to provide useful information on its pharmacology.

The ability to measure the hormone in the circulation and show its rise and fall after natural stimuli forms the vital first step in investigation of its physiology. In every case, the only available method of measurement sufficiently cheap, specific, and reliable is the radioimmunoassay (RIA). This technique depends on the precise quantitative reaction between an antibody and the hormonal peptide that forms the antigen. Unfortunately, the affinity of the binding site on the antibody is closely dependent on the molecule's tertiary structure. Thus, even slight changes in the ionic or hydrophobic environment alters the binding constant and influences the stoichiometry of the reaction. Thus, although antibodies are capable of detecting the tiny quantity of hormone present in the circulation (an assay test tube contains about 10^{-16} mole, which is only about one hundred million molecules), it is not a very reliable way of doing so. RIAs also suffer from the disadvantage that they measure a particular amino acid sequence rather than the biological potency of the molecule. Thus, biologically inactive forms are read identically to active ones. In some circumstances because large pro-hormonal forms are slowly cleared from the circulation, almost all the measurable "hormone" is inactive. This tends to be particularly true of measurements in the basal state. It is basic to the function of a regulating peptide that a mechanism for its rapid destruction must exist. Thus, most of the circulating hormones are easily degraded, producing further difficulties for the assayist. Many RIA problems are now being overcome by (a) scrupulous attention to the conditions of the assay to minimize nonspecific interference in antibody binding; (b) choice of antibodies that combine with the active site of the hormone and that therefore tend to accurately reflect biological activity; and (c) use of conditions that prevent hormone degradation. There is still much disagreement between laboratories concerning absolute concentrations of hormones, and it is clear that not all problems have been solved. There is now, however, a good consensus concerning the major stimuli for release or suppression of the established gut hormones and also some approximate idea of their true molar concentrations.

To establish a hormone's actual importance in everyday regulation is very difficult. The crudest method of investigation is to infuse into fasting volunteers an amount of hormone that mimics that seen after some physiological stimuli and then assess its effects in the light of known pharmacology. Although this does give useful information, it is certainly not physiology. The control of biological functions is usually a delicate balance between numerous agonists, antagonists, and modulators (for example, see Table 1). The isolated introduction of a single agonist will, therefore, have quite unphysiological effects. In order to truly ascertain the importance of one regulating substance in a complex control system, it is necessary to investigate the effect of a very small change in its concentration in the correct functional setting. This requires exquisitely accurate measurement systems and is, in most instances, beyond current methodology.

The final goal and purpose for such research is the understanding of human disease. Conversely, disease processes are natural experiments and the study of pathophysiology can yield very useful insight into physiology itself. It is impossible in a short chapter to survey all the gastrointestinal hormonal peptides; therefore, pancreatic polypeptide and motilin are examined in some detail as examples of the current investigative approach.

TABLE 1. *Some factors affecting gastric acid content*

Luminal	Neural
Nutrients	Cholinergic
pH	Adrenergic
	VIPergic
	Bombesinergic
	Substance Pergic
	Enkephalinergic
	Somatostatinergic
Hormonal	Paracrine
Gastrin	Somatostatin
Neurotensin	Histamine
Enteroglucagon	Serotonin
Motilin	Prostaglandins

INDIVIDUAL HORMONES

Pancreatic Polypeptide

Pancreatic polypeptide (PP) was first discovered quite accidentally by Kimmel (30) as a major peptide contaminant in semipurified chicken insulin. Subsequently, a similar peptide was found in the mammal (bovine) by Lin and Chance (33), who later showed that it had 36 amino acids (35) and that there were only three amino acid differences between bovine and human PP. They further reported that the last six amino acids constituted the active site and that this part of the sequence was identical in the PP of these two species. They were able to raise antibodies to human PP that allowed the localization of the producing cells (28,31) and also the development of an RIA (3). PP cells were localized both in the islets of Langerhans and between the acinar cells of the pancreas (28,31).

PP was found to be present in fasting blood and showed a dramatic rise in concentration after a meal, rivaling in magnitude the rise of insulin (3) (Fig. 1). In patients who had had a complete pancreatectomy no circulating PP was detectable, proving its pancreatic origin. It was initially thought that PP, like insulin, would be released after a meal directly by the rise in circulating nutriment concentrations. It was found, however, that infusions of glucose, fat (intralipids), or amino acids produced no significant change in PP concentrations. It was thus apparent that the postprandial PP release depended on an indirect signalling mechanism from gut to PP cells, and the concept of an entero-PP axis was introduced (2). After insulin-induced hypoglycemia, PP levels rose dramatically but this rise was absent in patients who had had a successful truncal vagotomy (2) (Fig. 2). Furthermore, in animals atropine administration blocked the postprandial PP rise. It was therefore concluded that the main mechanisms of postprandial PP release was via vagal activation (43). Further study of patients who had had a successful truncal vagotomy, however, showed a rise of PP

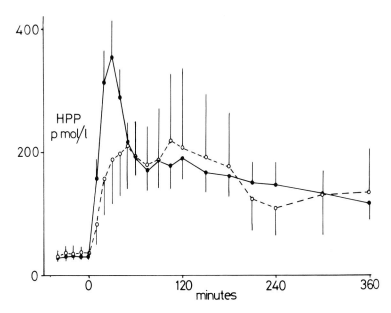

FIG. 1. Plasma pancreatic polypeptide (HPP) concentrations in 10 normal subjects after a standard lunch (———) and in 6 patients who had previously undergone a successful truncal vagotomy (———).

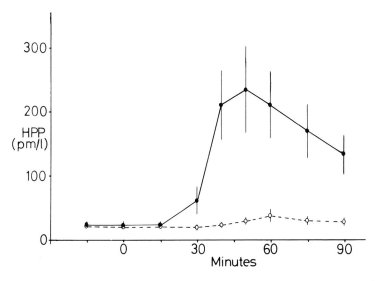

FIG. 2. Plasma pancreatic polypeptide (HPP) concentrations in 8 normal subjects (———) and 17 patients who had previously undergone a successful truncal vagotomy (———) during insulin (0.2 U/kg at time zero)-induced hypoglycemia.

after a meal that was not significantly different from normal controls (2), although the early phase was slightly reduced in magnitude (Fig. 1). Infusions of the impure hormone preparation, Boot's secretin, and cerulein released PP directly (4) (Fig. 3), but atropine blocked the effect (1). It was concluded that the control of PP release was in many ways analogous to the control of the gastric parietal cell. Here, three separate stimulants—histamine, acetylcholine, and gastrin— can all independently increase gastric acid secretion but are only effective in the presence of a background of the other agents (44). Thus, the PP cells appear to require cholinergic tone before they are capable of responding to changes in circulating hormone concentrations. The physiological importance of active release via the vagal innervation is demonstrated, however, by the rise of PP after sham-feeding (46) or gastric distension, although neither stimulus is nearly as effective as eating a meal.

There have been rather few reports on the pharmacological actions of PP but Lin and colleagues have shown that it can inhibit pancreatic enzyme secretions and gallbladder contractions at a very low dose, influence the output of pancreatic bicarbonate juice and gastric juice of a slightly larger dose, and, in greater amounts still, affect gastrointestinal motility (34,36). As PP remains a contaminant of many commercial insulin preparations (11), albeit in amounts below that likely to be pharmacologically active, it seemed of interest to study the effects of PP in man. This was made particularly relevant by the finding

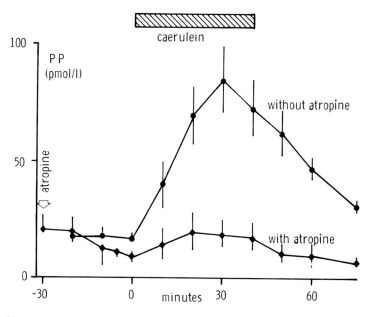

FIG. 3. Plasma pancreatic polypeptide (PP) concentrations during infusion of cerulein (100 ng/kg/hr) in five healthy subjects with and without prior intramuscular administration of 1.2 ng atropine.

that many insulin-dependent diabetics developed antibodies to this contaminant of insulin and that these antibodies reacted with high affinity with human PP (11). Thus, it was at least possible that the patients might have significant impairment of endogenous PP function. Studies of PP infusions in man were therefore initiated before obtaining abundant data in animals. No side effects of the infusions were noted, either subjective or objective (including hemodynamic, biochemical, hematological investigations, etc.). PP infusions at a dose that produced plasma concentrations approximately threefold higher than those seen after a normal meal did not affect levels of plasma glucose, insulin, glucagon, 3-hydroxybutyrate, free fatty acids, lactate, pyruvate, or alanine (5). Thus, the initial experiments in the bird, which had suggested that PP might have an effect on

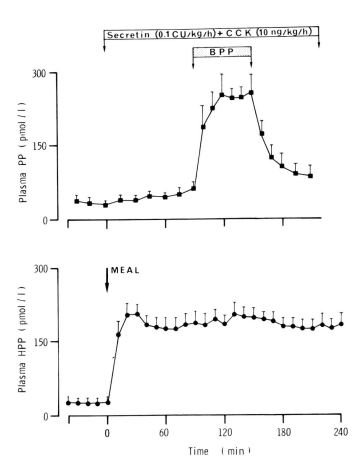

FIG. 4. Plasma pancreatic polypeptide (PP) concentrations. **Top:** Seven normal subjects during a 60-min bovine PP infusion at 65 pmoles/kg/hr superimposed on a secretin (0.1 U/kg/hr) infusion and a cerulein (CCK) infusion (10 ng/kg/hr). **Bottom:** Ten healthy subjects after eating a large (1,142 cal) breakfast.

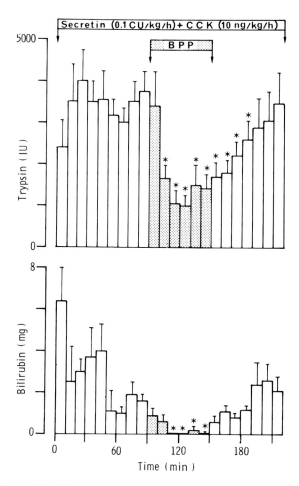

FIG. 5. The effect of the infusions shown in the upper panel of Fig. 4 on duodenal trypsin and bilirubin output in seven normal subjects. Stars indicate statistical significance.

lipid or carbohydrate metabolism (27), have not so far been reproduced in the mammal. In addition, no significant effect of this dose of PP was noted on gastric acid or pepsin secretion during submaximal pentagastrin stimulation (25). A significant reduction in duodenal juice volume, enzyme concentration, and bilirubin concentration was found and prompted further experiments using a smaller dose of PP to reproduce more precisely the normal postprandial concentrations (Fig. 4). A significant reduction in pancreatic enzyme output and bilirubin output was again demonstrated (26) (Fig. 5), but the latter effect was not seen in patients who had previously undergone a cholecystectomy, suggesting that it resulted from an inhibition of gallbladder contraction. Thus, the effects demonstrated so far in man suggest that PP has an action opposite to that of CCK on both pancreas and gallbladder. The physiological role of a hormone released by food [particularly fat and protein (3)] and that appears to impair digestion is difficult to understand. Pancreatic endocrine tumors frequently contain a considerable proportion of PP-secreting cells and these patients have chronically elevated plasma PP levels (38). To date no clinical correlation of this PP elevation has been noted. This may imply that other hormones readily overcome the effects of PP, but it is possible that PP exerts some unknown effect we have so far failed to detect.

Motilin

The peptide motilin, unlike PP, was discovered by searching for the hormonal mediator of an observed physiological effect. Brown and colleagues in 1966 (16) noted that stimulation of the duodenum produced gastric contractions, even in an isolated fundic pouch. They postulated a hormonal mediator and were able to show that impure intestinal extracts produced a similar biological effect (17). Motilin, a 22-amino acid peptide, was subsequently purified (15) and later synthesized. Pharmacological studies on this peptide demonstrated that it powerfully stimulated contraction of smooth muscle of the upper gastrointestinal tract. The development of a RIA indicated that motilin was produced solely by endocrine cells of the mucosa of the upper intestine. Furthermore, considerable concentrations were found to be present in human fasting plasma (14) (Fig. 6).

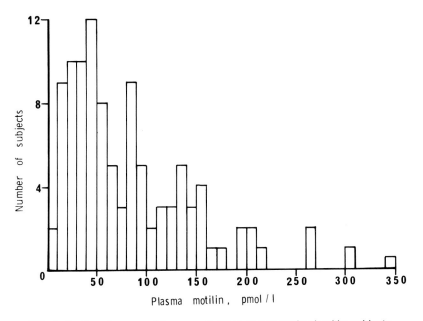

FIG. 6. Fasting plasma motilin concentrations in 110 resting healthy subjects.

The most potent stimuli to motilin release in man has been found to be the ingestion of a fat meal, a large volume of water, or rapid intraduodenal infusion of a supraphysiological quantity of acid (50 ml 0.1 M HCl) (20). Oral glucose was found to inhibit motilin release and protein to have no significant effect. Ingestion of a mixed meal thus does not provoke large changes of motilin though an early rise occurs, peaking at between 15 and 30 min, and is followed by a gentle decline to slightly below the initial basal concentrations at 2 to 3 hr. There is a wide variation of fasting motilin concentrations (14) (Fig. 6) and the absolute increment or decrement after a stimuli is in proportion to the basal concentration (21). Thus, if changes in motilin concentration are expressed as a percentage of basal levels, a quite uniform response becomes apparent. This can be seen, for example, in the very small standard errors illustrated in Fig. 7, in spite of the extremely wide variation in absolute motilin concentrations. The effect of intravenous nutriments (Fig. 7) was initially tested as a control for the subjects undergoing oral administration experiments (21). The surprising finding was that intravenous fat was as potent a motilin releasing agent as that given orally. Intravenous glucose caused a significant motilin suppression, similar to that seen with oral glucose. Intravenous amino acids suppressed motilin release, unlike the response to that seen after oral protein, where no change

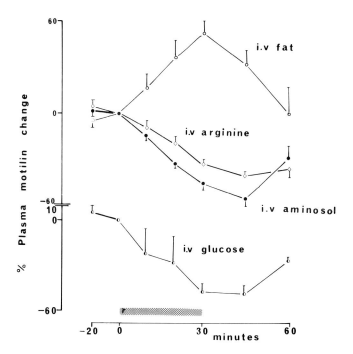

FIG. 7. Percentage change in plasma motilin concentrations after intravenous infusion of fat (8 g as 20% intralipid), amino acids (25 g as 250 ml 10% aminosol), arginine (0.5 g/kg), and glucose (20 g as 50% solution).

was observed. The discrepancy in this case might be explained by the relatively large volume of protein that had to be ingested to produce a similar caloric load and that might therefore have produced distension effects. The high concentration of fasting motilin, the considerable variation in concentration between individuals, and the lack of any very large response to the stimuli so far tested suggest the possibility that motilin may have its major role in the fasting state. This possibility was strengthened when the fasting motilin concentrations in man (47) and dog (29) were found to vary in a cyclical fashion with peak concentrations occurring just before the formation of a new interdigestive myoelectric complex.

Experimental motilin infusions in man initially were shown to produce a delay in gastric emptying (41). However, the dose used was relatively high and might be considered supraphysiological. Subsequent investigations have suggested that a lower dose of motilin (22) (Fig. 8), producing an 85% rise over basal fasting plasma concentrations, actually doubled the rate of initial gastric emptying of both liquids and solid particles (Fig. 9). Motilin infusions given fasting volunteers shortly after the cessation of an interdigestive myoelectric complex (a period when the bowel is normally quiescent) induced the formation of a premature new myoelectric complex (47). While this effect required a dose of motilin producing plasma concentrations in the upper physiological range, it was administered at a time when the bowel is normally refractory. No agent is yet available to inhibit specifically the release of motilin so that proper assessment of its importance in myoelectric complex formation is not at present possible. Investigations in disease states have shown an elevation of motilin in several conditions where the patient had active diarrhea at the time of the study (12), e.g., Crohn's disease, acute intestinal infection, irritable bowel syndrome, tropical

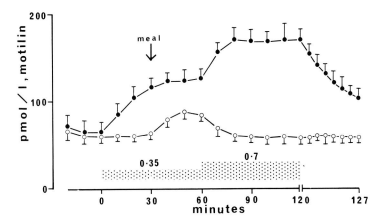

FIG. 8. Plasma motilin concentrations in five subjects after ingestion of a meal during saline infusion (○) and infusion of natural porcine motilin (●). The rate of infusion *(grid)* is indicated as pmoles/kg/min.

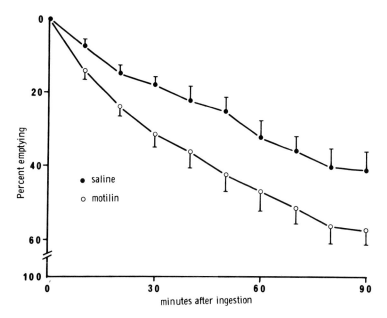

FIG. 9. Percentage of radioactive meal marker (^{129}Ce-Zr resin, 150 mesh) remaining in the stomach during saline infusion (●) and infusion of motilin (○), as in Fig. 8, plotted against time after meal ingestion.

sprue, and ulcerative colitis. In all these conditions, motor disorders of the gastrointestinal tract have been described and their study may therefore help in the understanding of motilin's physiological role.

Gastrin

Pharmacological effects of gastrin indicate a physiological role in controlling gastric acid secretion, mucosal growth, and possibly motor function (48). The evidence in favor of a physiological effect on gastric acid output is both circumstantial and also direct, using infusions producing physiological elevations in plasma gastrin (49). The trophic effects of gastrin have been demonstrated in animals but not in man, although gastric mucosal hypertrophy is seen in patients with gastrinomas. Much controversy exists on the motor actions of gastrin (particularly on the lower esophageal sphincter), and the consensus is that, although gastrin is not a major controlling influence, it is probably one of the relevant background factors (48). It has become obvious from studies with the new H_2 histamine receptor blocking agent as well as the older established effect of atropine, that control of gastric acid is complex. This is summarized in Table 1 and well illustrates the difficulty in unraveling physiology. Thus, although gastrin may be an important influence on acid secretion, it is only one of a number of factors and it is therefore not surprising that the correlation between plasma gastrin concentrations and acid secretion is unusually poor even in healthy individuals.

Secretin

As the first-named hormone, the role of secretin should be above suspicion. Nonetheless, it is proving extremely difficult in man to show any significant rise after a meal. It is also difficult to get unequivocable evidence of postprandial bicarbonate secretion in man, but nonetheless this does seem to be a likely response. When the duodenal pH is monitored, individual falls of pH are correlated with individual spikes of secretin release, and infusions of HCl into the duodenum certainly evoke a large and rapid secretin rise (19). Infusions of secretin itself, particularly on a background of CCK, does result in a significant bicarbonate response even with a rise in plasma concentration of only 1 pmole/liter. It is possible that as significant quantities of acid enter the duodenum only quite late after a meal, and with variable timing, the small individual rise of secretin that is necessary to stimulate the pancreas disappears when the data from many patients is meaned. Nonetheless, it remains an enigma that a significant secretin concentration is found in fasting plasma and that the mean concentration does not change significantly even late after ingestion of a normal meal.

Cholecystokinin

The RIAs for CCK have hitherto been unreliable and so investigation of its physiology has proved difficult (40). In addition, dog experiments have shown that the transplanted pancreas, while responding normally to exogenous CCK fails to respond to a meal, stressing the importance of neural influences (45).

Glucose-dependent Insulinotropic Peptide

Glucose-dependent insulinotropic peptide (GIP) has been shown in man to stimulate the release of insulin during hyperglycemia (24). A large rise in endogenous plasma occurs after ingestion of glucose or fat. Thus, GIP has been proposed as the main hormone of the entero-insular axis (23), which is the mechanism causing a much larger rise of insulin after oral nutriments than that evoked by intravenous feeding, and thereby accelerates metabolic disposal of food with a minimal disturbance of circulating metabolite levels. Unfortunately, there is considerable variation in the plasma concentrations reported by different laboratories. This may in part be due to the presence in the circulation of two molecular sizes of GIP (18) that are variably measured by different antibodies. In addition, the entero-insular axis can be shown to operate even when the rise of plasma glucose is too small to allow GIP stimulation of the β cell. Thus, while it seems quite possible that GIP is an important component of the entero-insular axis, the story is by no means complete.

Enteroglucagon

Enteroglucagon is the term used to describe glucagon-like immunoreactants released from the intestine by a single endocrine cell type (EG cell). There are two circulating molecular forms (large and small) and both are equally released by fat or glucose. Enteroglucagon has never been isolated in significant quantities (37) and therefore its pharmacology and physiology are unknown. A single enteroglucagon-producing tumor resulted in small intestinal mucosal hypertrophy (9) and enteroglucagon is elevated in pathological situations where there is an increase in mucosal growth (8), for example, in sprue, intestinal resection, or after intestinal bypass operations.

Neurotensin

Neurotensin is a 13-amino acid peptide released from endocrine cells in the mucosa of the ileum (39). Plasma concentrations rise after a meal and, the bigger the meal, the larger the rise. Pharmacologically, neurotensin inhibits gastric emptying (7) and gastric acid secretion (6). Nothing is yet known of its physiological role.

Vasoactive Intestinal Peptide

Considerable quantities of vasoactive intestinal peptide (VIP) are found in the nerves of the alimentary system. Pharmacologically, VIP is a potent smooth muscle relaxing agent and causes vasodilation. It also stimulates small intestinal secretion and is a causative agent of the Verner-Morrison syndrome (10) (watery diarrhea, hypocalcemia, and achlorhydria syndrome). VIP is thought to be one of the main neurotransmitters of the peptidergic branch of the autonomic nervous system, responsible for the nonadrenergic, noncholinergic inhibitory actions, a well-known physiological enigma. The physiological role of neuropeptides is even more difficult to ascertain than that of the hormones. VIP has been postulated as important in controlling sphincter relaxation and intestinal blood flow. Recently it has been shown that stimulation of the chorde tympani nerve to the salivary gland in the presence of atropine results in significant VIP release into the venous effluent, coinciding with the well-known salivary vasodilation that occurs. Intracarotid VIP infusions producing a similar concentration of VIP in the salivary venous effluent results in a closely similar vasodilation of the gland (13). Such experiments provide much support for the postulated neuro-transmitter role of VIP.

Somatostatin

Somatostatin is one of the most powerful inhibitory agents known, blocking the release of many gut hormones and independently causing additional direct inhibition of gastrointestinal secretions. The presence of large amounts of somatostatin throughout the gastrointestinal tract, localized to a particular type of endocrine cell, would suggest that a local, or paracrine role is most likely. Nonetheless, significant quantities of somatostatin have been reported in the circulation after appropriate physiological stimuli (42). Clearly, further work is required to validate this systemic release of somatostatin and to show that the concentrations achieved are likely to be effective biologically.

Bombesin

Bombesin, a peptide first extracted from amphibian skin, has now been found in significant quantities in the mammalian gastrointestinal tract. On infusion in man, it has effects that are mostly the opposite of those achieved by somatostatin. It stimulates gastric pancreatic secretion and is effective at releasing many different gut hormones, including gastrin, neurotensin, pancreatic polypeptide, motilin, and enteroglucagon (32). Unlike somatostatin, bombesin is localized in nerves; nonetheless, it is tempting to speculate that this exists in an agonist-antagonist control system.

Substance P

Substance P, the first substance to be localized both in brain and gut, is associated with pain transmission in the spinal cord. Pharmacologically, it stimulates contractions of smooth muscle, but its physiological role in the gut is unknown.

Endorphins

There are considerable amounts of both leucine- and methionine-enkephalin in the gastrointestinal tract. It is noteworthy that the opiates were first discovered because of their anti-diarrheal action. The physiological role of the enkephalins is nonetheless unknown. Progress is likely to be more rapid in this field, however, because of the availability of a highly specific inhibitor of enkephalin, naloxone. Most experiments so far have been performed with doses of naloxone sufficient to block circulating opiates, whereas the quantity likely to be effective against enkephalin released from synapses near the effector tissue is likely to be an order of magnitude greater.

SUMMARY

Our understanding of the physiology of gut hormones is in its early stage when compared with the mass of data available for other endocrine systems. However, the tools are now available, and only require further investigative effort for much of the problem to be solved. The investigation of the related peptidergic nervous system is likely to prove far more difficult. Nonetheless, it is now possible to see the major components of the gut control system and assess the true nature of the problem. Once a problem has been defined, mankind usually finds some way of quickly solving it.

REFERENCES

1. Adrian, T. E., Besterman, H. S., and Bloom, S. R. (1979): The importance of cholinergic tone in the release of pancreatic polypeptide by gut hormones in man. *Life Sci.,* 24:1989–1994.
2. Adrian, T. E., Bloom, S. R., Besterman, H. S., Barnes, A. J., Cooke, T. J. C., Russell, R. C. G., and Faber, R. G. (1977): Mechanism of pancreatic polypeptide release in man. *Lancet,* 1:161–163.
3. Adrian, T. E., Bloom, S. R., Bryant, M. G., Polak, J. M., Heitz, Ph., and Barnes, A. J. (1976): Distribution and release of human pancreatic polypeptide. *Gut,* 17:940–944.
4. Adrian, T. E., Bloom, S. R., Hermansen, K., and Iversen, J. (1978): Pancreatic polypeptide, glucagon and insulin secretion from the isolated perfused canine pancreas. *Diabetologia,* 14:413–417.
5. Adrian, T. E., Greenberg, G. R., Besterman, H. S., McCloy, R. F., Chadwick, V. S., Barnes, A. J., Mallinson, C. N., Baron, J. H., Alberti, K. G. G. M., and Bloom, S. R. (1978): Pancreatic polypeptide infusion in man—Summary of initial investigations. In: *Gut Hormones,* edited by S. R. Bloom, pp. 265–267. Churchill Livingstone, Edinburgh.
6. Andersson, S., Chang, D., Folkers, K., and Rosell, S. (1976): Inhibition of gastric acid secretion in dogs by neurotensin. *Life Sci.,* 19:367–370.
7. Andersson, S., Rosell, S., Hjelmquist, U., Chang, D., and Folkers, K. (1977): Inhibition of gastric and intestinal motor activity in dogs by (Gln) neurotensin. *Acta Physiol. Scand.,* 100:231–235.
8. Besterman, H. S., Sarson, D. L., Ghatei, M. A., and Bloom, S. R. (1979): Enteroglucagon in disease states. *J. Endocrinol.,* 81:153–154.
9. Bloom, S. R. (1972): An enteroglucagon tumour. *Gut,* 13:520–523.
10. Bloom, S. R. (1978): Vasoactive intestinal peptide, the major mediator of the WDHA (pancreatic cholera) syndrome: Value of measurement in diagnosis and treatment. *Am. J. Dig. Dis.* 23:373–376.
11. Bloom, S. R., Adrian, T. E., Barnes, A. J., and Polak, J. M. (1979): Autoimmunity in diabetics induced by hormonal contaminants of insulin. *Lancet,* 1:14–17.
12. Bloom, S. R., Christofides, N. D., and Besterman, H. S. (1978): Raised motilin in diarrhoea. *Gut,* 19:A959.
13. Bloom, S. R., and Edwards, A. V. (1979): The relationship between release of VIP in the salivary gland of the cat in response to parasympathetic stimulation and the atropine resistant vasodilatation. *J. Physiol. (Lond.),* 295:35P.
14. Bloom, S. R., Mitznegg, P., and Bryant, M. G. (1976): Measurement of human plasma motilin. *Scand. J. Gastroenterol.,* 11 (S39):47–52.
15. Brown, J. C., Cook, M. A., and Dryburgh, J. R. (1973): Motilin, a gastric motor activity stimulating polypeptide: The complete amino acid sequence. *Can. J. Biochem.,* 51:533–537.
16. Brown, J. C., Johnson, L. P., and Magee, D. F. (1966): Effect of duodenal alkalinization on gastric motility. *Gastroenterology,* 50:333–339.
17. Brown, J. C., Mutt, V., and Dryburgh, J. R. (1971): The further purification of motilin, a gastric motor activity stimulating polypeptide from the mucosa of the small intestine of hogs. *Can. J. Physiol. Pharmacol.,* 49:399–405.
18. Brown, J. C., and Otte, S. C. (1978): Gastrointestinal hormones and the control of insulin secretion. *Diabetes,* 27:782–789.
19. Chey, W. Y. (1978): Immunoreactive secretin and exocrine pancreatic secretion. *Gastroenterology,* 75:912–913.
20. Christofides, N. D., Bloom, S. R., and Besterman, H. S. (1978): Physiology of motilin II. In: *Gut Hormones,* edited by S. R. Bloom, pp. 343–350. Churchill Livingstone, Edinburgh.
21. Christofides, N. D., Bloom, S. R., Besterman, H. S., Adrian, T. E., and Ghatei, M. A. (1979): Release of motilin by oral and intravenous nutrients in man. *Gut,* 20:102–106.

22. Christofides, N. D., Modlin, I. M., Fitzpatrick, M. L., and Bloom, S. R. (1979): Effect of motilin on the rate of gastric emptying and gut hormone release. *Gastroenterology,* 76:903–907.
23. Creutzfeldt, W. (1979): The incretin concept today. *Diabetologia,* 16:75–85.
24. Dupre, J., Ross, S. A., Watson, D., and Brown, J. C. (1973): Stimulation of insulin secretion by gastric inhibitory peptide in man. *J. Clin. Endocrinol. Metab.,* 37:826–828.
25. Greenberg, G. R., McCloy, R. F., Adrian, T. E., Baron, J. H., and Bloom, S. R. (1978): Effect of bovine pancreatic polypeptide on gastric acid and pepsin output in man. *Acta Hepatogastroenterol. (Stuttg.),* 25:384–387.
26. Greenberg, G. R., McCloy, R. F., Adrian, T. E., Chadwick, V. S., Baron, J. H., and Bloom, S. R. (1978): Inhibition of pancreas and gallbladder by pancreatic polypeptide. *Lancet,* 2:1280–1282.
27. Hazelwood, R. L., and Turner, S. D. (1973): Spectrum effects of a new polypeptide (third hormone?) isolated from the chicken pancreas. *Gen. Comp. Endocrinol.,* 21:485–497.
28. Heitz, Ph., Polak, J. M., Bloom, S. R., and Pearse, A. G. E. (1976): Identification of the D_1-cell as the source of human pancreatic polypeptide (HPP). *Gut* 17:755–758.
29. Itoh, Z., Takeuchi, S., Aizawa, I., Mori, K., Taminato, T., Seino, Y., and Imura, H. (1978): Changes in plasma motilin concentration and gastrointestinal contractile activity in conscious dogs. *Amer. J. Dig. Dis.,* 23:929–935.
30. Kimmel, J. R., Pollock, H. G., and Hazelwood, R. L. (1968): Isolation and characterization of chicken insulin. *Endocrinology* 83:1323–1330.
31. Larsson, L.-I., Sundler, F., and Hakanson, R. (1976): Pancreatic polypeptide—A postulated new hormone: Identification of its cellular storage site by light and electron microscopic immunocytochemistry. *Diabetologia,* 12:211–226.
32. Lezoche, F., Ghatei, M. A., Carlei, F., Blackburn, A. M., Basso, N., Adrian, T. E., Speranza, V., and Bloom, S. R. (1979): Gut hormone responses to bombesin in man. *Gastroenterology,* 76:A1185.
33. Lin, T. M., and Chance, R. E. (1972): Spectrum gastrointestinal actions of a new bovine pancreas polypeptide (BPP). *Gastroenterology,* 62:A852.
34. Lin, T. M., and Chance, R. E. (1978): Spectrum of gastrointestinal actions of bovine pancreatic polypeptide. In: *Gut Hormones,* edited by S. R. Bloom, pp. 242–246. Churchill Livingstone, Edinburgh.
35. Lin, T. M., Evans, D. C., and Bromer, W. W. (1974): Action of a bovine pancreatic polypeptide (BPP) on pancreatic secretion in dogs. *Gastroenterology,* 66:A852.
36. Lin, T. M., Evans, D. C., Chance, R. E., and Spray, G. F. (1977): Bovine pancreatic peptide: Action on gastric and pancreatic secretion in dogs. *Am. J. Physiol.,* 232:311–315.
37. Moody, A. J., Jacobsen, H., and Sundby, F. (1978): Gastric glucagon and gut glucagon-like immunoreactants. In: *Gut Hormones,* edited by S. R. Bloom, pp. 369–378. Churchill Livingstone, Edinburgh.
38. Polak, J. M., Bloom, S. R., Adrian, T. E., Heights, P., Bryant, M. G., and Pearse, A. G. E. (1976): Pancreatic polypeptide in insulinomas, gastrinomas, VIPomas and glucagonomas. *Lancet* 1:328–330.
39. Polak, J. M., Sullivan, S. N., Bloom, S. R., Buchan, A. M. J., Facer, P., Brown, M. R., and Pearse, A. G. E. (1977): Specific localisation of neurotensin to the N cell in human intestine by radioimmunoassay and cytochemistry. *Nature* 270:183–184.
40. Rehfeld, J. F. (1978): Immunochemical studies on cholecystokinin. II. Distribution and molecular heterogeneity in the central nervous system and small intestine of man and hog. *J. Biol. Chem.,* 253:4022–4030.
41. Ruppin, H., Domschke, S., Domschke, W., Wünsch, E., Jaeger, E., and Demling, L. (1975): Effects of 13-Nle-motilin in man: Inhibition of gastric evacuation and stimulation of pepsin secretion. *Scand. J. Gastroenterol.,* 10:199–202.
42. Schusdziarra, V., Harris, V., Conlon, J. M., Arimura, A., and Unger, R. (1978): Pancreatic and gastric somatostatin release in response to intragastric and intraduodenal nutrients and HCl in the dog. *J. Clin. Invest.,* 62:509–518.
43. Schwartz, T. W., Holst, J. J., Fahrenkrug, J., Jensen, S. L., Nielsen, O. V., Rehfeld, J. F., Schaffalitzky de Muckadell, O. B. and Stadil, F. (1978): Vagal, cholinergic regulation of pancreatic polypeptide secretion. *J. Clin. Invest.,* 61:781–789.
44. Soll, A. H. (1978): Gastrin-histamine interactions in isolated canine parietal cells. In: *Gut Hormones,* edited by S. R. Bloom, pp. 149–150. Churchill Livingstone, Edinburgh.

45. Solomon, T. E., and Grossman, M. I. (1979): Effect of atropine and vagotomy on response of transplanted pancreas. *Am. J. Physiol.,* 236:186–190.
46. Taylor, I. L., Feldman, M., Richardson, C. T., and Walsh, J. H. (1978): Gastric and cephalic stimulation of human pancreatic polypeptide release. *Gastroenterology,* 75:432–437.
47. Vantrappen, G., Janssens, J., Peeters, T. L., Bloom, S. R., Christofides, N. D., and Hellmans, J. (1979): Motilin and the interdigestive migrating motor complex in man. *Dig. Dis. Sci.,* 24:497–500.
48. Walsh, J. H., and Grossman, M. I. (1975): Gastrin. *N. Engl. J. Med.,* 292:1377–1384.
49. Walsh, J. H., Isenberg, J. I., Ansfield, J., and Maxwell, V. (1976): Clearance and acid-stimulating action of human big and little gastrins in duodenal ulcer subjects. *J. Clin. Invest.,* 57:1125–1131.

Polypeptide Hormones, edited by
R. F. Beers, Jr. and E. G. Bassett.
Raven Press. New York © 1980.

38. Discussion

Moderator: Stephen R. Bloom

J. D. Gardner: I wonder if Gerry Smith could go over the feeding data in man. Maybe it is the way that data are analyzed, but it looked to me like a virtual superimposition of the experimental and control data.

G. P. Smith: The data essentially are that 9 out of 12 young men decreased their food intake during a lunch with infusion of CCK octapeptide. For the group, for all 12, the difference between the two saline infusion days and the octapeptide days is about 125 of almost 600 g of food.

So we are talking about something like a 15 or so percent inhibition for the group.

S. R. Bloom: The data you showed looked like the people who got the CCK stopped eating about a minute earlier.

G. P. Smith: Yes, that is true for 8 of the 12.

S. R. Bloom: Is that a physiologically significant difference?

G. P. Smith: I don't know. It is different in terms of the total amount of food eaten at that meal. If in fact one could replicate that for three meals a day, it would be very effective in cutting food consumption.

G. J. Dockray: I would like to add that in patients after vagotomy, there isn't an appreciable difference in their food intake and, therefore, do you think that the phenomenon you studied is physiologically significant?

G. P. Smith: I believe that something as complex as satiety is not going to be managed by only one signal.

The fact that vagotomy blocks the CCK effect in rats doesn't mean that other satiety signals can't be operating. The fact that vagotomized humans and animals show satiety, and the fact that, under certain test conditions, they will eat smaller meals than usual, doesn't really bear on the physiological implications of the vagal satiety factors.

In fact, the bombesin effect, that Gibbs has shown, escapes the vagotomy in the rat. That is, in the same animal model in which the satiety effect of CCK is abolished by vagotomy.

S. R. Bloom: Do you have any concept of the role of pancreatic polypeptide, which has been reported to be absent in the OB-OB and NZO mouse models and to be important for appetite control thereof?

G. P. Smith: I know of only the one report of using PP to inhibit food intake in those mouse models. There has been very little work done on it. We are planning to try some studies of this sort.

S. R. Bloom: The reason I asked is that we don't find any difference in the PP concentration in either species of mouse; nor during our infusions in man did we find any diminution of hunger in these volunteers who had to fast before the procedure, but perhaps that is a very crude experiment.

J. M. Polak: Dr. Dockray, you mentioned the molecular forms of gastrin and their presence in the antrum. You very nicely showed the G cells that you can detect with your three well-characterized antibodies.

You then said that they are not only in the same cell, but also possibly in the same granules. Would you explain to me what evidence you have for that and what in your view are the granules of the G cell?

G. J. Dockray: Yes. The current evidence is not overwhelming, but in all the cells that we have examined by means of these thin, serial sections, you get the same pattern of distribution of granules with all the antisera that we have used. We would thus be surprised if there were a substantial proportion of the granules containing only one molecular form or the other.

I think it is quite likely that there is a very small population of immature granules that contain predominantly precursor that hasn't been processed and they may have mainly G34.

So, I would say the distinction there was a quantitative rather than a qualitative one.

J. M. Polak: May I argue the point with you? You showed three G cells with negative nuclei packed throughout the entire cytoplasm with granules. In these cells, the patterns were identical but I don't think you are able to distinguish granules in this manner. What you should have done is compared serial sections under the electron microscope. The distribution of the secretory granules are mixed and you can then distinguish very small dotted granules from very large electrolucent granules.

G. J. Dockray: You have a problem even doing it at the EM level. The thickness of sections is such that you can't get more than two, at the most, serial sections through the same granule.

What you can do, though, is examine an area like the perinuclear area where there is a small rim of granules. When you look in that area, where they are not densely packed, I suppose you can distinguish the granules by the antisera used.

J. M. Polak: You nicely explained the different molecular forms of gastrin in the antrum and the intestine of animals.

I would like to ask if you have any experience concerning distribution of the molecular forms in the human antrum and intestine. How would this tally with our findings of two separate cell types containing gastrin in the antrum and the intestine?

G. J. Dockray: Most mammalian species have virtually no gastrin beyond the pylorus. Below mammals you don't find any gastrin at all and you have to talk exclusively about CCK. It is really only in mammals and birds that you actually have gastrin in the first place.

Human duodenal gastrin, in total amounts, are about 10 to 50% of those in the antrum mucosa and the ratio of molecular forms is quite different from that in the antrum. The antrum, as I showed, is about 5% big gastrin and 95% little gastrin. In the duodenum, it is more like 55% big gastrin and the rest little gastrin.

We can simply take this at face value and say there must be a difference in the processing pathway for the biosynthesis of gastrin. We could perhaps draw a parallel with the synthesis of CCK in the gut.

If you were to tell me that there are morphological differences between gastrin cells in the duodenum and those in the antrum, then I will say that is fair enough because there are also biochemical differences between them.

S. R. Bloom: This is not an unimportant question, as 10% of the male population has ulcers. After a meal in ulcer patients, gastrin rises higher than normal and this may be driving the higher acid output.

Dr. Dockray has studied the possible contribution of big (intestinal?) gastrin but has not, so far, found very dramatic differences.

J. D. Gardner: Julia, didn't you initially report that you couldn't find VIP in nerves in the gut? I thought you said VIP in the intestine was localized exclusively to cells and they were non-nervous cells.

J. M. Polak: Never. In the first report I did on the VIP in 1974, I looked explicitly in the mucosa. We didn't examine the rest of the bowel wall.

G. J. Dockray: But there are nerves in the mucosa. If you looked in the ileum in mammalian species, there are both endocrine cells and VIP nerves.

J. M. Polak: Yes. The early techniques were better at demonstrating cells but, with improvements in fixation, it was possible to show that the majority of VIP was localized in the nerves.

G. P. Smith: Would Dr. Dockray say whether bombesin circulates in the rat, an animal where it seems to be restricted only to nerves?

G. J. Dockray: My guess is that it doesn't.

I can say that there are high concentrations of circulating bombesin in the turkey, which has these endocrine cells, but we haven't looked in rat. In man, however, there are only low concentrations of immunoactive bombesin in the circulation. These appear not to change with feeding, where you might expect a hormonal substance to change.

I am inclined to think that in mammals it is acting as a neurotransmitter and not as a hormone.

H. O. J. Collier: Dr. Gardner showed a dose-response curve for amylase production against VIP that was far to the left of that for cyclic AMP formation. He quite easily explained that by the new concept of "receptor spareness."

Yesterday, Dr. Ramachandran showed a similar pair of curves for corticosteroid production by ACTH. He discussed at length really what was happening and concluded, as we did, to be rather worried about it.

So it was interesting to me that the concept of "receptor spareness" seems to make the whole thing simple. I don't know whether Dr. Gardner would like to comment on the concept of spareness to explain the difference in these two dose-response curves.

J. D. Gardner: Yes, I would. Spareness is a euphemism to hide a great deal of ignorance. That is the first thing to remember.

What is really being referred to is a discrepancy between a dose-response curve for some function and a dose-response for receptor occupation. When the dose-response curve for the function is to the left of that for receptor occupation, the term spareness is usually invoked.

What is important is not so much to recognize that spareness exists but to try to speculate and understand what sorts of mechanisms might be going on.

For many agents that act on cyclic AMP, it appears reasonably clear that the basis for this apparent spareness is for the cell to make more cyclic AMP than is necessary to produce a maximal biological response. That is not the case, however, for agents that act through other pathways, as illustrated with the calcium story. But that is not to diminish the complexity of this because we have a cascade of sequences that occur after the increase in cyclic AMP; so I was just more glib in covering up my ignorance than some of the previous speakers.

H. O. J. Collier: Dr. Bloom showed an enormous number of hormones and hormone-like substances that might interact in the control of gastric acid but I'm not sure I saw prostaglandin on the slide. Now, prostaglandins seem to be implicated in gut control, at least in some forms of diarrhea. I wonder if they form an interrelationship of peptides and hormone-like substances.

S. R. Bloom: In our most recent list we do have the prostaglandins, put in under paracrine. I wasn't quite sure, however, what category to put it under.

I am sure you are right that they are important, as well as several prostaglandin inhibitors exerting an effect on the stomach. One must assume they play an everyday role. Thus, I agree with the concept but how it fits in, I don't know.

H. O. J. Collier: In some interactions, prostaglandin release is sensitive to peptides.

Dr. Kendall: Drs. Polak and Dockray—correct me if I am wrong—were your EM photographs really localized using immune techniques?

I think that you would probably have to apply these at the EM level before you can make really relevant comments about the granule localization.

Are the antigenic determinants that Dr. Dockray finds in his three peptides going to be the same at the tissue level as in the circulating hormone?

Also, can you speculate as to the function of these peptides in the brain? Have you any evidence as to whether they are being secreted in the brain and to their localization?

J. M. Polak: You are absolutely right. At the moment we can't say with complete certainty that the large dense secretory granules we see do correspond to little gastrin.

We do direct cytochemistry but the PAP deposit, which we can detect with

EM, masks the secretory granules. However, in addition to that, there are other technical difficulties in the technique.

Establishing a parallel distribution by plotting the localization of particular types of secretory granules by EM and of particular hormone-producing cells by immunocytochemistry under light microscopy has been extremely valuable in the early days of plotting the endocrine cell in the gut. More recently, we have used semithin serial section technique and also direct immunoelectron cytochemistry.

G. J. Dockray: In immunocytochemistry, the antisera are used at lower dilution than in immunoassay and the first thing we found was that there were several different populations of antibodies, varying in specificity, in each of the antisera that was used.

Now we separated these different populations of antibodies out by immunoaffinity chromatography. To give you an example, the NH_2-terminal-specific, big gastrin antisera also has a minor population of antibodies in it that is specific for the COOH-terminus. These antibodies were of low titer and low affinity so they don't interact in the immunoassay but they nevertheless are involved in the immunocytochemical staining reaction. It is easy enough to get rid of them by simply taking the COOH-terminal fragment of gastrin and coupling it covalently to a support system, such as Sepharose beads and then passing your antiserum through it. The COOH-terminal antibodies stick to it and the rest go through.

In order to check antiserum, what we now do is analyze the binding of radioactive iodinated peptides at the same dilutions of antiserum that we are using in immunocytochemistry. We use the iodinated, intact forms of gastrin G17 and G34 as well as various COOH- and NH_2-terminal fragments and thereby monitor the presence of different antibody preparations.

That is the approach we have used to try to make sure that the specificity is matching up in the two systems and also that we are localizing only the antigenic determinant that we think we are localizing. I should say that, in addition, we do the normal sort of absorption controls that you would expect in immunocytochemistry.

As far as the role of these peptides in the brain is concerned, I can tell you that the octapeptide of CCK (with which we have been most intensely involved) is localized in synaptosomal fractions. You can release it by depolarization and show that the release mechanism is calcium-dependent.

I suppose one could say that this is consistent with a role as a neurotransmitter.

I wouldn't like to go any further in defining its physiological role in the brain at the moment.

B. W. Erickson: Dr. Smith, have you used your protocol in animals that have been surgically altered, such as by pancreatectomy, and might not have involved some of the many other agents that act on the stomach and perhaps feeding behavior? In other words, have you looked at animals that have been

surgically altered so that certain organs are not functional, such as pancreatec-
tomized animals?

G. P. Smith: I am not sure how useful this would be. It is not something
we have turned to because many of these major kind of alterations so alter
the feeding and nutritional status of the animal it invalidates the measurements.

The only alteration that we resorted to thus far has been the surgical preparation of the gastric cannula and the vagotomy procedures.

R. L. Suddith: Dr. Smith, I was particularly struck by your data for the
time course of the attenuation of feeding by the CCK octapeptide. Have you
considered the fact that this is really a secondary response? This question results
from our observation that both the octapeptide and the 33-amino acid forms
of CCK are very efficient at releasing pancreatic polypeptide. Therefore the
question is: Have you tried pancreatic polypeptide?

G. P. Smith: No, not yet.

J. Ramachandran: I would like to disagree with Dr. Collier's statement that
the situation vis-a-vis the adrenal is similar to that shown by Dr. Gardner.

First of all, in the adrenal, steroidogenesis is stimulated by ACTH at physiological concentrations. The rise in cyclic AMP is mostly seen with supraphysiological concentrations. Dr. Gardner is able to see amylase secretion from isolated
pancreatic acina cells at about 30 to 40% of the total cyclic AMP production,
whereas one can see steroid production without seeing any change in cyclic
AMP in the adrenal system.

Therefore, I am not convinced that you can simply extrapolate these results.

I agree there may be spareness as far as steroidogenesis is concerned. Spareness,
if you eliminate cyclic AMP; otherwise there are no spare receptors. They are
merely in excess.

I would also like to emphasize that Dr. Gardner's finding is important in
another way. That is, in the same system, amylase secretion can be induced
by a mechanism that is independent of cyclic AMP; this should also be kept
in view.

J. D. Gardner: I don't know if that was directed to me or a previous comment.
But you said one thing that I want to clear up: In our system, as well as
others, the cell makes more cyclic AMP than is necessary to cause maximal
change in the subsequent biological functions.

What is referred to as spareness between receptor occupation and the changes
in the subsequent biological functions is at the level of the mediator, in this
case, cyclic AMP. You don't have spare receptors as such. The dose-response
curve for occupation of the binding sites superimposes the dose-response curve
for the increase in cyclic AMP.

So, I wasn't trying to make a big point about spareness *per se* but to show
you the kind of results one obtains in studying the function of receptors in an
experiment designed to examine the relationship between receptor occupation
and the change in one or more biological functions.

J. Ramachandran: I agree. In fact, what I was trying to show yesterday was that there were no spare receptors in terms of cyclic AMP production. It seemed to correlate reasonably well. The only point was, in the adrenal system, that it is not yet fully established that cyclic AMP is the messenger. Calcium and cyclic AMP remain as very good candidates.

A. H. Surve: I would like to mention that at a meeting of the Endocrine Society earlier this week, Dr. R. H. Unger reported that they have extracted glucagon from various tissues. Of particular note is that the level in heart tissue was ten times the level in peripheral blood and the concentration did not follow changes in the circulation.

In the discussion that followed, the question was raised as to what this glucagon is doing in the heart muscle. The response suggested that perhaps all tissue has the potential genetic material to synthesize different hormones but some have a mechanism of secretion and others do not. Thus, I wonder about the detection of hormones by immunocytochemical techniques—are they really secreted and perform physiological functions?

S. R. Bloom: Every cell has every peptide, is what you are saying. There certainly seems to be a potential for tumors to produce every sort of peptide, but I don't think that the consensus of evidence would suggest your statement is correct. And I don't know that, for example, there is general agreement that this glucagon-like immunological activity, apparently extractable from cardiac muscle, is in fact true pancreatic glucagon synthesized there. Therefore, it may not be worthwhile speculating on its function if it was synthesized there, intriguing though the concept is.

Polypeptide Hormones, edited by
R. F. Beers, Jr. and E. G. Bassett.
Raven Press, New York © 1980.

39. Introduction to Section F: Thymic Hormones

Nathan Trainin

Department of Cell Biology, The Weizmann Institute of Science, Rehovot, Israel

Although most of the mysteries of thymic function have been solved in only the last 15 to 17 years, this organ was being actively investigated at the turn of the present century. As early as 1900, Maximow (5) elaborated on the interaction between thymocytes and the epithelial elements of the thymus and concluded that the thymus epithelium seems to attract wandering lymphoid cells which are induced to proliferate within the thymus' boundaries. This stimulating effect of the thymic epithelium on lymphoid elements was further stressed by Jolly, who assumed that thymic function was the result of a lympho-epithelial symbiosis (3).

The physiology of the thymus was still largely unknown in the early 1940s until Furth and co-workers established that thymic ablation prevented the appearance of lymphatic leukemia in AKR mice, whereas intact mice with thymus developed the disease and were killed by it (6).

Starting in 1954, Good described a few cases of a rare disease in man, characterized by a marked immunological deficiency accompanied by the development of a benign tumor of the thymus (2). Archer and Pierce in Good's laboratory observed that the removal of the thymus of young rabbits was followed by an impairment of antibody formation (1).

J. F. A. P. Miller (7) then succeeded for the first time in keeping newborn thymectomized mice alive and observed that extirpation of the thymus was followed by a series of dramatic changes in the anatomy of the lymphatic system that lead to the involution of the lymphoid organs; he noted that this was accompanied by a profound deficit in cell-mediated and humoral parameters of immunological function. Therefore, we adopted the hypothesis that thymic function is at least partially mediated by the secretion of a thymic hormone(s). By implanting cell-impermeable diffusion chambers containing thymic tissue into neonatally thymectomized mice, we observed that this procedure restored, to a considerable extent, the impaired immunological capacity created by ablation of the thymus (4).

These observations were confirmed in various laboratories and extended to numerous other species, establishing that the thymus—mainly known as a producer of lymphocytes—was also an endocrine gland and that its products regulated the function of the T-lymphocytes, the targets for hormonal activity. This opened up the field for very active research on the isolation, functional characterization, and chemical purification of thymic factors; as a result, various laboratories accepted the challenge. We have the privilege today of having with us many of the outstanding scientists who have contributed, through their personal endeavors, to the analysis and definition of these products which seem to be the mediators of the endocrine function of the thymus.

Finally, I would like to express my personal respect to Charles Gregoire and J. Comsa, who independently initiated in the 1930s a series of studies that established the foundations on which the whole concept of the thymus as an endocrine organ was built.

REFERENCES

1. Archer, O., and Pierce, J. C. (1961): Role of thymus in development of the immune response. *Fed. Proc.,* 20:26.
2. Good, R. A. (1954): Agammaglobulinemia: A provocative experiment of nature. *Bull. Univ. Minn. Hosp. Minn. Med. Found.,* 26:1–19.
3. Jolly, J. (1913): Sur les organes lympho-epitheliaux. *C.R. Soc. Biol. (Paris),* 74:540–543.
4. Levey, R. H., Trainin, N., and Law, L. W. (1963): Evidence for function of thymic tissue in diffusion chambers implanted in neonatally thymectomized mice: Preliminary report. *J. Natl. Cancer Inst.,* 31:199–217.
5. Maximow, A. (1909): Untersuchungen über Blut- und Bindegewebe. Über die Histogenese des Thymus bei Säugetieren. *Arch. Mikrosk. Anat.,* 74:525–621.
6. McEndy, D. P., Boon, M. C., and Furth, J. (1944): On the role of the thymus, spleen and gonads in the development of leukemia in a high leukemic stock of mice. *Cancer Res.,* 4:377–383.
7. Miller, J. F. A. P. (1961): Immunological function of the thymus. *Lancet,* 2:748–749.

Polypeptide Hormones, edited by
R. F. Beers, Jr. and E. G. Bassett.
Raven Press, New York © 1980.

40. Thymosin: Basic Properties and Clinical Application in the Treatment of Immunodeficiency Diseases and Cancer

Allan L. Goldstein, Teresa L. K. Low, and Gary B. Thurman

Department of Biochemistry, George Washington University School of Medicine and Health Sciences, Washington, D.C. 20037

INTRODUCTION

Thymosin fraction 5, a partially purified bovine thymic extract containing several hormonal-like factors, can partially or completely reconstitute immune function in animals and humans with primary immunodeficiency diseases and cancer (4,7,20,26,29). Sixteen of the polypeptide components of fraction 5 have been purified (29). Characterization of several of these by peptide mapping and sequence analysis have revealed that they are chemically distinct (26,29). Biological studies, using assay systems designed to measure T-cell differentiation and maturation, indicate that several of the active peptides are acting on different subpopulations of T-cells in the maturation sequence.

One of the most active peptide components termed thymosin α_1 (M.W. 3,108) is composed of 28 amino acid residues (15,27,28). Immunofluorescence studies, utilizing an antibody raised in rabbits, has revealed that this peptide is localized in the epithelial cells of the thymus (11,23,38). Studies by Freire et al. (12), utilizing a cell-free wheat germ system and messenger RNA isolated from calf thymus, indicate that α_1 is probably synthesized as a longer peptide chain of 16,000 daltons and is processed (or degraded) to form the smaller peptide detected in preparation of thymus tissues. The chemical synthesis of thymus α_1 has been achieved by several groups using both solution (6,39) and solid-phase (K. A. Folkers, *personal communication*) procedures.

As indicated in Fig. 1, thymosin α_1 acts primarily on prothymocytes to form helper T-cells (1,2). Two other peptides, β_3 (M.W. 5,500 and pI 5.2) and β_4 (M.W. 5,250 and pI 5.1), induce bone marrow T-cell precursors to mature into terminal deoxynucleotidyl transferase positive cells (prothymocytes) and thymocytes (22,31) and appear to act primarily on lymphoid stem cells at an earlier stage in T-cell differentiation (29) (see Fig. 1). An additional peptide, thymosin α_7 (M.W. 2,000 and pI 3.5), is a potent inducer of suppressor

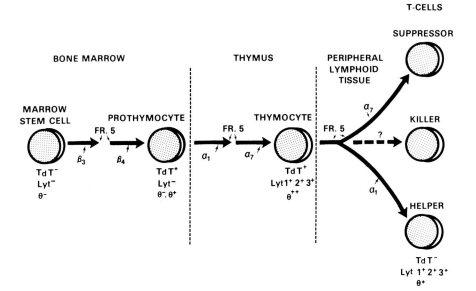

FIG. 1. Proposed sites of action of thymosin peptides on maturation of T-cell subpopulations.

T-cells (2,21). Ongoing studies with this peptide and others indicate quite clearly that the thymus produces a family of thymic hormones or factors that act on different pre-T and T-cell populations to maintain normal immunological balance and reactivity.

Clinical trials with thymosin fraction 5, the most extensively investigated of the thymic hormonal preparations, was initiated in April 1974 in patients with primary immunodeficiency diseases. Significant clinical improvement and partial immunological reconstitution have been observed in many of the children who have received thymosin (13,14,41). Similarly, treatment with thymosin of cancer patients undergoing radiotherapy or chemotherapy has resulted in improvement of several parameters of immunocompetence (9,13,32,33).

The need for larger quantities of thymosin fraction 5 for expanded clinical trials has required extensive scaling up of the purification procedure originally described by Hooper et al. (20). The development of methodologies for large-scale pharmaceutical production of thymosin fraction 5 has been achieved by Dr. Armin Ramel and his colleagues in the Biopolymer Laboratory of Hoffmann-La Roche, Nutley, New Jersey. Since January 1976, all of the thymosin fraction 5 utilized in clinical trials has been prepared by Hoffmann-La Roche. In this chapter we have summarized the current status of the chemical and biological characterization of the purified thymosin peptides and the clinical trials utilizing thymosin fraction 5.

CHEMISTRY OF THYMOSIN POLYPEPTIDES

Nomenclature

Thymosin fraction 5 is a mixture of perhaps as many as 60 heat-stable polypeptides that can be resolved by two dimensional gel electrophoresis or isoelectric focusing visualized by Coomassie blue staining. A number of the peptide components of fraction 5 are products of the thymic epithelial cells and can properly be termed thymic hormones. Other polypeptide components of thymosin fraction 5 are thought to be soluble products of thymic lymphocytes (hence, lymphokines), whereas still other peptides in the fraction 5 preparation (such as β_1 polypeptide) (17,27,28) are undoubtedly ubiquitous cellular components carried through the purification procedure and are without significant activity in terms of participating in homeostatic functions of the thymus.

A nomenclature for the thymosin peptides based on the isoelectric focusing pattern of thymosin fraction 5 in the pH range of 3.5 to 9.5 has been described (15) and is illustrated in Fig. 2. The separated polypeptides are divided into three regions: The α region consists of highly acidic polypeptides with isoelectric points below 5; the β region, 5.0 to 7.0; and the γ region peptides above 7.0. The subscript numbers α_1, α_2, β_1, β_2, etc., are used to identify the polypeptides from that region as they are isolated. The purified polypeptides are tested in various assay systems to study their biological efficacy. The active peptides are then given the prefix "thymosin"; the components that are inactive in our assay systems and are believed not to be involved specifically in controlling T-cell maturation and function are given the prefix "polypeptide," e.g., polypeptide β_1.

Purified Thymosin Polypeptides

Significant progress has been made in the chemical and biological characterization of polypeptide components of thymosin fraction 5, including sequencing of thymosin α_1 (15,27,28), polypeptide β_1 (27,28), thymosin β_3 and β_4 (Low and Goldstein, *in preparation*), and in the chemical synthesis of α_1 by both chemical solution synthesis and solid-phase methodologies (21,22,31). Properties of individual polypeptides that have been characterized to date are summarized below.

Thymosin α_1

Thymosin α_1 is the first polypeptide to be isolated from the highly acidic region of thymosin fraction 5. This peptide is a potent inducer of helper T-cells (Fig. 1) and is highly active in several bioassay systems (6,13,15,28,36, 39). Thymosin α_1 was isolated from fraction 5 by ion-exchange chromatography

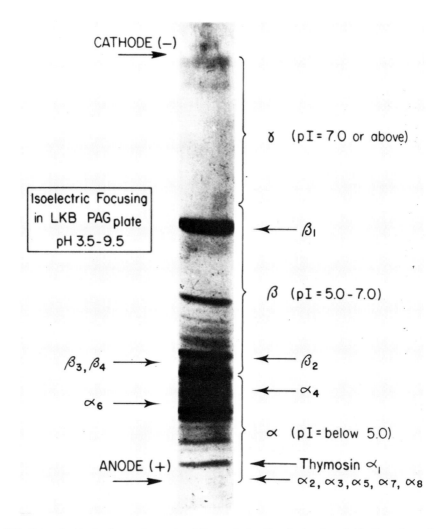

FIG. 2. Isoelectrically focused sample of thymosin fraction 5 showing distribution of mostly acidic peptide components. The α, β, and γ regions indicate segmentation of the gel based on isoelectric point (pl) ranges suggested for peptide nomenclature to facilitate interlaboratory comparison of purified thymic extracts.

on CM-cellulose and DEAE-cellulose, as well as gel filtration on Sephadex G-75 in guanidine hydrochloride (15,27,28). The yield of thymosin α_1 from fraction 5 is about 0.6%. Thymosin α_1, as illustrated in Fig. 3, is a polypeptide consisting of 28 amino acid residues with a molecular weight of 3,108. The NH_2-terminus of thymosin α_1 is blocked by an acetyl group.

Comparison of the sequence of thymosin α_1 with the published sequence of other thymic factors such as thymopoietin (34) and serum thymic factor (4)

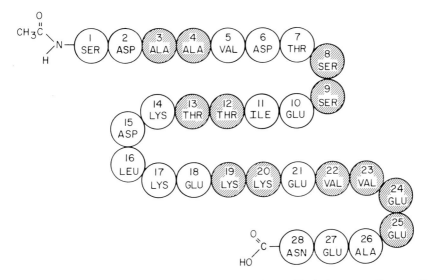

FIG. 3. Complete amino acid sequence of bovine thymosin α_1. *Shaded areas* are the repeating amino acid residues along the polypeptide chain.

reveals no homology. Computer analysis of the sequence of α_1 has established that α_1 bears very little homology to any of the 957 protein sequences that have been published to date (National Biomedical Research Foundation, *personal communication*).

Recently, Freire et al. (12) performed experiments to determine whether some of the reported thymic hormones are actually synthesized in the thymus gland. The translation of messenger RNA isolated from calf thymus was carried out in the cell-free wheat germ system. Some of the radioactive products that were immunoprecipitable with antisera against thymosin fraction 6 were analyzed and found to be identical to those expected for tryptic peptides from thymosin α_1. The results indicate that thymosin α_1 is synthesized in the thymus. Furthermore, α_1 is probably synthesized as a longer peptide chain of 16,000 daltons and is processed (or degraded) to form the peptide detected in preparations isolated from the thymus.

Thymosin α_7

Thymosin α_7 is purified from thymosin fraction 5 by ion-exchange chromatography on CM-cellulose and DEAE-cellulose and gel filtration on Sephadex G-75 (Low and Goldstein, *in preparation*). It is a highly acidic peptide with an isoelectric point around 3.5 and a molecular weight of approximately 2,200. The amino acid composition of this molecule revealed that this molecule does not contain any basic amino acid residues, but contains about 50% of aspartic acid (or asparagine) and glutamic acid (or glutamine). Ahmed et al. (2) observed that thymosin α_7 induces $Lyt^{1+,2+,3+}$ cells in the B layer of bovine serum albumin gradient-separated bone marrow cells and is a potent inducer of suppressor T-cells. Horowitz et al. (21) similarly found that thymosin α_7 reconstitutes suppressor cell function *in vitro* in lymphocytes of patients with systemic lupus erythematosus (SLE). These results suggest thymosin α_7 is acting on prothymocytes to form cells with suppressor function (Fig. 1).

Thymosin β_3 and β_4

Thymosin β_3 and β_4 are prepared from the 50 to 95% ammonium sulfate precipitate of thymosin fraction 3 by DEAE-cellulose and gel filtration on Sephadex G-75 (Low and Goldstein, *in preparation*). Thymosin β_3 has an isoelectric point of 5.2 and a molecular weight of approximately 5,500. Thymosin β_4 has an isoelectric point of 5.1 and a molecular weight of approximately 5,250. From the partial sequence obtained from these polypeptides (Low and Goldstein, *unpublished observations*), they appear to share an identical sequence through most of their NH_2-terminal part (about 45 residues) and differ in the COOH-terminal part (about 8 residues). Both preparations induce terminal deoxynucleotidyl transferase (TdT) positive cells *in vitro* and the A and B layers of bovine serum albumin gradient-separated nude mouse bone marrow cells (31). They also accelerate the repopulation of TdT-positive cells *in vivo* in thymocytes of hydrocortisone acetate-treated C57B1/6J mice (13). From these results, it has been postulated that thymosin β_3 and β_4 may be acting on stem cells to form prothymocytes (Fig. 1).

Purification of Non-Hormonal Peptides from Thymosin Fraction 5

To date, only one of the non-hormonal peptides, termed polypeptide β_1, has been purified from thymosin fraction 5. The polypeptide, which is present as the most prominent staining band in the β region of the isoelectric focusing profile, is a ubiquitous, non-histone chromosomal protein. Since it is devoid of significant functional activity in our assays, it is routinely used as a control protein. For purposes of classification, as it was isolated from the β region of fraction 5, it has been termed polypeptide β_1.

Polypeptide β_1

Polypeptide β_1 is the predominant band on the isoelectric focusing gel of fraction 5 (see Fig. 2). It was isolated from thymosin as previously described (28). It has a molecular weight of 8,451 and an isoelectric point of 6.7. The amino acid sequence of β_1 has been determined (27) and has revealed that this molecule is identical to ubiquitin (35) and a portion of protein A24, a nuclear chromosomal protein (30). Using a pyrogen-free preparation of β_1, we have not been able to substantiate the report that this protein termed "ubiquitin" induces cyclic AMP in lymphocyte cultures (17,28). Polypeptide β_1 does not show biological activity in our bioassay systems, indicating that it is not an important molecule for T-cell maturation.

SUMMARY OF CLINICAL TRIALS WITH THYMOSIN FRACTION 5

Over 100 children have received thymosin for a variety of primary immunodeficiency diseases (16,18,19,40,41). These patients have been treated with injections of thymosin up to 400 mg/m² for periods of over 6 years (usually daily for 2 to 4 weeks, then once per week). Most of the patients have received 60 mg/m² thymosin by subcutaneous injection. To date, there has been no evidence of liver, kidney, or bone marrow toxicity in this group due to thymosin administration. More than 80% of the pediatric patients who have responded *in vitro* in the E-rosette assay have also responded *in vivo*. A significant increase in T-lymphocyte number and function has been observed in over 40% of the patients studied who responded *in vitro* (E-rosette, MLR) (3,5,17,40,41). Significant clinical improvement has also been observed in a number of cases, particularly in children with thymic hypoplasia, DiGeorge Syndrome, and Wiskott-Aldrich Syndrome (3,5,17,40,41). *In vivo* treatment of patients with thymosin has also been found to induce appearance of serum thymic factor (10).

Phase I and Phase II Cancer Trials

More than 150 cancer patients have been treated according to phase I (9,10, 17,18,32) or phase II protocols (7,8,10,13,25). Cancer patients have been treated for periods of up to 4 years. As with pediatric patients, no major side effects have been seen in the majority of patients.

The first phase II randomized trial of thymosin has recently been completed in nonresectable small cell carcinoma of the lungs by Dr. Paul B. Chretien (National Cancer Institute) and Dr. Martin Cohen and associates at the Washington, D.C. Veterans Administration Hospital (8,25). In this trial, thymosin fraction 5 was found to significantly prolong the survival of cancer patients when given in conjunction with intensive chemotherapy. Mean survival time was increased from 240 days with chemotherapy alone to over 450 days with chemotherapy plus 60 mg/m² thymosin twice a week for the first six weeks of the chemotherapy induction period.

Six of the original twenty-one patients in the high dose thymosin group were alive and tumor-free at over 2 years (M. Cohen, *personal communication*).

Autoimmune Disease

To date, six patients with autoimmune diseases have been treated with thymosin fraction 5 in phase I study for periods ranging from 4 to 16 months (24).

Five of the patients had SLE and the sixth had rheumatoid arthritis. Thymosin administration resulted in improvement in immunological parameters and a major decrease in a cytotoxic serum factor that is present in the sera of many patients with autoimmune diseases. This heterologous factor causes the lysis of murine thymocytes in the presence of complement. Based on these encouraging findings, phase II randomized trials are planned to determine the efficacy of thymosin therapy in SLE. Although the mechanism of immune reconstitution with thymosin fraction 5 in persons with autoimmune disease is not as yet defined, it may be related, in part, to induction of a subpopulation of thymosin-activated suppressor or regulator T-cells.

CONCLUSIONS

Considerable progress has been made in the chemical and biological characterization of the thymosin peptides. Several of the peptide components of fraction 5 have been purified, sequenced, and studied in assay systems designed to measure T-cell differentiation and function. These studies indicate that a number of the purified peptides act on different subsets of T-cells to influence and perhaps control various steps in the differentiation and maturation of cells of the T-cell lineage (see Fig. 1). The thymosin peptides appear to play an important role in the overall maintenance of immune balance and homeostasis.

In the clinical area, pediatric and cancer trials completed to date would point to a potential significant role for thymosin in the treatment of diseases associated with thymic malfunctions, such as the immunodeficiency diseases, cancer and perhaps other so-called diseases of aging such as the rheumatic diseases.

It is becoming increasingly clear that immunological maturation is a process involving a complex number of steps and that a single factor initiating a single cellular event may not be reflected by any meaningful immunological reconstitution unless it is the only peptide lacking in the particular immunological disorder. Given the complexity of maturation of T-cells and the increasing numbers of T-cell subpopulations that are being identified, it would be surprising if a single thymic factor can control all of the steps and populations involved. Rather, it would appear that the control of T-cell maturation and function involves a number of thymic-specific factors and other molecules that rigidly control the intermediary steps of the differentiation process of T-cell lineage in an analogous manner to that established with the complement system.

ACKNOWLEDGMENTS

This study was supported in part by grants from the National Cancer Institute (CA 25017 and CA 24974), the Battelle Memorial Foundation, and Hoffmann-La Roche, Inc.

REFERENCES

1. Ahmed, A., Smith, A. H., Wong, D. M., Thurman, G. B., Goldstein, A. L., and Sell, K. W. (1978): *In vitro* induction of Lyt surface markers on precursor cells incubated with thymosin polypeptides. *Cancer Treat. Rep.,* 62:1739–1747.
2. Ahmed, A., Wong, D. M., Thurman, G. B., Low, T. L. K., Goldstein, A. L., Sharkis, S. J., and Goldschneider, I. (1979): T-lymphocyte maturation: Cell surface markers and immune function induced by T-lymphocyte cell-free products and thymosin polypeptides. *Ann. N.Y. Acad. Sci.,* 332:81–94.
3. Astaldi, A., Astaldi, G. C. B., Wijermans, P., Groenewoud, M., Schellekens, P. Th. A., and Eijsvoogel, V. P. (1977): Thymosin-induced serum factor increasing cyclic AMP. *J. Immunol.,* 119:1106–1108.
4. Bach, J.-F., Dardenne, M., and Pleau, J.-M. (1977): Biochemical characterization of a serum thymic factor. *Nature,* 266:55–57.
5. Barrett, D. J., Wara, D. W., Ammann, A. J., and Cowan, M. J. (1980): Thymosine therapy in the Di George syndrome. *J. Pediatr. (in press).*
6. Birr, C., and Stollenwerk, U. (1979): Synthesis of thymosin α_1, a polypeptide of the thymus. *Angew. Chem.,* 91:422–423.
7. Chretien, P. B., Lipson, S. D., and Makuch, R. (1978): Thymosin in cancer patients: *In vitro* effects and correlations with clinical response to thymosin immunotherapy. *Cancer Treat. Rep.,* 62:1787–1790.
8. Cohen, M. H., Chretien, P. B., and Ihle, N. C. (1979): Thymosin fraction 5 prolongs the survival of small cell lung cancer patients treated with intensive combination chemotherapy. *JAMA,* 241:1813–1815.
9. Costanzi, J. J., Gagliano, R. G., Loukas, D., Delaney, F., Sakai, H., Harris, N. S., Thurman, G. B., and Goldstein, A. L. (1974): The effect of thymosin on patients with disseminated malignancies: A phase I study. *Cancer,* 40:14–19.
10. Costanzi, J. J., Harris, N., and Goldstein, A. L. (1978): Thymosin in patients with disseminated solid tumors. Phase I and II results. In: *Immune Modulation and Control of Neoplasia by Adjuvant Therapy,* edited by M. A. Chirigos, pp. 373–380. Raven Press, New York.
11. Dalakas, M. C., Engel, W. K., McClure, J. E., and Goldstein, A. L. (1980): Thymosin α_1 in myasthenia gravis. *N. Engl. J. Med.,* 302:1092–1093.
12. Freire, M., Crivellaro, O., Isaacs, C., and Horecker, B. L. (1978): Translation of mRNA from calf thymus in the wheat germ system: Evidence for a precursor of thymosin α_1. *Proc. Natl. Acad. Sci. USA,* 75:6007–6011.
13. Goldstein, A. L. (1978): Thymosin: Basic properties and clinical potential in the treatment of patients with immunodeficiency diseases and cancer. *Antibiot. Chemother.,* 24:47–59.
14. Goldstein, A. L., Cohen, G. H., Rossio, J. L., Thurman, G. B., Brown, C. N., and Ulrich, J. T. (1976): Use of thymosin in the treatment of primary immunodeficiency diseases and cancer. *Med. Clin. North Am.,* 60:591–606.
15. Goldstein, A. L., Low, T. L. K., McAdoo, M., McClure, J., Thurman, G. B., Rossio, J., Lai, C.-Y., Chang, D., Wang, S.-S., Harvey, C., Ramel, A. H., and Meienhofer, J. (1977): Thymosin α_1: Isolation and sequence analysis of an immunologically active thymic polypeptide. *Proc. Natl. Acad. Sci. USA,* 74:725–729.
16. Goldstein, A. L., and Rossio, J. L. (1978): Thymosin for immunodeficiency diseases and cancer. *Compr. Ther.,* 4:49–57.
17. Goldstein, A. L., Thurman, G. B., Low, T. L. K., Rossio, J. L., and Trivers, G. E. (1978): Hormonal influences on the reticuloendothelial system: Current studies of the role of thymosin in the regulation and modulation of immunity. *J. Reticuloendothel. Soc.,* 23:253–266.
18. Goldstein, A. L., Thurman, G. B., Rossio, J. L., and Costanzi, J. J. (1977): Immunological reconstitution of patients with primary immunodeficiency diseases and cancer after treatment with thymosin. *Transplant. Proc.,* 9:1141–1144.
19. Goldstein, A. L., Wara, D. W., Ammann, A. J., Sakai, H., Harris, N. S., Thurman, G. B., Hooper, J. A., Cohen, G. H., Goldman, A. S., Costanzi, J. J., and McDaniel, M. C. (1975): First clinical trial with thymosin: Reconstitution of T cells in patients with cellular immunodeficiency diseases. *Transplant. Proc.,* 7:681–686.
20. Hooper, J. A., McDaniel, M. C., Thurman, G. B., Cohen, G. H., Schulof, R. S., and Goldstein,

A. L. (1975): The purification and properties of bovine thymosin. *Ann. N. Y. Acad. Sci.,* 249:125–144.

21. Horowitz, S., Borcherding, W., Moorthy, A. V., Chesney, R., Schulte-Wissermann, H., Hong, R., and Goldstein, A. (1977): Induction of suppressor T cells in systemic lupus erythematosus by thymosin and cultured thymic epithelium. *Science,* 197:999–1001.

22. Hu, S. K., Low, T. L. K., and Goldstein, A. L. (1979): *In vivo* induction of terminal deoxynucleotidyl transferase (TdT) by thymosin in hydrocortisone acetate (HcA) treated mice. *Fed. Proc.,* 38:1079 (Abstr. 4501).

23. Kater, L. Oosterom, R., McClure, J., and Goldstein, A. L. (1979): Presence of thymosin-like factors in human thymic epithelium conditioned medium. *Int. J. Immunopathol.,* 1:273–284.

24. Lavastiva, M. T., Rossio, J. L., Goldstein, A. L., and Daniel, J. D. (1979): *(submitted for publication).*

25. Lipson, D. S., Chretien, P. B., and Makuch, R. (1979): Thymosin immunotherapy in patients with small cell carcinoma of the lung (correlation of *in vitro* studies with clinical course). *Cancer,* 43:863–870.

26. Low, T. L. K., and Goldstein, A. L. (1978): Structure and function of thymosin and other thymic factors. In: *The Year in Hematology,* edited by R. D. Silber, A. S. Gordon, and J. LoBue, pp. 281–319. Plenum Press, New York.

27. Low, T. L. K., and Goldstein, A. L. (1979): The chemistry and biology of thymosin. II. Amino acid sequence analysis of thymosin α_1 and polypeptide β_1. *J. Biol. Chem.,* 254:987–995.

28. Low, T. L. K., Thurman, G. B., McAdoo, M., McClure, J., Rossio, J., Naylor, P. H., and Goldstein, A. L. (1979): The chemistry and biology of thymosin. I. Isolation, characterization and biological activities of thymosin α_1 and polypeptide β_1 from calf thymus. *J. Biol. Chem.,* 254:981–986.

29. Low, T. L. K., Thurman, G. B., Chincarini, C., McClure, J. E., Marshall, G. D., Hu, S. K., and Goldstein, A. L. (1979): Current status of thymosin research: Evidence for the existence of a family of thymic factors that control T-cell maturation. *Ann. N. Y. Acad. Sci.,* 332:33–48.

30. Olson, M. O. J., Goldknopf, I. L., Guetzow, K. A., James, G. T., Hawkins, T. C., Mays-Rothberg, C. J., and Busch, H. (1976): The NH$_2$- and COOH-terminal amino acid sequence of nuclear portein A24. *J. Biol. Chem.,* 251:5901–5903.

31. Pazmino, N. H., Ihle, J. N., McEwan, R. N., and Goldstein, A. L. (1978): Control of differentiation of thymocyte precursors in the bone marrow by thymic hormones. *Cancer Treat. Rep.,* 62:1749–1755.

32. Rossio, J. L., and Goldstein, A. L. (1977): Immunotherapy of cancer with thymosin. *World J. Surg.,* 1:605–616.

33. Schafer, L. A., Goldstein, A. L., Gutterman, J. U., and Hersh, E. M. (1976): *In vitro* and *in vivo* studies with thymosin in cancer patients. *Ann. N. Y. Acad. Sci.,* 277:609–620.

34. Schlesinger, D. H., and Goldstein, G. (1975): The amino acid sequence of thymopoietin II. *Cell,* 5:361–365.

35. Schlesinger, D. H., Goldstein, G., and Niall, H. D. (1975): The complete amino acid sequence of ubiquitin, an adenylate cyclase-stimulating polypeptide probably universal in living cells. *Biochemistry,* 14:2214–2218.

36. Thurman, G. B., Marshall, G. D., Low, T. L. K., and Goldstein, A. L. (1979): Recent developments in the classification and bioassay of thymosin polypeptides. *Proceedings of the 12th Leucocyte Culture Conference,* pp. 189–199. Academic Press, New York.

37. Thurman, G. B., Rossio, J. L., and Goldstein, A. L. (1977): Thymosin-induced enhancement of MIF production by peripheral blood lymphocytes of thymectomized guinea pigs. In: *Regulatory Mechanisms in Lymphocyte Activation,* edited by D. O. Lucas, pp. 629–631. Academic Press, New York.

38. Van den Tweel, J. G., Taylor, C. R., McClure, J., and Goldstein, A. L. (1978): Detection of thymosin in thymic epithelial cells by an immunoperoxidase method. *Program of the Sixth International Conference on Lymphatic Tissues and Germinal Centers in Immune Reactions,* Abstr. XXX.

39. Wang, S.-S., Kulesha, I. D., and Winter, D. P. (1978): Synthesis of thymosin α_1. *J. Am. Chem. Soc.,* 100:253–254.

40. Wara, D., and Ammann, A. (1978): Thymosin treatment of children with immunodeficiency disease. *Transplant. Proc.,* 10:203–209.

41. Wara, D. W., Goldstein, A. L., Doyle, W., and Ammann, A. J. (1975): Thymosin activity in patients with cellular immunodeficiency, *N. Engl. J. Med.,* 292:70–74.

Polypeptide Hormones, edited by
R. F. Beers, Jr. and E. G. Bassett.
Raven Press, New York © 1980.

41. Thymopoietin and Immunoregulation

Gideon Goldstein and *Catherine Lau

*Ortho Pharmaceutical Corporation, Raritan, New Jersey 08869; and *Ortho
Pharmaceutical Corporation, Don Mills, Ontario M3C 1L9, Canada*

INTRODUCTION

The evolution of life forms is associated with the development of progressively greater complexity and an accompaning proliferation of regulatory mechanisms. The nervous system and the endocrine system are the two traditional regulatory systems, and we now appreciate that the immune system constitutes another highly complex regulatory system devoted to the scrutiny of complex chemical signals within the body (antigens) and the triggering of appropriate effector mechanisms to deal with alterations from the normal. These three major regulatory systems each have their special spheres of influence (Fig. 1). For example, the nervous system is concerned, in general, with the more rapid regulatory responses pertaining to the *milieu extérieur* and also with rapid physiological responses within the body. The endocrine system is more involved, in general,

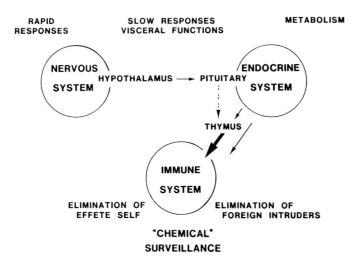

FIG. 1. Spheres of control in the regulation of the mammalian organism. The immune system constitutes an important system of control and regulation that is fully integrated with the nervous and endocrine systems.

with longer term metabolic regulations, whereas the immune system is concerned, as mentioned above, with the antigenic identity of cells, particles, molecules, and surfaces within the body. It is obvious, of course, that these divisions are artificial and that the systems act holistically and in an integrated fashion to regulate the entire organism.

This volume includes chapters emphasizing these integrations, with control of the endocrine system mediated via hypothalamic mechanisms and pari passu endocrine feedbacks on the nervous system itself. The immune system consists of networks of specialized cells that respond during an immune response by a number of mechanisms that are integrated by internal communications between these cells of the immune system (5). Thus, the immune system is highly regulated internally. We would like to develop the theme that this highly regulated system is, in turn, regulated by hormones and that thymic hormones are especially important in affecting the settings of the immunoregulatory networks.

To illustrate this theme, we will deal mainly with the thymic hormone thymopoietin since other chapters in this section will highlight other contributions to the field of thymic hormones. However, we should mention that facteur thymique serique (FTS), a nonapeptide whose structure was elucidated by Bach and colleagues (4), has been synthesized in our laboratories and found to act in a manner similar to, but not identical with, thymopoietin (3). Since thymopoietin and FTS have demonstrably different structures, these findings raise the possibility that the thymus may exert fine control of the immune system by secreting a number of thymic hormones, with overlapping but distinct actions on the various lymphocyte subsets.

RESULTS AND DISCUSSION

Isolation and Structure of Thymopoietin

Thymopoietin is a 49-amino acid polypeptide (17) whose complete sequence is shown in Fig. 2. The tridecapeptide corresponding to the thymopoietin residues 29–41 was synthesized and shown to have biological activity similar to the native molecule (18). Subsequently, a pentapeptide corresponding to residues 32–36 was shown to be the minimal fragment with biological activity (11), and we have focused our major efforts on studies of this pentapeptide, arginyl-lysyl-aspartyl-valyl-tyrosine (Arg-Lys-Asp-Val-Tyr), which we term TP5.

Our studies indicate that thymopoietin is a pleiotropic hormone with many sites of action and this is perhaps emphasized by the fact that it was isolated by its effects on neuromuscular transmission (1,8) rather than by its effects on the immune system. These neuromuscular studies were initiated in relation to study of the human disease, myasthenia gravis (6,9). In this disease, impaired neuromuscular transmission is associated with thymic abnormality; our studies led to the biological demonstration that the thymus exerts a hormonal activity

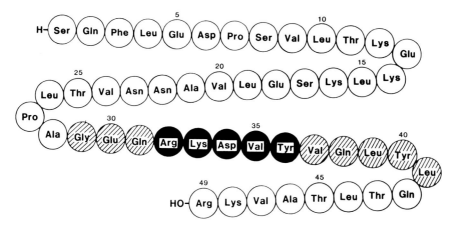

FIG. 2. Complete amino acid sequence of thymopoietin showing synthesized tridecapeptide *(cross-hatched)* and pentapeptide *(solid)* sequences that are biologically active.

effecting neuromuscular transmission (10) and subsequently to the development of a neuromuscular bioassay (7) that was used to monitor the fractionation of thymus extracts during the purification of thymopoietin (8). This purified thymopoietin was found to induce prothymocyte-to-thymocyte differentiation *in vitro* (1). Since the major function of the thymus is the regulation of T-cell differentiation, this finding established that thymopoietin was indeed a thymic hormone concerned in the primary functions of the thymus and not a fortuitously situated endocrine system in the thymus with actions restricted to neuromuscular physiology.

Control and Regulation of a Steady State Population

The lymphocytes, the major components of the immune system, are constantly replenished by progressive differentiation from hemopoietic stem cells. Thus, the maintenance of hemopoietic cells in the adult resembles, in some respects, the ontogenetic development of specialized tissues that occurs during embryogenesis. Hemopoietic stem cells replicate themselves and, at the same time, give rise by asymmetrical division to cells that develop progressive differentiative commitments to the various lines of hemopoietic cells. Cells committed to become T-cells (termed prothymocytes) are induced by thymopoietin to differentiate into thymocytes, and these continue to differentiate and give rise, by processes as yet poorly understood, to the functional subclasses of T-cells whose balanced compositions determine the eventual immune response of the host.

Regulation of such a system could theoretically involve control at a number of points and, again, analogies can be found with the ontogenetic processes that occur during embryogenesis. Certain commitment processes may occur stochastically, and such commitments may involve programs of differentiation not influenced by external signals. On the other hand, external signals could be used to mobilize the release of functionally active cells from reserves, to induce the differentiation of committed cells held in reserve, or to regulate the functional activity of mature cells. It is probable that most of these mechanisms are employed in immunoregulation and perhaps our greatest challenge in dissecting the chemistry of these signals is in devising the appropriate assay systems to detect these molecules.

Already, using chemically synthesized TP5, we can show that thymopoietin has pleiotropic actions, and probably effects immune function by a number of mechanisms including induction of differentiation of prothymocytes to thymocyte, inhibition of induction of B-cell differentiations, and actions on more mature cells that regulate the functional balance of the immune response.

Prothymocyte-to-Thymocyte Induction

Murine spleen and bone marrow contain a small population of cells that lack the surface molecules characteristic of thymocytes and that can be induced *in vitro* to differentiate and display such molecules within 2 hr (16). This forms the basis for the prothymocyte-to-thymocyte induction assay. In the mouse, a number of alloantigenic markers exist so that this transition can be documented in a well-controlled fashion, using antiserums and congenic mouse strains. The induction of T-cell differentiation, which is triggered by thymopoietin and TP5, involves a requirement for brief exposure of the cells to the peptide hormone, and a resultant cyclic AMP signal that is required for approximately 30 min; differentiation then progresses with the display of the surface alloantigens within 2 hr in a process involving transcription of messenger RNA and translation of protein, but not requiring replication of cellular DNA (20). A similar cyclic AMP-mediated inductive process is involved in early B-cell differentiation; these inductions can be used to test the specificity of putative hormonal signals, since a number of agents that elevate intracellular cyclic AMP will drive both differentiations in parallel. By these criteria, thymopoietin and TP5 are selective in inducing only T-cell differentiation and, in fact, inhibit B-cell differentiations (11,16). Similarly, FTS slows relative selectivity in the induction of T-cell differentiation (3).

The induction assay also provides a definition for prothymocytes; namely, they are cells that lack thymocyte surface antigens but can be induced, by exposure to thymopoietin, to display them. Using this operational criterion, it can be shown that prothymocytes are the cells in donor spleen or bone marrow that are responsible for eventual repopulation of the thymus in lethally irradiated recipients (2,12), and that in the normal bone marrow prothymocytes contain the major proportion of the enzyme terminal deoxynucleotidyl transferase (TdT) (19), this being an enzyme found mainly in thymocytes.

Thymopoietin and Peripheral T-Cells

Thymopoietin also affects peripheral T-cells and this can be shown most directly by its effect of elevating cyclic GMP levels in peripheral mononuclear cells (21). Indeed, the most interesting actions of thymopoietin are probably directed toward regulatory lymphocytes in the periphery. Thus, the focus of interest with thymopoietin has shifted from its original detection as a hormone affecting neuromuscular transmission, through studies of its action and specificity on prothymocyte-to-thymocyte differentiation, to its peripheral effects in regulating the immune response.

Unravelling the effects of thymopoietin on immunoregulation offers a great challenge, since the physiology of the cellular mechanisms involved in the regulation of this system is only beginning to be elucidated. Several principles, however, are emerging. First, thymopoietin can prevent some of the changes in lymphocyte subclasses, and corresponding functional changes that follow adult thymectomy (E. Goldberg et al., *unpublished observations*). Second, in the thymus-intact animal, thymopoietin does *not* act simply as an adjuvant that enhances the immune responses, nor does it act as an immunosuppressive agent depressing the immune responses. Rather, it appears to act as an optimizing agent of immunoregulation. Thus, immune responses to suboptimal antigenic stimulation are enhanced, whereas the immune response to optimal antigenic stimulation remains unaffected (14). In animals with depressed immune function, the immune response is enhanced (see below). In animals with exaggerated and abnormal immune responses, exemplified by autoantibodies, the autoimmune response is dampened (see below). Some years ago such claims would have really seemed preposterous, for we are used to agents having unidirectional functions. However, these seemingly contradictory actions of thymopoietin on the immune system, although not fully understood, are quite clear-cut experimentally, and the explanation probably lies in a mode of action directed toward regulatory cells that monitor the state of the immune network, and tend to restore it toward equilibrium. Cellular mechanisms of control networks in the immune system are currently being elucidated and the precise mode of action of thymopoietin remains to be worked out.

Most of the functional activities attributed to thymopoietin have actually been studied with synthetic thymopoietin pentapeptide (TP5) injected intraperitoneally, in some protocols as infrequently as once a week. One feature of these studies is particularly noteworthy. TP5 is especially susceptible to proteolytic enzymes found in plasma and its *in vitro* half-life in human plasma is less than 30 sec (22). Thus, a single injection into an animal provides a chemical stimulus which lasts a few min at most, yet triggers changes in lymphocytes that persist for a period of greater than a week.

Experiments directed toward studying the immunoregulatory actions of TP5 in disease have been directed toward three main areas: aging, autoimmunity, and cancer. Aged mice have well-characterized deficits of immune function and, in certain types of experiments, it can be shown that these are due to deficits or abnormalities in their T-cell population, since reconstitution with T-cells from young animals will largely reconstitute the immune response. TP5 has been shown to be effective in largely restoring the immune responsiveness of aged mice to the youthful pattern in certain protocols (23). Autoantibodies to mouse red blood cells can be provoked in certain mouse strains by injecting the animals with cross-reacting rat red blood cells (15). Injection of TP5 was shown to accelerate the elimination of such autoantibodies in the affected mice, whereas it did not affect the response to extrinsic antigens of rat red blood cells (13). In preliminary studies with transplantable mouse tumor lines, we have suggestive evidence that TP5 inhibits metastasis of Lewis lung carcinoma (C. Lau and G. Goldstein, *unpublished observations*).

Thus these experiments, which provide provocative directions for possible future therapies in man, reemphasize the action of TP5 in normalizing the immune response. In the case of aging and cancer models, impaired immune responses appear to be enhanced by thymopoietin, whereas in the case of autoimmune reactivity an exaggerated and inappropriate response is inhibited.

THE FUTURE

It is clear that we are only beginning to glimpse some features of the endocrine control of the immune system. The complexity of the immune system is best compared to that of the brain, and just as the chemical controls of the brain will need to be unravelled in parallel with understanding of the logic of its function, so will the endocrine control of the immune system need to be studied in parallel with dissection of the logic of immune networks. Already we have seen at this Symposium that there are a number of candidate thymic hormones. In the case of thymopoietin and FTS we see two molecules with quite distinct chemistries, acting in a similar fashion in certain assays yet dissimilarly in other assays. This suggests to us that fine control of the immune system may be exerted by a number of hormone signals with overlapping actions. Indeed, whilst the thymus is an obvious source of peptide signals affecting the immune system, it is to be expected that extra-thymic molecules will also play a part.

Clearly the advent of readily synthesized small molecules with such significant effects on the immune system offers new approaches to therapeutic intervention in man. Alterations of immune function probably occur in a large proportion of human diseases, and appropriate immunoregulation may thus provide therapeutic possibilities in these many diseases.

ACKNOWLEDGMENT

We thank Mrs. Dorothy Collins for typing and editing the manuscript.

REFERENCES

1. Basch, R. S., and Goldstein, G. (1974): Induction of T-cell differentiation *in vitro* by thymin, a purified polypeptide hormone of the thymus. *Proc. Natl. Acad. Sci. USA*, 71:1474–1478.
2. Basch, R. S., Kadish, J. L., and Goldstein, G. (1978): Hematopoietic thymocyte precursors. IV. Enrichment of the precursors and evidence for heterogeneity. *J. Exp. Med.*, 147:1843–1848.
3. Brand, A., Gilmour, D. G., and Goldstein, G. (1977): Effects of a nonapeptide (FTS) on lymphocyte differentiations *in vitro*. *Nature*, 269:597–598.
4. Dardenne, M., Pleau, J. M., Man, N. K., and Bach, J. F. (1977): Structural study of circulating thymic factor: A peptide isolated from pig serum. I. Isolation and purification. *J. Biol. Chem.*, 252:8040–8044.
5. Eardley, D. D., Hugenberger, J., McVay-Boudreau, L., Shen, F. W., Gershon, R. K., and Cantor, H. (1978): Immunoregulatory circuits among T-cell sets. I. T-helper cells induce other T-cell sets to exert feedback inhibition. *J. Exp. Med.*, 147:1106–1115.
6. Goldstein, G. (1966): Thymitis and myasthenia gravis. *Lancet*, 2:1164–1167.
7. Goldstein, G. (1968): The thymus and neuromuscular function. A substance in thymus which causes myositis and myasthenic neuromuscular block in guinea pigs. *Lancet*, 2:119–122.
8. Goldstein, G. (1974): Isolation of a bovine thymin. A polypeptide hormone of the thymus. *Nature*, 247:11–14.
9. Goldstein, G., and Hofmann, W. W. (1968): Electrophysiological changes similar to those of myasthenia gravis in rats with experimental autoimmune thymitis. *J. Neurol. Neurosurg. Psychiatry*, 31:455–459.
10. Goldstein, G., and Hofmann, W. W. (1969): Endocrine function of the thymus affecting neuromuscular transmission. *Clin. Exp. Immunol.*, 4:181–189.
11. Goldstein, G., Scheid, M. P., Boyse, E. A., Schlesinger, D. H., and Van Wauwe, J. (1979): A synthetic pentapeptide with biological activity characteristic of the thymic hormone thymopoietin. *Science*, 204:1309–1310.
12. Komuro, K., Goldstein, G., and Boyse, E. A. (1975): Thymus-repopulating capacity of cells that can be induced to differentiate to T cells *in vitro*. *J. Immunol.*, 115:195–198.
13. Lau, C., Freestone, J., and Goldstein, G. (1980): Effect of thymopoietin pentapeptide (TP5) on autoimmunity. I. TP5 suppression of induced erythrocyte autoantibodies in C3H mice. *J. Immunol. (in press)*.
14. Lau, C., and Goldstein, G. (1980): Functional effects of thymopoietin$_{32-36}$ (TP5) on cytotoxic lymphocyte precursor units (CLP-U). I. Enhancement of splenic CLP-U *in vitro* and *in vivo* following suboptimal antigenic stimulation. *J. Immunol.*, 124:1861–1865.
15. Playfair, J. H., Marshall-Clarke, S. (1973): Induction of red cell autoantibodies in normal mice. *Nature [New Biol.]*, 243:213–214.
16. Scheid, M. P., Goldstein, G., and Boyse, E. A. (1978): The generation and regulation of lymphocyte populations. Evidence from differentiative induction systems *in vitro*. *J. Exp. Med.*, 147:1727–1743.
17. Schlesinger, D. H., and Goldstein, G. (1975): The amino acid sequence of thymopoietin II. *Cell*, 5:361–365.
18. Schlesinger, D. H., Goldstein, G., Scheid, M. P., and Boyse, E. A. (1975): Chemical synthesis of a peptide fragment of thymopoietin II that induces selective T cell differentiation. *Cell*, 5:367–370.
19. Silverstone, A. E., Cantor, H., Goldstein, G., and Baltimore, D. (1976): Terminal deoxynucleotidyl transferase is found in prothymocytes. *J. Exp. Med.*, 144:543–548.
20. Storrie, B., Goldstein, G., Boyse, E. A., and Hämmerling, U. (1976): Differentiation of thymocytes: Evidence that induction of the surface phenotype requires transcription and translation. *J. Immunol.*, 116:1358–1362.
21. Sunshine, G. H., Basch, R. S., Coffey, R. G., Cohen, K. W., Goldstein, G., and Hadden, J. W. (1978): Thymopoietin enhances the allogeneic response and cyclic GMP levels of mouse peripheral, thymus-derived lymphocytes. *J. Immunol.*, 120:1594–1599.
22. Tischio, J. P., Patrick, J. E., Weintraub, H. S., Chasin, M., and Goldstein, G. (1979): Short *in vitro* half-life of thymopoietin$_{32-36}$ pentapeptide in human plasma. *Int. J. Pept. Protein Res.*, 14:479–484.
23. Weksler, M. E., Innes, J. B., and Goldstein, G. (1978): Immunological studies of aging. IV. The contribution of thymic involution to the immune deficiencies of aging mice and reversal with thymopoietin$_{32-36}$. *J. Exp. Med.*, 148:996–1006.

Polypeptide Hormones, edited by
R. F. Beers, Jr. and E. G. Bassett.
Raven Press, New York © 1980.

42. Role of Thymus Humoral Factor, a Thymic Hormone, in the Physiology of the Thymus

Nathan Trainin, Tehila Umiel, *Baruch Klein, and **Israel Kleir

Department of Cell Biology, The Weizmann Institute of Science, Rehovot, Israel

INTRODUCTION

Recent investigations have disclosed that the natural history of a T-lymphocyte starts in the bone marrow. There, its distant ancestor, a stem cell, circulates through the blood and on arrival at the thymus, this cell penetrates the cortical area of this organ. Meanwhile, a series of mitoses and intracellular changes have occurred, transforming it to a thymocyte and, subsequently, a T-thymocyte. The thymus is, therefore, the cradle of T-cell formation and differentiation. Removal of the thymus results in a depletion of cell numbers in particular areas of spleen and lymph nodes, in a decrease in the population of peripheral blood T-cells, and in a reduction in the number of circulating lymphocytes that can be obtained by cannulation of the thoracic duct. These structural defects are accompanied by impairment of lymphocytic activity that could be expressed across the whole gamut of immunological functions (27,28,30–33).

Participation of a thymus humoral factor (THF) in the induction of immunoreactivity has been demonstrated in our laboratory. Thus, partial recovery of cell-mediated and humoral immunological activities were observed in thymectomized mice implanted with thymus tissue contained in cell-impermeable chambers (20–23). It was subsequently demonstrated that administration of extracts of thymus tissue prepared from different species such as mouse, rat, rabbit, sheep, and calf, increases lymphopoiesis in the spleen and lymph nodes as well as the lymphocyte level in peripheral blood of intact and thymectomized mice (54). When thymus extracts were injected into neonatally thymectomized (NTx) mice, partial restoration of their ability to produce an immune response to sheep red blood cells (SRBC) as well as to reject skin and tumor allografts was observed (48,55–57,61). Furthermore, spleen cells from NTx mice gained the capacity to elicit an *in vitro* graft-versus-host (GvH) response when incubated in THF preparations (49,64,65,69). THF also increased the ability of thymocytes to manifest a helper capacity in the SRBC response

---

Present Address: *Department of Medicine, Hasharon Hospital, Petah Tikva, Israel; and **Department of Orthopedics, Beilinson Hospital, Petah Tikva, Israel.

under various *in vitro* and *in vivo* models (10,37). The accumulated information was thus compatible with the notion that the target cells for THF activity were younger elements within the T-cell lineage (26,66,70).

Experiments were performed more recently to further determine the identity of the target cells and the mechanism by which these cells acquire, under the influence of THF, the ability to participate in various immunological processes. We found that when spleen cells or thymocytes from intact mice were incubated for 24 hr in a THF-containing medium and then stimulated by concanavalin A (Con A) or phytohemagglutinin (PHA), a significant increase in the mitogenic activity of the cells tested was obtained. By utilizing a range of THF levels in the medium, it was possible to establish a differential effect on target cells: low concentrations of THF were relatively more effective on Con A reactivity, whereas higher ones increased the PHA response. These results suggested that progressive maturation of target cells by exposure to THF increases the number of cells responding to PHA, by permitting these cells to reach higher levels of maturation. On the other hand, it was observed that THF did not modify the response of spleen cells to LPS (*E. coli* lipopolysaccharide), a B-cell mitogen. Moreover, when spleen cells from nude mice were tested in parallel, no effect of THF on the T-mitogen responses was detected. Similarly, lymph node cells of normal animals showed no increase in mitogenic response after a THF treatment (36,43).

The mixed lymphocyte culture (MLC) is a model that represents the recognition phase of the homograft or of the GvH reactions. The one-way MLC system, in which the stimulating target cells are inactivated by pretreatment with mitomycin C, provides a model for the study of the behavior of cells that respond only to antigenic stimulation. Thus, responding cells from various lymphoid tissues were preincubated in THF for 1 hr and then admixed with mitomycin-treated stimulating cells. It was observed that THF increased the MLC competence of lymphocytes obtained from the spleen and thymus of intact mice and also the spleen of thymus-deprived mice. In contrast, no enhancing effect in the MLC response by THF treatment could be observed when bone marrow-derived spleen cells, cortisone-resistant thymocytes, or lymph node cells were used as the responder cells. These results confirmed our hypothesis that THF leads to differentiation of young thymus-derived (T) cells, promoting them to maturation, and thus to the acquisition of full immunocompetence (59,72,79).

It then became possible to test the effect of THF on tumor development. Indeed, extensive research performed by various groups in our laboratory led to the comprehensive hypothesis that the behavior of T-cells in response to tumor growth might represent a balance between two coexisting subpopulations of T-lymphocytes with opposed activities. One subpopulation seems to enhance tumor growth and to accelerate its evolution, whereas the other inhibits tumor cell multiplication, protecting the animal from the lethal effect of the tumor. We also demonstrated that the activity of the tumor-inhibiting lymphocytes was not apparent in the presence of the tumor-enhancing cells; this finding suggested that, during natural development of a tumor, the effect of the tumor-inhibiting cells may be masked by the activity of tumor-enhancing lymphocytes. These two subpopulations of T-cells could represent either two lines of cells totally distinct from beginning to end, or two successive stages in the maturation of T-cells. Investigations performed in our laboratory in the last 5 years permitted us to establish that an interaction between immature T-cells and syngeneic tumor cells leads to an acceleration and enhancement of tumor growth, whereas the same type of interaction with mature T-cells triggers an opposite response, leading to antitumor activity. When lymphocytes of various sources were sensitized *in vitro* in the presence of THF, increased antitumor activity was observed in both the *in vitro* and *in vivo* models. This led us to postulate that the increase in antitumor activity promoted by THF might involve essentially the same mechanism of cell maturation by which THF appears to confer competence on T-lymphocytes, e.g., the various parameters of cell-mediated immune responses described above. Under these circumstances, the role of THF may be manifested in one or both of the following alternate pathways: (a) the proportion of mature T-lymphocytes capable of participating in a cell-mediated response against the tumor may be increased by the presence of THF, or (b) the proportion of immature T-cells responsible for an enhancing effect on the tumor might be correspondingly reduced by the physiological effect of THF on T-cell maturation (3–5,9,14,40–42,50,53,67,68,75,78).

Another line of investigation at our laboratory that opened a new approach to the control of autoimmunity started with the finding that THF prevents sensitization against self-antigens. It was initially found that spleen cells of normal mice sensitized *in vitro* on monolayers of syngeneic fibroblasts demonstrated cytotoxicity against syngeneic tumor cells, and that the addition of THF to the cultures during the sensitizing period resulted in a striking inhibition of the cytotoxic activity. Moreover, it was observed that syngeneic GvH and syngeneic MLC activities (which were exhibited by spleen cells of normal mice after a period of sensitization on syngeneic fibroblasts) could be prevented by exposure of the lymphocytes to THF. The inhibitory action of THF on autoreactive lymphocytes was exerted before sensitization, during the course of sensitization, and even after sensitization has occurred. These observations also suggested that cells that lose autoreactivity as a result of exposure to THF are in the same immature stage as the cells that acquire, under the influence of THF, reactivity against nonself. Therefore, the results of these experiments were compatible with the unifying hypothesis that loss of reactivity against syngeneic tissue may also result from the maturation of lymphocytes that are under the influence of THF. These experiments also indicate that the thymus is involved in the discrimination between self and nonself and that this function seems to be at least partially mediated by THF, thus opening a new interpretation in the pathogenesis of autoimmunity and to its possible control (24,51,52,58).

Altogether, these experiments permitted us to classify the thymus as an endocrine organ, assigned with the role of production, differentiation, and maturation of T-cells. In a broader sense, the thymus could be compared with the ovaries and testes. Both the gonads and the thymus are the locus of an intensive and continuous production of germinal cells and T-lymphocytes, respectively, and both involve the hormonal milieu needed by their specific targets (71). This concept led us to explore the possibility of a feedback mechanism between the thymus and the bone marrow, as the latter is the source of cells populating the thymus after the earlier period of thymic embryogenesis.

Our investigations soon demonstrated that the thymus also plays a role in the regulation of hemopoiesis. This function was measured in terms of colony-forming units in vivo (CFU-S), the number of which were found to be reduced after neonatal thymectomy. Thus, when lethally irradiated mice were injected with bone marrow cells from NTx syngeneic donors, the number of hemopoietic colonies appearing in the spleen was significantly lower than the number observed in mice after administration of normal bone marrow. In addition, bone marrow cells from NTx or nude mice inoculated into lethally irradiated syngeneic recipients manifested a reduced radioprotective capacity. This was apparently due to a lower proliferative rate of hemopoietic cells originating in the bone marrow of thymus-deprived mice, since the rate of DNA synthesis in cells of colonies originating in the bone marrow of thymectomized mice was lower than that of colony cells derived from normal bone marrow. Moreover, by examination of the sensitivity of these cells to chlorambucil and by ^{3}H-thymidine "suicide" experiments, it was found that the number of CFU-S in spleens of thymectomized mice were indeed not developing at the same rate as normals. THF treatment of the bone marrow cells resulted in a restoration of the CFU-S capacity of bone marrow from NTx mice. Since the restorative action of THF was restricted to bone marrow cells of thymectomized mice, it is plausible that bone marrow of normal mice contains at least two subpopulations of CFU-S, one of which appears to depend on THF (35,62,86–88).

The investigations described above prompted us to examine the biochemical mechanisms by which THF confers immunological reactivity on noncompetent lymphoid cell populations, in the hope that an insight into the pathways leading to maturation of lymphoid cells will be provided. It was found that THF induces immunocompetence of thymocytes, or restores that of spleen cells of NTx mice, by activation of membranal adenylate cyclase, thus leading to a rapid elevation in intracellular cyclic AMP; further, that this effect is confined to thymus-derived cells only. Moreover, these biochemical changes under the influence of THF are early events that occur before antigenic stimulation, and are unrelated to antigenic challenge. The evaluation of intracellular levels of cyclic AMP in these cells was found to be an obligatory requirement for the cells to participate in an immune response. The fact that THF exerts its effect via cyclic AMP is in agreement with the concept that permits the classification of THF as a thymic hormone. THF could therefore be considered the first messenger acting on a specific target cell population of undifferentiated thymocytes or incompletely differentiated T-cells, whereas cyclic AMP is the second messenger acting at the intracellular level and becoming the tool for final differentiation toward the specific roles governed by these cell populations. In addition, our findings suggest that intracellular levels of cyclic AMP participate in the regulation of the immunocompetence of lymphoid cells. We found, actually, that the level of maturation of thymus-derived lymphocytes is correlated to, and can be assessed by, the levels of cellular cyclic AMP. In consequence, although THF increased cellular cyclic AMP levels and the immunocompetence of thymus-derived immature cells, it did not modify these parameters when lymphoid cell populations were tested (15–17,73,74).

In the light of the extensive research on the effect of THF on the immunological system in mice, and as a result of the information gained during these studies, we felt the urge to investigate whether these findings were reproducible when human cells were used as targets, with the eventual aim of using THF as a therapeutic tool in clinical conditions. Human lymphocytes were obtained from adult peripheral blood (PBL) or umbilical cord blood (UCBL). THF was found to increase strongly the reaction of these cells to PHA and Con A stimulation, as well as to improve their activity in an MLC assay. Injection of human lymphocytes preincubated with THF into immunosuppressed rats led to a striking increase in the capacity of these cells to mount a xenogeneic GvH reaction. Another model used for studying the effect of THF on PBL consisted of the *in vitro* measurement of their secondary response to varicella Zoster virus antigen, assessed by uptake of ^{3}H-thymidine by the stimulated cells. It was demonstrated that preincubation of normal PBL with THF resulted in a better response to this antigen. Finally, as in the mouse, human cells obtained from adult PBL or UCBL demonstrated a higher level of intracellular cyclic AMP after *in vitro* exposure to THF (8,12,29,36,38,44,47,63,82).

As a result of these human lymphocyte studies, preliminary trials of THF treatment in humans have been started in Israel. The parameters studied in patients receiving THF included the determination of total number of lymphocytes in peripheral blood and of lymphocytes capable of forming rosettes with SRBC (E-rosettes), the xenogeneic GvH reactivity of human lymphocytes mounted against immunosuppressed rats, the PHA and Con A reactivity, and the intracellular cyclic AMP level of lymphocytes. In addition, the macrophage inhibiting factor (MIF) index and the delayed hypersensitivity response to various antigens such as *Candida albicans,* purified protein derivative of tuberculin (PPD), *Trichophyton,* and streptokinase-streptodornase were performed. The first cases selected were those in which a T-cell deficiency, clearly established before initiation of treatment, was considered as an integral element of the physiopathology of such diseases. Therefore, they included patients with subacute sclerosing panencephalitis (SSPE), juvenile rheumatoid arthritis, Down's syndrome, and fulminant viral infections. After various schedules of THF injection, reconstitution of T-cell function was observed in most cases, and clinical improvement, sometimes dramatic, was often observed. The uneventful recovery of a group of children with acute lymphatic leukemia (ALL) or Hodgkin's disease, suffering from an intercurrent generalized varicella infection, suggests that THF therapy may be useful as an antiviral drug and as a supporting therapy to maintain immunocompetence in children with malignant neoplasms. In addition, more recent data suggesting a beneficial effect of THF in combination with chemotherapy in children affected with acute myelogenous leukemia (AML) is gaining evidence (6,7,11,46,80,81,84,85).

Regarding the chemical nature of THF, a procedure for isolation and characterization of the active principle of calf thymus has been described. It consists of homogenization, ultracentrifugation, and dialysis of the material. The active dialysate, which we call CTO (calf thymus outer material), is further purified by gel filtration on Sephadex G-10 and G-25 columns, followed by anion-exchange chromatography. The level of purification is assessed by isoelectric focusing on polyacrylamide gels. The isoelectric point is 5.6 to 5.9. The active principle, designated THF by us, is a polypeptide of M.W. 3,220. Determination of the amino acid composition revealed the presence of acidic residues. Pure THF is between 10 and 20 thousand times more active than CTO, as measured by the biological parameters described in the different models used. CTO and pure THF were used in the studies summarized above and others (18,19,83).

The experiments presented below are the result of a further endeavor to understand the intimacy of the steps that lead to the conferment of increased competence of T-lymphocytes by their interaction with CTO.

RECONSTITUTION OF THE LYTIC CAPACITY OF LYMPHOCYTES FROM THYMECTOMIZED MICE BY THF

Foreword

The *in vitro* MLC system consists of two sequential phases: (a) a proliferative step, which is considered to represent the recognition phase of the homograft response, and (b) an effector phase expressed by cell-mediated immune lysis (CML). Experiments performed in various laboratories suggested that T-cells proliferating in an MLC system may differ from those T-cells that become killers and are directly responsible for target lysis. More recently, the development of specific antisera to membranal T-lymphocyte markers has permitted a re-examination of this subject and has clearly established that cells involved in MLC and in CML represent two diverse subsets of the T-lymphocyte pool.

Using a semicrude preparation of thymus extract, we demonstrated a few years ago the capacity of this product to partially restore CML in lymphoid cells obtained from NTx or adult thymectomized (ATx) mice. The models used represented either a variation of an earlier technique that measures the lysis of tumor cells, or a more recent method of quantitating the lysis of Con A-induced (76) blast cell targets. With the development of a purer preparation of THF and of a more precise limiting dilution method of CML, we considered it worthwhile to use this system to reexamine the role of several thymus hormone preparations, with both *in vitro* and *in vivo* administration.

Materials and Methods

Mice

CBA/Lac (H-2^k), their homozygous athymic nude (nu/nu), and BALB/c (H-2^d) male mice bred at the Weizmann Institute Animal Breeding Center were used.

Thymectomy

Neonatal thymectomy was performed on mice up to 12 hr after birth and adult thymectomy was performed on 6- to 8-week-old mice, using CBA/Lac males for both procedures. Mice were anesthetized with ether (neonates) or nembutal (adults) and their thymuses were removed by suction. Mice later found to contain thymic remnants were discarded from the experiments.

THF

THF (CTO) was prepared as described above and added to the culture at a concentration of 4 ng/well. The control consisted of a nonactive fraction of thymic material obtained during the preparation of THF and used at the same concentration.

Cell Suspensions and Media

Spleens from 8- to 12-week-old mice were aseptically removed and dispersed by pressing through a stainless steel mesh into "standard medium" containing RPMI-1640 (Gibco, Grand Island, New York) supplemented with 10% heat-inactivated fetal bovine serum (FBS) (Rehatuin N.S.F., Reheis Chemical Co., Illinois), 25 mM Hepes buffer (Gibco, Grand Island, New York), 5×10^{-5} M 2-mercaptoethanol (2-ME) (Fluka AG, Buchs, Switzerland), 100 U/ml penicillin, 100 mg/ml streptomycin (Teva, Jerusalem, Israel), and 2 mM glutamine (Gibco, Grand Island, New York). Medium for the ^{51}Cr release test contained RPMI-1640 plus 10% FBS.

In Vitro Sensitization

Responder CBA/Lac spleen cells (Fig. 1) at dilutions of 500, 150, 50, 15, and 5×10^4 cells/ml were distributed in U-shaped microtiter plates (Greiner, Nürtingen, West Germany) in 0.1-ml volumes. Stimulator allogeneic BALB/c or autologous CBA/Lac TNP-modified spleen cells irradiated with 1,500 rad were mixed with CBA/Lac nu/nu cells (6×10^6 cells/ml and 4×10^6 cells/ml, respectively) and distributed in 0.1-ml volumes into each well. Nu/nu spleen cells were used as a source of non-T-cells needed to synergize with responder T-cells for elevation of the cytotoxic response without participating in the lytic

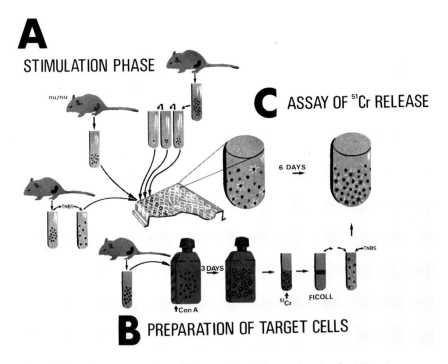

FIG. 1. Schematic representation of the experimental procedure for the ^{51}Cr release assay.

reaction. Control cultures in each experimental group contained stimulator and nu/nu spleen cells to which no responder spleen cells were added. Each experimental group contained a dozen cultures for each dilution tested and at least three dilutions were examined in each experiment. The cultures were incubated for 6 days at 37°C in a humidified atmosphere of 5% CO_2 in air.

TNP Modification

Coupling with TNP was done according to Shearer (45) by 10-min incubation of 10^8 stimulator and target cells in 2,4,6-trinitrobenzene sulfonic acid solution (Sigma Chemical, St Louis, Missouri) (17.36 mg in 5 ml RPMI-1640) at 37°C in 5% CO_2 in air. The cells were then washed three times and counted.

Target Cells (Fig. 1)

Target cells in the ^{51}Cr release assay were Con A-induced blasts of either BALB/c or CBA. Blast cells were prepared 3 days before the assay in tissue culture flasks having a 25 cm² growth area (Lux Scientific Corporation, Newbury Park, California). Each flask contained 1.5×10^7 spleen cells in standard media supplemented with 20% FBS and 10 μg Con A (Miles-Yeda, Rehovot, Israel). Labeling of the target cells for the ^{51}Cr release test was performed as follows. Target cells were washed once in the medium by centrifugation at 1,200 rpm for 10 min. The pellet was resuspended in 0.5 ml medium, labeled with 500 μCi ^{51}Cr as sodium chromate (Radiochemical Center, Amersham, England) and incubated for 2 hr at 37°C in 5% CO_2 in air. The labeled cells were washed once by centrifugation at 1,200 rpm, and the pellet layered in Ficoll-Hypaque gradient (Lymphoprep 1.0779 g/ml, Nyegaard and Co., AIS, Oslo, Norway) at a ratio of 4:3 and centrifuged at 2,000 rpm for 20 min. Blast cells in the interphase were collected, washed twice in medium, and counted. Target cells to be TNP-modified were first labeled with ^{51}Cr and then modified (45).

Micro ^{51}Cr Release Test

The microplates were centrifuged for 10 min at 2,000 rpm and the supernatant was removed by flipping over the microplates. The pellet was then mixed and a portion of the labeled target cell suspension (2×10^4 cells in 0.2 ml) was added to each well. The microplates were incubated for 4 hr at 37°C in a humidified atmosphere of 5% CO_2 in air. The plates were then centrifuged for 10 min at 2,000 rpm and 0.1 ml of the supernatant was transferred from each well into counting tubes and counted in an Auto-Gamma Scintillator 5260 (Packard, Downers Grove, Illinois). Control cultures containing stimulator and target cells were used to estimate the background ^{51}Cr release, which represented 5 to 10% of the total ^{51}Cr incorporated. The total releasable ^{51}Cr was estimated by placing 0.1 ml of the target cells into counting tubes, this usually giving 75 to 80% release. Under the labeling conditions described above, 2×10^4 cells gave 5,000 to 8,000 cpm.

A culture was considered positive when the cpm of the experimental cultures was two standard deviations above the mean of the cpm of control cultures. Quantitation of specific ^{51}Cr release was done by calculating the percentage of positive cultures.

Results and Discussion

The first experiment was performed to construct a dose-response curve for cytotoxicity according to increasing concentrations of responder cells. The limiting dilution assay permits the determination of the minimal number of cells required, under specific conditions, to achieve a positive response of cytotoxicity. Two different types of stimulator spleen cells were tested—one being allogeneic BALB/c (H-2^d) and the other TNP-modified CBA/Lac (H-2^k) cells. Responder cells in both cases were CBA/Lac spleen cells.

As seen in Fig. 2, there is a direct relationship between the number of responder cells and the level of cytotoxicity obtained; thus, 5×10^3 responder cells were

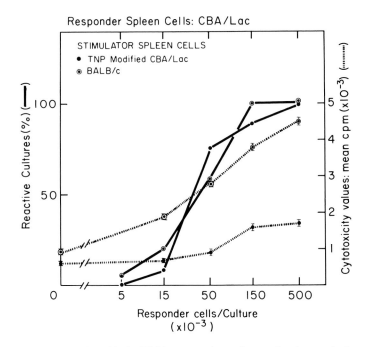

FIG. 2. Cell-mediated lysis (CML) assay using spleen cells of normal mice.

below the level of measurable cytotoxicity. The results indicate that self-modified stimulator cells induced, in general, a lower cytotoxicity than allogeneic stimulators in terms of intensity of the reaction. Yet, in both cases 100% of the cultures were reactive.

Since neonatal thymectomy has a long-lasting effect on the T-cell pool, we then attempted to determine the effect of thymus removal on T-cells participating in CML. Responder spleen cells from 8-week-old NTx were tested for their ability to be sensitized and to lyse target spleen cells of BALB/c or CBA/Lac TNP-modified origin. Figure 3 demonstrates that, over the cell concentration range used (5 to 50 × 10³), no measurable activity could be detected in any individual culture well. In the next experiment, THF (4 ng per well) was added to cultures containing NTx responder spleen cells for the 6-day period of the immunization phase. As seen in Fig. 3, a dramatic elevation in cytotoxicity against both allogeneic and TNP-modified autologous target cells by the NTx effector cells after *in vitro* THF treatment was obtained. As in the control experiments (Fig. 2), the lytic activity against TNP-modified target cells was also lower (85%) than allogeneic BALB/c targets (100%) at the highest cell concentrations.

Subsequently, NTx mice were injected systemically with THF for 12 consecutive days (0.1 μg/daily), while NTx controls were injected with an inactive material obtained during THF preparation (see Fig. 4). Restoration of the capac-

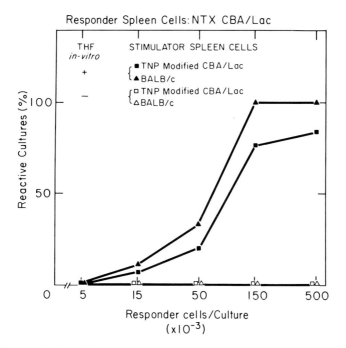

FIG. 3. Effect of *in vitro* THF treatment on CML response by spleen cells from neonatal thymectomized (NTx) mice.

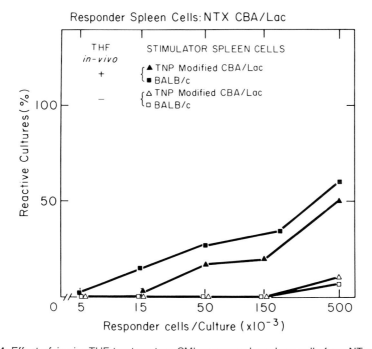

FIG. 4. Effect of *in vivo* THF treatment on CML response by spleen cells from NTx mice.

ity of spleen cells to induce lysis of respective allogeneic and self-modified target cells was observed only in the cells of THF-injected mice. Yet, it should be noted that the level of cytotoxicity (60%) obtained by *in vivo* treatment was lower than the *in vitro* treatment samples. In the next experiment we tested the ability of THF to modify the cytotoxic activity of spleen cells of adult mice obtained 3 months after thymectomy. Treatment consisted of adding THF (4 ng per well) to the cultures. Control cultures consisted of ATx responder cells to which was added an inactive material of thymic origin obtained during THF preparation. As seen in Fig. 5, no response could be detected in ATx responder cell cultures lacking THF. Again, at the highest concentrations of cells, THF addition elevated the response up to 100% in both the alloantigen and the TNP-modified model.

Recent experiments by Cantor and Boyse (1,2,13) have provided evidence favoring the concept that T-lymphocytes comprise several subclasses. Of the Ly cell surface antigens present in T-cells, there are at least two populations of mature T-lymphocytes, Ly_1 and Ly_{23}. The latter regulates cytotoxic or suppressive functions, whereas the former serves as a helper cell population to B antibody-forming cells and as an amplifier of the killer activity of Ly_{23} cells. Both mature sublines are derived from immature Ly_{123} ancestors and are not sequential stages of a single line of progression, but rather belong to different lines of differentiation. The same authors have shown that adult thymectomy produces

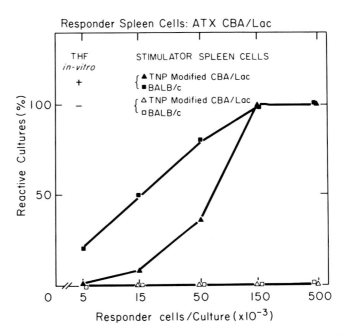

FIG. 5. Effect of *in vitro* THF treatment on CML response by spleen cells from ATx mice.

a rapid decline in the pool of Ly_{123} cells manifested in the spleen 3 to 4 weeks after performing this surgical procedure. In the light of these established concepts, the results of our previous and current studies point to THF as the hormone that modulates the natural differentiation of T-cells from their immature stage to total acquisition of competence in the absence of antigenic stimulation. Here we have evidence that THF, either by *in vivo* administration or added *in vitro* to the cultures, restores the impaired killer capacity of spleen cells from NTx or ATx mice. This repair is dramatic and, in some circumstances, the level of response exhibited by the spleen cells of normal animals is reached. Theoretically, this effect of THF in lytic models could be achieved by clonal expansion of either the Ly_1 population (which may help the cytotoxic function of Ly_{23} cells or of the Ly_{23} precursor killer cells) or by stimulating the differentiation of immature Ly_{123} cells toward maturation into both Ly_1 and Ly_{23} subpopulations. Of these two alternatives, it seems that the latter is more plausible, since our previous results have extensively demonstrated that THF stimulates the maturation of thymus cells bearing T-cell markers by acquiring properties that permit them to accomplish their role both as T-helper cells and T-cytotoxic cells. Finally, the present further strengthens our earlier observations as to the maturation of T-cells toward their role, under the influence of THF, as killer cells.

SHIFTING OF TUMOR-ENHANCING THYMOCYTES INTO TUMOR-INHIBITING CELLS BY THF

As mentioned earlier, the influence of T-cells on the outcome of tumor growth might represent the balance between populations with opposed activities. Indeed, two phases have been observed in the activities of spleen cells during the progression of syngeneic tumor growth in mice. In the first stage, tumor-inhibitory cells appeared shortly after tumor inoculation, but as the tumor progressed this population gradually declined, being replaced by an increasing population of tumor-enhancing cells. Separation of spleen cells from tumor-bearing mice by velocity sedimentation also revealed two antagonizing subpopulations of T-lymphocytes: One of them expressed tumor inhibitory activity whereas the other expressed tumor enhancement. However, when these two subpopulations were mixed, only enhancement of tumor growth was observed.

With the aim of tracing these cells back to their source, thymocytes from tumor-free donors were tested in similar experimental models. Earlier appearance and acceleration of growth of tumors were observed, thus suggesting that cells with the ability to enhance tumor growth are present in the thymus of normal animals. Since it has been well established that the thymus contains lymphocytes at various levels of differentiation, we undertook experiments to study the behavior of thymic cell subpopulations in relation to tumor development. It was recently found that exposure to peanut agglutinin (PNA) separates thymocytes into two subpopulations: the agglutinable cells, which represent approximately

90% of the total population, and the nonagglutinable thymocytes representing only 5 to 10%. It was also observed that PNA-agglutinable cells are related to the immature subpopulation of T-cells within the thymus, whereas nonagglutinable thymocytes represent the residual mature subpopulation having the competence to react immunologically in various models (34). On testing of thymocytes after separation of the two subpopulations according to their PNA agglutinability, we observed that the agglutinable immature cell (PNA$^+$) population accelerated the appearance of and enhanced tumor growth, whereas the nonagglutinable, mature (PNA$^-$) population disclosed properties inhibitory toward tumor development (25,77). These results prompted us to examine the effect of THF on the subpopulation of immature (PNA$^+$) thymocytes and to observe whether THF treatment modifies their tumor-enhancing properties.

Materials and Methods

Mice

C57BL/6 female mice were used throughout these experiments.

Thymic Cell Suspensions

Thymuses from 8- to 10-week-old mice were aseptically removed and dispersed by pressing through a stainless steel mesh in Eagle's medium (EM). Cells were washed several times in EM and the nucleated cells were counted.

Peanut Agglutinin

Peanut agglutinin (PNA) was kindly donated by Prof. N. Sharon, Department of Biophysics, The Weizmann Institute of Science, and stored in lyophilized form. Separation of the thymocytes by agglutination with PNA was carried out as described previously (34). Briefly, 2×10^8 cells in 0.25 ml of phosphate-buffered saline (PBS) (BDH Chemicals, Poole, England) were mixed with 0.25 ml PNA (1 mg/ml) in a small Falcon plastic tube, left at room temperature for 10 min, and then gently layered with a Pasteur pipette on the top of 50% fetal bovine serum (FBS) in PBS solution. When the agglutinated fraction settled on the bottom of the tube, it was carefully removed by aspiration with a Pasteur pipette. An upper layer of nonagglutinated thymocytes was similarly removed into another tube. The lectin was removed from both fractions by a 10-min incubation in 2 ml of 0.2 M D-galactose (BDH Chemicals). The separated cells were washed twice in PBS, resuspended in EM with 10% FBS, and brought to the required cell concentration. At all stages, the viability of cells was checked by trypan blue exclusion.

Tumor Cells

The Lewis lung carcinoma (3LL) tumor was used. This is a tumor that arose spontaneously in a C57BL mouse and has been maintained by serial passage in the same strain. Local 3LL tumors were aseptically removed, minced with scissors, washed twice in cold PBS, trypsinized for 30 min in a 0.25% trypsin solution, followed by filtration through a fine stainless steel mesh. The tumor cells were then centrifuged, washed twice in EM, and the viable cells were estimated by exclusion of trypan blue in a hemocytometer. Cell counts established that viability was always higher than 85%. Doses (0.2 ml volume) of 10^5 viable tumor cells were injected subcutaneously into mice that were periodically examined to determine the day of tumor appearance and the number of tumor takes.

THF (CTO) Treatment

PNA$^+$ thymocytes were mixed with 40 μg/ml THF and incubated for 3, 6, 16, 18, and 24 hr at 37°C in a humidified atmosphere of 5% CO_2 in air. It should be noted that thymocytes subjected to long periods (e.g., 16 to 24 hr) of incubation resulted in a 50% reduction of the total number of thymocytes, whether THF or EM was present. When testing cells after 16-, 18-, and 24-hr incubation periods, they were layered on Ficoll-Hypaque gradient at a ratio of 4:3 (cells:Ficoll) and centrifuged at 2,000 rpm for 20 min. The cells at the interphase were collected, washed twice in EM medium, and counted. This procedure was used to remove cell debris from the suspension. The THF-treated PNA$^+$ thymocytes were then mixed with tumor cells at a ratio of 1:100 (tumor cells:thymocytes) and injected subcutaneously into syngeneic recipients (Winn test).

Results and Discussion

The first set of experiments was aimed at detecting whether THF (CTO) can modulate membranal properties of immature PNA$^+$ thymocytes by observing the change in the percent of PNA$^+$ and PNA$^-$ cell populations after incubation with a THF preparation.

Figure 6 summarizes the results of such an experiment. It can be seen that the most dramatic effect of THF treatment was manifested after 24 hr of incubation. Only 24% of PNA$^+$ cells were detected in these cultures versus 95% PNA$^+$ cells in the original inoculum. Concomitantly, the percentage of PNA$^-$ cells was elevated, reaching 76% of the total counts. Thus, it could be concluded that THF is able to change the ratio between PNA$^+$ and PNA$^-$ cells in the thymic cell population. This is probably effected by maturational processes accompanied by membranal changes of the PNA$^+$ cells. It should be noted here that the transformation of PNA$^+$ into PNA$^-$ cells has also occurred under

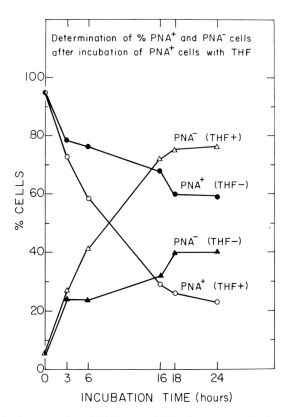

FIG. 6. Change in the proportion of PNA⁺ and PNA⁻ thymocytes after incubation with THF.

experimental conditions in the absence of THF; however, THF enhances the transformation.

Since PNA⁺ thymocytes enhance, while PNA⁻ thymocytes inhibit tumor growth, it was of interest to observe whether THF treatment, which causes membranal changes of PNA⁺ cells, also modifies their tumor-enhancing properties. Thus, PNA⁺ thymocytes treated or untreated with THF were mixed with 3LL tumor cells in a ratio of 100:1 (lymphocytes:tumor cells). Control mice were injected with 3LL tumor cells only, or with a mixture of tumor and PNA⁻ cells. The latter combination had been shown in previous experiments to delay tumor appearance and also to lower the rate of tumor growth. The incidence of tumor takes was determined in all the groups of mice. Figure 7 summarizes the results of such experiments. In mice injected with 24 hr-incubated PNA⁺ thymocytes mixed with 3LL tumor cells, the incidence of tumor was lower and the time required for tumor appearance was increased as compared with control mice that were injected with 3LL tumor cells only. This enhancing property was completely reversed in groups of mice injected with 3LL tumor cells admixed with PNA⁺ thymocytes previously treated with THF for 24 hr. As seen in Fig. 7, these cells behaved as PNA⁻ cells.

The method developed by Reisner et al. (34) has permitted the separation of two distinct populations of thymocytes in relation to their activities. The upper layer of nonagglutinated thymocytes (PNA⁻), representing no more than 10% of the total lymphocytic population of the thymus, has been characterized as possessing high H-2 and low θ (Thy-1) surface antigen levels, cortisone resistance, and high immune reactivities in both the GvH and the MLC reactions. On the other hand, the bottom layer is constituted by the majority of the lymphoid cell population of the thymus, and its components are characterized by high θ and low H-2 surface antigen levels, sensitivity to cortisone, and lack of reactivity in cell-mediated reactions. The experiments reported here demonstrate that, in the presence of THF, PNA⁺ thymocytes could be converted to PNA⁻ cells. However, experiments performed in the absence of PNA suggest that, under control conditions, there is a certain degree of spontaneous shifting of cells from PNA⁺ into PNA⁻ cells, thus indicating that the components of the culture medium (fetal calf serum, etc.) might serve as stimulators of this shift during the prolonged incubation. Whatever might be the cause of this process, spontaneous transformation occurs at a very slow rate, whereas THF causes a

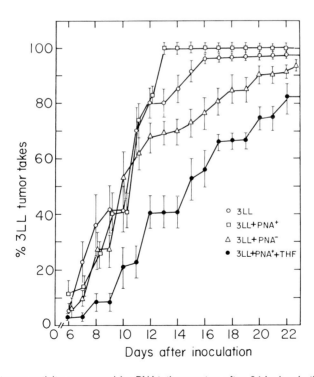

FIG. 7. Anti-tumor activity expressed by PNA⁺ thymocytes after 24-hr incubation with THF

dramatic change that starts soon after PNA$^+$ thymocytes are exposed to this hormone and involves the majority of the target cell population.

The above results resemble those earlier experiments in our laboratory: THF increases the hydrocortisone-resistant component of a thymic cell population by transforming hydrocortisone-sensitive cells into resistant ones, and this change is concomitant with thymocyte maturation relative to their behavior in cell-mediated immune models (60).

We have established that, under syngeneic conditions, the interaction between immature (PNA$^+$) T-lymphocytes and tumor cells accelerates tumor growth, while the same type of interaction with mature (PNA$^-$) T-cells leads to tumor inhibition. It was therefore important to determine whether the THF-induced shifting of PNA$^+$ thymocytes into PNA$^-$ was accompanied by a change in their properties vis-à-vis tumor growth. We have clearly confirmed this assumption, as PNA$^+$ cells exposed to THF had a small but consistent inhibitory effect on tumor growth. These experiments further strengthen the established concept that THF is a thymic hormone that leads to differentiation of thymocytes in the absence of antigenic stimulation. This differentiation is manifested in such membranal changes as hydrocortisone resistance, PNA agglutinability of thymic lymphocytes and in the functional behavior expressed by the known characteristics of maturation recognizable by cell-mediated phenomena.

REFERENCES

1. Cantor, H., and Boyse, E. A. (1975): Functional subclasses of T lymphocytes bearing different Ly antigens. I. The generation of functionally distinct T-cell subclasses is a differentiative process independent of antigen. *J. Exp. Med.,* 141:1376–1389.
2. Cantor, H., and Boyse, E. A. (1975): Functional subclasses of T lymphocytes bearing different Ly antigens. II. Cooperation between subclasses of Ly$^+$ cells in the generation of killer activity. *J. Exp. Med.,* 141:1390–1398.
3. Carnaud, C., Ilfeld, D., Brook, I., and Trainin, N. (1973): Increased activity of mouse spleen cells sensitized *in vitro* against syngeneic tumor cells in the presence of a thymic humoral factor. *J. Exp. Med.,* 138:1521–1532.
4. Carnaud, C., Ilfeld, D., Levo, Y., and Trainin, N. (1974): Enhancement of 3LL tumor growth by autosensitized T-lymphocytes independent of the host lymphatic system. *Int. J. Cancer,* 14:168–175.
5. Carnaud, C., Markovicz, I., and Trainin, N. (1974): The influence of a graft vs. host reaction on the incidence of metastases after tumor transplantation. *Cell. Immunol.,* 14:87–97.
6. David, M., Shohat, B., Feurman, M., and Trainin, N. (1980): Cell-mediated immunity in patients with mycosis fungoides in clinical remission. Effects of THF. *Cancer (in press).*
7. David, M., Shohat, B., Feurman, M., and Trainin, N. (1980): B & T lymphocytes in lymphoproliferative disorders of skin. Effects of THF. *Br. J. Dermatol.,* 102:145–148.
8. Douer, D., Shohat, B., Djaldetti, M., Trainin, N., and Kinkhas, J. (1978): Thymic humoral factor in the assessment of T-lymphocytes in a patient with T-cell chronic lymphocytic leukemia. *Isr. J. Med. Sci.,* 14:870–875.
9. Gabizon, A., Small, M., and Trainin, N. (1976): Kinetics of the response of spleen cells from tumor-bearing animals in an *in vivo* tumor neutralization assay. *Int. J. Cancer,* 18:813–819.
10. Globerson, A., Rotter, V., Nakamura, I., and Trainin, N. (1973): Thymus extracts induce differentiation of thymus derived cells. In: *Microenvironmental Aspects of Immunity,* edited by B. D. Jankovic and K. Isakovaic, pp. 183–189.
11. Handzel, Z. T., Dolfin, Z., Levin, S., Altman, Y., Hahn, T., Trainin, N., and Gadot, N. (1979):

Effect of thymic humoral factor on cellular immune functions of normal children and of pediatric patients with ataxia telangiectasia and Down's syndrome. *Pediatri. Res.,* 13:803–806.

12. Handzel, Z. T., Levin, S., Ashkenazi, A., Hahn, T., Altman, Y., Czernobilsky, B., Shechter, B., and Trainin, N. (1977): Immune deficiency of T system with possible T-cell regulatory activity defect. *Isr. J. Med. Sci.,* 13:347–353.

13. Huber, B., Cantor, H., Shen, F. W., and Boyse, E. A. (1976): Independent differentiative pathways of Ly1 and Ly23 subclasses of T-cells: Experimental production of mice deprived of selected T-cell subclasses. *J. Exp. Med.,* 144:1128–1133.

14. Ilfeld, D., Carnaud, C., Cohen, I. R., and Trainin, N. (1973): *In vitro* cytotoxicity and *in vivo* tumor enhancement induced by mouse spleen cells autosensitized *in vitro. Int. J. Cancer,* 12:213–222.

15. Kook, A. I., and Trainin, N. (1974): Hormone-like activity of a thymus humoral factor on the induction of immune competence in lymphoid cells. *J. Exp. Med.,* 139:193–207.

16. Kook, A. I., and Trainin, N. (1975): The control exerted by thymic hormone (THF) on cellular cAMP levels and on the immune reactivity of spleen cells in the MLC assay. *J. Immunol.,* 115:8–14.

17. Kook, A. I., and Trainin, N. (1975): Intracellular events involved in the induction of immune competence in lymphoid cells by a thymus humoral factor. *J. Immunol.,* 114:151–157.

18. Kook, A. I., Yakir, Y., and Trainin, N. (1975): Isolation and partial chemical characterization of THF, a thymus hormone involved in immune maturation of lymphoid cells. *Cell. Immunol.,* 19:151–157.

19. Kook, A. I., Yakir, Y., and Trainin, N. (1976): Isolation and partial chemical characterization of THF, a thymus hormone involved in immune maturation of lymphoid cells. In: *Immune Reactivity of Lymphocytes,* edited by M. Feldman and A. Globerson, pp. 215–220. Plenum Press, New York.

20. Law, L. W., Dunn, T. B., Trainin, N., and Levey, R. H. (1964): Studies of thymic function. In: *The Thymus,* edited by V. Defendi and D. Metcalf, pp. 105–120. Wistar Institute Press, Philadelphia.

21. Law, L. W., Trainin, N., Levey, R. H., and Barth, W. F. (1964): Humoral thymic factor in mice. Further evidence. *Science,* 143:1049–1051.

22. Levey, R. H., Trainin, N., and Law, L. W. (1963): Evidence for function of thymic tissue in diffusion chambers implanted in neonatally thymectomized mice: Preliminary report. *J. Natl. Cancer Inst.,* 31:199–217.

23. Levey, R. H., Trainin, N., Law, L. W., Black, P. H., and Rowe, W. P. (1963): Lymphocytic choriomeningitis infection in neonatally thymectomized mice bearing diffusion chambers containing thymus. *Science,* 142:483–485.

24. Levo, Y., Carnaud, C., Cohen, I. R., and Trainin, N. (1974): Increased incidence of urethan-induced lung adenomas by autosensitized lymphocytes. *Br. J. Cancer,* 29:312–317.

25. Linker-Israeli, M., Itzchaki, M., Umiel, T., Trainin, N., and Sharon, N. (1977): Separation of tumor enhancing murine thymocytes by agglutination with a peanut lectine (PNA). In: *Regulatory Mechanisms in Lymphocyte Activation,* edited by D. O. Lucas, pp. 515–517. Academic Press, New York.

26. Lonai, P., Mogilner, B., Rotter, V., and Trainin, N. (1973): Studies on the effect of a thymus humoral factor on differentiation of thymus derived lymphocytes. *Eur. J. Immunol.,* 3:21–26.

27. Mandel, T. (1969): Epithelial cells and lymphopoiesis in the cortex of guinea pig thymus. *Aust. J. Expt. Biol. Med. Sci.,* 47:153–155.

28. Mandel, T., Russel, P. J., and Byrd, W. (1972): Differentiation of the thymus *in vivo* and *in vitro.* In: *Cell Interactions, Proceedings of the Third Lepetit Colloquium,* edited by L. G. Silvestri, pp. 183–191. North-Holland, Amsterdam.

29. Michalevicz, R., Many, A., Ramot, B., and Trainin, N. (1978): The *in vitro* effect of thymic humoral factor and levamisole on peripheral blood lymphocytes in systemic lupus erythematosus patients. *Clin. Exp. Immunol.,* 31:111–115.

30. Miller, J. F. A. P. (1961): Immunological function of the thymus. *Lancet,* 2:748–749.

31. Miller, J. F. A. P., and Osoba, D. (1967): Current concepts of the immunological function of the thymus. *Physiol. Rev.,* 47:437–520.

32. Owen, J. J. T., and Raff, M. C. (1970): Studies on the differentiation of thymus-derived lymphocytes. *J. Exp. Med.,* 132:1216–1232.

33. Owen, J. J. T., and Ritter, M. A. (1969): Tissue interaction in the development of thymus lymphocytes. *J. Exp. Med.,* 129:431–437.

34. Reisner, Y., Linker-Israeli, M., and Sharon, N. (1976): Separation of mouse thymocytes into two subpopulations by the use of peanut agglutinin. *Cell. Immunol.,* 25:129–134.
35. Resnitzky, P., Zipori, D., and Trainin, N. (1971): Effect on neonatal thymectomy on hemopoietic tissue in mice. *Blood,* 37:634–646.
36. Rotter, V., Fink, A., and Trainin, N. (1978): *In vitro* allogenic response of human lymphocytes dependent upon dialysable plasma components and a thymic hormone, THF. *Cell. Immunol.,* 36:242–250.
37. Rotter, V., Globerson, A., Nakamura, I., and Trainin, N. (1973): Studies on characterization of the lymphoid target cell for activity of a thymus humoral factor. *J. Exp. Med.,* 138:130–142.
38. Rotter, V., Schlesinger, M., Kalderon, R., and Trainin, N. (1976): Response of human lymphocytes to PHA and Con A, dependent on and regulated by THF, a thymic hormone. *J. Immunol.,* 117:1927–1932.
39. Rotter, V., and Trainin, N. (1975): Increased mitogenic reactivity of normal spleen cells to T lectins induced by thymus humoral factor (THF). *Cell. Immunol.,* 16:413–421.
40. Rotter, V., and Trainin, N. (1975): Inhibition of tumor growth in syngeneic chimeric mice mediated by a depletion of suppressor T-cells. *Transplantation,* 20:68–74.
41. Rotter, V., and Trainin, N. (1975): Elimination of suppressor T-cells in mice undergoing a graft-versus-host reaction expressed by increased response to polyvinylpyrrolidone (PVP). *Cell. Immunol.,* 18:199–209.
42. Rotter, V., and Trainin, N. (1976): Depletion of suppressor T-cells in syngeneic chimeric mice. In: *Immune Reactivity of Lymphocytes,* edited by M. Feldman and A. Globerson, pp., 593–598. Plenum Press, New York.
43. Rotter, V., and Trainin, N. (1977): Effect of THF on the response of different lymphoid cell populations to T-mitogens. *Isr. J. Med. Sci.,* 13:363–370.
44. Rotter, V., and Trainin, N. (1979): Role of thymic hormone (THF) and of a thymic plasma recirculating factor (TPRF) in the modulation of human lymphocyte response to PHA and Con A. *J. Immunol.,* 122:414–420.
45. Shearer, G. M. (1974): Cell-mediated cytotoxicity to trinitrophenyl-modified syngeneic lymphocytes. *Eur. J. Immunol.,* 4:527–532.
46. Shohat, B., Spitzer, S., Topilsky, M., and Trainin, N. (1978): Immunological profile in sarcoidosis patients: The *in vitro* and *in vivo* effect of thymic humoral factor. *Biomedicine,* 29:91–95.
47. Shohat, B., Volah, B., and Trainin, N. (1979): Effect of thymic humoral factor (THF) *in vitro* on human bone marrow and blood cells from B-, T-, and null-cell ALL. *Cell. Immunol.,* 45:255–260.
48. Small, M., and Trainin, N. (1967): Increase in antibody forming cells of neonatally thymectomized mice receiving calf thymus extract. *Nature,* 216:377–379.
49. Small, M., and Trainin, N. (1971): Contribution of a thymic humoral factor to the development of an immunologically competent population from cells of mouse bone marrow. *J. Exp. Med.,* 134:786–800.
50. Small, M., and Trainin, N. (1975): Inhibition of syngeneic fibrosarcoma growth by lymphocytes sensitized on tumor cell monolayers in the presence of the thymic humoral factor. *Int. J. Cancer,* 15:962–972.
51. Small, M., and Trainin, N. (1975): Control of autoreactivity by a humoral factor of the thymus (THF). *Cell. Immunol.,* 20:1–11.
52. Small, M., and Trainin, N. (1976): Control of autoimmune processes by a thymic humoral factor (THF). In: *Immune Reactivity of Lymphocytes,* edited by M. Feldman and A. Globerson, pp. 659–664. Plenum Press, New York.
53. Small, M., and Trainin, N. (1976): Separation of populations of sensitized lymphoid cells into fractions inhibiting and fractions enhancing syngeneic tumor growth *in vivo. J. Immunol.,* 117:292–297.
54. Trainin, N. (1974): Thymic hormones and the immune response. *Physiol. Rev.,* 54:272–315.
55. Trainin, N., Bejerano, A., Strahilevitch, M., Goldring, D., and Small, M. (1966): A thymic factor preventing wasting and influencing lymphopoiesis in mice. *Isr. J. Med. Sci.,* 2:549–559.
56. Trainin, N., Burger, M., and Kaye, A. M. (1967): Some characteristics of a thymic humoral factor determined by assay *in vivo* of DNA synthesis in lymph nodes of thymectomized mice. *Biochem. Pharmacol.,* 16:711–719.
57. Trainin, N., Burger, M., and Linker-Israeli, M. (1967): Restoration of homograft response in neonatally thymectomized mice by a thymic humoral factor (THF). In: *Advances in Transplanta-*

tion, edited by J. Dausset, J. Hamburger, and G. Mathé, pp. 91–95. Munksgaard, Copenhagen.

58. Trainin, N., Carnaud, C., and Ilfeld, D. (1973): Inhibition of *in vitro* autosensitization by a thymic humoral factor. *Nature [New Biol.],* 245:253–255.

59. Trainin, N., Kook, A. I., Umiel, T., and Albala, M. (1975): The nature and mechanism of stimulation of immune responsiveness by thymus extracts. *Ann. N.Y. Acad. Sci.,* 249:349–361.

60. Trainin, N., Levo, Y., and Rotter, V. (1974): Resistance to hydrocortisone conferred upon thymocytes by a thymic humoral factor. *Eur. J. Immunol.,* 4:634–637.

61. Trainin, N., and Linker-Israeli, M. (1967): Restoration of immunologic reactivity of thymectomized mice by calf thymus extracts. *Cancer Res.,* 27:309–313.

62. Trainin, N., and Resnitzky, P. (1969): Influence of neonatal thymectomy on cloning capacity of bone marrow cells in mice. *Nature,* 221:1154–1155.

63. Trainin, N., Rotter, V., Yakir, Y., Leve, R., Handzel, Z. T., Shohat, B., and Zaizov, R. (1979): Biochemical and biological properties of THF in animal and human models, *Ann. N.Y. Acad. Sci. (in press).*

64. Trainin, N., and Small, M. (1970): Conferment of immunocompetence of lymphoid cells by a thymic humoral factor. In: *Ciba Foundation Study Group, No. 36 (Hormones and the Immune Response),* edited by G. E. W. Wolstenholme and J. Knight, pp. 24–41.

65. Trainin, N., and Small, M. (1970): Studies on some physicochemical properties of a thymus humoral factor conferring immunocompetence on lymphoid cells. *J. Exp. Med.,* 132:885–897.

66. Trainin, N., and Small, M. (1973): Thymic humoral factors. *Contemp. Top. Immunol.,* 2:321–337.

67. Trainin, N., and Small, M. (1978): T-lymphocytes and modulation of tumor growth. *Compr. Ther.,* 4:31–34.

68. Trainin, N., Small, M., and Gabizon, A. (1978): Combined effects of immune depression and carcinogenesis. In: *Proceedings Third International Congress Detection and Prevention of Cancer,* pp. 1621–1630.

69. Trainin, N., Small, M., and Globerson, A. (1969): Immunocompetence of spleen cells from neonatally thymectomized mice conferred *in vitro* by a syngeneic thymus extract. *J. Exp. Med.,* 130:765–776.

70. Trainin, N., Small, M., and Kimhi, Y. (1973): Characteristics of a thymic humoral factor involved in the development of cell mediated immune competence. In: *Thymic Hormones,* edited by T. D. Luckey, pp. 135–158. University Park Press, Baltimore.

71. Trainin, N., Small, M., and Kook, A. I. (1977): The role of thymic hormones in regulation of the lymphoid system. In: *B and T Cells in Immune Recognition,* edited by F. Loor and G. E. Roelants, pp. 83–102. Wiley, London.

72. Trainin, N., Small, M., Zipori, D., Umiel, T., Kook, A. I., and Rotter, V. (1975): Characteristics of THF, a thymic hormone. In: *The Biological Activity of Thymic Hormones,* edited by D. W. van Bekkum and A. M. Kruisbeek, pp. 117–144. Kooyker Scientific, Rotterdam.

73. Trainin, N., Yakir, Y., and Kook, A. I. (1979): Correlation between the cellular levels of cAMP, cell-mediated immunocompetence and the thymus humoral factor (THF): In: *Cell Biology and Immunology of Leucocyte Function,* pp. 201–211. Academic Press, New York.

74. Trainin, N., Zaizov, R., Yakir, Y., and Rotter, V. (1979): Thymic hormones: Characterization and perspectives. In: *Proceedings Serono Symposium,* edited by G. Doria and A. Eshkol, pp. 159–169. Academic Press, New York.

75. Treves, A. J., Carnaud, C., Trainin, N., Feldman, M., and Cohen, I. R. (1974): Enhancing T lymphocytes from tumor-bearing mice suppress host resistance to a syngeneic tumor. *Eur. J. Immunol.,* 4:722–727.

76. Umiel, T., Altman, A., and Trainin, N. (1976): Augmentation of cell-mediated lysis (CML) by THF. In: *Immune Reactivity of Lymphocytes,* edited by M. Feldman and A. Globerson, pp. 639–643. Plenum Press, New York.

77. Umiel, T., Linker-Israeli, M., Itzchaki, M., Trainin, N., Reisner, Y., and Sharon, N. (1978): Inhibition or acceleration of tumor growth by subpopulations of thymus cells separable by a peanut lectin. *Cell. Immunol.,* 37:134–141.

78. Umiel, T., and Trainin, N. (1974): Immunological enhancement of tumor growth by syngeneic thymus-derived lymphocytes. *Transplantation,* 18:244–250.

79. Umiel, T., and Trainin, N. (1975): Increased reactivity of responding cells in the mixed lymphocyte reaction by a thymic humoral factor. *Eur. J. Immunol.,* 5:85–88.

80. Varsano, I., Danon, Y., Jaber, L., Livni, E., Shohat, B., Yakir, Y., Shneyour, A., and Trainin,

N. (1976): Reconstitution of T-cell function in patients with subacute sclerosing panencephalitis treated with thymus humoral factor. *Isr. J. Med. Sci.,* 12:1168–1175.

81. Varsano, I., Schonfeld, T. M., Mathot, Y., Shohat, B., Englander, T., Rotter, V., and Trainin, N. (1977): Severe disseminated adenovirus infection successfully treated with a thymic humoral factor (THF). *Acta Paediatr. Scand. [Suppl.],* 66:329–331.

82. Yakir, Y., Kook, A. I., Schlesinger, M., and Trainin, N. (1977): Effect of thymic humoral factor on intracellular levels of cyclic AMP in human peripheral blood lymphocytes. *Isr. J. Med. Sci.,* 13:1191–1196.

83. Yakir, Y., Kook, A. I., and Trainin, N. (1978): Enrichment of *in vitro* and *in vivo* immunologic activity of purified fractions of calf thymic hormone (THF). *J. Exp. Med.,* 148:71–83.

84. Zaizov, R., Vogel, R., Cohen, I., Varsano, I., Shohat, B., Rotter, V., and Trainin, N. (1977): Thymic hormone (THF) therapy in immunosuppressed children with lymphoproliferative neoplasia and generalized varicella. *Biomedicine (Express),* 27:105–108.

85. Zaizov, R., Vogel, R., Wolach, B., Cohen, I. J., Varsano, I., Shohat, B., Handzel, Z. T., Rotter, V., Yakir, Y., and Trainin, N. (1979): The effect of THF in lymphoproliferative and myeloproliferative diseases in children. *Ann. N.Y. Acad. Sci. (in press).*

86. Zipori, D., and Trainin, N. (1973): Defective capacity of bone marrow from nude mice to restore lethally irradiated recipients. *Blood,* 42:671–678.

87. Zipori, D., and Trainin, N. (1975): Impaired radioprotective capacity and reduced proliferative rate of bone marrow from neonatally thymectomized mice. *Exp. Hematol.,* 3:1–11.

88. Zipori, D., and Trainin, N. (1975): The role of a thymus humoral factor in the proliferation of bone marrow CFU-S from thymectomized mice. *Exp. Hematol.,* 3:389–398.

Polypeptide Hormones, edited by
R. F. Beers, Jr. and E. G. Bassett.
Raven Press, New York © 1980.

43. Serum Thymic Factor: A Peptide Lymphocyte-Differentiating Hormone

J. F. Bach, M. A. Bach, M. Dardenne, J. M. Pleau, *P. Lefrancier, *J. Choay, **D. Blanot, and **E. Bricas

INSERM Unit 25, Necker Hospital, 75730 Paris, France; *Institut Choay, 92120 Montrouge, France; and **Peptide Laboratory, CNRS Institute of Biochemistry, Paris-Sud University, 91405 Orsay, France

INTRODUCTION

Lymphocytes represent a privileged tool for the study of cellular differentiation. Several pieces of evidence indicate that T-cell maturation may be divided into several steps, from the very immature lymphoid stem cell to the fully competent T-cell found in the periphery. The thymus, and more particularly its epithelium, plays a central role in this maturation. This differentiating action of the thymus appears to be mediated, at least in part, by various hormones. We describe in this chapter one of these hormones, the serum thymic factor (FTS) that is found in the thymus, like other thymic hormones, and also in the plasma from which it has been isolated. We have described elsewhere in detail the evidence in favor of the involvement of FTS in T-cell differentiation and discussed its possible target cell and mode of action (2,3). Rather, we shall present here the data giving FTS the status of a peptide hormone with all the relevant criteria.

DEFINITION

The initial experiment that led to the concept of FTS consisted in the demonstration that thymic extracts induce, after a short-term incubation, the θ (Thy-1) antigen marker on spleen cells from adult thymectomized (ATx) mice (5). The presence of a similar biological activity in normal serum [contrasting with its absence in the serum of thymectomized (Tx) mice] indicated that normal serum contained a thymus-dependent serum factor, inducing some T-cell characteristics on immature T-cells (4). The factor in question was shown to be a peptide produced by the thymus itself and endowed with a number of other biological activities. It was named "facteur thymique sérique." FTS is not the only described thymus-dependent serum factor. Astaldi et al. described a serum factor (SF) capable of stimulating cyclic AMP synthesis by thymocytes (1).

Rotter and Trainin reported a plasma factor of small molecular weight defined by its capacity to enhance lymphocyte proliferation in the presence of phytohemagglutinin (PHA) (21). White reported that prealbumin had a thymus-dependent activity on the rosette assay (10), but this latter activity may be due to the transport of FTS (see below). All these factors are probably different from FTS (although they may be carriers or degradation products of FTS). One should also note that thymopoietin (23) and α_1-thymosin have also been reported to be present in normal blood. The point is, however, not definitively proven either for thymopoietin (the definition of serum thymopoietin is indirect, based on a biological assay) or for α_1-thymosin [the negativity of the radioimmunoassay (RIA) in nude or Tx mouse sera has not been reported].

STRUCTURE

Porcine FTS has been purified from large amounts of pig serum ultrafiltrate using various steps of Sephadex and carboxymethyl cellulose (CMC) chromatography. FTS is sensitive to some proteolytic enzymes (e.g., pronase and trypsin) but resistant to ribonuclease. When pure, it is stable at 37°C for several hours; it can be stored at 4°C for several days and at −20°C (or lyophilized at room temperature) for several months without losing its activity. Its pI is 7.5 (11).

The amino acid sequence was obtained by the Edman degradation technique (19). Because the NH₂-terminal amino acid is blocked, the sequence was obtained only after treating the peptide with trypsin. The amino acid sequence is: <Glu-Ala-Lys-Ser-Gln-Gly-Gly-Ser-Asn. It is not known with certainty whether the native form has a pyroglutamic acid, or more likely a glutamine (transformed *in vitro* into pyroglutamic acid) as the NH₂-terminal residue.

Human plasma has been recently subjected to the same procedure as that

TABLE 1. *Structure and activities of FTS analogs*

FTS analogs						Biological activity[a]	Increased half-life[b]	Anti-genicity
Gln -Ala -Lys -Ser -Gln-Gly-Gly -Ser -Asn						+++	−	++
D-Gln ————————————						+++	+	++
—— D-Ala ———————————						++	−	++
———— D-Lys ——————————						++	++	+
——————— D-Ser ————————						−	−	−
————————— D-Gln —————						−	−	−
————————————— D-Asn						+	+	−
Ala —————————————						+	−	++
Lys ———————————						±	−	++
Ser ———————						−	−	−
———————————————— Ser						−	−	−

[a] − = >1 ng/ml; + = 0.1 to 1 ng/ml; ++ = 1 to 100 pg/ml; +++ = <1 pg/ml.
[b] Activity at 4 hr: − = <1:10³; + = 1:10³ to 1:10⁵; ++ = >1:10⁵.
From ref. 9.

TABLE 2. *Structure and activities of FTS analogs*

FTS analogs	Biological activity[a]	Increased half-life[b]	Anti-genicity
<Glu -Ala -Lys -Ser -Gln-Gly-Gly -Ser -Asn	+++	−	++
Gln ———————————————————	+++	−	++
Pro ———————————————————	+++	−	++
————— Orn —————————————	−	−	−
————— Hep —————————————	−	−	+
————— Arg —————————————	+	+	++
————— Har —————————————	+++	++	++
———— Nε-AcLys ————————————	+++	++	++
——————— Ala ——————————	−	−	−
——————————— Asn —————	++	+	−
——————————— Glu —————	+++	−	−
——————————— Nva —————	−	−	−
————————————— Ala ———	+	−	++
————————————————— Asn-NH₂	+	+	−
————————————————— Asp	−	−	−
————————————————— Gln	−	−	−
————————————————— βAla-NH₂	+	−	−

[a] − = >1 ng/ml; + = 0.1 to 1 ng/ml; ++ = 1 to 100 pg/ml; +++ = <1 pg/ml.
[b] Activity at 4 hr: − = <1:10³; + = 1:10³ to 1:10⁵; ++ = >1:10⁵.
From ref. 9.

used for porcine FTS. The amino acid composition of the isolated peptide proved to be identical to that of porcine FTS. This data fits with the recent report by Lacovara and Utermohlen (16) showing that a peptide with high activity in an human rosette assay was found in normal human plasma, and it had an amino acid composition very close to that of FTS.

Several analogs of FTS have been synthesized (8a,9). The study of their biological activity has shown that minor changes of the COOH-terminus altered the biological activity, whereas some changes could be made in the NH₂-terminus without influencing the biological activity (Tables 1 and 2). Note that the antigenic site is also located on the COOH-terminal portion of the molecule, as shown by a specific RIA (described below).

SITE OF PRODUCTION

Porcine FTS has been isolated from serum, and FTS has also been identified in other species by its presence in serum. Its dependence on the thymus is confirmed by its absence in congenitally athymic nude mice, its disappearance after thymectomy, and its reappearance after thymus grafting (4). More precisely, its dependence on the thymic epithelium is shown by the restoration of FTS levels seen after grafting low numbers of purely epithelial thymic cells, contrasting with the low restoring efficacy of lymphocyte-rich thymocytes (2).

Direct evidence for the thymic origin of FTS has recently been demonstrated by two experimental approaches. The first consisted in showing that thymic extracts contain an FTS-like material (as indicated by its molecular weight, its antigenicity as evaluated in a RIA, and its activity in the rosette assay) (2). Whether the extraction was performed by passage through an anti-FTS immunoadsorbent or by chemical fractionation guided by the rosette assay, it was shown that FTS is present in thymic extracts at concentrations higher than found in serum, which excludes a mere contamination of the thymus by blood (2). Recently, thymosin fraction 5 was purified on the basis of the rosette assay to purity. The substance present in fraction 5 and responsible for most (if not all) its rosette activity proved to be a peptide with a M.W. and especially, an amino acid composition very close to that of FTS (likely FTS itself).

An antiserum has been produced against the synthetic FTS coupled to bovine serum albumin (BSA). This antiserum was purified by the use of a FTS-gel immunoadsorbent in order to remove anti-BSA antibodies. The purified antibodies were shown to localize *in vitro* in the thymic epithelium by indirect immunofluorescence of rat thymus and cultures of mouse epithelium explants (17). The specificity of the anti-FTS antibody binding was assessed by its inhibition after the addition of 10 μg synthetic FTS and by the absence of binding to fibroblast cultures. It should be noted that the thymic lymphocytes were not labeled by the antibody.

RADIOIMMUNOASSAY—SERUM LEVELS

The antiserum produced against BSA-coupled FTS was used for performing a RIA. The specificity of the antibody for FTS was assessed by its capacity to eliminate FTS activity from serum *in vivo* and *in vitro*. Separation of free and bound FTS was achieved by incubation with activated charcoal (into which free, but not bound, FTS penetrates). The sensitivity of the RIA was of 10 to 50 pg with cold synthetic FTS. The specificity of the antibody for FTS was assessed by the absence of cross-reactivity with closely related synthetic analogs, differing by only one amino acid (Tables 1 and 2). The use of this RIA for the evaluation of serum FTS levels has been hampered by the presence of various interfering serum proteins. By using a complete extraction procedure (ultrafiltration on Amicon membranes followed by Sephadex chromatography), the presence of RIA-detectable levels of FTS was shown in normal (and not Tx) pig serum as well as in thymic (but not splenic) extracts (2). This procedure is, however, too time- and material-consuming to be applied routinely to serum samples for clinical use. A simpler method for FTS extraction is under development.

It is difficult, from these data, to evaluate accurately FTS serum levels. RIA data obtained after ultrafiltration, chromatography, and concentration indicate a value of the order of 50 pg/ml, but this certainly is underestimated due to the low yield of the procedure. Data from amino acid analyses suggest a content of 1 μg for 10 liter of serum ultrafiltrate, i.e., roughly 100 pg/ml, which is of the same order as the previous concentration, but again underestimated. Finally, it is likely, although not proven, that FTS serum levels range between 0.5 and 5 $\mu g/ml$.

SERUM INHIBITORS AND CARRIERS: PLASMA TRANSPORT

Circulating FTS is exposed to the action of several inhibitors that suppress its action in the rosette assay. These inhibitors have been characterized in human serum. Three molecules have been recognized, with approximate M.W.s of 3,000, 60,000 and 200,000 daltons, respectively. Their mode of action (FTS binding, pharmacological competition, etc.) is unknown.

There are several indications that FTS in serum exists in two forms. When one fractionates normal serum on Sephadex G-150 and examines activity in the rosette assay, two peaks may be observed: a major peak at the FTS (M.W. 867) and a minor one at the albumin-prealbumin zone (M.W. 60,000) (2). Both peaks are absent in profiles of Tx mouse sera but both appear after injecting synthetic FTS into such Tx mice, suggesting that the large M.W. peak material is directly related to FTS. This hypothesis is confirmed by the facts that the rosette activity of the proteins constituting this fraction is lost after its passage through an anti-FTS immunoadsorbent, and that the proteins can bind to FTS *in vitro*.

It is likely that these FTS-binding proteins play the role of carriers since the lower M.W. fraction significantly enhances the half-life of serum, as compared with the free FTS fraction. This hypothesis is also illustrated by the fact that when intact serum is injected into Tx mice, the half-life of FTS-like activity is of the order of 40 min, whereas that of free FTS is less than 10 min. It is interesting to note that FTS exhibits activity *in vivo* only when it has a sufficient half-life (for example, bound to CMC prior to injection). Recently synthesized long-lived analogs injected without a vehicle have shown biological activity (Tables 1 and 2) (8a,9).

MODE OF ACTION AT THE CELLULAR LEVEL

The cellular effects of FTS on T-cells have been examined at four levels: (a) receptors; (b) cyclic AMP synthesis; (c) induction of T-cell markers; and (d) induction of functions (true differentiation).

SPECIFIC FTS RECEPTORS ON T-CELLS

The first step in the action of a polypeptide hormone is the binding to specific receptors on its target cell. It is thus of utmost importance toward the understanding of the cellular mode of action of FTS to search for and characterize FTS receptors on lymphoid cells. To do this, we have applied the methodology (20) now well established for polypeptide hormones.

This effort was helped significantly by the finding of a lymphoblastoid T-

cell line (derived from cell cultures of patients with acute lymphoblastoid leukemia) that showed high levels of FTS binding. To demonstrate this, FTS was
labeled by tritium, using sodium borohydride, and cultured lymphocytes were
incubated for 90 min with labeled FTS. Twelve to 15% of the FTS was bound
to the cell line; the specificity of binding was assessed by observing a significant
inhibition of the binding after the addition of 10^{-8} M unlabeled FTS. In fact,
it was possible, after 90 min of incubation, to displace labeled FTS by a second
addition of unlabeled FTS. The production of FTS receptors by the T-cell line
was verified by their disappearance after trypsin treatment and their reappearance
after overnight incubation in a trypsin-free medium.

It is interesting to note that another T-cell line was shown to bind FTS,
whereas five B-cell lines and one null-cell line did not. Thus, the fact that
some T-cell lines did not bind FTS indicates that T-cells do not develop FTS
receptors during all stages of their differentiation. Preliminary data have shown
that normal human peripheral blood lymphocytes display FTS receptors when
they are preincubated in serum-free medium—probably, this treatment releases
any bound FTS. Finally, receptors with a high binding affinity for FTS
($K_D = 10^{-9}$M) appear on T-cells. Whether these receptors are associated with
the biological effects of FTS seems likely, but remains to be demonstrated.

The biological significance of the receptors is underlined by the high dissociation constant and the specificity (some FTS analogs, differing from FTS by only
one amino acid, lose most of their capacity to combine with the receptors).
The fact that not all T-cell lines have FTS receptors indicates that a minority
of T-cells bind FTS, and consequently that FTS acts only on a subpopulation
of T-cells. It is too early to determine the cell population(s) in question. However,
preliminary analyses of the membrane markers present on the FTS receptor-
bearing T-cell lines indicates that the FTS target cell is a relatively mature
T-cell, based on the presence of receptors for Fcμ and low rate of peanut agglutinin binding. This interpretation would fit well with the presence of FTS receptors
on some peripheral T-cells and with the preferential action of thymic factors
in T-cell-poor but not completely deprived mice (ATx or NZB mice).

CYCLIC AMP SYNTHESIS

The effect of thymic hormones on cyclic AMP and GMP remains a matter
of controversy and speculation. In brief, cyclic AMP and other substances that
increase its intracellular level mimic the induction of markers caused by thymic
factors (8,15,22). However, with the exception of THF, thymic factors do not
stimulate cyclic AMP synthesis, as evaluated directly at the total lymphocyte
level. Thymopoietin has been reported to increase the cyclic GMP level (13)
but this effect has not been found with other thymic extracts. The paradox
between indirect evidence suggesting cyclic AMP involvement and difficulties
in showing a direct cyclic AMP increase could relate (a) to the dilution of
thymic hormone target cells by other lymphoid cells (rendering impossible the

measurement of a modest increase in cyclic AMP level in such a minority of cells) and (b) to an effect restricted to a cytoplasmic or nuclear cyclic AMP pool. Studies in progress using the T-cell lines mentioned above should provide an interesting and new approach to that problem, since the cultured T-cells in question represent an homogeneous source of FTS-responsive cells.

INDUCTION OF T-CELL MARKERS

Marker studies indicate that the various types of T-cell antigens present during differentiation may be induced in precursor cells that are devoid of such markers. This was initially shown for the θ antigen in our laboratory, using various thymic extracts (3) and has now been confirmed and extended for Ly 1, 2, and 3 antigens, TL antigens, and xenogeneic antigens. In particular, FTS induces the theta and Ly antigens in the mouse and xenogeneic T-cell antigens in the human (2,14).

Other T-cell markers are induced by thymic factors. In particular, terminal deoxynucleotidyl transferase (TdT) expression is modified by incubation of immature lymphoid cells with FTS. Interestingly, the effects differ according to the cell type examined. TdT marker production in nude mouse spleen cells is increased by addition of thymosin (18) and decreased in BSA gradient-separated human bone marrow cells by synthetic FTS (14). Human E rosettes are seemingly increased *in vitro* and *in vivo* by all available factors (14).

INDUCTION OF FUNCTIONS

FTS is active on most T-cell functions (Table 3). Most strikingly, it enhances T-cell-mediated cytotoxicity in Tx mice. This effect is particularly clear in adult Tx mice using the Brunner assay (6). It is not known whether FTS directly stimulates the generation of the cytotoxic cells or enhances the function of a regulatory cell that could be the Ly 123^+ spleen cell. Similarly, FTS also acts on T-cells involved in delayed-type hypersensitivity induced by DNFB (12). It restores a normal response in ATx mice. Its effect on helper T-cells, as studied on anti-SRBC antibody, production is much less clear (we have not obtained major effects in a reproducible manner), perhaps due to a simultaneous action on suppressor T-cells.

In fact, FTS has recently proven to be remarkably active on suppressor T-cells in various *in vitro* and *in vivo* systems. Administered to normal mice, FTS suppresses the generation of allo-antigen reactive T-cells (6) or DNFB-sensitive T-cells (12). At 10 to 100 ng dosages, it may prolong skin allograft survival (2), or enhance the growth of MSV-sarcoma in T-cell-deprived mice (while at lower doses it stimulates its rejection). Lastly, *in vitro*, FTS impressively corrects the depressed capacity of most lupus patients to generate suppressor T-cells after Con A activation, as measured by pokeweed mitogen-driven immunoglobulin synthesis (R. Krakauer, *manuscript in preparation*).

TABLE 3. *Biological activities of FTS*

	In vitro[a]	In vivo[b]
Induction of T-lymphocyte markers		
Theta antigen	+	+
Xenogeneic T-cell antigen	+	
Autologous RFC (adult Tx and normal mice)	+	+
Antigen-binding receptors (thymus)	+	+
E-rosettes (T-cell depleted humans)	+	
PHA and Con A responsiveness	−	+
Reduction in TdT	+	
Effect on T-cell-mediated cytotoxicity		
Generation of anti-H-2 cytotoxic T-cells (adult Tx mice)		+
CML ("B" mice)	−	+
MSV sarcoma rejection ("B" mice)		+
Stimulation of helper T-cells		
Anti-SRBC antibody (PFC) ("B" mice)	−	±
+ Effects on autoimmunity (anti-DNA antibodies)		+
Enhancement of T-cell-mediated suppression or, less likely, depression of amplifier T-cells		
Decrease in PVP antibody production (NZB mice)		+
Depression of DNFB contact sensitivity (normal mice)		+
Depression of anti-H-2 cytotoxic T-cells (normal mice)		+
Retardation of skin allograft rejection (normal mice)		+
+ Effects on autoimmunity (Sjögren syndrome, hemolytic anemia)		+
Stimulation of Con A-induced T-cell suppression (humans)	+	

[a] 10^{-7} to 10^{-5} μg/ml.
[b] 0.1 to 1 ng/mouse.
From refs. 2,6,9,12,14.

This new, corrective effect of FTS probably has its counterpart for other thymic factors. It complicates the interpretation of the data observed in tests of various thymic functions, but widens the potential therapeutic applications. It appears, as far as FTS is concerned, that the suppressor effect is generally observed at high "pharmacological" doses of FTS, whereas other effects are seen at lower, presumably physiological doses. Whether this difference in dose is related to a difference in the cellular receptors of suppressor T-cells compared with helper or other T-cells, is not known. Whether this effect is related to a pharmacological stimulation of mature suppressor cells or to an induction or maturation of suppressor T-cell precursors has similarly not been determined. Note, however, that this represents a nonspecific inhibitory effect on immune responses is made unlikely, since pretreatment of recipient mice with low doses of cyclophosphamide (known to selectively inhibit suppressor T-cells in various systems) blocks this effect.

It is interesting to note that this effect of FTS on suppressor cells probably explains most of its preventive effects observed in NZB autoimmune mice [e.g., a decrease in anti-PVP antibody production and the blockade of Sjögren syndrome development (8)]. A simultaneous effect on helper T-cells probably explains the accelerated production of IgG anti-DNA antibodies also observed in these mice.

Finally, thymic factors show a large variety of effects on T-cell functions, especially in relatively mature cells, including suppressor T-cells. In addition to their effect on T-cell maturation, they seem to have a pharmacological effect on mature T-cells, and particularly suppressor cells that still possess receptors for thymic factors. A similar situation exists for corticosteroids which, at low doses, restore the various effects of adrenal insufficiency and induce dramatic and varied biological effects at higher, supraphysiological doses. In any case, the multiplicity of well-defined and well-controlled biological effects of purified or synthetic thymic peptides argues in favor of their important role in T-cell differentiation, at least in its late stages. Their action on the initial step of differentiation merits consideration if one hypothesizes that, at this stage and in high concentrations, they act only locally on cells in direct contact with the thymic epithelium.

POTENTIAL CLINICAL APPLICATIONS

FTS may have a clinical usage in the near future. Its diversified biological activities on T-cell functions, its availability in synthetic form, the knowledge of its pharmacology (including long-lived analogs), and its absence of detectable toxicity make it a good candidate for the treatment of a number of diseases that involve T-cell imbalance. In particular, patients having congenital T-cell deficiencies, viral infections, certain chronic bacterial infections, (e.g., lepromatous leprosy), and some malignant and autoimmune conditions could benefit from administration of FTS, as they seem to do from A. L. Goldstein's thymosin fraction 5 and N. Trainin's THF *(this volume)*. One should note that FTS is present in fraction 5 and could, to some extent, contribute to the biological activity of the latter. One should, however, mention that some difficulties may be predicted in view of the opposite effects observed during experiments with various T-cell subsets. It will be hard to predict, in a given case, whether helper or suppressor T-cells will be preferentially stimulated. In NZB and B/W mice, we have observed that some mice simultaneously improved in some parameters (e.g., Sjögren syndrome, hemolytic anemia) and worsened in others (e.g., glomerulonephritis and anti-DNA antibody production) (8). These difficulties that are identified with other thymic preparations are amenable to further investigation but necessitate caution in the first trials of thymic factor, particularly in studies of the autoimmune states.

REFERENCES

1. Astaldi, A., Astaldi, G. C. B., Schellekens, P. Th. A., and Eijsvoogel, V. P. (1976): Thymic factor in human sera demonstrable by a cyclic AMP assay. *Nature,* 260:713–715.
2. Bach, J. F., Bach, M. A., Blanot, D., Bricas, E., Charreire, J., Dardenne, M., Fournier, C., and Pleau, J. M. (1978): Thymic serum factor. *Bull. Inst. Pasteur,* 76:325–398.
3. Bach, J. F., Bach, M. A., Charreire, J., Dardenne, M., and Pleau, J. M. (1979): The mode of action of thymic hormones. *Ann. N.Y. Acad. Sci.,* 332:23–32.
4. Bach, J. F., and Dardenne, M. (1973): Studies on thymus products. II. Demonstration and characterization of a circulating thymic hormone. *Immunology,* 25:353–366.
5. Bach, J. F., Dardenne, M., Goldstein, A. L., Guha, A., and White, A. (1971): Appearance of T-cell markers in bone marrow rosette-forming cells after incubation with purified thymosin, a thymic hormone. *Proc. Natl. Acad. Sci. USA,* 68:2734–2738.
6. Bach, M. A. (1977): Lymphocyte-mediated cytotoxicity: Effects of ageing, adult thymectomy and thymic factor. *J. Immunol.,* 119:641–647.
7. Bach, M. A., and Bach, J. F. (1973): Studies on thymus products. VI. The effects of cyclic nucleotides and prostaglandins on rosette-forming cells: Interactions with thymic factor. *Eur. J. Immunol.,* 3:778–783.
8. Bach, M. A., Dardenne, M., and Droz, D. (1978): Effects of FTS on autoimmune disease in NZB and B/W mice. In: *Pharmacology of Immunoregulation,* edited by G. H. Werner and F. Floc'h, pp. 201–206. Academic Press, New York.
8a. Blanot, D., Martinez, J., Auger, G., and Bricas, E. (1979): Synthesis of analogs of the serum thymic nonapeptide, "facteur thymique sérique" (FTS). *Int. J. Peptide Protein Res.,* 14:41–50.
9. Blanot, D., Martinez, J., Sasaki, A., Auger, G., Bricas, E., Dardenne, M., and Bach, J. F. (1980): Synthetic analogs of serum thymic factor and their biological activities. In: *Proceedings of the Sixth American Peptide Symposium,* edited by E. Gross. Wiley, New York *(in press).*
10. Burton, P., Iden, S., Mitchell, K., and White, A. (1978): Thymic hormone-like restoration by human prealbumin of azathioprine sensitivity of spleen cells from thymectomized mice. *Proc. Natl. Acad. Sci. USA,* 75:823–827.
11. Dardenne, M., Pleau, J. M., Man, N. K., and Bach, J. F. (1977): Structural study of circulating thymic factor: A peptide isolated from pig serum. I. Isolation and purification. *J. Biol. Chem.,* 252:8040–8044.
12. Erard, D., Charreire, J., Auffredou, M. T., Galanaud, D., and Bach, J. F. (1979): Regulation of contact sensitivity to DNFB in the mouse: Effects of adult thymectomy and thymic factor. *J. Immunol.,* 123:1573–1576.
13. Hadden, J. (1978): Discussion. In: *Pharmacology of Immunoregulation,* edited by G. H. Werner and F. Floc'h, p. 380. Academic Press, New York.
14. Incefy, G. S., Mertelsmann, R., Dardenne, M., Bach, J. F., and Good, R. A. (1979): *In vitro* differentiation of human marrow precursor T-cells by the serum thymic factor (FTS). *Fed. Proc.,* 38:1212.
15. Kook, A. I., and Trainin, N. (1974): Hormone-like activity of a thymus humoral factor on the induction of immune competence in lymphoid cells. *J. Exp. Med.,* 139:193–207.
16. Lacovara, J., and Utermohlen, V. (1980): Isolation and asssay of a human "facteur thymique sérique." *Clin. Immunol. Immunopathol. (in press).*
17. Monier, J. C., Dardenne, M., Pleau, J. M., Deschaux, P., and Bach, J. F. (1979): Localisation dans le thymus par immunofluorescence indirecte (IFI) des Ac anti-facteur thymique sérique (FTS) (thymic localization by indirect IF of anti-FTS antibodies). *Soc. Fr. Immunol.,* p. 31.
18. Pazmino, N. H., Ihle, J. N., and Goldstein, A. L. (1978): Induction *in vivo* and *in vitro* of terminal deoxynucleotidyl transferase by thymosin in bone marrow cells from athymic mice. *J. Exp. Med.,* 147:708–718.
19. Pleau, J. M., Dardenne, M., Blouquit, Y., and Bach, J. F. (1977): Structural study of circulating thymic factor: A peptide isolated from pig serum. II. Amino acid sequence. *J. Biol. Chem.,* 252:8045–8047.
20. Pleau, J. M., Fuentes, V., Morgat, J. L., and Bach, J. F. (1979): Caractérisation d'un récepteur spécifique du facteur thymique sérique dans une lignée lymphocytaire T humaine. *C.R. Acad. Sci. [D] (Paris),* 288:445–448.
21. Rotter, V., and Trainin, N. (1979): Role of thymic hormone (THF) and of a thymic plasma recirculating factor (TPRF) in the modulation of human lymphocyte response to PHA and Con A. *J. Immunol.,* 122:414–420.

22. Scheid, M. P., Hoffmann, N. K., Komuro, K., Hämmerling, V., Abbott, J., Boyse, E. A., Cohen, G. H., Hooper, J. A., Schulof, R. S., and Goldstein, A. L. (1973): Differentiation of T cells induced by preparations from thymus and by nonthymic agents: The determined state of the precursor cell. *J. Exp. Med.,* 138:1027–1032.

23. Twomey, J. J., Goldstein, G., Lewis, V. M., Bealmear, P. M., and Good, R. A. (1977): Bioassay determinations of thymopoietin and thymic hormone levels in human plasma. *Proc. Natl. Acad. Sci. USA,* 74:2541–2545.

Polypeptide Hormones, edited by
R. F. Beers, Jr. and E. G. Bassett.
Raven Press, New York © 1980.

44. Thymus-Dependent Human Serum Factor: A Peptide Inducing Maturation of Thymocytes

A. Astaldi, G. C. B. Astaldi, P. Wijermans, *A. Facchini,
T. van Bemmel, C. J. M. Leupers, P. Th. A. Schellekens,
and V. P. Eijsvoogel

*Central Laboratory for the Netherlands Red Cross Blood Transfusion Service and
Laboratory for Experimental and Clinical Immunology, University of Amsterdam, 1006
AD Amsterdam, The Netherlands; and *Institute of Normal Human Anatomy,
Faculty of Medicine, University of Bologna, I-40126 Bologna, Italy*

INTRODUCTION

The development of immunocompetent T-cells appears to be at least partially under the influence of humoral factors controlled by the thymus. This hypothesis was suggested by the findings that (a) the immunocompetent cells in thymecto-mized mice bearing a grafted thymus are of host origin and the immunological reconstitution of thymectomized mice can be achieved by grafting a thymus enclosed in a diffusion chamber (16,45); (b) several soluble factors acting on T-cell maturation have been found in thymic extracts, in peripheral blood, and in supernatant fluids of thymic epithelial cultures (27).

Stutman et al. (44) proposed that T-cell precursors, which are the target cells for thymic factors, have already undergone some form of thymic influence, probably by passage through the thymus; consequently, he termed these cells post-thymic precursor cells (for reviews, see 42).

Mouse thymocytes can be separated into two subpopulations: One is mainly present in the cortex, is sensitive to hydrocortisone (HC^s), can be agglutinated by the lectin peanut agglutinin (PNA$^+$), and is immunologically immature; the other is HC-resistant (HC^r), PNA-nonagglutinating (PNA$^-$) and present mainly in the medulla (20,33). This latter subpopulation was reported to be as immuno-competent as mature T-cells, when tested with a graft-versus-host (GvH) assay *in vivo* (13).

Shortman et al. (36) suggested that most cortical thymocytes die within the thymus, whereas the medullary cells develop according to an independent path-way. Weissman (50), on the contrary, showed that at least some of the medullary thymocytes are derived from cortical cells. However, this does not mean that HC^r thymocytes are the source of thymic cell migrants, as shown by more recent experiments of Weissman et al. (51) and Stutman (42). Indeed, in recent studies on mouse T-cell ontogeny (34), no evidence was found for a maturation from PNA$^+$ to PNA$^-$ thymocytes; further, PNA$^+$ cells were also found in peripheral lymphoid organs.

Thus, it is conceivable that at least a part of PNA$^+$, HC^s thymocytes are exported by the thymus as relatively immunologically immature cells capable of further maturation in the periphery, as proposed by Stutman (42).

In this chapter, we discuss the possibility that immature thymocytes can be induced to immunological maturation by the serum factor (SF), a peptide present in normal human serum; this maturation process is probably controlled by the thymus, because SF is a thymus-dependent peptide.

RESULTS AND DISCUSSION

Thymus-Dependent Human Serum Factor

It is generally agreed that specific triggering of target cells by peptide hormones is accompanied by a rise in the level of cellular cyclic AMP (46). Furthermore, cyclic AMP itself and agents increasing intracellular cyclic AMP levels were found to induce T-cell maturation in a manner similar to that of thymic extracts (35). On these grounds, we formulated the hypothesis that a circulating thymic hormone, if any, would have also increased cellular cyclic AMP in specific target cells: Indeed, we found that normal serum contains a factor selectively increasing the level of cyclic AMP in thymocytes and we termed it "serum factor"; the factor was found to be distinct from nonspecific cyclic AMP-elevating agents (3,4). More recently, SF has been purified from large amounts of human blood and found to be a neutral peptide of low molecular weight (<500). SF has been isolated to a single spot by fingerprinting and sequencing experiments are currently being performed.

Thymus Dependency of SF

SF was found to be present in normal human donors between 0 and 90 years of age. The level of SF reaches its maximum in the third decade of life and decreases thereafter (52,56). Repeated determinations of SF activity before and after thymectomy revealed that SF decreases rapidly after thymectomy in humans, reaching very low levels within a few days (4,56). SF was found to be absent in most of the thymectomized myasthenia gravis patients tested, whereas normal levels occurred in non-thymectomized patients with this disease (3,4,56). SF was also found to be absent in several patients with thymus-dependent immunodeficiency diseases, such as Di George's syndrome (10). Treatment of such patients by means of transplanting a fetal thymus, transplanting cultured thymus epithelium or by administration of thymosin fraction 5 (a polypeptide extract of calf thymus) induced the prompt appearance of SF in the blood (6,8,10).

These data suggest that SF is produced directly by the thymus. Furthermore, THF, a peptide extracted from calf thymus, increases cellular cyclic AMP levels (25) as do SF. Thymic epithelial culture supernatant fluids (TES) (27) also increase cellular cyclic AMP levels and share several of the biological activities of SF (28,29). These findings provide indirect evidence for the thymic origin of SF. Since direct evidence of the thymic origin of SF is as yet lacking, we cannot rule out the possibility that SF is produced elsewhere in the body, under the control of the thymus. We conclude that SF is thymus-dependent, being either directly produced or controlled by the thymus.

Target Cell for SF

When tested on human and mouse cells, SF was found to act mainly on thymocytes, moderately on lymph node cells, and only marginally on bone marrow cells (3,54). The action of SF on bone marrow cells is restricted to cells of low specific gravity (54), i.e., to the lymphoid compartment (24). No activity of SF was found on other lymphoid and non-lymphoid cells except human cord blood lymphocytes (2,3,7,54). The target cell specificity of SF was confirmed by means of adsorption experiments (3): SF is completely adsorbed by thymocytes, not by other types of cells. We conclude that SF acts through a membranal site, probably a receptor, present mainly on thymocytes and distinct from the β-adrenergic receptor.

Additional evidence on the target cell specificity of SF was obtained by means of cell separation on density gradients (19). Human peripheral blood T-cells with a high specific gravity (heavy lymphocytes) were found to be more immature than T-cells with a low specific gravity (light lymphocytes) (19). However, no activity of SF was found on any of the peripheral blood T-cell fractions (19), and the activity of SF was found to be restricted to thymocytes. This is a difference with other thymic factors, such as TES and THF, as well as with nonspecific cyclic AMP-elevating agents that were also found to be active on peripheral blood T-cell populations (19,57).

These findings, indicating that target cells for SF are mainly among thymocytes, prompted us to investigate to which subpopulation of thymocytes target cells for SF belong and to characterize the target cells present in other organs. The activity of SF was found to be restricted to immunologically immature, PNA[+], HC[s] thymocytes (see introduction for our definition of thymocyte subpopulations); SF had no effect on immunologically mature, PNA[-], HC[r] thymocytes (1,2,7,9,54). The target cells for SF among thymocytes were further characterized as cells with high Thy-1 antigen density, low H_2 antigen density (55), and high levels at terminal deoxynucleotidyl transferase enzyme activity (5). Target cells for SF found in lymph nodes and bone marrow were also characterized as HC[s] cells with high Thy-1 antigen density (54).

These results indicate that the target cells for SF have several characteristics of the post-thymic precursor cells as defined by Stutman (42,43). However, because the thymus is the major source of the target cells for SF (54) and because most of our studies were performed on immunologically immature thymocytes (1,9), we cannot rule out the possibility that the target cells for SF are intrathymic predecessors of the post-thymic precursor cells.

Induction of Markers of Mouse Mature T-Cells

The effect of SF on the phenotypic expression of markers of mouse T-cells is summarized in Table 1. SF induces the phenotypic expression of markers of mouse mature T-cells (7,55). In brief, SF induces a decrease in the expression of the Thy-1 antigen and an increase in the expression of H_2 antigens, as demonstrated in both cytotoxicity and quantitative adsorption studies (55); in addition, SF induces an acquisition of resistance to the lytic action of HC (2). In contrast, SF has apparently no effect on the binding of PNA. As yet, there is no explanation for this: It might be caused by technical difficulties, but it is also possible that PNA$^-$ cells are not derived from PNA$^+$ cells, as suggested by Roelants et al. (34).

Induction of Markers of Human Mature T-Cells

A small subpopulation of human thymocytes lacks the T-cell receptor for sheep red blood cells (SRBC). Because a consistent increase in SRBC rosettes was observed after exposure to SF of human thymocytes (55), we partially purified the subpopulation of non-rosetting thymocytes. When this subpopulation was exposed to SF, the proportion of SRBC rosettes increased to values similar to those found in unseparated thymocytes (55).

Immunologically mature human T-cells have been shown to bear Fc receptors for IgG (Tγ) and for IgM (Tμ). Functional analysis has indicated a suppressor activity for Tγ and a helper activity for Tμ (32). Investigations on tissue distribution of Tγ and Tμ revealed the presence of at least one of these two subpopulations in all lymphoid tissues except the thymus (31). Incubation with SF induced

TABLE 1. *Effect of SF on the phenotypic expression of markers of mouse T-cells*

	Phenotypic expression in:			
Marker[a]	Immature T-cells	Immature T-cells treated with SF	Mature T-cells	Mature T-cells treated with SF
Thy-1	+++	+	+	+
H_2	+	+++	+++	+++
HC^s	+++	+	+	+
PNA$^+$	+++	+++	+	+
TdT	+++	+	−	−

[a] HC^s, sensitive to hydrocortisone; PNA$^+$, binding the peanut agglutinin; TdT, terminal deoxynucleotidyl transferase.

the appearance of the Fc receptor for IgM in about 9% of the thymocytes (7,55). No effect of SF could be observed on the induction of the Fc receptor for IgG. We conclude that SF induces also some phenotypic traits of immunocompetent human T-cells.

Decrease of Terminal Deoxynucleotidyl Transferase Levels

Terminal deoxynucleotidyl transferase (TdT), a DNA-polymerizing enzyme which catalyzes the addition of deoxyribonucleotides to a DNA primer in the absence of a template, was first described by Bollum (14). Under normal conditions, TdT is found only in precursors of immunocompetent T-cells, such as hydrocortisone-sensitive thymocytes and bone marrow cells, but not in fully immunocompetent peripheral T-cells (for reviews, see 12,15). These findings indicate that the final maturation of T-cells is associated with the disappearance of TdT activity and have led Baltimore (11) to suggest that TdT is a potential somatic mutagen, possibly involved in the generation of immunological diversity. SF induces a marked decrease of the TdT activity both in human and in mouse thymocytes (5) after 4 hr of exposure. We conclude that, if TdT is involved in the generation of immunological diversity, as proposed by Baltimore (11), SF might act either on fully diversified cells (and so induce their maturation) or on cells potentially capable of further diversification. Preliminary indications suggest that the second possibility might be correct.

Induction of Effector Function in the Graft-Versus-Host Reaction

A graft-versus-host (GvH) reaction occurs when the grafted cells are immunocompetent of reacting against the host, but the host is not immunocompetent of rejecting the graft. A typical situation of GvH reaction is achieved by the injection of homozygous parental (P) lymphoid cells into an F_1 hybrid mouse.

TABLE 2. *Effect of SF on the GvH reactivity of PNA$^+$ and PNA$^-$ B6 thymocytes injected into (B6 × C3H)F$_1$ newborn mice*

Thymocyte fraction from B6 mice	No. of thymocytes injected (× 10^6)	No. of mice injected	Response[a]
PNA$^+$, HC^s, untreated	1.25	9	1.62 ± 0.015
PNA$^+$, HC^s, SF-treated	1.25	8	1.75 ± 0.019
PNA$^-$, HC^r, untreated	0.625	10	1.84 ± 0.048
PNA$^-$, HC^r, SF-treated	0.625	7	1.83 ± 0.069
Unfractionated, untreated	1.25	17	1.66 ± 0.013
Unfractionated, SF-treated	1.25	27	1.77 ± 0.017
None	0	24	1.61 ± 0.010

[a] Expressed as log mg spleen/10 g body weight.

Simonsen (37) has developed a method for the bioassay of immunological activity in suspensions of lymphoid cells. The method is based on the finding that the degree of splenomegaly, which develops in the early stages of the GvH reaction, is directly correlated with the number of immunologically competent cells grafted into the host. It was shown (13) that the effector cells in this reaction are immunocompetent T-cells, and that HC^s thymocytes have a low activity.

Table 2 shows that SF increased the capacity of PNA$^+$, HC^s thymocytes to induce a GvH reaction; furthermore, treatment with SF had no effect on the capacity of immunocompetent PNA$^-$, HC^r thymocytes to induce the GvH reaction (9). We conclude that at least part of the immunologically immature thymocyte population can acquire properties of functionally immunocompetent cells under the influence of SF.

Early Intracellular Events Induced by SF in Thymocytes

The mode of action of SF at the intracellular level was evaluated by the study of the intracellular events associated with the appearance of markers and functions of immunocompetent T-cells.

Adsorption experiments (3) indicate that SF binds to a membranal site, probably a receptor, present on the thymocyte cell membrane. Within one min the binding is followed by an increase in the intracellular level of cyclic AMP, which reaches its maximum after 5 min and decreases thereafter (7,18,53). This type of kinetics renders it unlikely that SF might increase cyclic AMP by interfering with the degradation of cyclic AMP, thus indicating that SF does not act as an inhibitor of phosphodiesterases and suggesting a direct action of SF on the production of cyclic AMP. Therefore, we tested the effect of SF on thymocyte membranes and found that SF indeed stimulates adenylate cyclase that mediates the production of cyclic AMP. Because SF does not induce any changes in the level of intracellular cyclic GMP, we concluded that SF alters the cyclic AMP/cyclic GMP ratio in favor of cyclic AMP, an event associated with cell differentiation (49).

Protein synthesis was found to increase in thymocytes within 15 min after the binding of SF (53). The maximal stimulation of protein synthesis occurred after 2 to 4 hr (18,53). A similar stimulation has been reported to be induced by THF (26) and by thymopoietin (41). It was also suggested that the protein synthesis induced by thymic factors is followed by alterations at the level of the cell nucleus, such as a reduction in DNA synthesis (26), transcription of DNA, and translation of RNA (41). Furthermore, it has been shown that lymphocyte maturation requires synthesis of nuclear proteins (23). Several pieces of evidence (17,40) indicate that, among the nuclear proteins, the group of phosphorylated, nonhistone chromatin proteins (P-NHCP) contain macromolecules that are involved in the regulation of chromatin template activity. These findings prompted us to perform qualitative studies on the proteins synthesized in thymocytes under the influence of SF (18).

TABLE 3. *Effect of SF on the incorporation of ³H-leucine into protein fractions of thymocytes[a]*

Substances added	Total cell protein	Chromatin	P-NHCP	Histones	R-NHCP
			^{3}H-leucine (dpm $\times$ 10^{-5}) incorporated per milligram of:		
Control	3.3	3.4	15.3	1.8	0.5
SF	6.5	9.8	23.6	2.1	0.6

[a] Each value is the mean of four protein extractions.

Table 3 shows the effect of SF on the incorporation of ^{3}H-leucine into protein fractions of thymocytes after 30 min incubation with SF. At the chromatin level, SF induced a marked (2.9-fold) increase of incorporated radioactivity. When the distribution of radioactivity in the various nuclear proteins [phosphorylated nonhistone chromatin proteins (P-NHCP), histones, and residual nonhistone chromatin proteins (R-NHCP)] is compared, it is evident that the incorporation of ^{3}H-leucine was especially located in the P-NHCP, which represents only a small amount (8.8%) of the total nuclear proteins. SF induced a high incorporation of ^{3}H-leucine into the P-NHCP as early as after 15 min of culture (18). At the level of histones, which represent the highest amount of protein recovered from the chromatin (43.3%), SF also induced an increase of incorporation of ^{3}H-leucine, but the specific radioactivity was $\frac{1}{10}$ of that found in the P-NHCP fraction. The incorporation of ^{3}H-leucine into the R-NHCP fraction appeared to be only 3% of that found in the P-NHCP fraction. Because cycloheximide, a specific inhibitor of protein synthesis, fully prevented the increase in the incorporation of leucine by thymocytes exposed to SF (18,53), we concluded that SF stimulates protein synthesis rather than leucine transport in thymocytes.

Table 4 shows the effect of SF on the incorporation of ^{32}P into protein fractions of thymocytes after 30 min of culture. SF induced a 2.1-fold incorporation of ^{32}P in the total proteins. A similar factor of increase (2.2-fold) at the chromatin level was found to be induced by SF. When the distribution of radioactivity in the various nuclear fractions is compared, it is evident that the influence of

TABLE 4. *Effect of SF on the incorporation of ³²P into protein fractions of thymocytes[a]*

Substances added	Total cell protein	Chromatin	P-NHCP	Histones	R-NHCP
			^{32}P (dpm $\times$ 10^{-5}) incorporated per milligram of:		
Control	3.8	3.0	0.4	0.3	0.03
SF	8.0	6.8	1.1	0.4	0.04

[a] Each value is the mean of four protein extractions.

SF on the incorporation of ^{32}P was especially marked in the P-NHCP, in analogy with the findings on incorporation of ^{3}H-leucine. Cycloheximide reduced the incorporation of ^{32}P induced by SF into proteins of about 50%, indicating that part of the ^{32}P incorporation is due to protein phosphorylation and part is due to the increased protein synthesis. Indomethacin, an inhibitor of cyclic AMP-dependent protein kinases (22), reduced to about 30% the incorporation of ^{32}P induced by SF into total thymocyte proteins, further indicating that part of the ^{32}P incorporation reflects protein phosphorylation due to protein kinase activity (18).

Electrophoretic patterns in polyacrylamide gels of the P-NHCP fractions, extracted from the chromatin of the cells stimulated with SF, showed that proteins with molecular weights greater than 5×10^4 were synthesized to a larger extent as compared with synthesis in unstimulated cells (18).

We concluded that SF selectively stimulates synthesis and phosphorylation of high molecular weight NHCP (18). Since no substantial changes were observed at the histone level, these findings, taken together with the observation that SF does not stimulate thymocyte proliferation (9), are compatible with DNA transcription and RNA translation. Similarly, polypeptide hormones, such as insulin, prolactin, and chorionic gonadotrophin, as well as steroids (21,38,47) exert an action on nuclear protein phosphorylation of specific target cells.

In conclusion, the binding of SF to thymocytes stimulates adenylate cyclase with a subsequent rise in intracellular cyclic AMP levels; most likely, the increase in cyclic AMP leads to stimulation of protein kinases, since it is known that cyclic AMP regulates the activity of these enzymes (30,48); protein kinases are, in turn, responsible for the phosphorylation and synthesis of nuclear proteins. The P-NHCP would then be responsible for gene activation (39), which would result in the phenotypic expression of genetic information, as described in the first part of this chapter.

SUMMARY

It seems likely that SF acts on immunologically immature T-cells that have already undergone some form of thymic influence, because they bear the Thy-1 antigen and have high levels of TdT activity. These cells are found within the population of immature thymocytes, in lymph nodes, and in bone marrow. Because SF, a peptide present in normal human serum, can induce immunological maturation of these cells, we conclude that at least part of the immunologically immature T-cells present in the thymus and peripheral lymphoid organs are precursors of mature T-cells. This is in agreement with the concept of post-thymic maturation of T-cell precursors as proposed by Stutman (42,43).

In agreement with Weissman et al. (51) and Stutman (42), we also conclude that HC^r thymocytes are not the sole source of thymus cell migrants, since we find HC^s target cells for SF also in peripheral lymphoid organs.

Finally, because HC^s, PNA$^+$ thymocytes are the major source of the target cells for SF, we cannot rule out the possibility that at least part of the target cells for SF are intrathymic predecessors of the post-thymic precursor cells.

REFERENCES

1. Astaldi, A. (1979): Thymocyte maturation induced by a thymus-dependent serum factor. *Haematologia (in press)*.
2. Astaldi, G. C. B., Astaldi, A., Groenewoud, M., Wijermans, P., Schellekens, P. Th. A., and Eijsvoogel, V. P. (1977): Effect of a human serum thymic factor on hydrocortisone-treated thymocytes. *Eur. J. Immunol.,* 7:836–840.
3. Astaldi, A., Astaldi, G. C. B., Schellekens, P. Th. A., and Eijsvoogel, V. P. (1976): Thymic factor in human sera demonstrable by a cyclic AMP assay. *Nature,* 260:713–715.
4. Astaldi, A., Astaldi, G. C. B., Schellekens, P. Th. A., and Eijsvoogel, V. P. (1978): Is there a circulating human thymic factor that induces cyclic AMP synthesis? Reply. *Nature,* 271:666–668.
5. Astaldi, G. C. B., Astaldi, A., Wijermans, P., Bemmel, T. van, Schellekens, P. Th. A., and Eijsvoogel, V. P. (1979): A thymus-dependent human serum factor induces decrease of terminal deoxynucleotidyl transferase in thymocytes. *Immunol. Lett.,* 1:155–159.
6. Astaldi, A., Astaldi, G. C. B., Wijermans, P., Dagna-Bricarelli, F., Kater, L., Stoop, J. W., and Vossen, J. M. (1978): Experiences with thymosin in primary immunodeficiency disease. *Cancer Treat. Rep.,* 62:1779–1785.
7. Astaldi, A., Astaldi, G. C. B., Wijermans, P., Groenewoud, M., Bemmel, T. van, Schellekens, P. Th. A., and Eijsvoogel, V. P. (1979): Thymus-dependent human serum factor active on precursors of mature T-cells. In: *Cell Biology and Immunology of Leukocyte Function,* edited by M. Quastel, pp. 221–225. Academic Press, New York.
8. Astaldi, A., Astaldi, G. C. B., Wijermans, P., Groenewoud, M., Schellekens, P. Th. A., and Eijsvoogel, V. P. (1977): Thymosin-induced human serum factor increasing cyclic AMP. *J. Immunol.,* 119:1106–1108.
9. Astaldi, G. C. B., Astaldi, A., Wijermans, P., Schellekens, P. Th. A., and Eijsvoogel, V. P. (1980): A thymus-dependent serum factor induces maturation of thymocytes as evaluated by graft-versus-host reaction. *Cell. Immunol.,* 49:202–207.
10. Astaldi, A., Astaldi, G. C. B., Wijermans, P., Schellekens, P. Th. A., Kuis, W., Schuurman, R., Vossen, J. M., Weening, R. S., and Weemaes, C. M. (1980): Thymus-dependent human serum factor in primary immunodeficiency diseases. *Clin. Immunol. Immunopathol. (in press).*
11. Baltimore, D. (1974): Is terminal deoxynucleotidyl transferase a somatic mutagen in lymphocytes? *Nature,* 248:409–411.
12. Baltimore, D., Silverstone, A. E., Kung, P. C., Harrison, T. A., and McCaffrey, R. P. (1977): What cells contain terminal transferase? In: *The Generation of Antibody Diversity: A New Look,* edited by A. Cunningham, pp. 21–30. Academic Press, New York.
13. Blomgren, H., and Andersson, B. (1969): Evidence for a small pool of immunocompetent cells in the mouse thymus. *Exp. Cell Res.,* 57:185–192.
14. Bollum, F. J. (1960): Calf thymus polymerase. *J. Biol. Chem.,* 235:2399–2403.
15. Bollum, F. J. (1974): Terminal deoxynucleotidyl transferase. In: *The Enzymes, Vol. 10,* edited by R. D. Boyer, pp. 145–171. Academic Press, New York.
16. Daimasso, A. P., Martinez, C., Sjodin, K., and Good, R. A. (1963): Studies on the role of the thymus in immunobiology: Reconstitution of immunologic capacity in mice thymectomized at birth. *J. Exp. Med.,* 118:1089–1109.
17. Elgin, S. C. R., and Weintraub, H. (1975): Chromosomal protein and chromatin structure. *Annu. Rev. Biochem.,* 44:725–774.
18. Facchini, A., Astaldi, G. C. B., Cocco, L., Wijermans, P., Manzoli, F. A., and Astaldi, A. (1979): Early events in thymocyte activation. II. Changes in nonhistone chromatin proteins induced by a thymus-dependent human serum factor. *J. Immunol.,* 123:1577–1585.
19. Griend, R. J. van de, Astaldi, A., Wijermans, P., Doorn, R. van, and Roos, D. (1980): Changes in β-adrenergic receptor concentration in human T-cell ontogeny *(submitted for publication).*
20. Irlè, C., Piguet, P.-F., and Vassalli, P. (1978): *In vitro* maturation of immature thymocytes into immunocompetent T-cells in the absence of direct thymic influence. *J. Exp. Med.,* 148:32–45.

21. Jungmann, R. A., and Schweppe, J. S. (1972): Mechanism of action of gonadotrophin. I. Evidence for gonadotrophin-induced modifications of ovarian nuclear basic and acidic protein biosynthesis, phosphorylation and acetylation. *J. Biol. Chem.,* 247:5535–5542.
22. Kantor, H. S., and Hampton, M. (1978): Indomethacin in submicromolar concentrations inhibits cyclic AMP-dependent protein kinase. *Nature,* 276:841–842.
23. Kishimoto, T., Nishizawa, Y., Kikutani, H., and Yamamura, Y. (1977): Biphasic effect of cyclic AMP on IgG production and on the changes of non-histone nuclear proteins induced with anti-immunoglobulin and enhancing soluble factor. *J. Immunol.,* 118:2027–2033.
24. Komuro, K., and Boyse, E. A. (1973): *In vitro* demonstration of thymic hormone in the mouse by conversion of precursor cells into lymphocytes. *Lancet,* 1:740–743.
25. Kook, A. I., and Trainin, N. (1974): Hormone-like activity of a thymus humoral factor on the induction of immune competence in lymphoid cells. *J. Exp. Med.,* 139:193–207.
26. Kook, A. I., and Trainin, N. (1975): Intracellular events involved in the induction of immune competence in lymphoid cells by a thymus humoral factor. *J. Immunol.,* 114:151–157.
27. Kruisbeek, A. (1979): Thymic factors and T-cell maturation *in vitro:* A comparison of the effects of thymic epithelial cultures with thymic extracts and thymus-dependent serum factors. *Thymus,* 1:163–186.
28. Kruisbeek, A. M., and Astaldi, G. C. B. (1979): Distinct effects of thymic epithelial culture supernatants on T cell properties of mouse thymocytes separated by the use of peanut agglutinin. *J. Immunol.,* 123:984–991.
29. Kruisbeek, A. M., Astaldi, G. C. B., Blankwater, M. J., Zijlstra, J. L., Levert, L. A., and Astaldi, A. (1978): The *in vitro* effects of a thymic epithelial culture supernatant on mixed lymphocyte reactivity and intracellular cAMP levels of thymocytes and on antibody production to SRBC by Nu/Nu spleen cells. *Cell Immunol.,* 35:134–147.
30. Kuo, J. F., and Greengard, P. (1970): Cyclic nucleotide-dependent protein kinases. VI. Isolation and partial purification of a protein kinase activated by guanosine $3',5'$ monophosphate. *J. Biol. Chem.,* 245:2493–2498.
31. Moretta, L., Ferrarini, M., and Cooper, H. D. (1978): Characterization of human T-cell subpopulations as defined by specific receptors for immunoglobulins. *Contemp. Top. Immunobiol.,* 8:19–53.
32. Moretta, L., Webb, S. R., Grossi, C. E., Lydyard, P. M., and Cooper, H. D. (1977): Functional analysis of two human T-cell subpopulations: Help and suppression of B-cell responses by T-cells bearing receptors for IgM or IgG. *J. Exp. Med.,* 146:184–200.
33. Reisner, Y., Linker-Israeli, M., and Sharon, N. (1976): Separation of mouse thymocytes into two subpopulations by the use of peanut agglutinin. *Cell Immunol.,* 25:129–134.
34. Roelants, G. E., London, J., Mayor-Withey, K. S., and Serrano, B. (1979): Peanut agglutinin. II. Characterization of the Thy-1, Tla and Ig phenotype of peanut-agglutinin-positive cells in adult, embryonic and nude mice using double immunofluorescence. *Eur. J. Immunol.,* 9:139–145.
35. Scheid, H. P., Hoffmann, H. K., Komura, K., Hammerling, U., Abbot, J., Boyse, E. A., Cohen, G. H., Hooper, J. A., Schulof, R. S., and Goldstein, A. L. (1972): Differentiation of T-cells induced by preparations from thymus and by nonthymic agents: The determined state of the precursor cell. *J. Exp. Med.,* 138:1027–1032.
36. Shortman, K., Brunner, K. T., and Cerottini, J. C. (1972): Separation of stages in the development of the "T" cells involved in cell-mediated immunity. *J. Exp. Med.,* 135:1375–1391.
37. Simonsen, M. (1962): Graft versus host reactions: Their natural history and applicability as tools of research. *Prog. Allergy,* 6:349–467.
38. Spelberg, C. T. (1974): The role of nuclear acidic proteins in binding steroid hormones. In: *Acidic Proteins of the Nucleus,* edited by I. L. Cameron and J. R. Jeter, Jr., pp. 247–272. Academic Press, New York.
39. Stein, G. S., Chaudmury, S. C., and Baserga, R. (1972): Gene activation in WI-38 fibroblasts stimulated to proliferate: Role of non-histone chromosomal proteins. *J. Biol. Chem.,* 247:3918–3922.
40. Stein, G. S., Stein, J. L. Kleinsmith, L. J., Thompson, J. A., Park, W. D., and Jansing, R. L. (1976): Role of nonhistone chromosomal proteins in the regulation of histone gene expression. *Cancer Res.,* 36:4307–4318.
41. Storrie, B., Goldstein, G., Boyse, E. A., and Hammerling, U. (1976): Differentiation of thymocytes: Evidence that induction of the surface phenotype requires transcription and translation. *J. Immunol.,* 116:1358–1362.

42. Stutman, O. (1977): Two main features of T-cell development: Thymus traffic and post-thymus maturation. In: *Contemporary Topics in Immunobiology, Vol. 7,* edited by O. Stutman, pp. 1–46. Plenum Press, New York.

43. Stutman, O. (1978): Intrathymic and extrathymic T-cell maturation. *Immunol. Rev.,* 42:138–184.

44. Stutman, O., Yunis, E. J., and Good, R. A. (1969): Carcinogeninduced tumors of the thymus: IV. Humoral influences of normal thymus and functional thymomas and influence of postthymectomy period on restoration. *J. Exp. Med.,* 130:809–819.

45. Stutman, O., Yunis, E. J., Martinez, C., and Good, R. A. (1967): Reversal of post-thymectomy wasting disease in mice by multiple thymus grafts. *J. Immunol.,* 98:79–87.

46. Sutherland, E. W., Robinson, G. A., and Butcher, R. W. (1968): Some aspects of the biological role of adenosine-3',5'-monophosphate (cyclic AMP). *Circulation,* 37:279–306.

47. Turkington, R. W., and Riddle, M. (1969): Hormone-dependent phosphorylation of nuclear proteins during mammary gland differentiation *in vitro. J. Biol. Chem.,* 244:6040–6046.

48. Walsh, D. A., Perkins, J. P., and Krebs, E. G. (1968): An adenosine 3',5'-monophosphate-dependent protein kinase from rabbit skeletal muscle. *J. Biol. Chem.,* 243:3763–3774.

49. Watson, J. (1975): The influence of intracellular levels of cyclic nucleotides on cell proliferation and the induction of antibody response. *J. Exp. Med.,* 141:97–111.

50. Weissman, I. L. (1973): Thymus cell maturation: Studies on the origin of cortisone-resistant thymic lymphocytes. *J. Exp. Med.,* 137:504–510.

51. Weissman, I. L., Baird, S., Gardner, R. L., Papaioannou, V. E., and Raschke, W. (1976): Normal and neoplastic maturation of T-lineage lymphocytes. *Cold Spring Harbor Symp. Quant. Biol.,* 41:9–21.

52. Wijermans, P., and Astaldi, A. (1978): Effect of aging on thymus-dependent serum factor(s). *Ned. Tijdschr. Gerontol.,* 9:216–219.

53. Wijermans, P., Astaldi, G. C. B., Facchini, A., Schellekens, P.Th.A., and Astaldi, A. (1979): Early events in thymocyte activation: I. Stimulation of protein synthesis by a thymus-dependent human serum factor. *Biochem. Biophys. Res. Commun.,* 86:88–96.

54. Wijermans, P., Astaldi, G. C. B., Griend, R. J. van de, Leupers, C. J. M., and Astaldi, A. (1979): The thymus-dependent human serum factor SF: Studies on the target-cell specificity *(submitted for publication).*

55. Wijermans, P., Astaldi, G. C. B., Leupers, C. J. M., Bemmel, T. van, Schellekens, P.Th. A., and Astaldi, A. (1979): Effect of the thymus-dependent human serum factor (SF) on the phenotypic expression of markers of mouse and human lymphoid cells *(submitted for publication).*

56. Wijermans, P., Oosterhuis, H. J. G. H., Astaldi, G. C. B., Schellekens, P.Th. A., and Astaldi, A. (1980): Thymus-dependent serum factor in non-thymectomized and thymectomized patients with myasthenia gravis. *Clin. Immunol. Immunopathol.,* 16:11–18.

57. Yakir, Y., Kook, A. I., Schlesinger, M., and Trainin, N. (1977): Effect of thymic humoral factor on intracellular levels of cyclic AMP in human peripheral blood lymphocytes. *Isr. J. Med. Sci.,* 13:1191–1196.

Polypeptide Hormones, edited by
R. F. Beers, Jr. and E. G. Bassett.
Raven Press, New York © 1980.

45.   Discussion

Moderator: Nathan Trainin

A. Goldstein: Jean-Francois, I was very interested in your data suggesting the possibility that FTS was a part of fraction 5. If I understood you correctly, your active molecule has a pI of 7.3, so it may become the first γ-1-thymosin. But before it can be established as such, we need to have the sequence of FTS determined and confirmed. Of the 20 or so peptides that we have purified and examined for their sequence, we have not found a nonapeptide that is homologous with FTS. We have found, however, that the synthetic thymosin α_1 does induce rosettes in the mouse azathioprin assay, although not at the same level as FTS.

Have you attempted, using your RIA for FTS, to displace labeled synthetic FTS by thymosin fraction 5, and if so, what happened?

J. F. Bach: This is not an easy thing to do because in the RIA of such biological preparations, there are a number of molecules in common with those with fraction 5 (including the target which contains medium sized molecules), creating serious interferences in the RIA.

After separation of fraction 5 by incremental chromatography, and using it in its entirety, we could detect a displacement. We felt this was not specific, however, due to nonspecific differences in the RIA. The same problem occurs in RIA of serum.

Returning to the problem of thymic hormones, I would like to make one comment. It is a fact that substances can be classified into two categories: those that stimulate cyclic AMP production and those that do not. What puzzles us is that there are indirect arguments suggesting that thymosin, or thymosin peptides, or FTS stimulate the production of cyclic AMP, or work through this mechanism (and my wife wrote good arguments about this, showing in particular that there is a synergistic effect between cyclic AMP and FTS), while it is impossible to show a direct effect on lymphocytes. In a recent collaboration with A. I. Kook, we obtained preliminary data demonstrating that, when using the T-cell lines having FTS receptors, there is a small increase in cyclic AMP that we had not been able to observe when whole cell populations were used. This cyclic AMP technique might be one way of distinguishing between the various factors in addition, of course, to the chemical approach, which so far has proven very unproductive. It may be that in repeated experiments, our agent was more selective for T-cell subsets, whereas you may have factors acting at different stages. I would like to hear your comments about this.

N. Trainin: I would like to ask you, Dr. Bach, something else in relation to your very interesting observations on receptors in the lymphoblastoid cells. Did you get, in this association of FTS to lymphoblastoid cells, any expression of maturity, of differentiation, or indication that the association induces a change in the target cell?

J. F. Bach: This is not easy to do because these cell lines proliferate very rapidly and the cell cycle is associated with changes in the expression of a number of markers. So to do these studies, we first have to examine the behavior of the various markers and functions. Markers are complicated, but function is the worst—we still do not have data on this.

A. Astaldi: In view of your results, I wonder whether any of these cell lines is terminal deoxynucleotidyl transferase positive?

J. F. Bach: Most of them are.

N. Trainin: I think the consensus of this Symposium is that a series of factors are produced by the thymus gland, or found in circulation—but certainly of thymic origin—that have a series of functions that have been well established for the T-cell compartment of the lymphoid system. One basic difference, in addition to the fact that some of them are isolated from the thymus while others are collected from the blood, is the length of time of activity on the target. Particularly, this rapid exhaustion of activity of the material, as in the case of FTS. Dr. Astaldi, would you like to comment on your studies on the latency of serum factor activity, and the effective life of it?

A. Astaldi: These studies were done several years ago. Lacking the synthetic analogs, our results cannot be compared to those of J. F. Bach. As I mentioned, in humans, after thymectomy, the serum factor peptide of thymic origin disappears, indicating a half-life of approximately 6 to 8 hr; we found the same half-life for this peptide in certain strains of mice. The peptide has binding characteristics, as shown from studies in which we could adsorb the activity. The activation of cyclic AMP in a panel of cells was one of my slides. In those cells where we could turn on the cyclic AMP, they were very effective in adsorbing the serum factor peptide, while other cells did not adsorb it. After attachment of the peptide to the cell surface, we have been unable to detach it. Since we don't have a synthetic peptide with which to examine the system, we do not know what is really happening. Maybe it is bound—maybe it is consumed and no longer present. We have been unable to get it back.

N. Trainin: I would like to propose a thesis, according to experiments reported by all of the panel, that thymic hormones only act upon what Stutman termed "post-thymic" cells. Now, a "post-thymic" cell means a cell that has already undergone differentiation in the direction of maturation. Then, different thymic hormones, by inducing changes at the membrane of the target cells, trigger them towards maturation. Now, if we try to confront this information with the concept of Cantor and Boyse on the different subsets of populations, what is clear to me is that the Ly1, 2, and 3 cells of mice—and their equivalents in humans—are under the differentiating pressure of thymic hormones. This would favor the thesis that thymic hormones are a kind of general stimulator of a wide variety of T-cell subsets, in which the imprint of differentiation has already been established in the forefathers of these cells. Would some of you like to comment on this point?

J. F. Bach: I would like to comment about the difference between induction of markers and induction of functions.

There are data suggesting that one can induce Ly and, eventually, theta markers in fairly mature and nude mouse cells. One can hypothesize that thymic factors—including thymopoietin and FTS—could induce differentiation not only of stem cells, but also of very mature cells. On the other hand, when you look at functions, the only convincing data that have been reported deal with functions at the level of regulation in ATx or NTx mice. There is no valid data showing the acquisition of function in nude mice, for example, and I have not seen any good data showing functional acquisition in thymectomized, irradiated mice, with anti-θ serum-treated bone marrow cells, because the bone marrow cell population still contains T-cells.

There is a discrepancy—which I do not understand very well—between acquisition of markers and that of functions. That discrepancy should be taken into account when dealing with these concepts. But I would agree with you about the reservation on markers, and, as far as functions are concerned, all suggest that the Ly 1, 2, 3 cell is the target cell. Whether it has to be induced by thymic factor, or maintained in the presence of thymic factor and ultimately be transformed into Ly 1 or into Ly 2, 3 cells is still open to discussion.

A. Astaldi: I don't think that the site of action of the thymic factors is solely at the post-thymic cell. I think that since thymosin β_3 and thymosin β_4 can act at the level of the bone marrow TdT-negative cell and induce it into a TdT-positive cell, it indicates that at least two of the thymic factors are acting before the level of post-thymic cell is reached. Another point that has complicated this entire field is the fascination with surface markers. In many ways, many of us in the field of immunology have been chasing butterflies and making too much out of surface marker technology.

I would agree with J. F. Bach that the critical areas that we should be concentrating on in terms of the development of assays dealing with functional markers as well as with enzymes which are specific and doing something within the cell. The surface markers, surface Ly, theta, and the like, are really complicated by the fact that not only can thymic-specific molecules induce these markers, but a whole host of nonspecific agents can take over and activate them.

I think the fascination with these markers has held back the field and I am glad to see that there is now, at least, the beginning of a gathering of information on entities other than surface markers. For example, I was interested in Dr. G. Goldstein's mentioning that 2 weeks after administering TP5 to mice with Lewis lung tumors, there was a decrease in lung metastases. Dr. Goldstein, have you actually seen a difference in the survival of these animals and why did you terminate the experiment at the end of 2 weeks?

G. Goldstein: We are now repeating the experiment to examine this point. Previously, the animals were sacrificed for a metastases count.

A. Astaldi: Let us return to the question by Dr. Trainin regarding the target cells for thymic hormones. Actually, Dr. Trainin, that was more or less your hypothesis.

I tend to agree with Dr. Allan Goldstein that maybe it is too simplistic to assume that one thymic hormone acts on a whole array of T-cells. I think that pre-thymic T-cells cannot be fully converted from the pre-thymic state to the effector state by our thymic factor. Therefore, the so-called cell-to-cell interaction in the early stages of thymic cell differentiation could be the result of the presence of more than one thymic hormone in the system.

N. Trainin: I would like to add that when we started to inject hormone material into humans, one of the things which impressed us was the increase in the number of lymphocytes. We observed that before the increase in the number of rosettes appearing in the second week of injections, there is a rise in lymphocyte production. Since the children had a very severe reduction in the number of lymphocytes before our trials, this increase suggests that there is a kind of back stimulation to the bone marrow, which would be in agreement with Dr. Astaldi's comments.

B. W. Erickson: Dr. Trainin, you mentioned that you had a few cases involving juvenile rheumatoid arthritis and others with systemic lupus erythematosus. Did you have any success in treating patients under those conditions? Did you get any recovery or remission in those few cases involving these autoimmune diseases?

N. Trainin: The first case we treated was a 9-year-old child with severe juvenile rheumatoid arthritis, involving the joints, pericardium, and myocardium, complicated with hepatitis, pneumonitis, and agonising and moribund at the time we started THF administration. This child survived and 48 hr after the first injections of THF, there was a dramatic change in the situation. Initially, there was a reduction of temperature, and then progressively a reduction of all the objective symptoms. Now, a few weeks after daily injections, we reduced the amount of THF administered because we did not have enough material. In the third week, a second myocarditis developed. Then we doubled the dose, as we were able to produce more THF, and again, there was a remission. The same sequence happened three times. This child is alive, having received 500 injections of THF. She has very severe deformations, but does not have either mild pericarditis, myocarditis, or any other symptoms.

I would like to comment on this patient and on a few others in connection with experiments performed in our laboratory by Dr. Myra Small. The 9-year-old child, for example, was receiving 120 mg prednisone daily and one of her vertebra collapsed as a result of osteoporosis. It is impressive that doctors are not aware of the fact that cortisone, among many other side effects, destroys the source of the cells that could be differentiated to maturation by thymic hormones. Not until we very severely reduced the dose of prednisone, did we get improvement from the THF treatment. Myra Small has found that on injection of mice with the classic single dose of 5 ml cortisone per animal, one sees total destruction of the thymus and 10% of the population of mature cortisone-resistant cells remaining there. After 48 hr, you have a dramatic renewal of the population of very immature thymocytes, which is probably the result of the inner stimulation by thymic hormones.

A. W. Goldstein: I would like to add to Dr. Trainin's statement the results of a small phase I trial, conducted at the University of Texas Medical Branch in Galveston, with thymosin fraction 5. It was found that in treating, over a 2-year period, a group of five patients with SLE, and another group having rheumatoid arthritis with thymosin fraction 5, no toxicity was found and there was a marked normalization of immunological parameters in these patients, ranging from an increase in T-cell numbers (which were low in this particular group) to a very significant decrease in the level of cytotoxic antibody for murine thymocytes in the serum.

B. W. Erickson: Does this treatment increase the production of a new suppressor cell population?

A. W. Goldstein: Well, we are not sure if that is what happens *in vivo,* but *in vitro* thymosin fraction 5 and α_7 certainly are potent inducers of suppressor T-cells.

B. W. Erickson: Dr. Astaldi, would you comment on the composition or the possible chemical structure of your serum factor?

A. Astaldi: It is a peptide of 4 or 5 amino acids and we believe that most likely there is at least one aromatic amino acid. I do not believe one should try to synthesize the material until the sequence is determined. I might add that we have evidence that one of the internal amino acids is most likely methylated, but I think I wouldn't go any further with this, and spend too much time in speculation. I think that the data we have rule out the possibility that we are dealing either with TP5 or part of it, or that FTS is a part of our material. But, of course, the factor could well be one of the several components of thymosin fraction 5 or one of the components of THF.

E. Gross: Dr. Trainin, among the data from clinical trials, you showed that you had good recoveries in lymphoproliferative malignancies. Do I recall correctly that you mentioned Hodgkin's in this context, and can Hodgkin's disease be treated with THF?

N. Trainin: Our patients were children with lymphoma, malignant lymphoma, Hodgkin's disease, or acute lymphatic leukemia. They were not treated because of the disease, but because of intercurrent viral infections. These intercurrent viral infections were produced as a consequence of the disease plus chemotherapy, which, of course, is an immunosuppressor.

Subject Index